FINANCIAL MANAGEMENT

for Nurse Managers and Executives

FINANCIAL MANAGEMENT

for Nurse Managers and Executives

FOURTH EDITION

STEVEN A. FINKLER, PhD, CPA
Professor Emeritus of Public and Health Administration, Accounting, and Financial Management
Program in Health Policy and Management
Robert F. Wagner Graduate School of Public Service
New York University
New York, New York

CHERYL BLAND JONES, PhD, RN, FAAN
Associate Professor, School of Nursing
Research Program Consultant, Nursing Division UNC Hospitals
Research Fellow, Sheps Center for Health Services Research
University of North Carolina at Chapel Hill
Chapel Hill, North Carolina

CHRISTINE T. KOVNER, PhD, RN, FAAN
Professor, College of Nursing
Senior Faculty Associate, Hartford Institute for Geriatric Nursing
Nurse Attending, New York University Langone Medical Center
New York University
New York, New York

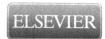

3251 Riverport Lane
St. Louis, MO 63043

FINANCIAL MANAGEMENT FOR NURSE MANAGERS AND EXECUTIVES   ISBN: 978-1-4557-0088-2

Notices

Knowledge and best practice in this field are constantly changing. As new research and experience broaden our understanding, changes in research methods, professional practices, or medical treatment may become necessary.

Practitioners and researchers must always rely on their own experience and knowledge in evaluating and using any information, methods, compounds, or experiments described herein. In using such information or methods they should be mindful of their own safety and the safety of others, including parties for whom they have a professional responsibility.

With respect to any drug or pharmaceutical products identified, readers are advised to check the most current information provided (i) on procedures featured or (ii) by the manufacturer of each product to be administered, to verify the recommended dose or formula, the method and duration of administration, and contraindications. It is the responsibility of practitioners, relying on their own experience and knowledge of their patients, to make diagnoses, to determine dosages and the best treatment for each individual patient, and to take all appropriate safety precautions.

To the fullest extent of the law, neither the Publisher nor the authors, contributors, or editors, assume any liability for any injury and/or damage to persons or property as a matter of products liability, negligence or otherwise, or from any use or operation of any methods, products, instructions, or ideas contained in the material herein.

Library of Congress Cataloging-in-Publication Data

Finkler, Steven A.
  Financial management for nurse managers and executives / Steven A. Finkler, Cheryl Bland Jones, Christine T. Kovner. — 4th ed.
    p. ; cm.
  Includes bibliographical references and index.
  ISBN 978-1-4557-0088-2 (pbk. : alk. paper)
  I. Jones, Cheryl Bland. II. Kovner, Christine Tassone. III. Title.
  [DNLM: 1. Financial Management—methods—United States—Nurses' Instruction. 2. Delivery of Health Care—economics—United States—Nurses' Instruction. 3. Nurse Administrators—United States. W 74 AA1]
  362.17'3068—dc23
                                                                                    2012010877

Senior Content Strategist: Yvonne Alexopoulos
Senior Content Development Specialist: Karen C. Turner
Associate Content Development Specialist: Emily Vaughters
Content Coordinator: Kit Blanke
Publishing Services Managers: Hemamalini Rajendrababu & Deborah L. Vogel
Project Managers: Prathibha Mehta & John W. Gabbert
Design Direction: Teresa McBryan

To our friends,
with great appreciation for all that we have learned
from you

SAF, CBJ, and **CTK**

Reviewers

Tammy S. Czyzewski, BA, BSN, MS, RN-BC, NEA-BC
Assistant Professor of Nursing
Sinclair Community College
Dayton, Ohio

Victoria Todd Durkee, PhD, APRN
Associate Professor
Nursing Department
University of Louisiana at Monroe
Monroe, Louisiana

Deborah Lessard, RN, BSN, MA, JD, CPHRM
Adjunct Faculty
Graduate Nursing
Carlow University
Pittsburgh, Pennsylvania

Connie Mullinix, PhD, MPH, MBA, RN
Clinical Associate Professor
MSN-Leadership Concentration
Department of Graduate Nursing Science
College of Nursing
East Carolina University
Greenville, North Carolina

Preface

We are extremely pleased to present the fourth edition of *Financial Management for Nurse Managers and Executives*. This edition builds on the successes of the first, second, and third editions and takes advantage of the many helpful comments that we have received over the years from colleagues and students. As we thought about writing the fourth edition of this book, we reflected on what has worked well in prior editions and the improvements that were needed. Much of the content has stood the test of time.

Nevertheless, we believed that substantial revisions were necessary for the fourth edition of the book to reflect the many changes that have occurred in nursing and health care. Of course, numbers and facts throughout the book required updating. In addition, we have made changes throughout this edition based on our own knowledge and perceptions of changes in the field, as well as feedback solicited from reviewers and current users of the third edition of the text.

First, we have updated the content in several chapters and added content on current issues in health care financing that cut across health care settings. Some of the revisions and additions include the following:

- **Chapter 2** was updated considerably to include details on health care reform—particularly the Patient Protection and Affordable Care Act—in relation to what it means for health care providers, managers, and executives. We also discuss nurses' roles in a reformed health care system. Federal government initiatives to stop paying hospitals and other providers for errors and preventable health care–acquired conditions are also explored. The concept of pay for performance, or value-based purchasing, is also introduced in this chapter, and the implications for nursing services are addressed. We also introduce content on the Institute of Medicine's *Future of Nursing* report (2011) in this chapter and reinforce it further in subsequent chapters.
- **Chapter 3** includes content on the role-transition of nurses from the bedside- or staff-nurse role to nurse manager or nurse executive. We emphasize the knowledge and skills required for this transition, including budgeting processes in centralized and decentralized organizations and the financial aspects of nurse manager and nurse executive roles. We also include a new section on nurse shared governance councils, and how they facilitate the involvement of staff nurses in organizational financing and cost containment initiatives.
- **Chapter 5** includes new content on quality, patient safety, health care costs, and financing. We focus particularly on the dilemma of balancing cost savings with quality and safety, a problem shared by all nurse managers and executives today. We also incorporate a focus on access, because of its relevance to discussions of quality and costs.

- **Chapter 9** was updated to include a discussion of nursing intensity weights, another approach for costing nursing services. This chapter outlines the advantages and disadvantages of using this approach.
- **Chapter 10** includes updated content on current nursing workforce issues, particularly recurring nursing shortages. We address financial-related issues that pertain to the shortage, such as why nurses leave, the importance of marketing to recruit nurses, and the recruitment of international nurses.
- **Chapter 14** was updated and streamlined. This content was viewed as important by our reviewers, who verified that nurse managers and executives are increasingly involved in the revenue side of health care organizational operations. Many reported being required to prepare revenue budgets and being held accountable for revenue.
- We reorganized **Chapter 15** and added new content to better illustrate how nurse managers and executives could use performance budgeting. We emphasize the potential for use in a pay-for-performance environment, a point that was validated by our reviewers. Examples were updated to reflect contemporary performance concerns faced by nurse managers and executives. Finally, we include a summary of the performance budgeting process.
- We have reorganized and expanded the section on variance analysis to include new material on alternative approaches to calculating variances. **Chapter 16** has been streamlined to present a computational approach for variance analysis that is more relevant to students, nurse managers, and nurse executives. **Chapter 17** was also streamlined considerably and elaborates on the topic of variance analysis by providing a more in-depth discussion of the causes of variances, the interpretation of variances, exception reports and how they are used, and caveats regarding acting on variances.
- **Chapter 18**, on benchmarking, productivity, and cost-benefit and cost-effectiveness analysis, has been reorganized. This edition includes comparative effectiveness research (CER), an approach for comparing two or more methods of care delivery. It will be important for students, nurse managers, and nurse executives to understand how this approach is used because it will likely become commonplace as the health care system considers ways to deliver more appropriate care in the future.
- **Chapter 19** was updated to expand the inventory discussion pertaining to economic order quantity. This is an important technique for nurse managers and executives to use in determining a balance between ordering costs and carrying costs, and avoiding stock outages.
- We have updated **Chapter 21** on forecasting to provide a more streamlined discussion on forecasting and its uses.

- In **Chapter 23**, we look to the future to consider directions in health care financing that we think will have important implications for nursing and nursing services. We examine the evolving role of financial management in nursing and how that evolving role will likely affect nurse managers and executives at all levels. We challenge nurse managers and executives to think about their roles in the evolving health care system in light of health care reform and the Institute of Medicine *Future of Nursing* report.

Those of you who are familiar with previous editions of this book will notice that two chapters—on computers and marketing—have been omitted from this edition. There are several reasons they are not included. First and foremost, the content in these chapters was peripheral to the focus of this book—that is, financial management. We do not diminish the importance of this content, but these are separate and distinct disciplines. Regrettably, we had to prioritize our content, and removing these chapters allowed us to expand discussions elsewhere on issues more pertinent to the core focus of the book. We hope that readers of this book will acquire a working knowledge of marketing and informatics through their academic coursework or other sources.

This edition also includes several online resources to accompany the text. There are discussion questions and financial problems available online that students can access. A test bank and solutions to the discussion questions and problems are also available online with access limited to instructors. The questions and problems can be used for homework assignments or for in-class discussion. We also have made PowerPoint class notes by chapter available online for instructors' use. Despite having made every effort to get this edition as near to perfect as possible, our past experience tells us that mistakes do happen. Thus, we expect to post errata online as they are discovered. To access these valuable resources, please visit our website at http://evolve.elsevier.com/Finkler/financial.

Our experience in the real world of health care shows us that nurse managers and executives are expected to understand a great deal about the financial management of organizations for which they work. What they know is often learned on the job—and often lacks a conceptual basis. Many nurse managers do not know a great deal about financial management, but it is our experience that most of them want to know more. They have found that an understanding of financial management would be a great asset to them in their managerial function.

This book is for nurses who want to know the questions to ask the finance department and what answers to give the finance department in response to its questions. Even more importantly, it is for nurses who want to manage and lead better. All levels of nursing management benefit from an improved understanding of financial management concepts. As more nurses develop their own practices or businesses, it is essential that they understand financial management.

We are often asked, "What about *Budgeting Concepts for Nurse Managers,*[1] written by Steven Finkler, one of this book's authors? Because that book exists, why is this particular financial management book needed?" The budgeting book is one of great depth but limited scope. It considers only issues related to budgeting. We believe that this book is needed because financial management extends beyond the realm of budgeting to issues such as financial statements, economics, policies, and business plans. We view these two books as complementary, with the *Budgeting Concepts for Nurse Managers* book focused more on budgeting per se and this book providing a broader, more inclusive text that covers budgeting and many other aspects of financial management that are of growing interest to nurses.

Why are the existing financial management texts written for business schools or even health care administration programs inadequate for this purpose? Our experience as teachers suggests to us that people learn concepts best when the examples are relevant to them. This book is not only about financial management but also about nursing and the problems and opportunities that confront nurses every day in providing nursing care. Business school courses often use "widget" production as the basis for their examples. Although the financial concepts of producing widgets are similar to those for the delivery of health care services, widgets are not people, and the examples are often disconnected to the world of nursing and health care. Producing widgets and treating patients are inherently, fundamentally different.

Making financial management concepts come alive to the reader requires some connection between the concept and its ultimate application. We have tried to make that connection in the nursing examples used throughout this book.

This book has been designed for use both as a textbook for graduate students and as a reference for practicing nurse managers, executives, and entrepreneurs who are seeking a better understanding of financial management. We cover topics in financial management areas that are important and relevant to nurse managers and executives at all levels.

As in any book, some areas are discussed in greater depth than others. The level of detail for each topic reflects our belief about the depth of knowledge required by today's nurse managers and executives. Each chapter has an extensive list of suggested readings for the reader who wants more depth in a particular subject area. In an attempt to provide a coherent whole, chapters refer to pertinent material in other chapters. However, each chapter is virtually self-contained, so the reader can choose to read a single chapter on a particular topic or read chapters in a different order than presented.

This book is not meant to prepare the nurse manager or executive to replace financial managers in health care organizations. Instead, it is intended to prepare nurse managers and executives for collegial relationships with financial managers. In fact, we believe that the financial managers should be the "best friends" of nurse managers and executives! For example, although the book covers business planning, it is not our expectation that every nurse manager or executive will single-handedly prepare a full 100-page business plan. Although entrepreneurs may need to complete a business plan, many nurse managers and executives are more likely to

---

[1]Finkler SA, McHugh M. 2007. *Budgeting Concepts for Nurse Managers,* 4th edition, Saunders, St. Louis.

participate in the development of business plans. As a nurse manager or executive, you may be aided by consultants, by your own staff, or by the organization's finance department. Nurse managers and executives need to know what a business plan is, why it is important, the components of a business plan, how to read a business plan, and how to make a decision based on it.

We envision that this book will be used in a graduate course in financial management for nurses. It is our expectation that a faculty member can use this book in the order it is written. However, we have attempted to allow flexibility in recognition of the fact that graduate programs prepare different levels of nurse managers and have different core course requirements. Some programs have prerequisites; others may provide an entire required course on some of the topics to which we devoted a chapter, such as the health care environment or economics. If students are already familiar with the content, it is not necessary to assign these chapters. We have attempted to prepare a book that can meet the needs of a variety of nursing programs, as well as those of practitioners. On the other hand, the chapters on topics such as economics (Chapter 4) do not provide the depth that one would find in an entire textbook written on those topics. In keeping with the financial management focus of this book, we attempted to provide an overview of those areas for students who have not yet taken a course in them and a refresher for those who have.

The topics covered in this book are appropriate for programs that prepare chief nurse executives (CNEs) and for programs that prepare first-line and midlevel nurse managers or advanced practice nurses. Instructors teaching courses in programs preparing different levels of managers may want to assign chapters that are most relevant to the level of student in their programs. Individual instructors also may choose to modify their coverage of chapters based on their students' specific needs.

Part I of the book includes chapters on the environment faced by health care organizations, how financial management fits in the health care organization, the fundamentals of applied economics, and current issues that pertain to the quality, costs, and financing of care. We believe that an understanding of the material in these chapters is fundamental to the study of financial management in health care. An instructor may choose to skip some or all of the chapters in this part if the material is a prerequisite for entry into the program or is covered elsewhere in the curriculum.

Part II discusses financial accounting, including accounting principles and analysis of financial statements. While we believe that the chapters in this section are appropriate for all levels of managers, instructors may want to target these chapters to fit within their programs. To understand costing and budgeting, it is important that the first-line and midlevel nurse manager be familiar with the basic accounting concepts in the first chapter in this part (Chapter 6). A thorough understanding of financial statements and financial statement analysis (Chapter 7) may be more appropriately targeted to the CNE level.

Part III discusses cost analysis. We believe that Chapters 8, 9, and 10 contain content essential for all levels of nurse managers and executives.

Part IV focuses on planning and control. The management role of making plans and then attempting to carry out those plans to the extent possible is central to the role of all managers and executives. The chapters in this part of the book therefore contain material with which all levels of nurse managers and executives should be familiar.

Part V deals with management of the organization's financial resources. It includes concepts such as management of cash, loans, and accounts receivable. This content may be of greater interest to managers approaching the nurse executive level.

Part VI takes a look forward at the future of financial management in nursing and health care and includes a chapter on the nurse entrepreneur. We believe this content should be read by all levels of nurse managers and executives.

The order of listed authors for this book—Finkler, Jones, and Kovner—reflects the relative contributions of each in terms of volume, with Steven Finkler providing the bulk of the writing. Nevertheless, we wish to emphasize that the entire book is a collaborative effort, with each author making important contributions throughout all chapters of the book.

We would like to express our thanks to the many people who helped with the preparation of this book. First we thank the many nurses who we have taught and with whom we have worked over the years. They have shared their knowledge and insights about the real world of financial management encountered by nurses in health care organizations. We have learned from them and have tried to address the important issues they raised.

We also very much appreciate the comments and suggestions made by the reviewers—Tammy S. Czyzewski, Victoria Todd Durkee, Deborah Lessard, and Connie Mullinix—who provided input on the previous edition and made thoughtful suggestions for the fourth edition.

We are also extremely indebted to our colleague, Professor Wendy Thomson, who prepared the PowerPoint slides for each chapter included in the online resource section of this book. Professor Thomson is an experienced educator who teaches health care finance to nurses. She may be reached at:

Professor Wendy Thomson, EdD, MSN, BSBA, RN, CNE
Director of Simulation Education and Research
O'Neill Family Foundation Clinical Simulation Center
Georgetown University, School of Nursing & Health Studies
3700 Reservoir Rd. NW
St. Mary's Hall
Washington, DC 20057
wt174@georgetown.edu

We are particularly grateful to the faculty and graduate students of the College of Nursing and the Robert F. Wagner Graduate School of Public Service at New York University and the University of North Carolina at Chapel Hill School of Nursing. We presented earlier versions of some of the examples used in this edition to them, and they let us know when the examples were not clear. We also discussed concepts that are used throughout the book. Our students' comments helped us to clarify our presentation in this edition.

We are grateful to Yvonne Alexopoulos, Karen Turner, Emily Vaughters, and John Gabbert at Elsevier for their efforts to transform our work from a raw manuscript to a published text.

Finally, we would like to thank our readers. We thank you not only for reading this book but also for helping to improve it. We encourage you to contact us with comments, suggestions, examples, or corrections.[1] All material we receive that is used in a subsequent edition will be acknowledged in that future edition.

Steven A. Finkler

Cheryl B. Jones

Christine T. Kovner

---

[1] Send all communications to Dr. Cheryl B. Jones at cabjones@email.unc.edu. Dr. Finkler may be contacted at steven.finkler@nyu.edu, and Dr. Kovner may be contacted at ctk1@nyu.edu.

About the Authors

STEVEN A. FINKLER, PhD, CPA

Steven A. Finkler is Professor Emeritus of Public and Health Administration, Accounting, and Financial Management in the Program in Health Policy and Management at New York University's Robert F. Wagner Graduate School of Public Service. At the Wagner School he teaches courses in budgeting and financial management. He is a past member of the National Advisory Council for Nursing Research at the National Institute of Nursing Research, National Institutes of Health, and recently completed seven years of serving as treasurer and board member of a large not-for-profit long-term care facility in New Jersey.

Professor Finkler has won a number of awards for his teaching, research, and textbooks. These include the 2002 Pioneering Spirit Award from the American Association of Critical-Care Nurses (AACN), the 2003 Sigma Theta Tau International Research Award in the Health Policy and Systems category, and the 2006 *American Journal of Nursing* (AJN) Book of the Year Award in the Nursing Management and Leadership category for *Accounting Fundamentals for HealthCare Management* (with David M. Ward).

In addition to this book, Professor Finkler has authored more than 200 publications, including *Accounting Fundamentals for Health Care Management* (second edition, 2013, with David Ward and Thad Calabrese), *Financial Management for Public, Health, and Not-for-Profit Organizations* (fourth edition, 2013 with Robert Purtell, Thad Calabrese, and Daniel Smith), *Finance and Accounting for Nonfinancial Managers* (fourth edition, 2011), *Budgeting Concepts for Nurse Managers* (fourth edition, 2007, with Mary McHugh), *Essentials of Cost Accounting for Healthcare Organizations* (third edition, 2007, with David Ward and Judith Baker); and articles in *The Journal of Nursing Administration, The New England Journal of Medicine, Nursing Economic$, Journal of Neonatal Nursing, Western Journal of Nursing Research, O.R. Nurse Managers' Network, Health Services Research, Medical Care, Healthcare Financial Management, Health Care Management Review,* and other journals; and a chapter in *Managing Hospitals: Lessons from the Johnson & Johnson–Wharton Fellows Program in Management for Nurses.*

Professor Finkler received a BS in Economics (summa cum laude) and an MS in Accounting (with highest distinction) from the Wharton School. His MA in Economics and PhD in Business Administration were awarded by Stanford University. Professor Finkler, who is also a Certified Public Accountant, worked for several years as an auditor with Ernst and Young and was on the faculty of the Wharton School before joining New York University. He was Editor of *Hospital Cost Management and Accounting* from 1984 through 1997, and was a faculty member of the Johnson & Johnson–Wharton Nurse Fellows Program for each of its 29 years.

CHERYL BLAND JONES, PhD, RN, FAAN

Cheryl Jones is an Associate Professor in the School of Nursing and a Research Fellow at the Cecil G. Sheps Center for Health Services Research at the University of North Carolina at Chapel Hill. She also holds the position of Research Consultant to the Nursing Division at UNC Hospitals. She is a recognized leader in nursing health services research, having devoted her career to studying micro- and macro-level issues in the nurse workforce to improve the work environment and executive practice and to address issues related to the cost and quality of health care. One of Dr. Jones' most recognized contributions has been the development, testing, and refinement of a method to measure nurse turnover costs. She has also studied other important and related nurse labor market issues, including nurse retention, wage differentials, employment patterns, migration and mobility. A study currently under way examines the personal, professional, employment, and job characteristics of nurses educated internationally and nurses education in the United States, as well as barriers and facilitators to the employment of internationally educated nurses in this country.

Throughout her career, Dr. Jones has been active in developing a nursing and health services research agenda to help advance our understanding of critical issues pertaining to health, health care delivery, and nursing practice. She also served as Senior Health Services Researcher at the Agency for Healthcare Research and Policy (AHRQ) and completed a policy fellowship in the U.S. Public Health Service. She has worked to build health services research capacity in nursing as a way to advance knowledge on critical issues in health, health care, and nursing practice. She acknowledges that one of her most personally satisfying experiences has been working with nurses, health care organizations, and systems to build staff nurse research capacity and programs of nursing research.

Dr. Jones is a member of many professional organizations such as the American Academy of Nursing, the American Nurses Association, Sigma Theta Tau (the national honor society for nursing), AcademyHealth (the professional organization for health services research), and the American Organization of Nurse Executives. She also actively serves on national research review and expert panels and has consulted with health care organizations, professional groups, and the federal government on matters related to health care delivery and the health care workforce. Cheryl has taught health economics, finance, policy, and administration at undergraduate and graduate levels. She obtained her BSN at the University of Florida and her master's and doctoral degrees at the University of South Carolina.

CHRISTINE T. KOVNER, PhD, RN, FAAN

Christine Kovner is a Professor in the College of Nursing New York University, where she has worked for over 25 years. She also holds the positions of Senior Faculty Associate, Hartford Institute for Geriatric Nursing, also at the College, and Nurse Attending, New York University Langone Medical Center (NYULMC). She was the first Agency for Health Care Policy Research (AHCPR)/American Academy of Nursing Senior Scholar. She is the author of numerous journal articles and book chapters.

Her research interests are the cost and use of health personnel. Dr. Kovner is the principal investigator for a study funded by a grant from the Robert Wood Johnson Foundation examining the career trajectories of newly licensed registered nurses over the first ten years of their careers. She has published numerous peer-reviewed articles, and has served as a grant reviewer for government agencies and foundations. She serves as the Senior Associate Editor of *Policy, Politics, & Nursing Practice* and as a reviewer for many health-related journals. In addition to these roles, Dr. Kovner is an advisor to government and private sector; for nine years she was a member of the New York State Hospital Review and Planning Council and she is on the Steering Committee for New York's Nursing Workforce Center.

At NYU she teaches courses on the organization and delivery of nursing care, including issues of cost, quality (including patient safety), and the nursing workforce. She is a member of many professional organizations, such as the American Academy of Nursing, the American Nurses Association, and Sigma Theta Tau, the national honor society for nursing. She was awarded the Distinguished Nurse Researcher award from the Foundation of New York State Nurses Association in 1994.

Dr. Kovner earned her baccalaureate degree in nursing BSN from Columbia University, her master's degree from the University of Pennsylvania, and her PhD from NYU. She completed a three-year post-doctoral fellowship in the cost of nursing care funded by the National Center for Health Services Research and Health Care Technology and was a senior Scholar at the Agency for Healthcare Research and Quality.

Contents

PART II

FINANCIAL ACCOUNTING

PART VI

LOOKING TO THE FUTURE

❋ A FINANCIAL MANAGEMENT FRAMEWORK

The framework presented in Part I provides a structure for the book and a preview of the book's contents. More importantly, however, this framework provides a foundation that is necessary for understanding and applying financial management concepts in nursing and health care. Chapter 1 highlights the major sections and chapters of the book and their contents. Chapter 2 focuses on the environment within which health care organizations (HCOs) exist, including the key participants in the health care system, the different roles of these key participants, the inner workings of the health care financing system, the mechanisms for paying health care providers, and the approaches that have been introduced to constrain the growth of health care costs. Chapter 2 also describes health care reform efforts—specifically, the Patient Protection and Affordable Care Act—and the expected impact of this legislation on the health care environment.

Chapter 3 provides a look into HCOs and how financial management pertains to the structure of HCOs. This chapter discusses the financial management function that is critical to health care managers and executives today, including the roles played by financial managers, nurse managers and executives, staff nurses, and nurse shared governance councils, and the interconnectedness of these roles. The structural hierarchies common in HCOs are introduced, including centralized and decentralized approaches and formal as well as informal lines of authority. Understanding the inner workings of any organization or collection of organizations can be challenging, but understanding complex HCOs can be particularly daunting, especially to new managers. The nature of HCOs is therefore discussed, along with the importance of networking with individuals and groups, both inside and outside of the HCO.

Chapter 4 introduces the fundamentals of applied economics—content that grounds the study of financial management in health care. This chapter covers major economic concepts and principles, including economic goods and services, utility, supply and demand, the functioning of free markets, elasticity of demand, economies of scale, market efficiency, and market failure. The role of incentives in economic behavior is considered, along with the economic view of the market for nurses and periodic nursing shortages.

Finally, Chapter 5 presents current issues that pertain to quality, costs, and financing of care. Quality, costs, and financing issues are critically important in health care today and are intricately related, as reflected by increased public awareness about quality and patient safety issues in HCOs and the interest generated from groups both within and outside of health care. The chapter provides a basic discussion of quality and how it is measured along with an overview of the impetus for integrating quality, cost, and financing issues. Incentives inherent in the financing system that support and deter quality are discussed, including the current focus on achieving value in health care through pay-for-performance or value-based purchasing initiatives. The use of report cards in health care is also considered. This is a strategy that is increasingly being used to inform consumers about the providers from whom they receive care and to encourage quality improvements in HCOs. Two initiatives—the Magnet Recognition Program® and the Malcolm Baldridge National Quality Award—are presented because of their potential role in influencing hospital quality. The chapter also addresses the important issue of access to care and the linkages among cost, quality, and access. Finally, the chapter concludes with a discussion of the concept of a business case for quality and how nurse managers and executives may use the business case to support investments in quality and to evaluate trade-offs between the costs and quality of care.

Introduction and Overview

CHAPTER GOALS

The goals of this chapter are to:

- Provide the reader with an introduction to financial management
- Clarify the components of financial management

- Give the reader a road map for the study of financial management

✱ INTRODUCTION

Few professionals have seen as dramatic a change in role over the past several decades as nurse managers and executives. The nurse managers and executives of the 1960s were predominantly clinical managers. The role focused on ensuring the adequacy of the clinical care provided to patients, and the manager or executive was expected to accomplish the delivery of clinical care with the resources provided.

Today's nurse managers and executives still must accomplish this primary clinical function; it remains the essence of nursing. The responsibilities of the job, however, are much different and much more expansive. Managers and executives must be able to determine the resources they will need and then argue convincingly to get their share of resources from a limited total amount available to the organization.

The accuracy with which resource needs must be projected and the efficiency with which care must be provided are much greater in today's health care environment. Health care services cost more than ever, and the pressures to control costs are tremendous. As a result, the financial aspects of the roles of nurse managers and executives are growing and becoming increasingly sophisticated. Nurse managers and executives are expected to understand and use financial and forecasting tools to develop and justify budgets and to minimize the cost of staff and supplies.

Many of the nonclinical managerial aspects of nursing relate to the financial management of the nursing unit, the department, and the health care organization (HCO) itself. This book is divided into six major sections or parts; within each part, chapters are included that delve into a wide range of related financial management topics. Each aspect of the book is designed to meet the needs of nurse managers and executives at all levels of the HCO. However, some readers may wish to selectively choose topics and chapters that are most relevant to their personal learning needs and their current or future roles.

✱ A FINANCIAL MANAGEMENT FRAMEWORK

Part I of this book is designed to set the stage for the study of financial management. It contains five chapters. This overview chapter provides an in-depth guide to the book and should aid readers in making an informed choice in approaching the subject matter. Chapter 2 discusses some of the essential elements of the environment of HCOs. Chapter 3 establishes the relationships among nurse managers and executives, financial managers, and the organizations within which they work. Chapter 4 provides a fundamental discussion of the principles and tools of microeconomics. Chapter 5 discusses the interrelationship of health care quality, costs, and access.

The Health Care Environment

Every organization must act within the confines of an existing environment. Some HCOs are the sole providers of health care services in their geographic region; others have substantial competition. These geographic differences may mean that it is easier to hire new staff in certain areas of the country than in others.

Who are the key players in the health care industry? Who buys services? Who sells them? Who pays for them? What legal bodies make regulations that affect what HCOs can do? Answers to questions such as these are key in putting together the pieces to appreciate the complex financial issues inherent in the health care environment.

The health care industry is also subject to legislation and is heavily regulated. This has created an especially complex and difficult environment in which to operate an organization. Before one can begin to address the financial management of HCOs, it is important to tackle issues related to government, policy making, regulation, and competition. Particularly relevant are laws that introduce large or even seemingly small changes to the system. These laws typically impact the key players in the system, including purchasers, providers, and recipients of care. Pending these changes, it is not uncommon for considerable political "jockeying" to occur as various entities try to position themselves in the best light, so that they benefit from any proposed changes. It is critical for nurse managers and executives to understand such issues, because they are often in positions to influence the outcomes for nurses.

Organizations that exist to provide and manage care are here to stay. These organizations are discussed in Chapter 2 to provide a foundation for nurse managers and executives to use in first identifying the relevant issues and then integrating them in subsequent application of specific financial management techniques. The chapter also discusses recent events and trends, including alternative payment approaches, the concept of pay for performance, and the Medicare prescription drug plan.

Financial Management and Nursing Leadership in Health Care Organizations

In addition to understanding the environment within which HCOs operate, it is useful for nurse managers and executives and those who aspire to these roles to understand the structure of organizations within which they might work and how financial management is related to that structure.

Health care organizations are generally structured as hierarchies. Too many people work in most organizations for them all to report to one person. Therefore a "pyramid" structure is often established in which caregivers report to a manager, who in turn reports to another manager higher in the "pyramid" or organizational structure.

Increasingly, HCOs are also using matrix management. A matrix organizational structure is a cross-functional system in which a manager has responsibility that cuts across departmental lines. For example, the service line structure is now common. A health care service line represents all units that provide care to a specific type or group of patients, such as cardiology. A manager is responsible for the service line, including all products, services, and caregivers needed to provide care to patients in that service line. This requires a cooperative relationship among the service line manager, the staff within the service line, and the managers and staff of all areas and departments in the organization. The staff members in a service line need to respond to both the service line manager or executive and their unit or departmental manager. Although matrix organizations are becoming more common in HCOs, the reality is that these are very complex structures, and research is still needed to address the most effective models.

Despite the use of matrix management in some HCOs, the traditional hierarchical management structure is prevalent in many HCOs. Much of the discussion in Chapter 3 focuses on issues related to the degree of centralization—the locus of decision making—created by such a structure. It also considers the official and actual authority of specific individuals filling key roles within the organization. Equally critical is the discussion of the distinction between the line and staff roles in organizations. Within that context, the role of finance is discussed. The roles of the chief financial officer and the finance department staff are explained and compared with the roles of nurse managers and executives at various levels in the organization. The transition of

nurses from the bedside to nurse manager or executive roles is presented, and the knowledge and skills required to address financial management issues during this transition are discussed. Although nurse managers and executives in practice have varying levels of education, the expectations for most are commensurate with graduate-level education, supplemented through on-the-job and continuing education.

Key Issues in Applied Economics

Accounting and finance are applied areas of microeconomics. The theory of economics forms the foundations upon which all financial management is ultimately built. The essence of economics is that society has a limited amount of resources, with competing demands for them. The economic system attempts to allocate those resources in an optimal fashion.

Chapter 4 introduces the building blocks used in economics. The critical building blocks—economic goods, marginal utility, marginal cost, supply and demand, and economies of scale—are discussed. This leads into an examination of the workings of a free enterprise system.

In the free enterprise system, one cannot separate human motivation from the actions of human beings. The economic system will always be the result of the interplay of resource allocation with the actions of people. As a result, it is necessary to consider the issue of incentives and their role in achieving market efficiency.

The economic system, even a free enterprise system, cannot always be relied upon to generate a perfect outcome. In fact, there may be times when the system simply fails to achieve a socially optimal result. The existence of monopolies, the absence of full information, the impact of insurance systems, and other factors may lead to less-than-desirable outcomes. Chapter 4 addresses these issues of market failure and of society's attempts to intervene to generate a more equitable outcome.

Economics has a bearing on nursing. It forms the framework from which resources are allocated. Chapter 4 also specifically addresses issues related to the market for nursing labor: Why do nursing shortages occur from time to time and then diminish? Is there some logic or rationale that can explain how the economic system leads to such shortages and then resolves them? This chapter provides nurse managers and executives with a foundation for engaging in related labor market discussions and planning for nursing workforce needs.

Quality, Costs, and Financing

Chapter 5 addresses the delicate balance among costs, quality, and access in today's health care environment. Increasing media attention has brought increased public awareness about quality and patient safety in HCOs. This movement has been spurred by groups within and outside of health care and supported to a degree by an evolving body of research.

An understanding of the dilemmas presented by this movement is critically important for today's nurse managers and executives. Nurse managers and executives are in leadership positions within HCOs that must pay close attention to new and constantly changing patient safety and quality requirements and initiatives. In many respects, organizational leaders look to nurses for help in identifying creative solutions to address these requirements. Nurse managers and executives must also oversee aspects of care delivery that are ultimately reported in quality report cards and other public reporting mechanisms for HCOs. It is therefore extremely important for nurse managers and executives to understand the connection between nursing and the information that gets presented in these reports, as well as the larger role that nursing plays in today's quality reporting process. More importantly, the financial resources available to an HCO today are dependent on its performance on quality and patient safety indicators, and many of these indicators are related to the care delivered by nurses.

Access to care is also an important issue in the financing of health care because of the increasing number of people who lack health insurance and/or cannot pay for the care they receive. When such uninsured persons receive care, they may not receive it until they need emergency care or are critically ill. Ultimately the care they receive may be more costly than it might have been if a more basic level of care, such as preventive care, had been available to them. Thus, the lack of access may actually add costs to an already costly system.

The key reason for nurse managers and executives to develop a strong understanding of the relationship between cost and quality is the ever-present challenge of balancing the costs and quality of nursing care in an environment of constrained nursing and financial resources. They face this challenge on a daily basis when they make decisions about nurse staffing, scheduling, or resource use. We use the issue of nurse staffing in Chapter 5 to highlight the complexities of managing nursing services while engaging in the delicate act of balancing the costs and quality of care.

✳ FINANCIAL ACCOUNTING

Accounting has often been referred to as "the language of business." One needs to be conversant with the basic principles of accounting to conduct any of the various aspects of financial management. Part II focuses on these basic accounting issues.

The two principal areas of accounting are managerial accounting and financial accounting. *Managerial accounting* refers to the generation of any financial information that would be useful to managers and executives in their roles overseeing an organizational unit, department, or division. Most of this book focuses on managerial accounting issues. The nurse manager or executive also needs to understand financial accounting. Part II contains two chapters on financial accounting issues. *Financial accounting* provides the foundations of accounting. It focuses on generating financial information about the results of operations and the financial condition of the organization.

Financial accounting originated largely to provide information to outsiders who were lending money to an organization or investing in it, but the information generated is extremely useful for the organization's internal managers as well. Nurse managers and executives who can assess and use this information will be at an advantage. Chapter 6 looks at the basic principles of accounting, and Chapter 7 provides a more advanced look at the analysis of financial statements.

Accounting Principles

Accounting does not represent a science. In fact, accounting professors teach that accounting is closer to an art than a science. No fundamental laws of nature govern accounting. One generally agreed-upon principle forms the keystone on which all accounting is built, however: The books must balance.

This concept has become so pervasively known and accepted that readers of this book likely take it for granted. Everyone knows you must balance the books. But what does that really mean? Does it mean that you must break even, that you must balance the revenues against the expenses of each organization or individual? No. Clearly, some organizations make money, and others lose money. What does it mean when one says that the books must balance?

Balancing the books refers to the basic equation of accounting that describes the relationship between the valuable resources possessed by the organization and the claims on those resources by creditors and owners of the organization. That equation becomes the basis for ledgers and journals and the other technical elements of an accounting system. Chapter 6 introduces readers to the equation of accounting and to the concepts of assets, equities, revenues, expenses, journal entries, ledgers, and generally accepted accounting principles. These concepts affect every manager and executive in most HCOs. A fundamental understanding of these concepts is essential to understand financial management.

Financial Statement Analysis

At higher levels of management, the focus of a manager's interest in financial management must broaden. The tools of financial management become not only an integral element for being able to efficiently manage a unit or department but also the messengers of the general financial well-being of the organization.

Can the organization afford to provide nurses with substantial raises? Can the organization reasonably be expected to replace old intensive care unit monitors with new ones? Is the organization acting in a prudent manner that will allow for its continued existence? These are just a few examples of the types of issues that become relevant as one moves up through the ranks of nursing management. The answers to these questions require information about the general financial condition of the organization.

Chapter 7 focuses on issues of analysis of the information contained in financial statements (also called *financial reports* or *financials*). What do the income statements and balance sheets of organizations really tell the reader? Are other elements of information also important? Are there ways to use raw financial statement information to make it more informative? What is the difference between the audit and other financial reports? Chapter 7 builds on these concepts by discussing the appropriate uses of financial reports. This knowledge is particularly important to nurse managers, executives, and entrepreneurs when faced with the task of securing financing for capital and operational needs.

✳ COST ANALYSIS

One of the most critical areas of financial management is the analysis and control of costs. The surplus (profit) or deficit (loss) of an organization each year depends on both its revenues and its costs. Both elements—revenues and costs—require managerial thought and attention. Increasingly, cost management has become an essential role of nurse managers and executives at all organizational levels. Part III examines issues related to costs.

Cost Management

The first chapter in Part III, Chapter 8, deals with basic issues of cost management. All levels of management encounter these issues in their normal activities.

The chapter introduces definitions of critical terms. The concepts of fixed, variable, marginal, and relevant costs are discussed at some length. The nature and behavior of costs are covered, with emphasis on the relationship between patient volume and costs. As volume changes over time, managers and executives must be able to understand and predict the impact that such changes will have on costs. Techniques are provided for such prediction or estimation of future costs.

The health care industry has evolved over the past several decades to become much more entrepreneurial. In an effort to find the resources to subsidize services offered at a loss, many HCOs, even not-for-profit organizations, are constantly searching for profitable ventures. The last section of Chapter 8 provides a method to determine when a program or project or service will have sufficient volume to break even (i.e., to be financially self-sufficient). Such an approach is frequently used by organizations to determine whether to undertake a proposed new venture.

Determining Health Care Costs and Prices

Chapter 9 moves from basic cost concepts to the broader issue of cost measurement with two primary focuses. One is on how HCOs collect cost information by unit or department and assign those costs to patients. The second is on how to determine the cost of nursing care.

The Medicare step-down cost-finding and rate-setting method is presented in Chapter 9 and compared with more recently developed costing methods. Attention is also paid to understanding product-line costing. Issues of patient classification systems and staffing are considered. Standard costing techniques are also discussed.

Determining the cost of nursing is a topic of much interest to nurses, nurse managers, and nurse executives. As HCOs are forced to operate in a constrained financial atmosphere and as organizational reimbursements become increasingly dependent on outcomes sensitive to nursing care, nurse managers and executives at all levels are taking a greater role in managing and controlling costs. To do this, nurse managers and executives need a better understanding of the costs of providing nursing care. Such an understanding can also be useful to the advanced practice nurse, who must set a price for care. The current focus on pay for performance, or value-based care, is discussed, along with how this system might affect nursing. This system presents opportunities and challenges for nurse managers and executives. Understanding how the costs of nursing services might be influenced by or take advantage of these new reimbursement models will be key to successful nurse manager and executive practice in the future.

Recruiting and Retaining Staff

Chapter 10 addresses a concern that peaks during recurring nursing shortages but requires managerial attention regardless of whether there is a shortage of nurses. That is the issue of measuring and managing the costs of recruiting and retaining staff and the costs associated with vacant nursing positions.

There is little question that personnel is the single greatest cost in health care. Attracting and retaining qualified staff are essential to maintaining a desired quality-of-care level. Because of the high cost of recruiting nurses, the aging of the nursing workforce, and chronic nurse shortages, the recruitment and retention of nurses have become financial management issues. Nurses from other countries have been recruited to work in HCOs to relieve staffing shortages, and there are many more who are willing to do so. The global nurse labor market can provide nurse managers and leaders with strategies for filling vacant positions (including those that are particularly hard to fill) and providing staffing flexibility, but there are associated costs. High rates of nurse turnover and high nurse vacancy rates have their own costs, and these must be balanced against retention costs.

What can management do to keep nurse satisfaction high? What are the tools and approaches an organization can use in attracting new nurses? What alternative sources of personnel are there? How much does nurse recruitment cost, and how does one measure that cost? How do expanding nurse employment opportunities in emerging sectors of the health care industry—beyond hospitals in areas such as long-term care, home care, rehabilitation care, community care, hospice care, and independent practice—affect the ability of nurse managers and executives to attract, recruit, hire, satisfy, and retain nurses? These emerging employment opportunities for nurses could cause problems for managers and executives because they provide nurses with so many employment options. It behooves nurse managers and executives in both existing and emerging settings to develop competitive recruitment initiatives and build systems to retain nurses to avoid problems with nurse turnover. These are just a few of the issues on which Chapter 10 focuses.

✳ PLANNING AND CONTROL

Planning and control are elements central to the success of any organization. Planning helps the organization to know where it wants to go and to develop a plan to get there. Control helps to ensure that the adopted plan is carried out.

Part IV devotes eight chapters to this important topic. These chapters specifically address strategic management and planning, budgeting concepts, preparation of operating, revenue and performance budgets, the control of operating results and variance analysis, benchmarking, productivity, cost-benefit analysis, and cost-effectiveness analysis.

Strategic Management

Strategic planning is an outgrowth of the long-range planning movement of the 1950s. *Strategic management* is the process of integrating strategic thinking throughout the management process. Organizational success largely depends on the care with which the organization acts strategically. Knowing an organization's strengths and weaknesses and being aware of its opportunities and threats are critical elements upon which the field of strategic management has been built.

Strategic planning is discussed in Chapter 11. How are strategic plans defined? Why are they prepared? What benefits can the organization hope to achieve from strategic management? What are continuous quality improvement (CQI) and rapid CQI, and how do they relate to strategic management? The chapter also discusses long-range plans and program budgets.

Budgeting Concepts and Budget Preparation

The budgeting aspect of planning is explored in four chapters: Chapter 12 provides an overview of the various types of organizational budgets and of the budget process; Chapter 13 goes into greater depth on the preparation of the operating budget; Chapter 14 builds on and expands the revenue budgeting section included in earlier editions of this book; and Chapter 15 addresses performance budgets.

The types of budgets examined include operating, long range, capital, product line, program, zero base, cash, and special purpose. Each type of budget has an integral role in planning for HCOs.

The budget process is much broader than the actual preparation of each unit's budget. The process includes preparing a timetable; doing an environmental review; and developing goals, objectives, assumptions, and priorities. It also includes budget negotiation and revision.

Capital budgeting has become more complicated in the health care industry. HCOs must examine the financial implications of capital acquisitions more closely. The technical appendix to Chapter 12 discusses sophisticated analytical approaches to capital budget evaluation. The methods discussed include the present cost approach, net present value, and internal rate of return.

Chapter 13 looks at specific issues related to preparation of operating budgets. The starting point for preparing the operating budget is the estimated workload. First, however, the likely number and mix of patients must be considered before a determination can be made of the resources needed to care for those patients.

The largest and most complicated element of the budgeting process relates to personnel costs. The major part of Chapter 13 is devoted to examining the issues related to staffing and to calculating labor costs. Costs of services other than personnel services are also covered. The last section of the chapter deals with budget implementation. A budget loses much of its value if it is largely ignored after being approved. It is vital that nurse managers and executives think specifically of the actions that must be taken to implement their budgets. Often, they must weigh the costs of adding nursing personnel against the safety problems averted.

Chapter 14 examines specific issues related to the preparation of revenue budgets. Revenues, obviously critical to the survival of every HCO, must be adequate to cover all the costs of providing services during the current year and great enough to provide a profit. In a growing number of situations, nurse managers and executives are required to prepare revenue budgets and are held accountable for revenue. This chapter introduces basic issues related to revenues and revenue management, and it includes detail on the calculation of revenues as they relate to nursing. The chapter concludes with a discussion of managed care revenues, with a particular emphasis on issues pertaining to revenues from capitation arrangements.

Health care budgeting focuses to a great extent on the resources needed to provide a certain volume of services. This is a one-dimensional view of health care. Managers and executives generally attempt to achieve many objectives. Rather than simply trying to provide care to a specific number of patients, managers and executives try to keep patients satisfied, improve the quality of care, control costs, keep staff and other clients happy, and achieve other ends. Performance budgeting, discussed in Chapter 15, is a technique that examines the things that a department or organization is trying to achieve. With this technique, the nurse manager or executive can develop a budgeted level of performance and cost for each of a number of objectives of the organizational unit. As health care continues to evolve to a performance-based reimbursement system, performance budgeting may become more widely used.

Controlling Operating Results and Variance Analysis

Implementation of the budget, however, does not mean that everything will come out according to plan. This topic is discussed in two chapters. Chapter 16 discusses the provision of specific tools of variance analysis, which are used to help managers discover variations from the original plan and keep outcomes as close to the plan as possible. Chapter 17 elaborates on the topic of variance analysis and discusses interpretations, exceptions, and caveats.

Traditional variance analysis compares the actual results with the budgeted plan. Information is provided for each line item of each budget for the most recent month and cumulatively for the year to date. Chapter 16 also introduces the concept of flexible budgeting, a variance analysis technique that provides better insight into the likely causes of observed variances. By subdividing variances into their underlying components, the manager or executive is able to identify the major influences that generated the variation from the budget.

Chapter 17 provides additional information on the use of variance analysis along with examples. Exception reports and their benefits are discussed. The causes of variances are explored, and the interpretation of variances is discussed, particularly with respect to staffing patterns and patient acuity. Guidance is given to help nurse managers know when variances are large enough to warrant further attention and investigation. The relationship between variance analysis and performance budgeting is addressed.

Benchmarking, Productivity, and Analysis of Costs

Chapter 18 introduces nurse managers and executives to tools of benchmarking—strategies by which the performance of units, departments, and organizations can be compared against other similar organizational entities and targets. Benchmarking is widely used in health care today to determine organizational and clinical "best practices" and effectiveness on the basis of both internal and external sources of data. Productivity and its measurement are also addressed in this chapter. Finally, two methods are presented—cost-benefit analysis and cost-effectiveness analysis—that can be used by nurse managers and executives to evaluate alternative projects under consideration by the unit or organization and to determine the value and efficiencies in nursing care delivery.

❋ MANAGING FINANCIAL RESOURCES

All managers and executives of HCOs manage resources. Determining which personnel and other resources to use and how to use them is a managerial function. Organizations have many types of resources. The people working for any HCO are a valuable resource, as is the organization's reputation for quality. The financial resources of the organization—specifically, its money—is another. To the same extent that clinical resources must be carefully used, financial resources must be managed efficiently.

Decisions concerning where and how to get money are important considerations in managing financial resources. Some resources in proprietary organizations come from investments in the organization by its owners. In not-for-profit organizations, a common source of financial resources is the issuance of bonds. Profits are a potential source of financial resources for all types of HCOs. It has also become common for HCOs to borrow much of the money they need.

Organizations have financial resources that they must manage efficiently. Decisions must be made concerning how much cash to have on hand. Management techniques must ensure that cash is received as promptly as possible. In addition, managers and executives must ensure that cash is available when needed for payrolls or interest payments. The need to have control over the inflow and outflow of cash necessitates careful management of receivables, inventories, marketable securities, payables, and leases.

It is likely that readers of this book do not assume that the management of financial resources is the strict domain of financial managers. However, others may not value or understand the importance of this aspect of nurse managers' or executives' roles, and may believe that financial resources should be managed by financial managers. However, financial management done by nurse managers and executives is critical. For example, a financial manager can do little to control inventory levels. The nurse manager or executive is in a much better position to make determinations regarding necessary inventory levels and to enforce policies established to avoid unnecessary stockpiling of inventory. Inventory usage directly affects the amount of money available to the organization. Nurse managers and executives must work together with financial managers in the management of financial resources to arrive at an optimal outcome for the organization. It is often necessary for nurse managers and executives to communicate this aspect of their roles to others in the organization, especially to nurses, who may not appreciate the value of having them represent their financial interests.

Part V of this book is divided into two chapters. Chapter 19 focuses directly on the management of the short-term financial resources of the organization. Chapter 20 is concerned with the long-term financing of HCOs. Understanding both of these areas is essential to contemporary nurse manager and executive practice.

Short-Term Financial Resources

Short-term resources appear in the current asset and current liability sections of the balance sheet (which is discussed in Chapter 6). Such resources generally provide or require cash within a relatively short time, usually less than a year. These short-term resources and short-term sources of resources are referred to as the organization's *working capital*. Working capital is discussed in Chapter 19.

Long-Term Financial Resources

Management of long-term financial resources relates to the alternatives the organization has for acquiring financial resources that will not have to be repaid for more than a year. To acquire capital assets such as buildings and equipment, the organization must be able to acquire money that does not have to be repaid in a short time. The choices it makes regarding such long-term financing can have dramatic effects on the ability of the organization to provide health care services and to compete in the health care marketplace. The aspects of financial management related to long-term financing are discussed in Chapter 20.

❋ LOOKING TO THE FUTURE

The health care sector has rapidly become complex. To keep up, nurse managers and executives must constantly expand and improve their capabilities. Part VI of this book examines some additional management tools that can help nurse managers and executives to cope with the complicated environment of health care.

The chapters in this part focus on the future: forecasting and other methods for decision making, nurse entrepreneurship, and future directions for nursing relative to health care financial management. Each of these may be thought of as peripheral to traditional financial management, yet each represents an important topic for nursing managers and executives, today and in the future.

Forecasting

An essential role of nurse managers and executives is to make decisions. Forecasting methods can be used to provide nurse managers and executives with information about the future that can be used to make a variety of decisions. Chapter 21 discusses a number of quantitative and qualitative approaches to forecasting. These include computerized techniques as well as the less high-tech but often equally effective Delphi and Nominal Group approaches. The use of spreadsheets in forecasting is highlighted.

Chapter 21 also provides an explanation of expected value. This technique is important for generating information for managerial decision making that has proved effective over a period of years and a range of applications.

The Nurse as Entrepreneur

At the end of the 20th century, *entrepreneur* became a common word in nursing. Nurses have developed their own businesses, such as private clinical practices and home health agencies, and have developed companies to support and address various health information technology needs in organizations. The breadth and variety of entrepreneurial options available to nurses have expanded greatly. Chapter 22 describes the characteristics of nurse entrepreneurs and identifies opportunities for nurses to engage in business development. A critical element of any entrepreneurial activity—the development of a business plan—is discussed, and the steps of the process are outlined.

Nursing and Financial Management: Current Issues and Future Directions

The role of nurses in HCOs has been rapidly evolving over the past several decades. Few nurse managers and executives who left the profession in the past 20 or 30 years would recognize it or the expanding role of nurse managers and executives today. The level of responsibility for issues of financial management has increased dramatically for nurses at all levels of HCOs, particularly for nurse managers and executives.

We doubt that the rate of change confronting nurse managers and executives will decrease in the near future. The share of the total economy consumed by health care services is large and growing. The pressures to control health care spending grow stronger. Discussions about reforming, transforming, and re-envisioning the health care system of the future are commonplace. Innovations are introduced on what seems like a daily basis. These changes translate into more and more pressure on nurse managers and executives to provide high-quality care in a cost-effective manner.

Nurses will respond to the need for greater efficiency by becoming more knowledgeable about and by taking on an ever-expanding financial management role. To be able to control costs, nurse managers and executives need to understand those costs, their origin, and the way they can be managed. They need timely and accurate cost information.

Chapter 23 relates to issues of the future. What will be the evolving role of financial management in nurse manager and executive practice? How will financial management issues affect the nurse executives? First- and midlevel nurse managers? Nurse policymakers? We believe that we are just beginning to see the roles take shape that nurse managers and executives may play in the financial management of HCOs today and in the future. It is an exciting time for nurses in these roles and those who aspire to these roles. The content presented in the chapters of this book provides a solid foundation for nurse managers and executives to build on in changing the landscape of nursing and health care.

The Health Care Environment

CHAPTER GOALS

The goals of this chapter are to:

- Describe the health care system
- Describe the Patient Protection and Affordable Care Act and its impact on the health care environment
- Explain the role of each major participant group in the health care system
- Explain the financing system for health care services

- Explain how different health care providers are paid for the services they provide
- Discuss approaches developed over the past several decades to stem the growth in health care costs
- Analyze the implications of the health care environment for nurse managers

❋ INTRODUCTION

Before the specific tools of financial management are discussed, it is important to provide an overview of the health care system to help readers better understand the intricate relationship between the health care environment and the care patients receive. This context is foundational to relating the techniques of financial management to the organizations that use them.

The health care system is based on relationships among a number of different participants. The participants are extremely varied, including not only those who give care and those who receive health care services but also those who regulate the care that is provided and those who provide payments that supplement those made by the consumers. The actions of the participants in the health care system are affected by the economic and regulatory environment at local, regional, and national levels. The economic and regulatory environment changes frequently and is influenced by political, economic, and social factors. These factors interplay with technological and other scientific advances in the capabilities of health care organizations (HCOs) to, hopefully, provide the highest level quality of care possible within budget constraints.

The traditional interplay among the nurse, the physician, and the patient is just a small part of the larger health care system. There are many different types of care providers. Some are individually based, such as nurses and physicians; some are institutionally based, such as hospitals and long-term care facilities; some are organizationally based, such as health maintenance organizations (HMOs) and home care agencies; and some are societally based, such as government-sponsored programs of care for veterans and the military.

The health care system also must take into account the needs of a broad base of consumers, from the typical acute care hospital patients to those in need of drug rehabilitation, extended convalescent care, permanent nursing home care, mental health care, dental care, rehabilitative therapy, home care, and a myriad of other health care services.

The care that providers supply to consumers is subject to a complex web of regulations. For the most part, such regulations stem from an intention to protect consumers. Professional nurses, similar to other health professionals, often get frustrated because they are skilled clinicians and believe they know what care is needed for their patients and how to best provide that care. The regulatory environment often seems to be an unneeded intrusion of politicians into an area in which they have little knowledge and even less expertise. The reason for the regulations is not generally to control the activities of competent, trained individuals but rather to protect consumers from untrained or incompetent ones. In providing care in accordance with regulations, nurses and other health professionals must consider what untrained, unqualified providers of care might do in an unregulated environment.

Care is paid for in a complex manner under a set of changing rules by a diverse group of payers. We have already reached the point at which the cost of care is too great for most individuals to bear. One hospitalization can easily wipe out the life savings of a family. Therefore, we have developed an insurance system that uses pooled resources, with many individuals each contributing some money so that the tremendous costs of a serious illness can be paid for with those pooled resources. The system we have created, however, has fallen short in terms of providing care to many others who need it and has carried a high burden for providers in terms of paperwork and administrative costs.[1]

Nurse managers and executives can benefit greatly by being aware of the economic, regulatory, political, and social environments as well as the constraints and opportunities within them. Financial decisions that pertain to the delivery of nursing and other health care services must take into account not only the current environment but also anticipated changes that may affect that environment in the future. Although there may be limitations on changes that nurse managers or executives can make to run their units and departments in a more efficient manner, over time regulations change, and current constraints may fade away, only to be replaced by other regulations that pose new challenges. This point has never been more relevant than today, as the first major reform of our health care system—since the enactment of Medicare and Medicaid in the mid-1960s—is being implemented. These efforts are intended to transform our health care system by emphasizing a more integrated, coordinated, and seamless system of care and providers.

This chapter focuses on the health care environment, including a brief review of recent health care reform legislation, followed by a description of the major participants in

the health care system. Next it addresses the principal issues related to the financing of health care. Several current approaches to controlling the costs of health services are addressed. The development and growth of managed care organizations (MCOs) are discussed, along with accountable care organizations (ACOs) and other approaches that focus on paying providers for quality and not simply what it "costs" them to deliver care.

✳ HEALTH CARE REFORM

The health care environment and the financing of the health care system cannot be discussed without providing context for the discussion via recent U.S. health reform legislation. The Patient Protection and Affordable Care Act (P.L. 111-148, hereafter Affordable Care Act [ACA])[2] was passed in 2010. The major components of this legislation are outlined in Table 2–1. The impetus behind this legislation was to reduce the number of uninsured and underinsured Americans while at the same time reducing health care costs; thus, the legislation necessarily takes aim at all aspects of the health care industry and all key participants (discussed in the next section). Some of the key

---

[1]Woolhandler S, Campbell T, Himmelstein D. 2003. Costs of health care administration in the United States and Canada. *N Engl J Med* 349(8):768-775.

[2]For a summary of the legislation, see The Kaiser Family Foundation. 2011. *Focus on Health Reform: Summary of New Health Reform Law.* Retrieved July 6, 2011, at http://www.kff.org/healthreform/upload/8061.pdf. For the law itself, see The Patient Protection and Affordable Care Act, Mar. 23, 2010, PL 111-148, Government Printing Office, available at http://www.gpo.gov/fdsys/pkg/PLAW-111publ148/pdf/PLAW-111publ148.pdf.

✳ **TABLE 2–1** *Selected Highlights of the Patient Protection and Affordable Care Act (P.L. 111-148)**

Focus	Overview
Individuals	**Expand access through required coverage:** Require health insurance coverage for most Americans through state-based Health Benefit Exchanges.
Employers	**Coverage for employees:** Employers with ≥50 employees must provide coverage. Employers with <50 employees are exempt.
States	**Expand Medicaid:** Coverage to all non-Medicare eligible individuals younger than age 65 years with incomes up to 133% of the federal poverty level. **Expand CHIP:** Maintain current eligibility; CHIP-eligible children who cannot enroll because of enrollment caps will be eligible for tax credits via state exchanges. **Create health benefit exchanges:** States must create a Health Benefit Exchange and a Small Business Health Options Program through which eligible individuals and small businesses can purchase health coverage.
Health plans	**Simplify administrative requirements:** Adopt single set of operating rules for determining eligibility, claims status, payments, and referrals.
Federal government	**Revise Medicare** ■ Restructure payments to Medicare Part C: Higher payments for areas with low fee-for-service rates; lower payments for areas with high rates. ■ Establish Independent Payment Advisory Board to propose ways to reduce rate of growth in Medicare spending in excess of target growth rate. ■ Reduce Medicare payments to hospitals to account for excess preventable hospital readmissions and for HACs. ■ Pharmaceutical companies to provide discount on brand-name drugs filled in coverage gap; federal subsidies for generic drug prescriptions in gap. ■ Provide a bonus to primary care physicians and general surgeons practicing in health professional shortage areas. **Revise Medicaid** ■ Increase Medicaid drug rebate for certain drugs. Extend drug rebate to Medicaid managed care plans. ■ Reduce aggregate Medicaid disproportionate share hospital allotments. ■ Withhold payments to states for health care-acquired conditions. **Prescription drugs:** Authorize FDA to approve generic versions of biologic drugs; allow manufacturers 12 years sole rights before generics developed. **Reduce waste, fraud, abuse:** Review providers and suppliers; freeze enrollments in areas of high fraud; require establishment of compliance programs.

✳ **TABLE 2–1** *Selected Highlights of the Patient Protection and Affordable Care Act (P.L. 111-148)—cont'd*

Focus	Overview
Health care system	**Improve quality and system performance:** Establish nonprofit Patient-Centered Outcomes Research Institute (PCORI). **Medical malpractice:** Evaluate and implement alternates to tort litigation. **Medicaid** ■ Create demonstration projects for bundling payments for episodes of care. ■ Allow certain enrollees to designate a provider as health home. **Primary care:** Increase Medicaid payments in fee-for-service and managed care for primary care services provided by primary care doctors; pay bonuses to primary care physicians in Medicare. **National quality strategy:** Develop national priorities for improvements in health care delivery, patient outcomes, population health; establish program to support consortiums of providers to coordinate and integrate health care services for low-income uninsured and underinsured individuals. **Disparities:** Require enhanced collection and reporting of data on race, ethnicity, gender, primary language, disability, and underserved rural and frontier populations. **Disclose financial relationships:** Require disclosure of financial relationships among health entities (e.g., physicians, hospitals, suppliers). **Develop national strategy:** Establish National Council to coordinate federal efforts. Establish fund for research and screening.
Prevention— wellness	**Coverage of preventive services** ■ Authorize Medicare coverage of personalized prevention plan services. ■ Health plans to provide highly rated preventive services and recommended immunizations without cost sharing. **Spread wellness programs:** Provide grants and technical assistance to small employers to establish wellness programs. Offer employee rewards for joining wellness program and meeting health standards.
Long-term care	**Implement Community Living Assistance Services and Supports (CLASS) Act:** Establish a national, voluntary insurance program for purchasing community living assistance and supports. **Medicaid** ■ Provide states new options for offering home- and community-based services through Medicaid state plan; permit states to extend full Medicaid benefits to individual receiving home- or community-based services under a state plan. ■ Establish a community-first choice option in Medicaid to provide community-based attendant and support services to individuals with disabilities who require an institutional level of care. **Skilled nursing facility services:** Require facilities under Medicare and Medicaid to disclose ownership information, accountability requirements, and expenditures. Publish standardized information on a website for Medicare enrollees to compare facilities.
Workforce	**Improve workforce training and development** ■ Establish Workforce Advisory Committee to develop a national workforce strategy. ■ Increase the number of GME training positions; priority given to primary care and general surgery, and to states with the lowest resident physician-to-population ratios; promote training in outpatient settings; ensure availability of residency programs in rural/underserved areas. ■ Increase capacity for nurse education and training programs, provide loan repayment and retention grants, create a career ladder to nursing. ■ Support training programs that focus on primary care models, such as medical homes, team management of chronic disease, and the integration of physical and mental health services.
CHCs and SBCs	**Improve access to CHCs and SBCs:** Increase funding to community health centers (CHCs) and the National Health Service Corps; establish new programs for school-based centers (SBCs) and nurse-managed health clinics.
Trauma care	**Build capacity in emergency department, trauma care:** Establish a new trauma center program; fund research on emergency medicine, including pediatric emergencies; develop demonstration programs to design, implement, evaluate innovative models for emergency care systems.
Non-profit hospitals	**Additional Requirements:** Conduct community needs assessment every 3 years and adopt implementation strategy to meet needs; publicize financial assistance policy on free/discounted care, how to receive it; limit charges to patients who qualify for federal assistance to the amount generally billed to insured patients.

*Various components of this legislation are scheduled to be implemented at different times, ranging from 2010 to 2020. For more detailed information on the law, see The Patient Protection and Affordable Care Act, March 23, 2010, PL 111-148, Government Printing Office, available at http://www.gpo.gov/fdsys/pkg/PLAW-111publ148/pdf/PLAW-111publ148.pdf. For a timeline outlining when specific components are implemented, see *Understanding the Affordable Care Act: Timeline: What's changing and when*, retrieved July 6, 2011, at http://www.healthcare.gov/law/timeline/index.html.
CHC, Community Health Center; CHIP, Children's Health Insurance Program; FDA, U.S. Food and Drug Administration; GME, Graduate Medical Education; HAC, hospital-acquired condition; SBC, School-Based Center.
Adapted from The Kaiser Family Foundation: *Focus on health reform: Summary of new health reform law* (website). www.kff.org/healthreform/upload/8061.pdf. Accessed July 6, 2011.

participants may benefit under the legislation (e.g., patients, nurses, primary care physicians, and general surgeons), but others (e.g., individual consumers, employers, health plans, hospitals) will be penalized if they fail to comply with certain aspects of the legislation. More comprehensive aspects of the law include potentially expanding health care coverage to an estimated 32 million people who would not otherwise have it by providing strong incentives for employers to provide health insurance and for individuals without coverage through an employer to get health insurance (the so called "individual mandate"); potentially reducing waste, fraud, and abuse in the health care system by addressing poor quality and systems inefficiencies; providing more preventive care; and promoting research to compare treatment options.

Not all components will be implemented at one time. Instead, various components of the ACA are scheduled to be phased in over several years beginning in 2010 and spanning as far into the future as 2020.[3] Thus, although some aspects of the legislation will be put into place immediately, the overall impact of the legislation will not be known for some time yet to come.

❋ THE KEY PARTICIPANTS IN THE HEALTH CARE SYSTEM

Essentially, there are five key groups of participants in the health care system, as shown in Table 2–2. Providers are persons and organizations that deliver health care services to

---

[3]For a detailed timeline, see the Implementation Timeline, available through the Kaiser Foundation at http://healthreform.kff.org/timeline.aspx.

patients. Suppliers are the manufacturers and distributors of the equipment and supplies used in the process of providing care. Consumers are persons who receive health care services (or would if they had adequate access to care). Regulators are bodies that create rules with which health care suppliers and providers must comply. Finally, payers are persons and organizations that pay for the care provided. This section discusses these five important groups of health care system participants in more detail.

Providers

The providers of health care services include all persons and organizations that produce and distribute health care services. Included among providers are health professionals such as nurses and physicians and HCOs such as hospitals, long-term care facilities, and home health agencies. The government is also a major provider of health care services.

In discussions of the health care environment, providers are often grouped together as if they were one entity. However, providers often have different and competing interests, as well as financial incentives. The traditional providers and those about whom the most have been written are nurses, physicians, hospitals, and the government. We begin by discussing these providers and then discuss others who currently play—and will continue to play—an important role in a reformed health system.

Nurses

Most nurses work for hospitals, but many work in other settings, such as long-term care facilities, home care agencies, surgical centers, clinics, HMOs, physician offices, hospices, and schools.

❋ TABLE 2–2 *Key Participants in the Health Care System*

Key Participants	Role
Providers	Professionals and entities that deliver care to patients
Nurses	Licensed individuals who deliver nursing care to patients. Includes RNs, APRNs, and LPNs
Physicians	Licensed individuals who deliver medical care to patients. Includes MDs and DOs who focus on general and specialty medical practice
Hospitals	Institutions that employ individuals (e.g., nurses, physicians, and other staff) to deliver nursing and medical care to patients who are ill, injured, or seeking treatment for which specialized equipment, procedures, or services are required
Governments	Local (e.g., schools), state (e.g., health departments), and national (e.g., Department of Veterans Affairs) entities supported through public funds to deliver a variety of health care services to patients
Others	Licensed (e.g., pharmacists, dentists, physician assistants) and unlicensed (nursing and medical assistants) individuals and institutions (e.g., home health care, long-term care, mental health facilities) that provide a specific type and scope of health care to patients
Suppliers	Entities that make and distribute materials, goods, pharmaceuticals, and equipment used in the provision of health care
Consumers	Individuals who receive health care services; this refers to patients and clients to whom care is provided, as well as their families
Regulators	Entities that make the rules and regulations that govern the delivery of health care
Payers	Entities that pay for the delivery of health care
Individuals	Entities who receive care and also pay for it
Insurers	Entities that pay for health care services delivered to individuals under covered plans by pooling risk
Employers	Entities that pay a portion or the entire amount of health care insurance or health care services delivered to its workforce
Governments	Local (e.g., health clinics), state (e.g., Medicaid), and federal (e.g., Medicare) entities that pay for care delivered to citizens who meet certain requirements through public funds

APRN, advanced practice registered nurse; DO, Doctor of Osteopathic Medicine; LPN, licensed practical nurse; MD, Medical Doctor; RN, registered nurse.

Nurses affiliated with hospitals generally work on nursing units that are part of specialty areas within the greater nursing department. A chief nursing officer (or chief nurse executive) oversees nursing departmental operations and generally reports to the hospital's chief operating officer or chief executive officer. The organizational structure of nursing within HCOs is addressed in Chapter 3.

The primary role of the staff nurse is to provide direct, hands-on care to patients, although that role has evolved over the years. In addition to hands-on care, nurses today plan, coordinate, and oversee the care that patients receive. They also act in a supervisory capacity, managing other individuals, such as unlicensed assistive personnel and licensed practical nurses, who provide care directly to patients. The many professional activities that fall within the domain of nurses and nursing are well known to most of the readers of this book. Nurses often believe that only educated health professionals can assess the type and quality of care that should be or is being provided to patients, and they generally believe that nursing should have autonomy over its own professional practice.

Nurses have traditionally been employees of HCOs, with their income related to the amount of time they work rather than to the number of care episodes they provide. This relationship of income and work must be considered to fully understand nurses' incentives in the provision of care. The commonly touted need to control costs in HCOs and the health care system has often taken a lower priority for nurses at the point of care delivery than providing excellent patient care. From a professional perspective, nurses have typically seen their role as providing the best possible care. They considered it the role of other managers in the organization to find the resources necessary for nurses to provide that care. On the other hand, the financial management of resources has been a key component of nurse managers' and executives' roles, and many have felt caught between staff who deliver care and other health care administrators who allocate financial resources—or they feel caught between focusing on quality or cost aspects of care.

Today the nursing profession—including nurse managers—is in a very different position. The passage of health reform legislation—the ACA—in 2010 opened the door for nurses to fill expanded roles in a variety of health care settings. On the heels of this legislation, the landmark Institute of Medicine (IOM)–Robert Wood Johnson Foundation report, *The Future of Nursing: Leading Change, Advancing Health* (2011), outlined opportunities for nurses to contribute in a transformed health care system. This report proposed a set of key messages and recommended strategies (shown in Table 2–3) that are already shaping the future roles for nurses at local, state, and federal levels. As the federal government also puts efforts in place to stop paying hospitals and other providers for errors and preventable health care–acquired conditions, the importance of nurses in patient surveillance and error prevention at the point of care has become evident. Nurses are now viewed as key to ensuring safety and, in turn, hospital reimbursements.[4] Although the combined effects of these efforts hold great promise for the future of nursing, realizing that promise will take time and require a change not only in the health care system itself but also in the mindset of all of key participants in the health system, including nurses, as they begin working together in new approaches to care delivery.

Although a majority—62%—of nurses work in acute care hospitals,[5] they have a variety of options when it comes to selecting a work setting. Each opportunity has its own specific characteristics, advantages, and disadvantages. For example, the salaries paid to nurses working as employees in physicians' offices have often been lower than those paid in other settings. The working hours tend to be better, however, and the level of job-related stress has been lower. Some nurses work as consultants. They tend to work longer hours and earn higher salaries, but they may lose most, if not all, patient contact. Some nurses work for insurers or MCOs evaluating claims. They may also lose patient contact, but they work stable, 9-to-5 hours with less overtime and stress. Other nurses work as independent

---

[4]Retrieved July 12, 2011, at http://www.aannet.org/files/public/ippswhitepaper.pdf.
[5]Retrieved July 11, 2011, at http://bhpr.hrsa.gov/healthworkforce/rnsurveys/rnsurveyfinal.pdf.

✳ **TABLE 2–3** *Key Messages and Associated Recommendations from the Institute of Medicine–Robert Wood Johnson Foundation's The Future of Nursing Report*

Key Messages	Recommendations
Nurses should practice to the full extent of their education and training.	Remove scope-of-practice barriers.
Nurses should achieve higher levels of education and training through an improved education system that promotes seamless academic progression.	Implement nurse residency programs. Increase the proportion of nurses with a baccalaureate degree to 80% by 2020. Double the number of nurses with a doctorate degree by 2020. Ensure that nurses engage in lifelong learning.
Nurses should be full partners with physicians and other health care professionals in redesigning health care in the United States.	Expand opportunities for nurses to lead and diffuse collaborative efforts. Prepare and enable nurses to lead change to advance health.
Effective workforce planning and policymaking require better data collection and an improved information infrastructure.	Build an infrastructure for the collection and analysis of interprofessional health care workforce data.

Adapted from Institute of Medicine: *The future of nursing: leading change, advancing health,* Washington, DC, 2011, National Academies Press. Reprinted with permission from the National Academies Press, Copyright 2011, National Academy of Sciences.

nurse practitioners or entrepreneurs, setting their own time schedules.

As nurses' roles expand with health reform, their employment options will likely expand. As a result of the ACA, ACOs, patient-centered medical (or health) homes, community health centers, and nurse-managed health centers will bring opportunities for nurse employment. The salaries paid to nurses and the hours they work will likely change, such that the characteristics, advantages, and disadvantages noted previously may change. For example, some insurers have begun reimbursing physician practices higher payments so that nurses can be hired to fill roles as care coordinators for patient follow-up and care management. Thus, there are potentially great changes ahead for nurses in terms of where they work, the roles they fill, and how they are paid, and these changes provide a great opportunity for nurses to emphasize the value they bring to their work. Chapter 22 discusses the expanding opportunities for nurses as entrepreneurs. In all of these cases, there are tradeoffs of employment whereby nurses must select the job, hours, salary, level of patient contact, setting, and stress level that best fits with their personal lives and helps them achieve their career goals.

Nurse managers and executives will see their roles change, too. They will be under increasing pressure to balance human resources, particularly nurse staffing and models of care, with quality of care metrics. Given that health care–acquired conditions have been closely linked to nurse staffing and nursing care, investments to improve nurse staffing and the work environment may be the best quality improvement strategies available to HCOs.[6]

Physicians

Physicians provide health care both in and outside of the hospital. They are generally paid for each episode of care they provide, although frequently they are paid a fee per month no matter how much care they provide. The two predominant locales for the provision of care by physicians are their offices and hospitals.

In their offices, physicians are generally owners or co-owners, although sometimes they are employees working for another physician or for a hospital that has purchased their practice. Often the structure of the physician's office is corporate. By forming a corporation, the physician acts to limit personal liability. The corporation owning the practice is liable for paying for equipment, rent, supplies, and salaries. If the corporation fails, the owner is not personally liable to pay the debts of the business.

Some essential health care procedures and supplies are used by physicians in their offices regardless of cost. For example, they always use sterile needles. On the other hand, physicians often add services and facilities to their office practice only if they believe they are financially justified. That is, an internist's office will add an x-ray machine for taking chest radiographs only if it is seen as a profit enhancement; otherwise, patients will be referred to a radiologist.

Traditionally, most physicians have been considered "guests" at or affiliated with a hospital rather than employees. This relationship created an unusual set of incentives for both physicians and hospitals. Most technological improvements in the quality of care offered by the hospital are paid for by hospitals. The same physician who might not replace an existing office x-ray machine with the latest model available is still likely to demand that the hospital purchase the latest equipment. The hospital's acquisition of such equipment does not cost the physician anything, but it gives the hospital some assurance that the physician will admit patients to the hospital to receive the service. The hospital will then charge patients for the service afforded by the purchase of the new equipment. In some cases, the equipment can reduce physicians' time treating each patient, allow physicians and hospitals to treat more patients, or allow physicians and the hospital to provide additional types of treatments based on their clinical findings from using the equipment, enhancing both physicians' and the hospital's income.

Today, physicians are increasingly becoming hospital "employees." They are assuming a variety of roles, including hospitalist (i.e., physicians hired specifically to care for patients while they are admitted to hospitals), care team member (as a primary care provider or specialist), and organizational manager or executive. In some cases, entire physician practices are being purchased, and subsequently all practice employees become hospital or health system employees. In other cases, physicians are becoming owners of health care delivery entities, such as surgical centers, putting them in direct competition with hospitals. Employee, competitor, or guest, physicians are duly motivated to ensure that their patients receive the best care possible. In fact, the federal government has provided incentives to report on physician care via the Physician Quality Reporting System.[7] The value-based purchasing movement (discussed later) will increasingly place pressure on physicians to focus on the quality of care delivered to patients because their payment will depend on it.

Being an employee or guest rather than an owner has implications for physicians' views of the financial structure of the hospital. For example, it has always been in physicians' best interests for their affiliating hospitals to stay in business, but there was often little perceived reason not to convince the hospitals to acquire the latest technology so that patients received the presumed best quality of care. As they become hospital employees, hospital managers, partners, or competitors, their view on acquiring the latest technology regardless of cost may be more restrained.

Physicians also stand to benefit under the ACA. The legislation provides a 10% bonus to primary care physicians and general surgeons working in health professional shortage areas and 100% reimbursement for providing preventive service in

---

[6]Litvak E, Buerhaus PI, Davidoff F, et al. 2005. Managing unnecessary variability in patient demand to reduce nursing stress and improve patient safety. *Jt Comm J Qual Patient Saf* 31(6):330-338.

[7]Retrieved July 11, 2011, at https://www.cms.gov/PQRS.

outpatient settings. However, it also requires physicians to disclose financial relationships with suppliers and manufacturers, including pharmaceutical companies, to minimize potential unethical behaviors.

Physicians can be extremely persuasive because of their role in advising patients where to go for treatment. The physician represents the primary source of patients for most hospitals. A physician affiliated with two or three hospitals, as many have been in the past, had the ability to steer patients toward any of those hospitals. In most cases today, physicians affiliate with a particular hospital because of certain characteristics or indicators that make it most suitable for their patients' needs, and in many cases, because of contractual arrangements.

As more and more physicians become hospital employees, they too will likely begin selecting hospital employers in ways that are very similar to those used by nurses; that is, they will seek out hospitals in which to work based on the offering of competitive salaries and benefits, good schedules and back-up coverage, professional advancement opportunities, and good working environments. Incentives being what they are, however, physicians in certain roles can still use their control over patient admissions to gain specific concessions from hospitals.

The power that physicians have over hospital admissions is one of the most important forces in the hospital industry. Their control over admissions also affects long-term care and admissions, home care agency patient referrals, and referrals to other physician specialists. In trying to understand the actions of participants in the health care system, it is essential to understand this key role that physicians play in directing patients where to go for their care.

Hospitals

Hospitals serve two primary functions. They house sophisticated technological equipment, and they are locations where patients can receive 24-hour-per-day nursing and medical care for acute episodes. Society centralizes services, locating essential pieces of equipment and skilled personnel resources in specific locations: acute care hospitals. Patients with acute health problems go to hospitals for diagnostic tests and for treatment. A wide range of health care professionals can make use of sophisticated clinical supplies and technologies in hospitals to provide patient care.

The hospital is an organizational entity with an existence apart from the individual professionals who provide care within its walls. Some hospitals are organized as for-profit companies, and many of these are publicly traded corporations whose stock can be bought and sold on national exchanges. Some hospitals are owned by governments. A majority of hospitals in the United States (~80%) are established as voluntary agencies; that is, they are not-for-profit organizations and are not run by corporations or government agencies. Any profits that they earn are reinvested for the benefit of the local community. Some hospitals are established as subsidiaries of larger not-for-profit organizations, such as religious organizations or universities.

The hospital's leadership typically consists of health care executives, professionals, and a board of directors or trustees. The board is generally made up of respected members of the community, many who often are not health care professionals, as well as physicians, health care leaders, and other health professionals.

The hospital's professional leadership, together with the board, establishes overriding goals and directions for the organization and provides oversight to ensure that the organization acts to achieve those goals. Most hospitals have as part of their primary mission the provision of the highest quality of care possible. Hospitals, however, also have limited resources. In recognition of that fact, the achievement of all goals is tempered by the need to stay in business. If the hospital fails financially and stops providing services, the result will be less desirable than providing only acceptable care rather than the highest quality care.

Hospitals today are rarely the stand-alone, sole organizational entities of the past. More than ever before, they are part of integrated systems or networks formed to deliver care to patients along a continuum of care. There are also specialty hospitals dedicated to providing care to specific groups of patients, such as children's hospitals, which focus on pediatric care; cancer hospitals, which provide specific care and treatments to oncology patients; psychiatric hospitals, which care for patients' mental health care needs; and rehabilitation hospitals, which care for patients with certain physiologic and orthopedic needs. Within integrated systems, there may be organizational entities ranging from primary care facilities to acute care hospitals, specialty hospitals, and long-term care facilities. This approach reflects the industry's attempt to better organize, coordinate, and consolidate care. Although the approach, in principle, seems innovative, cost-effective, and patient-centered, in some cases, it may have the undesired effect of driving up costs, fragmenting care, and shutting out independent providers.

Hospitals will also be affected by the ACA. Hospitals that receive Medicare Disproportionate Share Hospital payments (i.e., payments for providing uncompensated care) will see that amount reduced initially but subsequently adjusted based on the percent of unpaid care delivered to uninsured individuals. Other notable impacts will be that, beginning October 1, 2012, Medicare payments to individual hospitals will be reduced to account for the occurrence of preventable hospital readmissions; in 2015, Medicare payments to hospitals will be reduced by 1% for hospital-acquired conditions (HACs). Similar to physicians, hospitals will also be required to disclose relationships with other key health system participants (e.g., suppliers or physicians) and will be subject to value-based purchasing programs, or programs that reward hospitals based on quality measures.[8] These issues are discussed in greater depth later in this chapter, but because of the implications of the ACA, they are addressed as appropriate throughout the book.

Government

The three levels of government—local, state, and national—are large providers of health care services. The federal government provides health care and operates significant hospital systems

---

[8]Retrieved July 12, 2011, at http://www.kff.org/healthreform/upload/8061.pdf.

for the active duty military, for veterans, and for the federal prison system. State governments often operate a variety of health care facilities, including hospitals for mental health and clinics and hospitals for prisoners. Public hospitals have existed for many decades in the United States. Local governments have often become actively involved as providers of health care services because many cities and counties own hospitals, long-term care, and outpatient facilities.

The government generally provides only services that it believes will not otherwise be available, and it generally does so by supporting a variety of public health services and programs. For example, it aids in preventing the spread of diseases through vaccination programs; protects against environmental hazards through the study and issue of warnings against toxins such as lead exposure; prevents commonly occurring injuries through programs such as teen motor vehicle accident prevention; encourages healthy behaviors through such programs as smoking cessation and obesity prevention; responds to disasters that affect community health, such as floods and hurricanes; and provides access to health services through programs, such as the training of health professionals through the Public Health Service Commissioned Corps.[9]

The government also has a role as a payer for care. That role is partly intended to ensure adequate access. Nonetheless, there are clearly situations in which access is still not adequate without the direct intervention of the government as a provider of care, and in some cases, the government directly provides the care. However, as local, state, and federal budgets have become constrained to deal with mounting budget deficits, some of these services have been severely curtailed. For example, one area that has received serious cutbacks at local, state, and federal levels is the provision of government-supported mental health services.

Other Providers

Many other types of providers of health care services are not discussed in detail here. These include other professionals, such as pharmacists, as well as entities that employ professionals and in which nurses have a significant role, such as long-term care facilities, home care agencies, and primary care clinics. There are also providers in which nurses have little or no role, such as dental offices. Each type of provider has unique perspectives, incentives, and problems.

Many providers share commonalities and have differences from those described above. For example, physical therapists may work for a salary at a hospital or rehabilitation facility, as nurses do, or be paid on a per treatment basis, as physicians are. Pharmacists play an important role in the dispensing and delivery of pharmaceuticals and in patient counseling to prevent medication errors and drug interactions. They are generally salaried employees in hospitals, drugstores, retail pharmacies, and pharmaceutical companies, although a small number are still self-employed and own local pharmacies.[10]

Other types of providers, such as home health agencies, may have a goal of making profits or may be not-for-profit voluntary organizations.

A newer type of provider, the "minute clinic," represents a movement to provide health services for routine care more quickly than waiting to be seen at an emergency department or for a physician appointment and at a lower cost than one might incur in these other settings. Minute clinics are often extended hour, or in some cases, round-the-clock, for-profit entities, owned or operated by pharmaceutical chains, other large retailers, or health systems.[11] These clinics offer employment opportunities for nurse practitioners, who are typically employed as the primary provider of care in the minute clinic. Not only are nurse practitioners skilled in providing these kinds of services, but they are also less costly to employ than physicians. This model provides a "one-stop shopping" approach to care delivery because retailers offering health services can get customers "in the door" to purchase the health service plus pharmaceuticals, groceries, school supplies, and other goods and services.

It is important to note the variety of providers with competing goals and interests. Even some providers working for other providers may have conflicting interests in the area of finance: Physicians may make money if the hospital expends resources and loses money. For example, the addition of a lithotripter machine will probably increase the income of urologists at a hospital, but the machine may be so expensive that the hospital loses money on lithotripsy procedures.

Other conflicts arise in the area of quality of care. Faced with declining reimbursements, hospitals may look to cut the number of professionals or professional hours (or both) of care provided per patient day. On the other hand, nursing staff, concerned about widely publicized reports of errors in health care delivery, patient safety, and nurse staffing levels, may be unable to achieve their primary goal of increasing the quality and safety of patient care. The differences in the underlying goals of each provider may carry over to the strategies that each provider uses to achieve its goals.

Suppliers

The second key participant in the health care system is the supplier. This group includes the manufacturers and distributors of all pharmaceuticals, supplies, and equipment used in HCOs.

Often suppliers are not considered in discussions of the key participants in the health care system. They are virtually always for-profit corporations that are part of the general industrial complex. Are they related to health care? Suppliers play an important role in the production of health services and make billions of dollars of sales each year. For example, in 2009, 10% of U.S. health care spending went to pharmaceuticals, and 3% went to durable (e.g., wheelchairs and hearing aids) and nondurable (e.g., over-the-counter drugs) goods.[12] Although

---

[9]Retrieved July 11, 2011, at http://www.health.gov/phfunctions/public.htm.
[10]Retrieved July 11, 2011, at http://www.bls.gov/oco/ocos079.htm#emply.

[11]Retrieved July 11, 2011, at http://www.chcf.org/~/media/Files/PDF/H/PDF%20HealthCareInTheExpressLaneRetailClinics.pdf.
[12]Retrieved June 25, 2011, at http://www.cms.gov/NationalHealthExpendData/downloads/PieChartSourcesExpenditures2009.pdf.

these percentages sound small, they amounted to more than $300 billion! Thus, one cannot ignore their role.

Suppliers do not just provide the health care industry with the items that providers need to care for their patients. Suppliers also invent new technologies, such as new drugs and computerized equipment. That innovative role is a significant issue in understanding the environment in which the health care system operates.

Often new technologies are extremely expensive. The suppliers have therefore taken an active role that, on the one hand, may improve the quality of care that can be provided and the quality of life for individuals but on the other hand may increase the costs of providing it.

Consumers

Consumers are the individuals who use health care services.[13] Consumers use a variety of services, ranging from preventive and advisory services to diagnostic, therapeutic, and rehabilitative care and in some cases to monitoring or custodial care.

Consumers are becoming increasingly knowledgeable about the services they want from health care providers. Access to the Internet has dramatically increased information available to consumers. Nevertheless, there is still a gap in knowledge between the health care professional and the consumer of health care services. As a result, individual consumers often rely heavily on health care professionals to advise them.

Most nurses view consumers as patients and their families. Nurses are educated to encourage consumers to participate actively in their care. Therefore, nurses work with patients to select treatment options and to choose where care will be provided.

This may not always be the case with other providers. Physicians in particular have tremendous power over consumers because of the physicians' specialized knowledge. Physicians can use this to their advantage—and perhaps their patients'—by convincing hospitals to provide resources in exchange for patient admissions, as discussed earlier. However, these power distinctions may change as health care systems, consumer and physician relationships evolve. Given the emphasis on patient-centered care in quality and safety initiatives, the role of patients and their families will likely grow even more prominent in the future.

Although one usually thinks of patients as individuals, in recent years, consumers have become increasingly involved in collective action. Consumer groups such as the American Association of Retired Persons (AARP) have actively lobbied for better health care options that are ostensibly in the interest of the represented group. Because many of these groups represent constituencies of voters, governments often respond to them.

Regulators

The regulatory environment in which the health care system exists is dominated by rules and regulations that affect the actions and activities of health care providers, payers, and consumers. Some regulations even regulate the activities of regulators in a technical tangle of rules that often seems to distract the health care system from the activity of providing health care services.

Regulations are generally thought of in terms of a government order that has the force of law. The government, at local, state, and federal levels, as part of its role to protect the public, has an interest in maintaining the public's health. To achieve that end, a number of regulations are issued. Although regulations are generally not laws, they are often promulgated by government agencies to carry out laws. Health care providers must obey the regulations or be subject to specific legal sanctions. In some instances, the sanctions have strong implications for reimbursement. This would be the case, for instance, if a hospital were not eligible to receive Medicaid payments if it failed to comply with a certain state regulation.

The U.S. Constitution identifies the federal government's responsibility to protect the health and welfare of the people. In recent years, this has been broadly interpreted by the federal government to develop increasing safeguards for the public's health, including regulating pharmacologic agents and monitoring communicable diseases.

In its role as a payer for health services (discussed later in this chapter), the federal government has developed regulations for providers of health care services that are paid for with federal dollars. For example, the federal government has created a number of regulations that specify who can participate in Medicare. These regulations affect providers, consumers, and even organizations that the federal government contracts with to process Medicare claims for payment. Beginning in 1998, advanced practice nurses could be paid directly by Medicare.

The state regulatory function varies widely from state to state. In part, this regulatory influence is derived from the state's function to regulate those services for which it pays, such as those provided under Medicaid. The regulations also derive from the state's interest in protecting the public through the licensure of those professionals and organizations that provide health care. Regulations vary, ranging from rules that decree the square footage of patient rooms in hospitals, to the ratio of nurses to patients in an intensive care unit, to the information that must be provided to patients before they are discharged from hospitals.

Licensure is one of the widely applied regulations. It is not without controversy, however. Every state has laws concerning the licensing of health professionals and HCOs that provide care. Some economists have argued that such licensing is unnecessary. Instead, they suggest disclosure. HCOs would have to provide consumers with information about the training or credentialing of professionals employed, their experience, and their care outcomes. Then consumers could decide what providers to use and how high a price they are willing to pay. Although some of this information is available today, such as certain outcomes of hospital care, licensure remains prominent in our society. The arguments in favor are that licensure ensures the public of minimum practice levels for various professionals and providers.

---

[13]The term *consumer* is viewed broadly to include patients, their families, and others who use health care products and services.

Furthermore, the damage that could be done by an untrained, unexamined provider is too great to warrant the risk. There is little consensus on whether regulation is positive or negative for the health care system, but protection of the public is the general position of policymakers. How that protection plays out depends on the information available to the public and the political positions prevalent in our society.

Local government regulations often cover areas related to construction, fire safety, and how to handle a death. For example, in many states, regulations do not allow nurses to declare a patient dead. Often such regulations result from lobbying efforts by special interest groups such as the American Medical Association (AMA) rather than from an underlying need to protect the consumer.

Because the government is a large provider of health care services, it is interesting to realize that the government in some instances is regulating itself. Often the federal government is exempt from local law. Therefore, the building codes and licensing regulations that affect a voluntary hospital may not affect a military hospital. Only the government has the legal authority to issue regulations and to mandate adherence to them. However, health providers are also subject to the regulations of voluntary accreditation and certification bodies, such as The Joint Commission (formerly the Joint Commission on Accreditation of Healthcare Organizations). Although adherence to the standards of these organizations is voluntary, societal and fiscal pressures are such that few hospitals elect not to be accredited by The Joint Commission, and few surgeons choose not to be certified by their specialty board.

Nurse managers and nursing associations can do a number of things to influence the adoption of regulations at all levels of government and by associations such as The Joint Commission and the Institute for Healthcare Improvement (see Chapters 5 and 23). Change is slow, however, and satisfying the wishes of individual provider groups is not always possible.

It is essential that nurse managers and executives become familiar with the various regulations that affect their profession, organization, department, and unit. They must reflect on how those regulations affect not only day-to-day operations but also the management decisions they can make. Because regulations vary so much from state to state, it is important for nurse managers to know the regulations in the state in which they practice.

Payers

In the U.S. health care system, often the consumer of health care services does not pay for them directly. The most common payers are individuals, insurance companies, employers, and government.

The single largest payer group for health care services is the government. Among Medicare, Medicaid, and other direct government payments for health care services, the government paid for about 42% of the care provided in 2009.[14] Table 2–4 illustrates the projected national health expenditures for the year 2013 by

✳ **TABLE 2–4** *National Health Care Expenditures*

	2013*	
	$ in Billions	**Percent**
Private	1,484	49
Federal	1,131	37
State and local	410	14
Total	3,025	100

*Projected.
Abstracted from Center for Medicare & Medicaid Services, Office of the Actuary. *National Health Expenditure (NHE) Amounts by Type of Expenditure and Source of Funds: Calendar Years 1965-2019 in PROJECTIONS Format.* Retrieved at http://www.cms.gov/NationalHealthExpendData/03_NationalHealthAccountsProjected.asp.

source of funding. As shown here, the federal and state governments combined are projected to contribute just over half (51%) of all funding for the health care system by 2013.

Insurers and employers were the next largest payer for care followed by individuals paying for their own care. About 32% of health care costs were paid for by private insurance and 7% by other third-party payers and programs, such as worksite health care and other private and charitable sources. About 12% of all personal health expenditures were paid for by individuals "out of pocket." In 2009, health care expenditures amounted to approximately $8,086 per person, with individuals spending on average about $975 out of pocket.[15] The services and goods purchased out of pocket included over-the-counter medications, prescriptions, physician services, private duty nursing service, and institutional care. Figure 2–1 illustrates where the health care dollars came from in 2009.

The ACA will change the incentives, constraints, and behaviors of payers. However, the extent to which each type of provider is affected will be better understood as the reforms evolve and as various initiatives are put into place.

Individual Consumers

In most aspects of our society, individuals are obligated to pay for the resources they consume. In health care, however, that is only the case for the minority of payments. Most of the money paid to health care providers does not come directly from individuals.

Given the high cost of health care services, this should not be surprising. For example, if a $300,000 house burns down, it is unlikely that it will be rebuilt with money directly from the owner. It is much more likely that the owner was paying an annual insurance premium to protect the house in case of a fire. Many people pay premiums to the insurer, but only a few houses burn down. The insurance company then pays the $300,000 to rebuild the house. Similarly, individuals who have health insurance call upon their insurance to pay for major health care services. What about an individual who has not been paying premiums and does not have insurance? If your

[14]Centers for Medicare and Medicaid Services. *The Nation's Health Dollar: Where It Came From.* Retrieved June 30, 2011, at https://www.cms.gov/nationalhealthexpenddata/02_nationalhealthaccountshistorical.asp.

[15]*Ibid.*

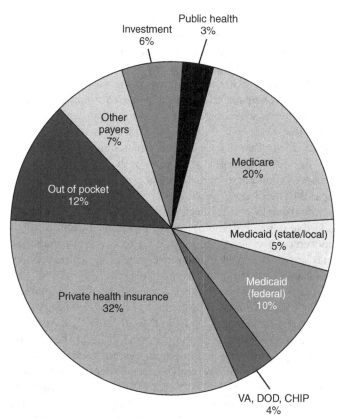

FIGURE 2–1. Health care spending: Where the money came from, 2009. (Data from Centers for Medicare & Medicaid Services, Office of the Actuary, National Health Statistics Group. Available at https://www.cms.gov/NationalHealthExpendData/.)

house burns down and it is uninsured, there are two main choices: Rebuild it with your own money if you have it or do without a new house if you do not.

Individuals who pay providers directly for health care services are referred to as *self-pay* patients. They are often charged the highest rates. They are also the most likely to default on their payment obligations because the high cost of care is beyond their personal means.

Approximately 50.7 million Americans—or almost 19% of the non-elderly population—had no health insurance in 2009 and were forced to pay for all their care or seek care from public facilities that do not require payment.[16] Many uninsured individuals are older than 18 years of age, ineligible for support through Medicaid or other public sources of funding, and younger than 65 years of age, when Medicare coverage becomes available. A large and growing segment of the uninsured population is young adults. For example, approximately 57% of individuals younger than 34 years of age lack health insurance, with 40% of uninsured individuals being between the ages of 19 and

34 years.[17] Moreover, individuals of racial and ethnic minority groups represent a disproportionate share of the uninsured population; whereas about 21% of Blacks, 28% of American Indians/Alaska Natives, and 32% of Hispanics lack health insurance, only 13% of Whites lack health insurance.[18] These uninsured individuals inevitably receive care in the health care system at some point in time that must be paid for in some way. Other Americans, even though they have insurance for some health care costs, may be "underinsured" because they have to pay for certain kinds of care that their insurance does not cover. This often includes preventive care, such as annual gynecologic examinations or mammograms; eyeglasses; medications, both prescription and nonprescription; and many home health services.

One of the more controversial aspects of the ACA is the "mandate" that individuals must obtain health coverage or face a penalty. Although some exceptions can be made because of hardship, the penalty for individuals without insurance coverage is $95 or 1% of taxable income in 2014, escalating to $695 or 2.5% of taxable income in 2016; beyond that, the penalty escalates according to cost of living adjustments.[19] Because this law requires individuals to have health insurance coverage or be penalized, it has been challenged in court. One of the principal arguments against the act is the contention that the federal government cannot impose the requirement because health insurance is regulated at the state level. Others argue that the law is a "valid exercise of legislative power by Congress under the Commerce Clause."[20] The rationale for the latter view is that individuals who do not purchase health insurance still impact the health care system through the use of its services. Legal experts anticipate that this issue ultimately will be decided by the U.S. Supreme Court.[21]

Any payers other than the individual consumers who receive care are often called *third-party payers*. This term means that the care provided to an individual is paid for not by the primary parties involved in the transaction—the consumer and the provider—but by a third party. The most common third-party payers are insurers, employers, and the government.

Insurers

Insurance companies take money from individuals and employers, pool the money, and then pay providers or reimburse insured individuals for part of their outlays when they consume health care services. Some insurance companies operate as for-profit corporations. Other insurers are not-for-profit organizations, existing to provide service rather than to profit from the provision of that service. Still other insurers are formed as mutual companies, returning any profits earned to their insured population in the form of dividends or reduced premiums.

[16]The Kaiser Commission on Medicaid and the Uninsured. 2011. *The Uninsured: A Primer.* Retrieved February 2, 2012, at http://www.kff.org/uninsured/upload/7451-07.pdf.
[17]*Ibid.*

[18]*Ibid.*
[19]The Kaiser Family Foundation. 2011. *Focus on Health Reform: Summary of New Health Reform Law.* Retrieved July 6, 2011, at http://www.kff.org/healthreform/upload/8061.pdf.
[20]Retrieved July 12, 2011, at http://www.medscape.com/viewarticle/745897.
[21]*Ibid.*

Many insurers are able to demand discounted rates from health care providers. If hospitals or other providers refuse to negotiate a discount, the insurer can tell its insured members that they will not be paid for all or a certain amount of the care received from that provider. Losing payments for all patients who are covered by an insurer can present a substantial financial blow to a health care provider; thus, it is in their interest to negotiate discounted rates with insurers.

The negotiated discount from normal charges becomes formalized through a contract drawn up between the insurer and the health care provider. The discount is referred to as a *contractual allowance* because it is a discount from standard rates, as allowed for in the contract between the payer and the provider.

In the 1990s and early 2000s, insurance was increasingly provided by MCOs such as Oxford Health Plans or Aetna. A backlash by consumers (related to choice and plan complexity) and providers (related to reimbursement and red tape) brought about transformation in the provision of coverage by MCOs and other insurers.[22]

Managed care set the stage for insurers today to negotiate with providers. For example, the creation ACOs under the ACA evolved from managed care and retained some of the principles established by the managed care movement. Unlike managed care, however, ACOs cannot restrict patients from seeing providers outside of the "network" by requiring them to pay higher fees. ACOs also require providers to share the risks and profits. This can result in losses for the providers if care is more costly than anticipated or if quality care is not provided.

Private insurers will face a very different set of requirements and constraints under the ACA. One of the most notable requirements is that insurers must cover individuals with pre-existing conditions, and they cannot restrict coverage limits or deny coverage for policyholders who get sick. They must also offer coverage to the dependent children of policyholders until they are 26 years of age, and they must provide a "minimum" level of coverage to policyholders, which includes certain types of preventive services (e.g., covering immunizations). The waiting period for individuals to obtain insurance coverage is also limited to 90 days. Finally, insurers must put certain consumer protections in place, such as providing Web access to coverage information and simplifying the administrative and financial transactions related to coverage.

Employers

Employers, especially larger ones, have included health care benefits as a fringe benefit for many years. To a great extent, this benefit used to consist of buying health insurance for the employee. For large companies, however, there are often enough employees to reasonably anticipate likely claims. In such cases, employers provide health care insurance benefits to the employees without contracting with an insurance company to take the risk.

Consider if the employer had decided to offer its employees fire insurance. If the employer has 20,000 employees, it might reasonably determine from historical patterns that in any given year between 5 and 10 houses will burn down among its 20,000 employees. Rather than buying insurance for each employee, the company may find it cheaper to simply reimburse the employees whose houses burn down. Suppose, hypothetically, that there is an average $300,000 loss when a house burns down. Ten fires would cost the company $3 million. Paying $1,000 for a policy for each of the 20,000 employees, however, would cost the company $20 million. It is cheaper to bear the risk directly.

Most employers, however, are small companies and cannot afford to reimburse employees for the health care services they consume—it is simply too costly. In this case, the employer may provide a health insurance benefit to employees by purchasing a group policy from an insurer.

The cost of insurance coverage has escalated for employees. In 2010, approximately 69% of employers provided health benefits to their employees, up from 60% in 2005.[23] This increase reflects a 13% increase in the provision of health benefits by small firms with three to nine employees, but these figures may be inflated because many small businesses went out of business during the same period. The cost of insurance coverage has also continued to escalate for employers, and they, in turn, have shifted the costs of health insurance to employees through reduced coverage and higher premiums, deductibles, coinsurance, and co-pays. Whereas the average single and family insurance premiums have increased 114% since 2000, the employee's contribution has increased 147%—from $4,819 in 2000 to $9,773 in 2010. Between 1999 and 2010, inflation and wages grew only 31% and 42%, respectively.[24]

Many aspects of health care insurance and claims are complicated. Was the treatment patients received appropriate? Was it provided by a qualified provider? Is the charge appropriate? Because of these complexities, insurance companies generally work for employers under contract and serve as a conduit of payments from employers to health care providers.

Insurance companies use their expertise to process health insurance claims, and the employer pays the insurance company an administrative fee for processing the claims. The employer pays its portion of the actual costs for the claims, which gives the employer a strong incentive to limit benefits covered, encourage employees to restrain their use of health care services, and shift more health care costs to employees. Under the ACA, employees with more than 50 employees that do not offer health coverage will be assessed fees under

---

[22]Mechanic D. 2004. The rise and fall of managed care. *J Health Soc Behav* 45(suppl):76-86.

[23]The Kaiser Family Foundation and Health Research & Educational Trust. 2010. *Employer Health Benefits: 2010 Annual Survey*. Retrieved June 29, 2011, at http://ehbs.kff.org/pdf/2010/8085.pdf.

[24]*Kaiser/HRET Survey of Employer-Sponsored Health Benefits, 1999-2010*. Bureau of Labor Statistics, Consumer Price Index, U.S. City Average of Annual Inflation (April to April), 1999-2010; Bureau of Labor Statistics. *Seasonally Adjusted Data from the Current Employment Statistics Survey, 1999-2010* (April to April). Retrieved June 29, 2011, at http://facts.kff.org/chart.aspx?ch=1681.

certain conditions, but employers with more than 200 employees must enroll employees in an employer-based health plan. Employers with fewer than 50 employees are exempt from penalties.[25]

Government

Governments, in addition to regulating care and providing care, are also the largest payer for care. The most notable areas of government involvement are Medicare and Medicaid. Medicare services are paid for by the federal government, and Medicaid services are paid for by a combination of federal and state payments. Through the Public Health Service Act, the government also supports Federally Qualified Health Centers (FQHCs), which are community-based programs that provide health care to medically underserved populations and areas, including migrants and homeless individuals, and provide public housing programs for residents in program areas.[26] There are also many other smaller federal, state, and local programs that pay health care providers for services.

Both federal and state governments contribute considerable amounts to the provision of health care.[27] The federal government pays for and provides all health care, including dental care, for members of the active duty military through the Military Health System (Department of Defense), and provides a more limited range of benefits for veterans through the Veterans Health Administration (Department of Veterans Affairs). Veterans' coverage is substantial if obtained at Veterans Administration facilities. The U.S. Department of Health and Human Services oversees 11 agencies, including the Indian Health Service, which provides health care for Native Americans, and it is charged with protecting the health of all Americans and providing essential human services for the most vulnerable people in our society. The federal government also provides health care for federal prisoners through the Federal Bureau of Prisons (U.S. Department of Justice). On a more limited basis, the federal government provides health care in a variety of special situations, such as hospital care at the Hospital Center of the National Institutes of Health.

Most state governments provide and pay for health care in institutions for developmentally disabled and mentally ill individuals. Many city and county governments provide and pay for health care in locally owned hospitals and clinics that have historically provided care to medically indigent individuals. In addition, most local governments provide minimal services to citizens, including immunizations and treatment of sexually transmitted disease. Some jurisdictions provide care for children and treatment of communicable diseases. However, in many cases, these services have been curtailed and in some cases eliminated because of the budget cuts imposed by state

and local governments, likely brought about by the Great Recession of 2007–2009.

Other programs are usually directed at vulnerable or at-risk populations such as substance abusers, pregnant women, persons infected with human immunodeficiency virus (HIV), and children at high risk. These programs are also subject to the whims of local political forces and do not have the breadth of coverage and permanence of programs such as Medicare and Medicaid.

As a payer for health care services, the government takes money, usually raised from taxes, and uses it to pay for health services. In a sense, this is a pooling of money, similar to an insurance system, except that there is often a redistributive element. Most of the taxes are paid by individuals who do not directly benefit from the government's health care expenditures at the time the taxes are paid. In other words, the government has adopted a "pay-as-you-go" philosophy in which current employees pay for the health care received by Medicare and Medicaid beneficiaries. Government payments to providers are only for covered groups that the government has specifically identified.

Federal and state governments are also impacted by the ACA. Although it is beyond the scope of this book to cover all of these issues in great detail, the most immediate impact is the requirement for states to create health insurance exchanges through which qualified consumers can purchase insurance to meet the individual mandate. Medicaid expansions will also bring increased funding into states initially, gradually declining to 90% federal funding by 2020. States will also be required to continue providing coverage to children through the Children's Health Insurance Program (CHIP) to eligible children and families. Incentives will be provided for states to cover preventive services (e.g., immunizations). On a more controversial note, federal funds cannot be used to pay for abortions except to save the life of the woman or in cases of incest; states also cannot use federal funds in this manner but may use other funds for this purpose if they so choose. The federal government will also prohibit payments to states via Medicaid for health care–acquired conditions.[28]

✳ FINANCING THE HEALTH CARE SYSTEM

Many individuals and organizations provide health care services because they want to help people stay healthy or get well. However, the economic reality is that most providers would not be able to provide care unless they were compensated. As is the case for other consumer goods and services, health care services represent a product that must be paid for. Thus, it is important for nurse managers and executives to understand the costs of providing health care and the major sources of revenues for health care providers.

Nurse managers and executives also need to understand aggregate health care expenditures and how aggregate trends impact health care and, in turn, their organization. For example,

[25]Retrieved July 12, 2011, at http://www.kff.org/healthreform/upload/8061.pdf.

[26]Retrieved July 12, 2011, at http://bphc.hrsa.gov/about/.

[27]Martin A, Lassman D, Whittle L, et al; the National Health Expenditure Accounts Team. 2011. Recession contributes to slowest annual rate of increase in health spending in five decades. *Health Aff* 30(1), 11-22.

[28]Retrieved July 12, 2011, at http://www.kff.org/healthreform/upload/8061.pdf.

in 2004, national health expenditures were almost $2.5 trillion. The rate of increase in spending for health care services stabilized in the mid 1990s but accelerated again near the turn of the century. The rate of health care spending grew 4% in 2009, the slowest rate of increase in 5 decades.[29] Figure 2–2 shows where the U.S. health care dollars went in 2009. Of the total amount spent on health care in 2009, about 31% ($759 billion) went to hospitals. The remainder of 2009 health care spending went to physicians and clinics (20%); prescription drugs (10%); dental and other professional services (7%); government administration (7% each); investments such as research, structures, and equipment (6%); long-term care facilities and continuing care (6%); medical goods and supplies (3%); home health (3%); government-supported public health activities (3%); and other health, residential, and personal care such as residential care facilities, ambulance providers, and community and senior citizen centers (5%).[30]

There is tremendous pressure to contain the growth in health care costs. Before the passage of Medicare in 1965, health care consumed just 4% of every dollar earned. By 2009, nearly 18% of all U.S. society's earnings was spent on health care.[31] This is not merely the result of inflation. Although more money is spent on health care services, a much larger share of all money earned is also spent on health care. For example, in 1965, an individual earning $15,000 spent $600 on average for health care services. In 2009, if the same individual were earning $60,000 (because of

increases in wage rates), the money spent on health care would not increase proportionately to $2,400 but would have risen to $10,800! This amount includes direct payments by the individual, payments for insurance, and taxes paid to the government to support programs such as Medicare and Medicaid. Much of the growth in costs is related to innovations that have allowed the health care system to do more things to provide care and to provide care in different ways. However, as much as 26% of hospital spending has been reported to be from administrative costs, with administrative costs in for-profit hospitals representing about 36% of spending compared with 23% in not-for-profit hospitals.[32] The costs of health care are expected to continue growing to represent about 19.3% of gross domestic product (GDP) by the year 2019, likely increasing pressures to contain health care costs in the future.[33]

The pressure to contain costs has been the driving force behind U.S. health care reform. It is therefore not surprising that the two largest government-sponsored care delivery and financing programs—Medicare and Medicaid—will undergo some of the most sweeping changes.

The Medicare and Medicaid Programs

By far the most pervasive role of government in the payment for health care is as a third-party payer. This role is primarily a result of Titles 18 and 19 of the Social Security Act of 1965. These laws created Medicare and Medicaid, which commenced in 1966.

[29]Martin et al. 2011.

[30]Centers for Medicare & Medicaid Services, Office of the Actuary, National Health Statistics Group. Retrieved June 29, 2011, at http://www.cms.gov/NationalHealthExpendData/downloads/tables.pdf.

[31]Martin et al. 2011.

[32]Woolhandler S, Himmelstein DU. 1997. Costs of care and administration at for-profit and other hospitals in the U.S. *N Engl J Med* 336(11):769-774.

[33]Truffer CJ, Keehan SK, Smith S, et al. 2010. Health spending projections through 2019: The recession's impact continues. *Health Aff* 29:522-529.

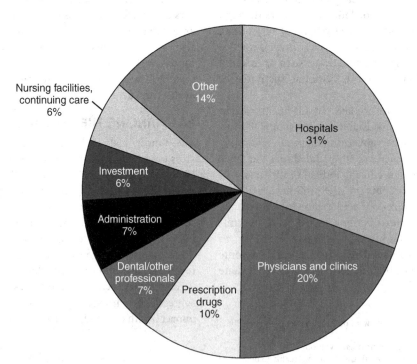

FIGURE 2–2. Health care spending: Where the money went, 2009. (Data from Centers for Medicare & Medicaid Services, Office of the Actuary, National Health Statistics Group. Available at https://www.cms.gov/NationalHealthExpendData/.)

Under Title 18, the federal government administers *Medicare*, an insurance program for individuals age 65 years and older, individuals with certain disabilities younger than the age of 65 years, and individuals of all ages with end-stage renal disease.[34] The Medicare program is administered by the Centers for Medicare and Medicaid Services (CMS) (discussed later). The actual payment system is carried out through the assignment of a number of *fiscal intermediaries*. These organizations receive an administrative fee from the government for processing bills received from providers. The intermediary receives money from CMS and pays it to the providers based on approved claims. Often insurance companies such as Blue Cross act as intermediaries, benefiting from their own expertise in processing health care claims.

Medicare is divided into four separate elements: Parts A, B, C, and D. Part A of the program provides payment for hospital care, hospice care, and some home health care. Part B is the medical care portion of the program that provides payment for physician and outpatient services. Part C provides for some Medicare patients to participate in managed care programs. Part D is a prescription plan for Medicare beneficiaries.

Part A, which is financed by taxes on individual earnings, covers all Medicare members. The amount of payments is decided at the federal level.

Part B is optional. It is financed by premiums from beneficiaries. In 2009, member premiums for Part B coverage ranged from about $96 to more than $300 per month, depending on beneficiary income; beneficiaries with incomes at or above $85,000 for individuals or $170,000 per couple paid higher premiums. The deductible was about $135 per year, and most coinsurance payments were about 20%.[35]

Part C, made available to Medicare recipients through the Tax Equity and Fiscal Responsibility Act (TEFRA),[36] was called the Medicare+Choice and, more recently, the Medicare Advantage (or MA) Plan. This is Medicare's managed care plan offered through private, Medicare-approved insurance companies. Beneficiaries enrolled in these plans receive all of the same Medicare benefits offered through Parts A and B (except hospice care) and often have extra benefits such as vision or dental care that are available through specific managed care plans (including HMOs, or preferred provider organizations [PPOs], and private fee-for-service plans). Under this plan, Medicare pays insurers a fixed amount per enrollee per month, and beneficiaries may also pay a monthly premium, depending on the plan selected. In 2003, enrollees in Part C totaled about 4.6 million beneficiaries and accounted for about 11% of Medicare spending (~$31 billion); more recent figures indicate that enrollees in Part C totaled about 11 million beneficiaries and accounted for about 22% of Medicare spending (~$116 billion).[37] Unfortunately, this plan has

proved to be very expensive because it actually pays plans—or overpays them—at a higher rate than traditional Medicare plans. The research on quality of care under MA plans is also inconclusive.[38] Medicare Part C has become known as a "failed attempt at savings."[39] The ACA brings cost-sharing requirements for benefits offered under Part C plans in line with the traditional fee-for-service program,[40] which represents a significant cut in MA plan payments.[41]

Part D was created through the Medicare Prescription Drug Improvement and Modernization Act of 2003 and is the prescription drug plan offered by Medicare. This insurance plan for prescription drug coverage is also administered by Medicare-approved private insurers in each state. Early in its implementation, Medicare Part D accounted for about 8% of Medicare expenditures; that number has grown to about 11% of spending, covering about 28 million beneficiaries in 2010.[42] Enrollment is voluntary, but beneficiaries must have coverage from another source that is at least as good as Part D or incur a penalty of about 1% of the national benchmark beneficiary premium set by CMS for each month beneficiaries delay enrollment in the plan.[43,44] In 2011, the average monthly payment was about $41 per enrollee, the deductible was $310, and the coinsurance remained at 25% up to the initial coverage limit of $2,840; the catastrophic coverage limit was $6,448.

The ACA addresses several criticisms of Medicare Part D. Beneficiary payments will gradually decrease when they reach the "donut hole,"[45] from paying 100% of the coinsurance rate to paying only 25% of the gap by 2020. In 2011, enrollees who reach the gap will also receive a 50% discount from drug makers on the cost of brand name drugs plus government subsidies of 25% to be phased in between 2013 and 2020. Federal subsidies of 75% will also be phased in for generic drug costs by 2020.[46]

Under Title 19, the federal government also runs the *Medicaid* program for medically indigent individuals. The program is financed by federal general tax revenues (and borrowing) and state contributions. The percentage share paid by the federal government varies from state to state, with poorer states receiving more than wealthier states. The program is optional for states, but all states are currently participating.

[34]Centers for Medicare and Medicaid Services. Retrieved June 26, 2011, at http://www.cms.hhs.gov/MedicareGenInfo/.

[35]Kaiser Family Foundation. 2008. *Medicare At a Glance*. Retrieved July 7, 2011, at http://www.kff.org/medicare/7067/ataglance.cfm.

[36]McGuire TG, Newhouse JP, Sinaiko AD. 2011. An economic history of Medicare Part C. *Milbank Q* 89(2):289-332.

[37]Kaiser Family Foundation. 2010. *Medicare Fact Sheet*. Retrieved July 5, 2011, at http://www.kff.org/medicare/upload/1066-13.pdf.

[38]Kaiser Family Foundation. 2003. *Medicare Fact Sheet: Medicare+Choice*. Retrieved July 7, 2011, at http://www.kff.org/medicare/upload/Medicare-Choice-Fact-Sheet-Fact-Sheet.pdf.

[39]McGuire et al. 2011.

[40]Kaiser Family Foundation. 2003.

[41]McGuire et al. 2011.

[42]Kaiser Family Foundation. 2010.

[43]Staff writer. May 17, 2006. Medicare drug plan covers 38 million people. *Wall Street Journal*, p. A10.

[44]Kaiser Family Foundation. 2010.

[45]When Medicare Part D was implemented in 2006, beneficiaries could reach a gap in coverage that became known as the *donut hole*. The gap was reached when beneficiaries had exceeded their initial coverage limit of $2,250 but had not reached the catastrophic coverage limit of $5,100, when their payments would decline again. Beneficiaries were responsible for 100% of drug costs when they reached the donut hole.

[46]See the July 2006, January 2010, and Fact Sheet reports available at the Kaiser Family Foundation, Retrieved July 6, 2011, at http://www.kff.org/medicare/1066.cfm.

States that choose to participate must pay for a minimal level of services for eligible participants. States may also cover other services in addition to the federally mandated minimum. Services paid for under this title vary widely from state to state. Reimbursement rates are decided by each state and also vary widely. Unlike Medicare, in which participation in managed care is optional, some states mandate that patients receiving Medicaid receive care through an MCO.

In 2010, about 60 million low-income Americans—including children, families, and senior citizens—were covered under Medicaid. During the recession of the late 2000s, Medicaid became the safety net for individuals who lost jobs and health coverage.[47] Interestingly, a recent study indicates that per capita Medicaid spending varied considerably across states. For example, per capita spending in the 10 highest spending states was $1,650 above the average national, and a large proportion of this—72%—was attributable to the volume of services delivered. Per capita spending in the 10 lowest spending states was about $1,160 below the national average, and only 58% was attributable to the volume of services delivered. The mid-Atlantic region spent the most among all regions, and the South Central region spent the least.[48] Another study reported that Medicaid recipients are more likely to receive health services, have fewer out-of-pocket medical expenses and acquired debt, and report being in better physical and mental health than those who are uninsured.[49]

As with Medicare, the ACA will change Medicaid considerably. Some of the changes include covering individuals up to 133% of the federal poverty level ($18,310), offering a benchmark set of essential benefits for newly eligible adults (similar to those available in the newly created health exchanges), and increased funding to states (with 100% federal financing for new enrollees in 2014 to 2016, and gradually leveling to 90% in 2020 and beyond).[50] Although expanding Medicaid will be challenging because of national and state budget pressures, it is anticipated that an additional 16 million people will be covered under this new law. In fact, the changes brought about by the ACA health reform law will ". . . establish Medicaid as the coverage pathway for low-income people in the national framework for near-universal coverage. . . ."[51]

In the nearly 50 years that the Medicare and Medicaid programs have existed, their presence has had a dramatic effect on shaping the way health care is delivered. The original intent was to improve access to care for indigent and elderly groups, which are two underserved populations. Through these programs, the government, as a major payer, has gained increasing control of what care is provided to whom and how it is provided. These programs have also had a major influence on other payers and their practices, with most insurers taking their lead from these programs. However, many believe that these two programs have been the most important factor in the rising health care costs since their inception.

The Insurance System

Insurance is a major source of financing for the health care system, second only to the government in terms of the amount of money it pays to health care providers. Most Americans (61%) have private health insurance, usually provided by employers.[52] Some individuals buy their own health insurance, but the cost of doing so can be prohibitive.

In some cases, insurance companies take the risk of high claims. In other cases, employers assume the risk and retain insurance companies to just process the claims; sometimes providers such as physicians share the risk. In any event, consumers are provided some degree of protection by insurance because resources from a large number of people are pooled together, and not everyone in the pool will need coverage (or the same level of coverage) at the same time.

Thus, insurance is an organized way to share the risk of the costs associated with undesirable events. An insurance *premium* is paid to buy protection against a negative event, or "loss." If a negative event occurs, the insurer provides payment to cover the loss. In this way, the risk of a major financial loss is transferred from the person insured to the insurer, spread among all who are paying premiums into the system, and only those who require health care services use this pooled money.

There are several requirements of an ideal insurable risk.[53] First, there must be large numbers of people who pay into the insurance program. Second, the loss should be accidental or unintentional. Third, the loss or the chance of a loss must be measurable. Fourth, the loss should not be catastrophic, or large numbers of people should not be affected in the same way and at the same time. Finally, the premium should be affordable from a practical standpoint (although many might claim that this last requirement is not met in health care).

A phenomenon, called adverse selection, occurs when people at high risk for a certain disease (e.g., cancer) purchase insurance coverage for the disease but individuals at low risk do not. Unless an insurance company can overcome this problem through its underwriting practices and variable premium rates, it is likely to experience higher-than-expected losses on those policies.[54] This process is similar to individuals' choosing to purchase insurance based on age—younger adults may choose not to purchase health insurance because they do not

[47]Kaiser Family Foundation. 2010. *Medicaid and the Uninsured: The Medicaid Program at a Glance.* Retrieved July 7, 2011, at http://www.kff.org/medicaid/upload/7235-04.pdf.

[48]Gilmer TP, Kronick RG. 2011. Differences in the volume of services and in prices drive big variations in Medicaid spending among U.S. states and regions. *Health Aff 30*(7):1316-1324.

[49]Retrieved July 12, 2011, at http://www.rwjf.org/humancapital/product.jsp?id=72587&cid=XEM_205596.

[50]Kaiser Family Foundation. 2010. *Medicaid and the Uninsured: The Medicaid Program at a Glance.* Retrieved July 7, 2011, at http://www.kff.org/medicaid/upload/7235-04.pdf.

[51]*Ibid*, p. 2.

[52]State Health Access Data Assistance Center. 2011. *State-Level Trends in Employer Sponsored Health Insurance.* Robert Wood Johnson Foundation. Minneapolis MN: University of Minnesota. Retrieved July 8, 2011, at http://www.rwjf.org/files/research/72528shadac201106.pdf.

[53]Rejda GE. 2010. *Principles of Risk Management and Insurance.* Upper Saddle River, NJ: Prentice Hall.

[54]*Ibid*.

perceive to be at risk for health problems; older individuals, however, will likely purchase insurance to cover health problems that generally come with age because they perceive a higher risk. From an insurers' perspective, it is to their advantage to have a greater number of younger, lower risk adults in their plans or to address this problem by charging higher premiums or offering limited services to older adults; if they purposefully enroll younger or healthier, lower cost individuals, it is known as "skimming" or "cherry-picking."

One reason that the ACA imposes penalties on those who do not acquire health insurance is to minimize adverse selection. If young, healthy individuals do not have to buy insurance, then the insured pool will include too many of those who are older and sick. Worse yet, because the ACA does not allow insurance companies to reject individuals based on pre-existing medical conditions, individuals could potentially wait until they are sick before acquiring insurance. That would create an extreme and destructive adverse selection scenario.

Health insurance most often covers services (benefits) rather than being an *indemnity* plan, which provides a dollar amount for a specific medical condition. The policy states that the insurer will provide payment for specified procedures and activities of specified health care providers. Historically, insurers provided a standard set of benefits. Currently, employers negotiate with insurers to provide an array of benefits for a set price. This price is usually based on the previous experience of the group being insured *(group-rated)*.

In *community-rated* plans, the premium is based on the general experience of the community rather than a specific group. Some argue that community rating is the only fair way to share risks. Otherwise, there will be an attempt to load high insurance costs on a small group with a high expense experience. To some extent, this defeats the purpose of insurance. Others argue that community rating is inherently discriminatory, making persons at low risk pay for the high losses experienced by distinctly different groups. Sometimes insurers handle this problem by using community rating but adding surcharges for persons at high risk, such as smokers.

Beneficiaries often complain that "my health plan won't cover that," or nurses complain that "the insurance company won't pay for a nurse to do that procedure." Although it may be accurate that the insurance company will not pay for certain services, it is important to remember that the decision about benefits is made based on the costs of coverage. If more items are included, the costs to the insurer, employer, and consumer will be higher, and the premium will have to be raised.

Moral Hazard

In theory, insurance is an ideal way to deal with the random risk of large losses. Even though some people pay a premium year after year and never collect, they benefit from the peace of mind of knowing that they are protected from a devastating loss.

In practice, however, there are a number of problems with health insurance. Most problems relate to a phenomenon known as *moral hazard*. A moral hazard reflects the fact that after becoming insured, an individual's behavior may change.

Consider an extreme example: Why buy a home fire extinguisher when your house is insured against fire? This example is extreme because it is unlikely that fire insurance can ever adequately reimburse someone for the loss of a home. Personal items may have little dollar value but are meaningful to their owner. Therefore, it is unlikely that an individual would fail to own a fire extinguisher just because the house is insured. Yet fire insurance companies often offer a discount on the premium for working fire alarms or extinguishers. Apparently, even in this extreme situation, insurers have found that moral hazard exists.

In health care, the problems are significantly greater. We might argue that no one is likely to smoke simply because they know they have the safety of insurance to cover treatment for lung cancer. Yet there are other ways that health insurance policyholders can influence to some extent the number and cost of undesirable events that befall them.

Many health care services may be optional, such as some types of mental health services, some elective procedures, or even whether to go to a doctor because of a cold. Health insurance creates a problem related to buying in an economical fashion. The person who has to pay for services is likely not to consume services unless they are worth the price. If a physician charges $100 for an office visit and the patient must pay that out of pocket, the patient will think twice as to whether it is really necessary to see the physician. But when the patient has insurance, the price for the visit could drop to $0. At that price, all the individual is giving up is time, and the individual may be more likely to see the physician. There is a moral hazard effect because the individual changes behavior from what it would be without insurance.

Sometimes insurers turn this to the advantage of all concerned. Some dental plans may pay 100% benefits for routine preventive care but lesser percentages for other types of treatments. The theory behind this is that if full coverage is provided for dental cleanings and examinations, more people will follow a plan of routine oral examinations, reducing the likelihood of larger dental claims for more extreme treatment later. However, some plans will not cover small costs, such as routine preventive care, that have a high likelihood of occurrence because the administrative costs may be too high.

Coinsurance, Deductibles, and Co-payments

In an effort to overcome the problems of moral hazard, insurance companies often require that beneficiaries pay *coinsurance,* a *co-payment,* or a *deductible* to make consumers bear enough of a portion of the cost of health care services so that they do not use the services as if they were free. All of these fees have increased in recent years, leaving patients to pay a higher dollar amount for the care they receive.

A deductible is an amount of money the consumer must pay before the insurer will pay anything for care. For example, an insurer may require the consumer to pay the first $500 for care each year before becoming eligible for any benefits. This can forestall unneeded trips to health care providers for minor complaints. However, if a serious condition arises, the individual is likely to seek care even if he or she must pay the first several hundred dollars of cost. Deductibles vary by insurer, but it is common for deductibles to be $2,500 or higher.

A co-payment is a dollar amount that must be paid each time a service is used. This approach is common among HMOs. Co-payments are usually small enough (e.g., $35, $40, or $50) that the consumer is unlikely to fail to seek care when really needed, but they are a reminder that care is not free. Some believe that even a small co-payment discourages unnecessary patient use of health care services.

Coinsurance is a portion of each health care payment that is the responsibility of the consumer. It is similar to a co-payment but tends to be more substantive. Generally, coinsurance is stated in terms of a percentage of the cost of a health care procedure or service that the consumer must pay, typically from 20% to as high as 50%.

Insurers and the businesses that pay for insurance use these mechanisms to decrease the use of "unnecessary care." They believe that if the beneficiary must pay some of the cost, he or she will not seek care for conditions that are self-limiting or do not require medical or nursing care. Others argue that these mechanisms prevent people from seeking care early when treatment could be effective and could prevent more expensive care later.

When there is no deductible, co-payment, or coinsurance, the insurer must pay all health care claims that are valid. This is referred to as *first dollar coverage.*

Two types of plans that allow individuals to either defer taxes or purchase certain health services tax-free are health savings accounts (HSAs) and flexible spending accounts (FSAs). HSAs are options available to insured individuals that allow them to set aside a certain portion of their income to pay for health care–related expenses tax free.[55] The advantage of HSAs is that they are investment accounts that can grow if unused and can be rolled over from one year to the next if the funds are not expended. One of the problems is that individuals have used these accounts to pay for health care services that do not qualify for payment (i.e., would not qualify for a medical tax deduction). The ACA law will impose a 20% tax on such payments made by individuals for services in the future.[56] FSAs, on the other hand, are funds that individuals can deduct from their paychecks to be used for a broader range of health care–related expenses, such as dependent care and certain over-the-counter medical items.[57] FSAs are not subject to payroll taxes, which makes them appealing. However, any funds not expended at the end of the plan year or some designated period are lost to the policyholder. FSAs will also be affected by the ACA beginning in 2013, when the amount of annual contribution to an FSA is limited to $2,500 per year (adjusted thereafter based on cost-of-living adjustments).[58]

Customary and Reasonable Charges

Whether first dollar coverage is in effect or not, insurers often place some limitations on how much they will pay for services. This is most commonly accomplished through use of limitations at the level of customary and reasonable charges and, more recently, negotiated rates between the provider and the insurer.

Customary charges are based on surveys of what providers in an area are charging. Insurance companies can carry out these surveys simply by reviewing all bills that they receive over a period of time from a particular geographic region. The insurance company decides that any bills that exceed the average charge by a certain amount are excessive. The company then only reimburses up to a level that it determines is reasonable.

In some cases, insurance policies contain specific limitations on payment amounts. For example, it is common to have a 50% coinsurance rate for mental health care benefits *and* a limit of $40 per visit. In a high-cost area such as New York City, psychiatrists commonly charge $250 to $300 per session. At these rates with a $40 cap and 50% coinsurance, the benefit paid would be only $20, and the patient would be responsible for the remaining $230 to $280. It is not clear to what extent this is because insurers believe there is great moral hazard in the utilization of mental health care services or because mental health services are not seen as being as valuable or necessary as acute care hospital treatment or even a physician office visit for a runny nose. Regardless, the high costs of mental health services often means that individuals go without the care they need. This same mechanism also allows other specialists to charge high fees, limits the insurer's responsibility, and places the responsibility for the bulk of payment on individuals.

Other Sources of Financing

Government and insurance payments accounted for approximately 81% ($1.9 trillion) of the money that went into the health care system in 2008.[59] Of the remaining 19% spent on health care (~$449 billion), about 12% is attributable to consumers' out-of-pocket expenditures, and 7% is attributable to other private sources, including philanthropic gifts.

Many payments are small and include those for over-the-counter drugs or prescriptions, an occasional physician visit, uninsured dental care, and routine eye care and eyeglasses. Such charges are paid for out of pocket by the large majority of persons. A 2009 report[60] indicates that among consumers with private health insurance, approximately 42% of their health care expenditures were out of pocket (i.e., items not covered by the policy or deductibles, co-payments, and coinsurance). When individuals pay out of pocket for their own care, they are referred to as *self-pay patients.*

Self-pay dollars for hospital and other expensive care generally come from the lower and upper classes of society; the rich

[55]Robinson JS. 2005. Health savings accounts—the ownership society in health care. *N Engl J Med* 353:1199-1202.

[56]Retrieved July 12, 2011, at http://www.kff.org/healthreform/upload/8061.pdf.

[57]Retrieved July 12, 2011, at http://www.healthcare.gov/law/provisions/fsa_hra/.

[58]Retrieved July 12, 2011, at http://www.kff.org/healthreform/upload/8061.pdf.

[59]Truffer et al., *Op. cit.*

[60]Kaiser Family Foundation. 2009. *Trends in health care costs and spending.* Retrieved July 8, 2011, at http://www.kff.org/insurance/upload/7692_02.pdf.

tend to pay for many items that health insurance finds beyond the customary and reasonable limits. The working poor often have inadequate health insurance. They are too well off to benefit from many programs designed for the indigent but not well off enough to have a comprehensive health insurance plan. Many workers have no health insurance at all. It has been estimated that about 61% of uninsured families have at least one member working full time.[61]

The last major source of funding for health care services is philanthropy. Historically, the charitable sector of society considered health care services to be one of its most important concerns. A lot of dollars still flow into HCOs from philanthropic sources, although this represents a much smaller share of the total than it once did, estimated to be only 3% of health spending.[62] The reason for the decline has largely been because of the growing role of the government and insurance. An additional factor has been the growth of the for-profit sector in health care. In 2004, 16% of hospital beds[63] and 17% of hospitals were investor-owned (for-profit).[64] Most of those beds are owned by large multi-hospital for-profit corporations.

As the industry has become more for-profit oriented and as other sources of funding have increased, the role of philanthropy as a major financer of health care services has gradually declined. The economic recession of 2007–2009 has also likely had an impact on health care philanthropy, with 77% of hospital fundraisers indicating that the recession would have a negative impact on charitable giving and 11% anticipating the impact to be very negative.[65]

Alternative Payment Approaches

The complexity of our health care financing system naturally begs the question: *Is there a better way?* Decision makers, politicians, and scholars have struggled to answer this question with limited success. The U.S. health care system is the most expensive in the world, yet leading indicators point out that health care in the United States is not the best in the world. The Canadian and U.S. systems are often contrasted because of their geographic proximity, because of the relative ease of movement between the two countries, and because the Canadian health care system is socialized versus the U.S. model of public and private coverage.

The Canadian system, also called Medicare, is funded solely through taxes and covers most health care needs with a few exceptions (routine dental and eye care for adults and prescription drugs). Funding is provided to provinces, which in turn bill the government for health care services provided to citizens in accordance with the Canada Health Act. The total, per capita, and out-of-pocket health care expenses are less in Canada than in the United States. In 2009, per capita health care expenditures in Canada totaled $4,363, versus $7,960 in the United States and about 9.5% of Canada's GDP versus 17.4% in the U.S.[66] When these figures are broken down between public and private spending, however, about 71% of funding in the Canadian system comes from public funds versus 47.4 in the United States. Interestingly, among advanced and emerging countries, the share of public funds spent on health care in the United States is among the lowest, second only to Chile.[67]

There are advantages to both the Canadian and U.S. health care systems. The Canadian system provides the same level of care to all of its citizens, has lower overall costs (including the costs associated with administration, billing, marketing, and malpractice),[68] has much lower drug prices, and funds education for health professionals. A recent study also reported that U.S. physicians spend almost four times as much time as their Canadian counterparts to interact with payers and meet payer requirements.[69] The U.S. system typically has shorter waits for seeing providers and allows more choice in provider selection.[70] Physicians in the United States generally earn higher wages and salaries, but they also pay much more for malpractice insurance.[71] In an overall ranking of health system performance, the United States ranked 37th of 190 countries, and Canada ranked 30th.[72]

Despite spending less on health care, Canadians have better outcomes on leading health indicators than Americans, including life expectancy (81 vs. 78 years in the United States), infant mortality rate (5 vs. 7 per 1,000 live births in the United States),[73] and overall mortality (7.7 vs. 8.2 per 1,000 population in the United States).[74] The United States has higher cancer

[61]The Kaiser Commission on Medicaid and the Uninsured. 2011. *The Uninsured: A Primer.* Retrieved February 2, 2012, at http://www.kff.org/uninsured/upload/7451-07.pdf.

[62]Cowan CA, Hartman, MA. 2005. Financing health care: Businesses, households, and governments, 1987-2003. *Healthcare Finan Rev* 1(2):1-26. Retrieved July 8, 2011, at https://www.cms.gov/NationalHealthExpendData/downloads/bhg-article-04.pdf.

[63]Congressional Budget Office. 2006. *Non-profit Hospitals and the Provision of Community Benefits.* Retrieved July 8, 2011, at http://www.cbo.gov/ftpdocs/76xx/doc7695/12-06-Nonprofit.pdf.

[64]American Hospital Association. 2011. *AHA Hospital Statistics 2009 Edition.* Chicago: AHA.

[65]Kreimer S. 2009. Philanthropy. More than ever, big donors want to see value for their dollars. *Hosp Health Netw* 83(6):20. Retrieved July 9, 2011, at http://www.hhnmag.com/hhnmag_app/jsp/articledisplay.jsp?dcrpath=HHNMAG/Article/data/06JUN2009/0906HHN_Inbox_philanthropy&domain=HHNMAG.

[66]OECD Health Data 2011. *How Does Canada compare?* Retrieved July 10, 2011, at http://www.oecd.org/dataoecd/46/33/38979719.pdf.

[67]*Ibid.*

[68]Woolhandler S, Campbell T, Himmelstein D. 2003. Costs of health care administration in the United States and Canada. *N Engl J Med* 349(8):768-775.

[69]Morra D, Nicholson S, Levinson W, et al. 2011. U.S. physician practices versus Canadians: Spending nearly four times as much money interacting with payers. *Health Aff* 30(8):1443-1450.

[70]Davis K, Schoen C, Schoenbaum SC, et al. 2010. *Mirror, Mirror on the Wall: How the Performance of the U.S. Health Care System Compares Internationally.* Retrieved July 10, 2011, at http://www.commonwealthfund.org/Search.aspx?search=Enter+keywords http://www.commonwealthfund.org/usr_doc/1027_Davis_mirror_mirror_international_update_final.pdf.

[71]Smith M, Walker E. *Special Report: Canada and the U.S.—Comparing Key Practice Parameters.* Retrieved July 10, 2011, at http://www.medpagetoday.com/PublicHealthPolicy/PublicHealth/15931.

[72]World Health Organization. 2000. *Health Systems: Improving Performance.* Retrieved July 10, 2011, at http://www.who.int/whr/2000/en/whr00_en.pdf.

[73]Retrieved July 10, 2011, at http://www.who.int/gho/en/.

[74]Retrieved July 10, 2011, at http://new.paho.org/hq/dmdocuments/2009/BI_ENG_2009.pdf.

survival rates (almost 92%) than Canada (82.5%), but there is less variability in the range of cancer survival rates across provinces in Canada (ranging from 79% to 85%) than across states in the United States (ranging 78% to 90%).[75] Interestingly, Canadians also rate their health care system higher than Americans with regard to their overall view of the system, out-of-pocket spending, quality of physician care,[76] care coordination and communication,[77] and satisfaction.[78] Americans tend to give higher ratings to issues that pertain to access to care and waiting times.[79]

Differences in these two contrasting systems may be partially explained by differences in lifestyle between the two countries. For example, in 2008, the rate of obesity, a widely recognized health problem in the United States was 24% among adults in Canada but 33% in the United States.[80] Canada and the United States have similar rates of tobacco consumption (at 16.2% and 16.1%, respectively),[81] but Canadians consume slightly less alcohol than Americans (8.2 vs. 8.8 L per capita). These lifestyle differences reflect differences in the social values and beliefs that exist between the two countries, which, in turn, play out in our respective health care policies, including each country's willingness to accept high numbers of uninsured individuals and limits on access to care.[82]

❋ PAYING HEALTH CARE PROVIDERS

The preceding section addressed the issue of where the resources come from to pay health care providers. We now turn our attention to the payment systems for providers. We will focus in particular on hospitals, the segment of the health care industry that receives the largest share of health care dollars.

In most industries, goods and services are produced at a certain cost to the provider. Providers then add a "profit" for the cost of doing business and to cover their investment. The cost plus the profit is used to establish a charge. Consumers then choose to buy or not buy the product. If a company is making a large profit, other potential providers may decide to enter the industry. Competition increases, and prices are lowered (see a discussion of this process in Chapter 4). If prices become too low, some providers will no longer be able to make

a profit and will leave the industry. Eventually, equilibrium is reached at a stable set of prices, with additional competitors neither entering nor leaving the industry.

Hospital Payment

Hospital prices are not set by the process of market economics just described. People who buy health care services do not have the detailed level of knowledge needed to choose among providers the way consumers can choose among hotels. Once in a hospital, consumers do not have the knowledge to choose which tests they should have as they might choose which services to order in a hotel. The need for health care services is often sudden and unexpected and does not involve a choice.

Furthermore, prices are also controlled to a great extent by the government reimbursement. Both Medicare and Medicaid impose their own pricing on hospitals. In the past 2 decades, there has been a dramatic shift in focus on the part of Medicare payments nationwide and Medicaid payments in states. This movement is from a cost-based system of hospital payment to a prospective payment system and now to a system that pays for performance. Discussed next is the prospective payment system, which is used to pay for most Medicare inpatient care as well as some other hospital patient care, and the pay-for-performance, or value-based purchasing, system that has evolved and will continue to do so in the coming years. The principles of managed care have led to new payment approaches based on negotiated rates. This trend will be discussed. This section also addresses the issue of charity care.

Prospective Payment Systems

After implementation of Medicare and Medicaid in 1966, the cost of hospital care began to escalate dramatically. Because government was paying a large share of these costs, it was in the government's (and taxpayers') interest to slow this escalation of costs. In 1983, Congress authorized the Health Care Financing Administration (HCFA) (renamed the Centers for Medicare and Medicaid Services [CMS] in 2001) to pay hospitals for care of Medicare inpatients on the basis of an inpatient prospective payment system (IPPS) called *Diagnosis Related Groups* (DRGs). Each DRG has an associated payment weight, based on the average resources used to treat Medicare patients in that DRG.[83] Similar systems were created under the Balanced Budget Act of 1997 (BBA) for care of hospital outpatients (known as the Ambulatory Payment Classification [APC]) and for home care (known as Home Health Prospective Payment System [HHPPS]). In fact, prospective payment systems are associated with hospice, inpatient psychiatric facilities, inpatient rehabilitation facilities, long-term hospital care, and skilled nursing facilities. With *prospective payment*, a hospital or other entity has predetermined prices for services, rather than simply being reimbursed for whatever costs are incurred.

[75]Coleman MP, Quaresma M, Berrino F, Lutz JM, De Angelis R, et al. Cancer survival in five continents: a worldwide population-based study (CONCORD). *Lancet Oncol* 9(8):730-756. Retrieved July 10, 2011, at http://www.lshtm.ac.uk/eph/ncde/cancersurvival/research/concord/concord_article__tables_and_figures.pdf.

[76]Schoen C, Osborn R, Doty R, et al. 2007. Toward higher-performance health systems: Adults' health care experiences in seven countries. *Health Aff* 26(6):W717-W734.

[77]*Ibid.* See also Schoen C, Osborn R, Squires D, et al. 2010. How insurance design affects access to care and costs by income, in eleven countries. *Health Aff (Millwood)* 29(12):2323-2334.

[78]*Ibid.* See also Blendon R, Schoen C, DesRoches C, et al. 2003. Common concerns amid diverse systems: Health care experiences in five countries. *Health Aff* 22(3):106-121.

[79]Schoen et al., *Op. cit.*

[80]OECD Health Data 2011. *How Does Canada compare?* Retrieved July 10, 2011, at http://www.oecd.org/dataoecd/46/33/38979719.pdf.

[81]OECD. *StatExtracts*. Retrieved July 10, 2011, at http://stats.oecd.org/index.aspx.

[82]*Ibid.*

[83]Retrieved July 14, 2011, at https://www.cms.gov/AcuteInpatientPPS/01_overview.asp.

The classification system known as Diagnosis Related Groups categorizes similar types of patients into groups that reflect the amount of care required. These groups were constructed to reflect similar medical diagnoses requiring about the same amount of hospital time. Medicare DRGs are based on factors including patient age, principal and secondary medical diagnoses, whether an operating room procedure was performed, complications, and comorbidity.

It should be noted that a DRG is not assigned to a patient until the patient is discharged. The DRG assigned is based on the illness that required the admission. In most cases, a good estimation of what the DRG will be can be made at admission.

Under the IPPS, hospitals are not paid on the basis of the cost of care but on a predetermined amount based on the DRG. If a patient's hospital stay costs the hospital more than the DRG rate, the hospital loses the difference. If the stay costs less than the rate, the hospital keeps the surplus. The rates paid are based on the national costs of each DRG, adjusted for annual inflation, local wage rates, and expected productivity gains.

As a result of the Deficit Reduction Act (DRA) of 2005, Medicare has put several regulations in place to refine its system for paying hospitals. On October 1, 2007, Medicare implemented an updated DRG payment system, the Medicare Severity DRG (or MS-DRG) to better account for patients' severity of illness and resource consumption based on three levels of severity: a major complication or comorbidity (MCC), which greatly affects a patient's severity of illness; a complication or comorbidity (CC), which has some effect on a patient's

severity of illness; and a noncomplication or comorbidity (non-CC), which has no significant effect on a patient's illness.[84] This system introduced 745 new MS-DRGs to replace the previous 538 DRGs.[85]

Also part of the Deficit Reduction Act of 2005, on October 1, 2008, CMS stopped paying hospitals for care provided to patients who experience 1 of 10 HACs, or conditions that are high-cost or high-volume conditions and not "present on admission" (POA), result in the assignment of a higher paying DRG as a secondary diagnosis, and could have been prevented through the application of evidence-based guidelines.[86] These 10 conditions ("adverse events" that result from care) are outlined in Table 2–5 along with their associated MS-DRGs.[87] Under this ruling, hospitals are required to report on these HACs, and they will no longer receive ". . . additional payment for cases in which one of the selected conditions was not present on admission. That is, the case [will] be paid as though the secondary diagnosis were not present."[88] Medicare also prohibits hospitals from

[84]Retrieved July 8, 2011, at https://www.cms.gov/MLNProducts/downloads/AcutePaymtSysfctsht.pdf.

[85]Retrieved July 8, 2011, at http://www.aannet.org/files/public/ippswhitepaper.pdf.

[86]Retrieved July 8, 2011, at http://www.cms.gov/HospitalAcqCond/01_Overview.asp#TopOfPage.

[87]Retrieved July 15, 2011, at http://www.cms.gov/HospitalAcqCond/Downloads/HACFactsheet.pdf.

[88]Retrieved July 9, 2010, at https://www.cms.gov/hospitalacqcond/.

✳ TABLE 2–5 *Hospital-Acquired Conditions Subject to Payment Denial*

Hospital-Acquired Condition	MS-DRG
Foreign object retained after surgery	998.4 (CC); 998.7 (CC)
Air embolism	999.1 (MCC)
Blood incompatibility	999.60–999.63; 999.69 (all CC)
Catheter-associated UTI	996.64 (CC); plus others excluded as CC/MCC
Stage III and IV pressure ulcers	707.23 (MCC) 707.24 (MCC)
Vascular catheter–associated infections	999.31 (CC)
Surgical site infection, mediastinitis after CABG	519.2 (MCC); plus one of these procedure codes: 36.10–36.19
Falls and trauma	CC/MCC in the following ranges:
■ Fractures	800–829
■ Dislocations	830–839
■ Intracranial injuries	850–854
■ Crushing injuries	925–929
■ Burns	940–949
■ Electric shock	991–994
Manifestations of poor glycemic control	
■ Diabetic ketoacidosis	250.10–250.13
■ Nonketotic hyperosmolar coma	250.20–250.23
■ Hypoglycemic coma	251.0
■ Secondary diabetes with ketoacidosis	249.10–249.11
■ Secondary diabetes with hyperosmolarity	249.20–249.21
Surgical site infections after certain orthopedic surgeries (spine, neck, shoulder, elbow)	996.67, 998.59 (CC); plus one of these procedure codes: 81.01-81.08; 81.23–81.24; 81.31–81.38; 81.83, or 81.85
Surgical site infection after bariatric surgery (laparoscopic gastric bypass; gastroenterostomy; and laparoscopic gastric restrictive surgery)	278.01; 998.59 (CC); plus one of these procedure codes: 44.38, 44.39, or 44.95
Deep vein thrombosis and pulmonary embolism after total knee replacement or hip replacement	415.11 (MCC) 415.19 (MCC) 453.40–453.42 (MCC); plus one of these procedure codes: 00.85–00.87; 81.51–81.52; or 81.54

CABG, coronary artery bypass graft; CC, complications and comorbidities; MCC, major complications and comorbidities; UTI, urinary tract infection.
Modified from http://www.cms.gov/HospitalAcqCond/Downloads/HACFactsheet.pdf. Retrieved July 19, 2011.

charging beneficiaries for the care required to treat the HAC, but it will pay for physician care and certain items and services needed to treat the beneficiary who experiences a HAC, including post-discharge care and follow-up that would not have been otherwise needed.

Although certain specialty hospitals (e.g., critical access, pediatric, oncology) are exempt from these requirements, for the most part, DRGS and now MS-DRGs are dominant forces in hospital payments, particularly if the hospital cares for many Medicare patients. These IPPS changes have drastically changed the way hospitals approach care delivery. They can no longer expect to be paid for the highest-cost condition for which a Medicare patient might need care. Instead, they have had to anticipate how care might go wrong; examine how it does go wrong; put systems in place to prevent these events from occurring; and if one of these events does occur, determine how to appropriately mitigate their losses. This is discussed in greater detail in Chapter 5.

Negotiated Rates

Hospitals may also provide care based on negotiations for a percentage discount of the hospital's normal rates. Sometimes a flat charge per patient day is agreed to regardless of services provided. In some cases, MCOs negotiate capitated rates, which are a flat monthly payment per member regardless of his or her consumption of medical services.

Operating under either prospective payment or negotiated rates means that the rules governing the payment of care have changed for nurses. The total revenue to the hospital for many patients is fixed regardless of the costs incurred in treating these patients. It *does* matter how many catheter kits are used, and it *does* matter if the patient has one more x-ray because those items may not be reimbursed and may cost the hospital money. Most importantly, it matters how long the patient stays in the hospital. The most important predictor of hospital cost is the patient's length of stay. If on average it costs $3,000 per day to stay in a hospital, the patient who stays 2 extra days will cost the hospital as much as $6,000 more than the patient who stays fewer days. Consequently, there is increasing pressure on nurse managers and executives to decrease patient length of stay. In organizations where the nurse manager is fiscally accountable for the unit, it is vital for the manager to understand the importance of the reimbursement system. For patients whose care is paid according to a negotiated rate, using fewer resources means more profit for the hospital.

Pay for Performance

Introduced in the early 2000s, pay for performance is a system that pays hospitals and health care providers based on their *performance*, rather than on the costs providers incur to provide specific services or the diagnoses of the patients they treat. Although provider performance can be assessed in different ways (e.g., financial performance, patient outcomes, or internal processes), the focus under pay-for-performance systems is quality. Pay-for-performance systems—also known as P4P and *value-based purchasing*—offer incentives to reward providers according to their performance on quality indicators.

The CMS started using this approach to reward providers with the passage of the Medicare Prescription Drug, Improvement, and Modernization Act of 2003, which provided incentives for Medicare-eligible hospitals to participate in the Hospital Quality Initiative.[89] This initiative based hospital payment on the submission of data on an initial set of 10 quality measures.[90] Hospitals submitting the required data received full DRG payments. The CMS Premier Hospital Quality Incentive Demonstration project, an initiative that began in 2003, was a partnership with a nonprofit hospital group, Premier Inc., involving more than 200 hospitals nationwide to evaluate the impact of rewarding participating hospitals based on the submission of data on more than 30 quality measures.[91] Similar programs are available for physicians and integrated health systems.

Although participation in the Hospital Quality Initiative was voluntary, hospitals were motivated to report data on the 10 quality measures because failure to do so would result in a 0.04% reduction in Medicare payments. This may not sound like much, but given that Medicare payments represent about 30% of hospital payments[92] and private payers have initiated similar pay-for-performance structures, the possibility of a reduction in payments was, for many hospitals, enough to encourage them to participate in the program. Although very little research remains available on the effects of pay-for-performance systems on quality improvement, recent systematic reviews show that results are inconclusive.[93]

The CMS Hospital Quality Initiative has evolved into what is now known as the Hospital Value-Based Purchasing Program (effective October 1, 2012). Similar to the Hospital Quality Initiative before it, this program offers incentive payments to hospitals based on their performance or their improvement (relative to baseline) on a set of quality measures. Hospitals with higher relative performance or improvement will receive higher payments for the fiscal year. The list of quality measures that hospitals' performance will be based on include 12 clinical process of care measures (for acute myocardial infarction [AMI], heart failure [HF], pneumonia [PN], health care–associated infections, and surgical care improvement) and patient experience of care measures from the Hospital Consumer Assessment of Healthcare Providers and Systems Survey (HCAHPS). Additional outcome measures will be added in 2014 to include 30-day

---

[89]Retrieved June 26, 2011, at http://www.cms.hhs.gov/apps/media/press/release.asp?Counter=1343.

[90]Retrieved July 15, 2011, at http://www.cms.gov/HospitalQualityInits/downloads/HospitalOverview.pdf.

[91]Retrieved July 10, 2011, at http://www.cms.gov/HospitalQualityInits/Downloads/HospitalPremierPressRelease-FactSheet.zip [HospitalPremierFactSheet2010].

[92]Truffer et al., *Op. cit.*

[93]See, for example, Blusteink J, Weissman JS, Ryan AM, et al. 2011. Analysis raises questions on whether pay-for-performance in Medicaid can efficiently reduce racial and ethnic disparities. *Health Aff* 30(6):1165-1175; Friedberg, MW, Safran, DG, et al. 2010. Paying for performance in primary care: Potential impact on practices and disparities. *Health Aff* 29(5):926-932; and Grossbart SR. 2005. What's the return? Assessing the effect of "pay-for-performance" initiatives on the quality of care delivery. *Med Care Res Rev* 63 (1 suppl):29S-48S.

mortality (for patients diagnosed with AMI, HF, and PN), certain Patient Safety Indicators and Inpatient Quality Indicators Composite Measures developed by the Agency for Healthcare Research and Quality, and eight HACs.[94]

Other efforts also exist that encourage providers to focus on quality improvement. In 2005, a Web-based tool, Hospital Compare, was launched by CMS and was made available to consumers. This tool[95] allows consumers to examine and compare specific hospital information on care provided to patients with certain conditions. The Joint Commission has a similar Web-based tool, Quality Check,[96] which can be used by consumers to gather quality and safety information about organizations accredited by The Joint Commission.[97] Although these tools do not directly affect provider payments, some of the data that populate these sites—especially the Hospital Compare site—help determine provider payments. More importantly, these data may be used by patients and influence patients' choice of provider, which in turn could influence the dollars that flow to providers. In other words, patients can use these data to "vote with their feet."

Charity Care

In our society, hospitals are not permitted to turn away patients in need of emergency care. There have been unfortunate examples of hospitals that used extremely narrow definitions of what represents an emergency episode that requires hospital care and then used that definition to turn away patients. Other hospitals have been more open in admitting all patients who truly are in need of care. Patients who either could not pay (indigent) or did not pay (bad debts) have created financial problems that were addressed in a number of ways, including government subsidies, philanthropy, and cross-subsidization.

Hospitals with high rates of poor and uninsured patients are also known as *safety net hospitals*. Many state and local governments have developed *disproportionate share arrangements* with these hospitals, which provide extra payments to hospitals for "uncompensated" care. Often these arrangements have been financed by taxing hospitals with fewer poor patients to provide a subsidy to those hospitals with more poor patients. Philanthropy also covers some of the cost. However, as the government role has increased, the role of philanthropy in paying for care has declined.

Charges in excess of cost for some insured and self-pay patients may result in enough revenues to offset the losses on bad debts and charity care. This is often referred to as *cross-subsidization*. Payments from one group of patients cover unrecovered costs for another group of patients. Many argue that the costs of poor patients should be borne by society through a general tax. In the cross-subsidization approach, only individuals who are hospitalized are taxed for care of the poor.

Some financial reporting requirements for hospitals focus on charity care. Each year hospitals must indicate on audited financial statements the amount of charity care they have provided. This should reveal the extent to which hospitals provide care to needy individuals as well as some information on how that care is financed. The ACA will initially reduce the payments to disproportionate share hospitals by 75% and thereafter base payments on the hospital's percent of uninsured patients and the amount of uncompensated care provided.[98]

Although some skeptics do not believe that hospitals provide much charity care, in some cases, the burden of charity care has overwhelmed hospitals, and a number of hospitals have had to merge or close.

Nurse Payment

According to the 2008 National Sample Survey of Registered Nurses,[99] about 62% of nurses work in hospitals. Most staff nurses working in hospitals are paid an hourly wage by their employers. Overtime is generally paid at a higher rate for hours worked in addition to base hours. Nurse managers and executives are likely to be paid a salary rather than an hourly wage. In general, they are not paid overtime but may be given compensatory time off. Many nurse managers and executives, however, work far more than their scheduled hours without additional compensation.

Some hospitals have experimented with alternative payment systems for staff nurses. These include paying nurses a salary with no additional compensation for overtime, paying nurses a salary plus bonus based on the productivity of the nursing unit, and paying a group of nurses a set amount of money to provide care for a specified period of time. Similar to the pay-for-performance, or value-based, system of paying hospitals, some hospitals also use a pay-for-performance, or value-based, system to reward employees. This system rewards employees based on meeting some predetermined level of performance standards. For example, hospitals could reward groups or teams of employees—such as a nursing unit or team—based on the receipt of consistently high patient satisfaction and important quality outcome scores (e.g., relevant HACs) that exceed performance standards. Under such an arrangement, employees on the unit may receive a bonus or pay increase for the role each plays in achieving the performance standard or for the output of the team. Hospitals may also reward individual employees for performance, such as providing bonuses to nurse managers for putting strategies in place to decrease turnover or retain staff on their unit. These plans work well if they are clear and consistent with organizational goals; do not punish individuals who have performed well despite unit or team outcomes; or do not reward unhealthy competitiveness among individuals, teams, or units.[100] As hospital

---

[94]For a more complete list of measures, see http://www.gpo.gov/fdsys/pkg/FR-2011-05-06/pdf/2011-10568.pdf.

[95]Available at http://www.hospitalcompare.hhs.gov.

[96]Available at http://www.qualitycheck.org/consumer/searchQCR.aspx.

[97]Available at http://www.qualitycheck.org/index.htm.

[98]Retrieved July 14, 2011, at http://www.kff.org/healthreform/upload/8061.pdf.

[99]U.S. Department of Health and Human Services, Health Resources and Services Administration (2010). *The Registered Nurse Population: Findings from the 2008 National Sample Survey of Registered Nurses*. Retrieved July 15, 2011, at http://bhpr.hrsa.gov/healthworkforce/rnsurveys/rnsurveyfinal.pdf.

[100]Burns L, Bradley E, Weiner B. 2011. *Shortell and Kaluzny's Health Care Management: Organization Design and Behavior*, 6th edition. Albany, NY: Delmar.

management attempts to increase productivity, alternative methods of payment and reward systems are expected to expand.

Many nurses work in organizations other than hospitals. In most cases, they are employees working for an annual salary or an hourly wage. For example, nurse practitioners working in primary care or specialty care physician practices are typically paid an annual salary and may also have profit-sharing arrangements and/or bonuses. Nurse practitioners working in "minute clinics" are typically paid an hourly wage. Nurses working in some settings, such as home health care, are paid on a per-visit basis. Nurses employed by organizations are rarely paid directly by insurers or consumers of care. Most often these payments are made to their employing organization, which pays the nurse.

Some nurses are self-employed and receive payment directly from patients or insurers. Private duty nurses are often paid directly, as are nurse psychotherapists. Advanced practice nurses, including nurse practitioners, nurse midwives, and certified registered nurse anesthetists, are sometimes paid directly by insurers. Professional nurses have been lobbying to expand third-party reimbursement for nurses. Nurses argue that they should be reimbursed in the same way physicians are because they provide the nursing care for which patients come to hospitals. They argue that they should be able to authorize care and should be reimbursed directly for it.

Substantial evidence indicates that when nurses provide care that would otherwise be provided by physicians, money is saved (and quality is improved). Examples are prenatal care and well-child care. The concept of direct payment to nurses has been met with resistance from both physicians and payers alike. Physicians may believe that nurses are providing services that should be provided by (and paid to) physicians. Payers may believe this care will be additive and will increase total health care costs rather than lowering them.

It should be noted that the benefit structure of employees' health insurance is determined by the employer, not the government. Therefore, if employers wanted the benefit of cost savings that could be provided by nurses and were willing to pay for it, their insurers would provide it. Nursing could make substantial progress in the area of payments for nursing services if it lobbied more effectively. Effective lobbying led to Medicare's directly paying advanced practice nurses.[101]

Physician Payment

Physicians have traditionally been paid by patients, either directly or through the patient's insurance company. Their income is usually directly related to the number of care episodes they provide. In recent years, however, a number of changes in physician payment have occurred.

First, the percentage of physicians who are salaried employees has been growing dramatically. Physicians have long been salaried employees in some hospitals, such as some academic medical centers. However, as the costs of opening a practice continue to increase, fewer physicians have opened their own practices. It is very likely that the majority of physicians will be salaried employees in the future.

Another major change in physician payment was introduced by Medicare early in the 1990s. This change, known as *resource-based relative value scale* (RBRVS), reoriented the payment scale for different types of physicians. The intent was to reemphasize the importance of cognitive skills and to de-emphasize the importance of procedures. Medicare hoped to provide higher payments to physicians for making diagnoses and lower payments to physicians for performing surgery and other high-tech procedures. It has become common for physicians to be paid either a rate per patient per month without regard for the amount of care provided or a fee per episode of care. For example, a specialist such as a psychiatrist might be paid $2,000 to treat an episode of depression rather than a fee for each patient visit.

The ACA may also impact physician payment. If ACOs are formed as proposed, many physicians may become a part of and receive payments through an ACO. Also, Medicare will establish pilot programs to examine the "bundling" of payments to hospitals, physicians, and others involved in an "episode" of care, which begins before patient admission and extends beyond patient discharge. Physicians will also be fully reimbursed for preventive services delivered in outpatient settings. These incentives will change physician behaviors by changing the structure and focus of care delivery.

Home Health Agency Payment

Home health agencies are paid by government, by insurers, and directly by patients. Before October 1, 2000, most agencies billed for services based on a per-visit basis for professional nursing services and on an hourly basis for unskilled aide care. In essence, the agency would calculate its allowable costs, divide by the number of visits, and calculate a per-visit charge. Assuming that this reimbursement per-visit covered their costs, it was in the agency's interest to provide more rather than fewer visits.

Because of escalating home health care costs, the BBA of 1997, as amended by the Omnibus Consolidated and Emergency Supplemental Appropriations Act of 1999, called for the development and implementation of a prospective payment system for Medicare home health services.[102] This evolved into Medicare's HH PPS, which went into effect on October 1, 2000. It is common for private insurers and MCOs to also negotiate payments for episodes of care for home health agencies. In such cases, the agency is paid a set fee to care for the patient without regard for the number of visits provided. Under the ACA, plans will be developed to implement value-based purchasing programs in home health.[103]

Certified home care agencies provide skilled nursing care and other services. They are authorized to receive direct payment from Medicare for the services they provide; in addition, they

[101]Wong ST. 1999. Reimbursement to advanced practice nurses (APNs) through Medicare. *J Nurs Scholar* 31(2):167-173.

[102]Retrieved June 19, 2006, at http://www.cms.hhs.gov/HomeHealthPPS/.
[103]Retrieved July 17, 2011, at http://www.kff.org/healthreform/upload/8061.pdf.

receive payment from Medicaid, from insurers, and directly from patients. Also under the ACA, states providing home health–related services (including care management, coordination, and health promotion) will receive incentives for doing so.[104]

Home care agencies that are not certified to receive payment from Medicare may receive payments from Medicaid, from other third-party payers, and directly from patients. Both certified and noncertified agencies are usually reimbursed by third-party payers on a prospective basis.

With the implementation of the HH PPS, home health agencies, similar to hospitals, are paid based on a predetermined amount adjusted for the Medicare beneficiary's health condition, care needs, and geographic differences in wages for home health agencies across the country. If the care provided costs the home health agency more than the HH PPS rate, the agency loses the difference. If the care costs less than the rate, the home health agency keeps the surplus. Agencies may not be able to cover their costs because of these cost constraints or because certain costs are not allowable by the third-party payers. Some agencies also lose money because they provide care to people who have no insurance and cannot pay.

Nurses, aides, physical therapists, and others who work for home health agencies may be paid a salary or be paid for each home visit they make, similar to the way physicians are paid.

Hospice Payment

Hospice is a philosophy about end-of-life care. The goal of hospice is to deliver "humane and compassionate care for people in the last phases of incurable disease so that they may live as fully and comfortably as possible."[105] Hospice is care delivered near the end of a patient's life (usually 6 months or less), but unlike general hospital care, it is not focused on curing a disease. Instead, hospice is palliative care, focusing on the patient and family, symptom management (especially pain management) and quality of life. Hospice care is typically delivered by a team of providers, including physicians, nurses, counselors, aides, and others, who work with the patient and family to ensure that their needs—physical, spiritual, and emotional—are met.

Hospice care can be and often is delivered in the patient's home; however, there are also special hospital units devoted to hospice care, and hospice care may be given in long-term care facilities or in a free-standing hospice facilities. It is a round-the-clock commitment, so patients who receive hospice care at home must have family or loved ones available to provide some of the care needed.

Hospice care payments come from Medicare, Medicaid, the Veterans Affairs, many private insurance plans, MCOs, and patients and families themselves. Both Medicare and Medicaid patients must meet certain requirements, such as the individual must have a terminal illness with a prognosis of 6 months or less, assuming an illness runs an expected course.[106] There

are also typically restrictions on the coverage provided. For example, Medicare will pay for physician and nursing care, as well as related supplies and equipment, but it will not pay for care delivered in an emergency department or inpatient care facility unless the care is arranged by the hospice care team or the care is unrelated to a patient's terminal illness.[107]

Medicare pays a daily rate to hospice agencies based on the level of care required by the beneficiary and family. It pays for routine home care, continuous (round-the-clock) home care, inpatient respite care, and general inpatient care.[108] Payment rates to individual facilities are adjusted using the hospice wage index to adjust for wage differences among local markets and the hospital market basket to adjust for goods and services relative to a fixed index for those goods and services.[109]

Nurses who work for hospice are generally paid on a per-visit basis to deliver care to patients in their homes or on an hourly basis to work on a hospice specialty unit. Nurses who are in administrative roles in hospice are generally salaried employees, and advanced practice nurses who work in hospice may be salaried, hourly, or paid on a per-visit basis.

Nursing Home Payment

Although nursing homes (also known as skilled nursing facilities) provide short-term care for patients recovering from injuries such as a hip fracture, most nursing home residents are institutionalized for an average of approximately 2 years. Paying for long-term care is a major and evolving national policy issue. Most nursing home care is paid for by Medicaid. However, most people are not eligible for Medicaid until they have used up all their savings and become impoverished. Medicare pays for very limited nursing home care, and similar to inpatient, outpatient, and home health care, nursing home payments are made on a prospective basis. The shift from retrospective to prospective payment for nursing homes occurred in 1998 as a result of the BBA of 1997. Resource utilization groups (RUGs) are used to set beneficiary payments under Medicare, and payments are adjusted for case mix (i.e., patient characteristics and conditions) and geographic variation in wages. Technically, nursing homes are paid the costs of providing covered skilled nursing facility services, including routine and ancillary care, and capital costs, but the payments provided by Medicare and the time period of coverage are limited. Because Medicare and Medicaid funding for nursing home care is limited and because many managed care plans do not cover the costs of nursing home care, the responsibility for paying nursing home care often falls to individuals. For these reasons, more and more people are purchasing long-term care insurance through private sources to cover nursing home care.

Funding of Nurse Education

Much of the funding for nurse education comes from students' tuition and fees and through philanthropic efforts. Beyond

[104]*Ibid.*

[105]Retrieved July 17, 2011, at http://www.cancer.org/acs/groups/cid/documents/webcontent/002868-pdf.pdf.

[106]Retrieved July 17, 2011, at http://www.cms.gov/MLNproducts/downloads/hospice_pay_sys_fs.pdf.

[107]*Ibid.*

[108]*Ibid.*

[109]Retrieved July 17, 2011, at http://www.cms.gov/MedicareProgramRatesStats/downloads/info.pdf.

these sources, however, the funding of nurse education is a complex issue. On the one hand, nurses are necessary to provide access to needed services in almost every type of health care setting, and in some ways, nurses could be considered a "public good" (i.e., everyone needs access to a nurse at one time or another), but the payment for the education of nurses has not always been done in the public's best interest. The education of health professionals—and particularly physicians and nurses—has generally been accomplished through Title VII and Title VIII of the Public Health Services Act (P.L. 78-410, enacted in 1944).[110] Title VII (enacted in 1963) provides funding to encourage health professionals to practice in underserved areas (creating, e.g., the National Health Service Corps) or specialize in primary care, recruit health care professionals from minority and disadvantaged groups, and increase the number of health professions faculty. Title VIII (enacted in 1964) provides funding to support the training of advance practice nurses, the recruitment of minorities and disadvantaged students into nursing, and the retention of nurses through career development opportunities and improvements in the nursing work environment.[111] These funds are primarily distributed through the Health Resources and Services Administration (HRSA).

Interestingly, Medicare is also a major funder of nursing education, albeit indirectly, through Graduate Medical Education (GME) payments made to hospitals for training physicians and nurses. Aiken and colleagues report that, in 2006, Medicare payments to hospitals for nursing education funding were about $152 million (about 6% of *total* GME payments to hospitals in 2006), and Title VIII funding for nursing education was about $150 million.[112] The irony is that most of the funding through this mechanism was included in the initial Medicare legislation (i.e., in 1965) and goes to support programs preparing only about 5% of the nursing workforce—hospital-based (i.e., diploma) nursing programs and licensed practical nursing programs. These funds do not support community college or university programs,[113] which prepare 80% of the nursing workforce with their initial nursing education![114] More importantly, these funds cannot be used to prepare advanced practice nurses and master's prepared nurse leaders, who will be key in the provision and oversight of services in a reformed health care environment. Thus, U.S. policies are needed to "redirect" funds to prepare a nursing workforce that better meets the needs of society.

❋ METHODS USED TO CONTROL PAYMENTS FOR CARE

With the rapid rise of health care costs over the nearly 50 years since the introduction of Medicare and Medicaid, there has been a growing push to control spending. This has given rise to a number of approaches. Most prominent among them is the development of managed care, which includes HMOs, PPOs, and other efforts aimed at controlling costs.

Managed Care

Managed care—sometimes called "managed cost"—is a term used to refer to a system for paying and delivering care through organizations such as HMOs and PPOs that attempts to control the consumption of health care resources. More formally, managed care is a cost-management system in which someone acts as an intermediary between the patient and many providers of services, such as specialist physicians and hospitals. The primary care physician is viewed as the gatekeeper or the point of entry through which the patient must pass to acquire health care services. In a managed care system, a designated person (often called the case manager) rather than the physician may be the one who authorizes the provision of the services. Many nurses and social workers fill the roles of case manager in HCOs and with insurers, and they have responsibility for overseeing patients' utilization of services.

Most insurance companies now have some form of managed care or use managed care principles. They may require prior approval for all but emergency care and may refuse to pay for care that was not authorized. Managed care programs often require a second opinion for surgical procedures and may require that only certain facilities and providers be used.

Although a major goal of managed care is to decrease costs by decreasing unnecessary services, case management can also ensure that patients get appropriate and timely care. Among the current criticisms of HMOs, PPOs, and other managed care insurers is that patients are being unduly restricted to care that may jeopardize their health. However, managed care is also responsible for the reduction in the number of unnecessary and potentially dangerous procedures and surgeries. Research has documented considerable geographic variation in use and subsequent costs of care across different types of managed care plans. Studies from researchers at the Dartmouth Atlas, for example, and others note that managed care has certainly slowed the growth of costs in certain areas, but it cannot explain the extent of the variation.[115]

Health Maintenance Organizations

Health maintenance organizations provide health care services to individuals or groups in exchange for a monthly payment. The payment is the same whether the individual uses services or not. This contrasts with the fee-for-service approach, in which an individual pays specifically for health care services consumed. HMOs were first popularized in the 1960s as a way to contain health care costs and to improve health. However, the basic type of organization had existed for many decades before the 1960s. Two noteworthy examples are

[110]Retrieved July 17, 2011, at http://www.apha.org/NR/rdonlyres/13E647B5-E51B-4A47-91A8-652EE973A2DB/0/TitleVIIandTitleVIII.pdf.

[111]*Ibid.*

[112]Aiken LH, Cheung, RB, Olds DM. 2009. Education policy initiatives to address the nurse shortage in the United States. *Health Aff WebExclusive* W646-W656.

[113]*Ibid.*

[114]Retrieved July 17, 2011, at http://bhpr.hrsa.gov/healthworkforce/rnsurveys/rnsurveyfinal.pdf.

[115]See, for example, Baker LC, Bundor MK, Kessler DP. 2009. HMO coverage reduces variation in the use of health care among patients under age 65. *Health Aff* 29(11), 2068-2074 and Fisher ES, Bynam JP, Skinner JS. 2009. Slowing the growth of healthcare costs—lessons from regional variation. *N Engl J Med* 360:849-852.

the Kaiser-Permanente Health Plan, which is a dominant force in the West, and the Health Insurance Plan (HIP) in New York. The developers believed that the insurance system was designed to pay for "sickness care." Most insurance pays only for care for people who are sick. Why not develop an insurance system that would pay to keep people well?

In HMOs, preventive care is paid for, and there is an emphasis on keeping people well and out of the hospital. Not only should HMOs improve care, but they also have the potential to lower costs by eliminating unnecessary care and by detecting health problems early.

For the HMO system to work, there need to be incentives for primary care physicians (the *gatekeepers)* to use less expensive outpatient care (e.g., fewer specialty referrals) and to hospitalize patients only when necessary. The incentive is money. In most HMOs, physician groups are paid on a *capitation* basis; that is, they are paid a flat fee per patient regardless of the amount of care that the patient consumes.

Patients pay a flat premium, or capitation charge, called the PMPM (per member per month) charge. If the population stays well and does not use a lot of health services, the physician group shares in the money that is not spent. However, the physicians are at risk. If the patient population consumes a lot of health care resources, physician payments are lower.

From the HMO patients' point of view, there is usually little or no charge for most health care visits. Preventive care is encouraged, and patients do not have to pay doctors and then be reimbursed. However, if patients do not stay with one plan long enough, they may not see the results of preventive care.

There are two principal types of HMOs: the group model and the individual practitioner association (IPA) model. In the group model, all of the HMO's physicians are employees of the HMO. They provide care only to patients of the HMO who receive care in HMO-owned facilities and affiliated hospitals. All HMO members get their care from a physician who is part of the group. This substantially limits choice in selecting a physician.

In the IPA model, physicians have their own private practice and treat many of their non-HMO patients on a traditional *fee-for-service* basis; that is, they charge patients for each episode of care and each service provided. However, for members of the IPA HMO that chose the physician as their primary provider, the physician provides the care in exchange for a portion of the HMO's PMPM charge. The IPA model keeps the physicians at risk. They earn less if the covered HMO members consume a lot of health care services; they earn more if HMO members consume relatively few services.

Individual practitioner associations tend to have far more affiliated physicians than group model plans. In the group approach, the HMO must have enough members to keep its physicians busy. The IPA model allows the physicians to have their own non-HMO patients. Therefore, an HMO with the same number of members can offer a much larger number of physicians. This provides more choice to members of the HMO. Furthermore, it uses the physicians' office space. Therefore, the HMO does not have to make nearly as large an investment in clinical offices and equipment.

However, some observers think that IPA doctors are not as committed to the ideals of the HMO approach as are members of a group model HMO. There is a large rift in the industry between dedicated HMO physicians who believe that HMOs not only can be less expensive but can also provide more appropriate care and physicians who view HMO IPA affiliation as just another way to get more patients into their offices.

Most HMOs have arrangements with specific hospitals to provide care. Often the HMO negotiates a discounted rate for hospital care. In such cases, patients' choice of hospitals is limited. Many consumers do not like HMO restrictions on choices of physicians and hospitals. Even though HMOs are less expensive than other types of plans, these restrictions may have influenced employers' move away from HMOs to other types of plans. In 2004, about 25% of the employed population was enrolled in HMOs; that level is expected to drop to about 19% of the employed population being enrolled in HMOs in 2010.[116]

Preferred Provider Organizations

While HMO enrollment has been declining, PPO enrolment has been increasing, although a recent study by the Kaiser Family Foundation reported that approximately 58% of the employed workforce was enrolled in PPO plans in 2010, down slightly from 60% in 2009.[117] PPOs are arrangements between providers (e.g., physicians, hospitals) and third-party payers. The providers agree to provide care for set prices, usually less than the current prevailing rate. The payers agree to steer large numbers of patients to that provider. Incentives are given to insured individuals that encourage them to receive their health care services from these preferred providers.

Arrangements for discounts from preferred providers are most often made by insurers or employers. In some cases, state governments negotiate PPO arrangements for state employees, Medicaid recipients, or other groups for whom care is paid for by the state.

If clients choose to receive care from a preferred provider, they often have lower out-of-pocket expenses. For example, the coinsurance for each episode of care may be 0% or 10% if the preferred provider is used but 30% if the preferred provider is not used (if care is received by an "out-of-network" provider). Sometimes deductibles are waived if care is from the preferred provider. Although the systems restrict the provider options for patients, many employers prefer this method because it lowers expenses. Insurers (and the employers who pay their premiums) believe that PPOs decrease costs.

There is a saying in the PPO industry that "if you've seen one PPO, you've seen one PPO." Each arrangement tends to be unique, which makes it difficult to make generalizations about PPOs.

[116]The Kaiser Family Foundation and Health Research and Educational Trust. 2010. *Employer Health Benefits: 2010 Annual Survey.* Retrieved July 17, 2011, at http://ehbs.kff.org/pdf/2010/8085.pdf.
[117]*Ibid.*

Point of Service

In the latter half of the 1990s, one of the most rapidly growing forms of managed care was point of service (POS) plans. However, enrollment in POS plans has declined from 24% of enrolled workers in 1999 to 8% of enrolled workers in 2010.[118] Typically, these plans offer a choice of in-network or out-of-network care. In-network care often operates as an HMO, with HMO-type coverage. Out-of-network benefits allow choice of provider but reimburse patients as if they were in a PPO and chose not to use the preferred provider.

Other Variations on Managed Care

There is no doubt that we will continue to see managed care evolve, especially plans that make use of managed care principles. For example, ACOs—networks of doctors, hospitals, and other health care providers, including advanced practice nurses—are a part of the ACA. These organizations will provide care to groups of Medicare patients and are required to be "accountable" for the overall care of Medicare beneficiaries. They will also share in the cost savings for the Medicare program if they meet certain quality thresholds.[119]

Interestingly, a sector of the insurance market with the largest growth in 2010 was plans with a high deductible and a savings option. These plans grew from 8% of covered employed workers in 2009 to 13% in 2010. It is likely that these kinds of plans will continue to increase as the cost of care is shifted to employees.

❋ IMPLICATIONS FOR NURSE MANAGERS AND EXECUTIVES

The purpose of this chapter was to present the various elements of the health care system to provide an explanation of the environment in which nurse managers and executives work. There are a number of key players or participants in the health care system. These not only include the providers of care and the patients but also the health care suppliers, regulators, and payers. In health care, much of what an organization and professional can or cannot do is influenced by forces external to the organization. These forces may be government regulatory bodies, insurance companies, accrediting bodies, or consumer groups. Changes in legislation and payment systems to HCOs have implications for how care is provided. Changes in the regulation of health professionals have implications for what ancillary workers can and cannot do. Without considering the role of each participant and the relationships among all the

participants, one risks making decisions that do not take all relevant factors into account.

Many things are done by health care providers that may not make obvious sense. Some of these things can be understood if the manager considers the system of financing the health care system. Health care providers have become dependent on revenues from Medicare, Medicaid, insurance, and self-pay patients. However, the payments being made have placed a great stress on the economy.

In reaction to increasing health care expenditures, the government has focused on prospective payment, managed care, and better coordination of care. Insurers have placed hurdles such as coinsurance, deductibles, co-payments, and limits on customary and reasonable charges, as well as restrictions on the specific care that will be reimbursed. With decreasing funding from philanthropic sources, providers must be ever more diligent to carefully remain financially solvent. The main payers are attempting to restrict payments while at the same time providers see a growing number of patients who are not covered, even by government programs for indigent individuals, because they cannot afford to pay for their care or choose not to buy health insurance. Either way, growing numbers of uninsured patients continue to stress the health care system and our payment structures.

In further response to the need to control health care costs, more programs have been created to manage these costs. The most prominent among these are managed care plans, or plans based on managed care principles, including HMOs, PPOs, POS, and ACOs. Potentially, in most health care provider organizations, the nurse manager or executive will have to deal directly with each of these cost containment alternatives. There is likely to be a growing need for nurse managers and executives to have financial information that can be used in negotiations and decisions that relate to HMOs, PPOs, POS plans, ACOs, and other managed care efforts.

Today, nurses are viewed as key players in the health care system certainly because nursing services plays an important role in the delivery of care to patients and communities. However, they are becoming increasingly important because of the role they play in hospital reimbursements, which are now tied to the prevention of HACs—urinary tract infections, catheter-associated blood stream infections, ventilator-associated pneumonias, pressure ulcers, and hospital readmissions, to name a few. Therefore, nurse managers and executives need to be more conscious than ever of the costs of running units and departments and the financial impact of their operational decisions on other units, their department, and the organization. They need strong financial and political skills to advocate for the additional resources that may be needed to staff nursing units and to demonstrate how these costs will offset the loss of reimbursement caused by adverse events such as HACs.

---

[118]*Ibid.*

[119]Retrieved July 17, 2011, at http://www.kff.org/healthreform/upload/8061.pdf.

✳ KEY CONCEPTS

Key participants   Major groups involved in the organization and delivery of health care are the providers, suppliers, consumers, regulators, and payers.

> **Providers**   Health workers such as nurses or physicians and HCOs such as nursing homes or hospitals that dispense health care services to people. The most important providers of care are hospitals, nurses, physicians, and the government. However, many other types of providers are essential to providing the total range of health care services. Different providers have different goals, incentives, and perspectives.
>
> **Suppliers**   Manufacturers and distributors of supplies, equipment, and pharmaceuticals used by health care providers. Suppliers have a dramatic impact on the health care industry as a result of their development on new technologies.
>
> **Consumers**   Individuals who receive health care services. Generally, consumers of health care are less knowledgeable about health care purchases than they are about the purchase of other goods and services.
>
> **Regulators**   Federal, state, and local governments have the legal authority to regulate the health care industry as part of their function of protecting the public. Health providers are also subject to the regulations of voluntary accreditation and certification bodies such as The Joint Commission.
>
> **Payers**   Individuals or organizations that pay for health care services provided to consumers. The most common groups of payers are individuals, insurers, employers, and the government.

Third-party payer   Organization or government ("third parties") that pays for health care services consumed by individuals.

Contractual allowances   Discounts from normal charges that are given to large payers of health care services.

Health care financing   Government is the largest payer for health care services, providing about 46% of the funding. Insurers and employers are the next largest group, followed by individuals.

Medicare and Medicaid   Government programs that pay for health care services for elderly individuals, permanently disabled individuals, and some indigent individuals. The Medicare program is administered by the CMS, and payments to providers are made through fiscal intermediaries.

Insurance system   Most people in the United States have private health insurance. In exchange for a premium, often paid for by an employer, individuals receive health insurance coverage. The premium rates are set based either on the experience of a specific group (group rated) or the community as a whole (community rated). To discourage unnecessary use of health care services, insurance usually has deductibles, co-payments, and coinsurance.

Adverse event   Harm to a patient that results from the health care they receive.

Hospital-acquired conditions (HACs)   High-cost or high-volume conditions that are not "present on admission," result in the assignment of a higher-paying DRG as a secondary diagnosis, and could have been prevented through the application of evidence-based guidelines.

Present on admission (POA)   A health condition that exists at the time a patient is admitted to the hospital.

Deductible   Amount the individual must pay each year before insurance begins to pay for care. This payment is usually several hundred dollars.

Co-payment   Dollar amount that must be paid by the individual each time a health service is used. For example, some pharmaceutical plans require that a $10 or $15 fee be paid for each generic prescription and $20 or $50 for a brand name drug.

Coinsurance   Percentage of charges that must be paid by the beneficiary, usually 20%.

Out-of-pocket expense   Money the individual must expend directly for health care services not covered by insurance or other third-party sources.

Customary and reasonable charges   Limits set by insurers on the amount that they will consider for payment based on surveys of typical charges in the community.

Cost-based reimbursement   Payments made to providers based on reimbursement to the provider for the cost incurred in providing care.

Prospective payment   Payments made to providers based on a fixed price for each specific type of patient. Payments are not made in advance of treatment.

Pay-for-performance   System of paying hospitals and health care providers based on quality performance rather than on the costs incurred to provide specific services for patients with a particular diagnosis. Also known as *value-based purchasing*.

Diagnosis Related Groups (DRGs)   Medicare prospective payment system. Patients are placed in specific groups (DRGs) based on their principal diagnosis, surgical procedure, age, and other factors. Payment for each patient within a specific group is the same. The payment is a predetermined fixed amount and is not dependent on the costs incurred in treating the patient.

Health maintenance organization (HMO)   Health Care Organization (HCO) that agrees to provide health care on a capitation basis. The HMO is paid a set fee per member per month to provide all specified health care services to enrolled patients.

Preferred provider organization (PPO)   Organization that agrees to provide care for a group of individuals, such as an employee group, based on a negotiated set of fees. These fees are often lower than the prevailing fees in the community. In contrast with HMOs, the providers are paid on a fee-for-service basis.

Point of service (POS) organization   Organization that offers members either in-network, HMO-type coverage with low coinsurance and deductible rates but limited choice or out-of-network care with greater choice but higher deductible and coinsurance rates.

Managed care   System for organizing the delivery of care in which someone other than the provider of care controls the services the patient uses. These systems are usually used to control and limit the use of services. However, they are also used so that people do not receive unnecessary care, which subjects the patient to unnecessary risk.

Fee-for-service   Traditional approach whereby patients are charged and providers are paid based on each episode of care and each service provided.

Capitation   Managed care approach that pays providers a flat fee per patient regardless of the amount of care that the patient consumes.

Bad debt   Operating expenses related to care provided to patients who ultimately do not pay their bills. Amounts included in revenues but never paid are balanced by the charge to bad debts.

Charity care   Care provided to patients who are not expected to pay because of limited personal financial resources.

✳ SUGGESTED READINGS

Aiken LH, Cheung RB, Olds DM: Education policy initiatives to address the nurse shortage in the United States, *Health Aff (Web Exclusive)*:w646–w656, 2009.

American Hospital Association: *AHA hospital statistics, 2009 edition.* Chicago, 2011, AHA.

Baker LC, Bundor MK, Kessler DP: HMO coverage reduces variation in the use of health care among patients under age 65, *Health Aff* 29(11):2068–2074, 2009.

Blendon RJ, Schoen C, DesRoches C, et al: Common concerns amid diverse systems: health care experiences in five countries, *Health Aff* 22(3):106–121, 2003.

Blusteink J, Weissman JS, Ryan AM, et al: Analysis raises questions on whether pay-for-performance in Medicaid can efficiently reduce racial and ethnic disparities, *Health Aff* 30(6):1165–1175, 2011.

Borger C, Smith S, Truffer C, et al: Health spending projections through 2015: changes on the horizon. *Health Aff (Millwood)* 25(2):w61–w73, 2006.

Burns L, Bradley E, Weiner B: *Shortell and Kaluzny's health care management: organization design and behavior,* ed 6, Albany, NY, 2011, Delmar.

Campbell C, Schmitz H, Waller L: *Financial management in a managed care environment (Delmar's health information management series),* Albany, NY, 1998, Delmar.

Campbell S: The newest gatekeepers: nurses take on the duties of primary care physicians, *Health Care Strateg Manage* 15(3):14–15, 1997.

Coleman MP, Quaresma M, Berrino F, et al: Cancer survival in five continents: a worldwide population-based study (CONCORD), *Lancet Oncol* 9(8):730–756, 2008.

Congressional Budget Office: *Non-profit hospitals and the provision of community benefits* (website), 2006. www.cbo.gov/ftpdocs/76xx/doc7695/12-06-Nonprofit.pdf. Accessed July 8, 2011.

Cowan CA, Hartman MA: Financing health care: businesses, households, and governments, 1987–2003, *Healthc Finan Rev* 1(2):1–26, 2005. Available at www.cms.gov/NationalHealthExpendData/downloads/bhg-article-04.pdf. Accessed July 8, 2011.

Davis K, Schoen C, Schoenbaum SC, et al: *Mirror, mirror on the wall: how the performance of the U.S. health care system compares internationally* (website), 2010. http://www.commonwealthfund.org/~/media/Files/Publications/Fund%20Report/2010/Jun/1400_Davis_Mirror_Mirror_on_the_wall_2010.pdf. Accessed July 10, 2011.

DeNavas-Walt C, Proctor B, Lee C: Income, poverty, and health insurance coverage in the United States: 2004. In *Current population reports P60-229,* Washington, DC, 2005, U.S. Department of Commerce, Economics and Statistics Administration. Available at www.census.gov/prod/2005pubs/p60–229.pdf. Accessed June 23, 2006.

Finkler S: Cost containment. In Kovner A, Knickman J, editors: *Jonas and Kovner's health care delivery in the United States,* ed 8, New York, 2005, Springer, pp 628–659.

Fisher ES, Bynam JP, Skinner JS: Slowing the growth of healthcare costs: lessons from regional variation, *N Engl J Med* 360:849–852, 2009.

Friedberg MW, Safran DG, Coltink K, et al: Paying for performance in primary care: potential impact on practices and disparities, *Health Aff* 29(5):926–932, 2010.

Gilmer TP, Kronick RG: Differences in the volume of services and in prices drive big variations in Medicaid spending among U.S. states and regions, *Health Aff* 30(7):1316–1324, 2011.

Gordon S: *Nursing against the odds: how health care cost cutting, media stereotypes, and medical hubris undermine nurses and patient care,* Ithaca, NY, 2005, Cornell University Press.

Grimaldi P: Managed care glossary update, *Nurs Manage* 28(8):22–25, 1997.

Grossbart S: What's the return? Assessing the effect of "pay-for-performance" initiatives on the quality of care delivery, *Med Care Res Rev* 63(Suppl 1):S29–S48, 2005.

Kovner A, Knickman J, editors: *Jonas & Kovner's health care delivery in the United States,* ed 10, New York, 2011, Springer.

Kreimer: Philanthropy. More than ever, big donors want to see value for their dollars, *Hosp Health Netw* 83(6):20, 2009. Available at www.hhnmag.com/hhnmag_app/jsp/articledisplay.jsp?dcrpath=HHNMAG/Article/data/06JUN2009/0906HHN_Inbox_philanthropy&domain=HHNMAG. Accessed July 9, 2011.

Litvak E, Buerhaus PI, Davidoff F, et al: Managing unnecessary variability in patient demand to reduce nursing stress and improve patient safety, *Jt Comm J Qual Patient Saf* 31(6):330–338, 2005.

Martin A, Lassman D, Whittle L, et al: Recession contributes to slowest annual rate of increase in health spending in five decades, *Health Aff* 30(1):11–22, 2011.

McGuire TG, Newhouse JP, Sinaiko AD: An economic history of Medicare Part C, *Milbank Q* 89(2):289–332, 2011.

Mechanic D: The rise and fall of managed care, *J Health Soc Behav* 45(Suppl): 76–86, 2004.

Morra D, Nicholson S, Levinson W, et al: U.S. physician practices versus Canadians: spending nearly four times as much money interacting with payers, *Health Aff* 30(8):1443–1450, 2011.

OECD: *Health data 2011: how does Canada compare?* (website). www.oecd.org/dataoecd/46/33/38979719.pdf. Accessed July 10, 2011.

Rejda GE: *Principles of risk management and insurance*, Upper Saddle River, NJ, 2010, Prentice Hall.

Rich VL, Porter-O'Grady T: Nurse executive practice: creating a new vision for leadership, *Nurs Admin Q* 35(3):277–281, 2011.

Robinson JS: Health savings accounts—the ownership society in health care, *N Engl J Med* 353:1199–1202, 2005.

Rodwin V: A comparative analysis of health systems among wealthy nations. In Kovner A, Knickman J, editors: *Jonas & Kovner's health care delivery in the United States,* ed 8, New York, 2005, Springer.

Rosenberg C: *The care of strangers,* New York, 1987, Basic Books.

Rosenthal M, Frank R, Li Z, Epstein A: Early experience with pay-for-performance: from concept to practice, *JAMA* 294(14):1788–1793, 2005.

Safiiet B: Health care dollars and regulatory sense: the role of advanced practice nursing, *Yale J Regul* 9(2):417–488, Summer 1992.

Schoen C, Osborn R, Doty R, et al: Toward higher-performance health systems: adults' health care experiences in seven countries, *Health Aff* 26(6): w717–w734, 2007.

Schoen C, Osborn R, Huynh P, et al: Primary care and health system performance: adults' experiences in five countries, *Health Aff (Millwood)*: w4-487–w4-503, 2004.

Schoen C, Osborn R, Huynh P, et al: Taking the pulse of health care systems: experiences of patients with health problems in six countries, *Health Aff (Millwood)*:W5-509–w5-525, 2005.

Schoen C, Osborn R, Squires D, et al: How insurance design affects access to care and costs by income, in eleven countries, *Health Aff* 29(12):2323–2334, 2010.

Smith C, Cowan C, Heffler S, et al: National health spending in 2004: recent slowdown led by prescription drug spending, *Health Aff* 25(1):186–196, 2006.

Smith M, Walker E: *Special report: Canada and the U.S.—comparing key practice parameters* (website). www.medpagetoday.com/PublicHealthPolicy/PublicHealth/15931. Accessed July 10, 2011.

Stahl D: The phases of managed care: where does subacute care fit? *Nurs Manag* 27(Suppl):8–9, 1996.

Thorpe K: The health system in transition: care, cost and coverage, *J Health Polit Pol Law* 22:355, 1997.

Truffer CJ, Keehan SK, Smith S, et al: Health spending projections through 2019: the recession's impact continues, *Health Aff* 29:522–529, 2010.

U.S. Department of Health and Human Services, Health Resources and Services Administration: *The registered nurse population: findings from the 2008 National Sample Survey of Registered Nurses* (website), 2010. bhpr.hrsa.gov/healthworkforce/rnsurveys/rnsurveyfinal.pdf. Accessed July 15, 2011.

Weinberg D: *Code green: money-driven hospitals and the dismantling of nursing,* Ithaca, NY, 2003, Cornell University Press.

Wong ST: Reimbursement to advanced practice nurses (APNs) through Medicare, *J Nurs Scholar* 31(2):167–173, 1999.

Woolhandler S, Campbell T, Himmelstein D: Costs of health care administration in the United States and Canada, *N Engl J Med* 349(8):768–775, 2003.

Woolhandler S, Himmelstein DU: Costs of care and administration at for-profit and other hospitals in the U.S., *N Engl J Med* 336(11):769–774, 1997.

World Health Organization: *Health systems: improving performance* (website), 2000. www.who.int/whr/2000/en/whr00_en.pdf. Accessed July 10, 2011.

The Role of Financial Management and Nurse Leadership in Health Care Organizations

CHAPTER GOALS

The goals of this chapter are to:

- Explain the role of nurse managers and executives in the financial well-being of health care organizations
- Explain the role of organizational structure in theory and practice
- Distinguish between formal and informal lines of authority, and between line and staff roles of managers
- Describe the role of nurse councils in the nursing department
- Assess advantages and disadvantages of centralized and decentralized management approaches

- Describe the role of financial managers in health care organizations
- Describe the financial responsibilities of the chief nurse executive, nurse managers, and other nurses
- Discuss the interactions between nurse managers and executives and financial managers in health care organizations
- Explain the concept of responsibility accounting, including cost and revenue centers
- Discuss issues of politics in budget determinations
- Describe the role of networking

✳ INTRODUCTION

The primary role of nurses is the delivery of patient care. Historically, anything to do with money or financial resources was seen by most nurses as the purview of administration. Most nurses did not know about budgets or organizational resources and did not want to know about them. They wanted to keep people healthy and provide nursing care to those in need and to those who could not care for themselves. They did, however, want resources to be available to support patient care—whatever they needed, whenever they needed it. By default, some nurses had to become involved with money; they became nurse administrators. These nurses were viewed by some in nursing as having abandoned clinical nursing and patient care. Even worse, when some of these nurse administrators became hospital administrators, they were characterized as having completely "sold out."

There has been increasing pressure for health care organizations (HCOs) to control costs and to provide care efficiently. In the past, many HCOs tried to accomplish this with as little involvement as possible from nurse managers and executives in the area of resource management. Financial managers would simply provide nursing departments with a budget and tell nurse managers and executives to hold to the budgeted level of spending. That approach largely failed.

Managers and executives who are accountable for spending know the most about the resources that are needed and how

they will be used. This is in keeping with the philosophy that those closest to the problem are in the best position to solve the problem. Managers and executives must be involved in the planning process if the budget is to be realistic. To control costs, nurse managers and executives—in hospitals, long-term care facilities, home health agencies, ambulatory care facilities, or nurse-managed clinics—must be directly involved in a wide array of financial activities. In some organizations, this means that nurses are taking on an increasing burden of financial calculations. In other organizations, nurses are hiring nonclinical persons with MBA degrees to work for them as staff members. Those individuals do the financial calculations and provide nurses with essential financial information. In either case, nurses are ultimately responsible for the content of those calculations. Nurse managers and executives must have sufficient financial skills either to develop or to supervise the development of financial information needed to run their organizations. This is necessary not only to provide acceptable quality of care but also to provide that care on a cost-effective basis.

In the past, nurses were able to isolate themselves from financial issues. Today that is simply not possible or even advisable. The complex health care environment of the 21st century requires that nurses know about financial issues and apply that knowledge to address the organization's financial concerns. This responsibility should not rest solely with nurses in leadership positions. Nurses at all levels of the organization must understand where the organization's money comes from and where it goes to be effective and efficient in the delivery of nursing care, to articulate the economic value of nursing, and to influence the use of more creative and innovative models of care delivery. In other words, nurses have the knowledge to help translate patient care into dollars and vice versa; this ability is a unique domain of nursing. Health care administrators are looking to nurses at all levels for solutions to problems that have an impact on organizational finances. This has spurred a growing number of undergraduate and graduate programs in schools of nursing to include financial management in their programs.

This chapter explains the role of financial management in the structure of organizations and how nursing, nurse managers, and nurse executives fit into that organizational structure from a financial management perspective. To accomplish that, issues that affect nurses' ability to be effective and savvy stewards of financial resources are discussed, such as lines of authority, formal and informal organizational linkages, interrelationships among managers and executives, and the role of politics and power in HCOs.

✳ THE ROLE OF MANAGEMENT

Health care organizations include a wide variety of providers of health care services, such as hospitals, long-term care facilities, home health agencies, hospice, and nursing centers. Regardless of the type of organization, certain management functions must be carried out. Three of the most important of these are planning, control, and decision making.

Planning is essential for the efficient management of the organization. Through planning, managers and executives consider possible options available to the organization and steer its path. Without planning, the organization drifts like a rudderless ship. With planning, the organization is able to set a direction; determine, allocate, or obtain resources to get there; and then move forward. Strategic planning and budgeting, two topics covered in this book, are essential elements of the planning process.

Control is a critical management task. After the plan has been established, it must be implemented. *Control* refers to the managerial tasks related to ensuring that the plans of the organization are carried out as closely as possible. Control is necessary for carrying out the plans, assessing progress, evaluating related income and expenditures, and determining what can be done when progress is not satisfactory. Control, however, does not mean blind allegiance to a plan gone awry!

Decision making is perhaps the overriding role of management. Plans will not carry any weight unless someone makes decisions that are necessary to carry them out. Control will lack authority if no one makes decisions to correct problems that arise when the plan is not met or when the plan needs modification. Organizations do not progress without change. Change cannot occur without someone having the authority to make decisions and exercising that authority.

These basic elements of the role of management apply to all managers and executives within the organization. Only when they apply these principles can organizations most efficiently achieve their goals. Other skills are also needed to ensure financial success, such as vision and innovation at all levels of staff and management within the organization.

✳ THE HIERARCHY OF HEALTH CARE ORGANIZATIONS

To make plans, control the implementation of plans, and make and carry out decisions, each organization has a managerial structure that reflects its *hierarchy*. The hierarchy establishes the authority and responsibility that different individuals have within the organization.

Organizations typically have a governing board, referred to as the board of trustees or board of directors, composed of respected individuals from the community, health care, and business. Although some board members may be affiliated with the organization, most of the board members are *not* full-time employees of the organization.

The board has the ultimate responsibility for organizational decisions and, in turn, the financial condition of the organization. The board has the final approval over adoption of the annual budget and provides the direction for setting that budget. The board adopts a mission statement that sets the overall direction of the organization. It also adopts goals and objectives that tell the organization's managers what they should be doing to accomplish the mission. The highest-level administrator, often called the chief executive officer (CEO) or president, reports to the board and is responsible for managing the organization. As is typical in bureaucratic organizations, a variety of managers report to the CEO.

The Top Management Team

It is unusual to find any moderate-to-large sized organization that can be run by one manager; too many different functions must be carried out. As a result, there are many managers, each with a specialized set of responsibilities and scope of authority. For the single top manager to know what each manager is doing requires a hierarchy of managers. Instructions may be passed down through the hierarchy along with the authority to carry out the instructions. To facilitate this process, many organizations form a top management or executive team, which acts together to make major organizational decisions. Information flows up through the hierarchy so that the top manager is aware of issues and concerns at other levels in the organization, including the point of service. For example, nurse managers often directly observe events about which the higher levels of management should be informed. This information gets passed up through the hierarchy to the management team and top manager.

Many large organizations have an associate administrator as part of this team, often called the chief operating officer (COO) or executive vice president for operations, who is responsible for the day-to-day operations of the organization. The team typically includes a chief financial officer (CFO), who is responsible for the financial aspects of running the organization. The CEO, the COO, and the CFO usually attend board meetings. The CEO is often a member of the board. Some organizations also have a chief information officer (CIO), who is responsible for overseeing and integrating organizational information systems.

In the past, the chief nurse executive (CNE) was known as the director of nursing. More recently, the titles vice president for nursing, vice president for patient services, and senior vice president for nursing or patient care services have gained widespread use. The titles CNE and chief nursing officer (CNO) are also used to denote the top-level nurse in the organization.[1] In some organizations, however, there may still be a wide gap between the role these chief (or "C") titles convey (i.e., the CNE as a key member of the top management team consisting of the CEO, COO, CFO, and CNE) and the actual role of the CNE as functioning on par with a number of other department heads who report to a member of the top management team. Although in the past, the role of the CNE was diminished as organizations reorganized and downsized to contain costs, today many organizations have revamped and enhanced the CNE role because of the recognized need for a top nursing voice within the organization.

The essence of these issues is captured in the following quote from a landmark Institute of Medicine (IOM) report titled *Keeping Patients Safe: Transforming the Work Environment of Nurses*[2]:

> *Clinical nursing leadership has been reduced at multiple levels, and the voice of nurses in patient care has diminished. Hospital reengineering initiatives often have resulted in the loss of a separate department of nursing (Gelinas and Manthey, 1997). At the same time, nursing staff have perceived a decline in chief nursing executives with power and authority equal to that of other top hospital officials, as well as in directors of nursing who are highly visible and accessible to staff (Aiken et al., 2000). These changes— along with losses of chief nursing officers without replacement; decreases in the numbers of nurse managers; and increased responsibilities of remaining nurse managers for more than one patient care unit, as well as for supervising personnel other than nursing staff (e.g., housekeepers, transportation staff, dietary aides) (Aiken et al., 2001; Sovie and Jawad, 2001)—have had the cumulative effect of reducing direct management support available to patient care staff. This situation hampers nurses' ability to fix problems in their work environments that threaten patient safety (Tucker and Edmondson, 2002).*

Therefore, one of the important recommendations from this IOM report is a call for the inclusion of nurses at all levels of executive decision making. Others include the use of transformational leadership and evidence-based management, both of which necessitate strong nursing leadership.

Today as organizational leaders come to understand the relationship between nursing care and the organization's financial health, the trend is recognition of the special role played by the CNE, who controls approximately half of most HCOs' budgets and an even greater share of the organizations' salaries. In home care agencies, the CNE controls almost the entire budget. In more and more HCOs, the CNE is an active member of the top management team, attends board meetings, and participates in making some of the organization's most important decisions.

As the CNE becomes part of the top management team, the responsibility of that position shifts from responsibility for and management of *the nursing department* to responsibility for and management of *the organization*. Instead of looking downward at the nursing department, CNEs are starting to look outward at the overall actions of the organization and how they affect the organization as a whole. The result is that nursing is gaining in prestige as a member of the inner circle of management. The CNE is privy to more information and is a key player in the most important decisions of the organization. However, some argue that the role that CNEs serve in such situations lessens their ability to be an advocate for the needs of nursing in the organization. The role removes the CNE even further from patients and from an awareness of the needs of staff nurses.

We believe that the new role of the CNE is appropriate and very much needed in HCOs. The organizational resources controlled by nursing are too great for it to be excluded from the key decisions that affect those organizations or to relegate these important decisions to others. This role is also critical to advance the *Future of Nursing* initiative[3] introduced in Chapter 2. Involvement at this level in the HCO also provides an extraordinary opportunity for CNEs to represent nursing to organizational leadership; to articulate the role of nursing in the health care value chain; to represent an organization at national and international levels; and to use the skills of planning, control, and decision making at a high level to garner resources for acquiring nursing expertise and improving care delivery.[4] However, the CNEs must be cognizant of the difficult position in which this trend places them and make special efforts to ensure that the needs of the organization are balanced with the needs of the nursing department and its managers and staff. These efforts are often achieved through the CNE's reliance on a hierarchy of organizational nurse leaders and on shared governance structures. Through these structures, the day-to-day responsibilities for managing nursing services are carried out by organizational nurse leaders. Shared governance structures play a central role by using nurse councils to give nurses a voice in decisions that pertain to nursing practice, quality of care, education, and research. Shared governance structures and nurse councils have become prominent in HCOs as they strive to achieve Magnet Recognition® (discussed in Chapter 5).

Line versus Staff Authority

To carry out its mission, goals, and objectives, the organization has a hierarchy of managers who ultimately report to the CEO,

---

[1]In this book, the titles CNE and CNO are used interchangeably.

[2]National Research Council. Keeping Patients Safe: Transforming the Work Environment of Nurses. Washington, DC: The National Academies Press, 2004, p.4.

[3]Institute of Medicine. 2011. *The Future of Nursing: Leading Change, Advancing Health.* Washington, DC: National Academies Press.

[4]*Ibid*, p. 16.

the top management team, or both. The types of managers that exist in an organization can be divided into two major classes based on their *line function* or *staff function*. The line function is the element of running an organization that is related directly to the production of its goods and services. In the case of HCOs, the line function is carried out by the managers who oversee departments that provide patient care. Most nurse managers are considered *line managers*. Their managerial efforts are directed at overseeing the day-to-day operations of providing direct care to patients, including the management of line staff (i.e., nurses, other direct care providers, and ancillary care personnel).

In contrast, the staff function focuses on the provision of auxiliary assistance or indirect service to the line managers and their departments. Finance officers are *staff managers*. The role of finance is, as a staff department, to carry out necessary functions for running the organization that are indirect to the provision of care. Finance makes sure that there is money to buy the things that the organization needs and to pay for them. It also provides necessary information about the finances of the organization.

Line managers do not report to staff managers. For example, the finance officer and department do not have authority over any line operations of the organization. However, the information provided by finance is often used by line managers to help them make more effective managerial decisions. Nurse managers and executives must understand the staff role played by the finance department and make use of its departmental staff as a resource.

To better understand the distinction between staff and line authority, one must understand the framework of both formal and informal lines of authority and responsibility within an organization.

Formal Lines of Authority

Organizations have formal chains of command that define lines of authority and responsibility. Of interest to readers of this book is how the nursing department fits within the overall organizational structure and its relationship to the organization's financial management. Also of interest is the nursing organization, whether a small nurse-run clinic or a large temporary nurse agency. As new models of delivering and financing care have evolved, nursing organizations have also evolved to include new ways of delivering nursing services, often through contracting.

The formal lines of authority for most organizations are specified in the form of an organizational chart. An organizational chart is simply a diagram of organizational interrelationships represented by boxes and lines. Each position on the chart supervises the departments or positions below it and reports to those above it, as denoted by the solid lines. Other positions on the same level of the chart are on a similar level of the organizational hierarchy. There is often communication among individuals on the same level, but there is not a direct reporting relationship. Whereas organizational charts that are more vertical (i.e., taller) tend to have more levels of reporting and are therefore more complex to navigate, organizations that are more horizontal (i.e., flatter) tend to have fewer levels of reporting and are somewhat less complex.

It is also common to have formal relationships that do not represent the same degree of authority or control. For instance, a manager at one level in the organization may report to a manager directly above. The director of the dietary department may report to the COO but may also communicate on a regular basis with the CNE, who is concerned about the impact of nutrition on the quality of patient care and the interactions between the two departments that are needed to improve it. However, the CNE is not the supervisor of the dietary manager and has limited ability to make decisions and give instructions in that area. Such formal but limited relationships may or may not be indicated on organizational charts by dashed lines.

Informal lines of authority and relationships may also exist. These are completely outside the official policy of the organization and do not appear on the organizational chart, but they may be very important because they often reflect political alliances.

Figure 3–1 shows a sample organizational chart for a community hospital of moderate size. Solid lines indicate direct paths of formal authority and responsibility. As shown here, the CNO reports to the president, who reports to the board of trustees. The CNO is on the same level as the five other members of the senior management staff. It is worth noting that although the CFO is highly placed in the organization, only financial departments report to that individual. None of the direct providers of care report to the CFO.

Figure 3–2 shows the organizational chart for a major medical center. The CNO, who is a Senior Vice President, reports to the COO, who is the Executive Vice President. In this type of structure, there will be a CNO, and often an associate CNO, and nursing directors for each of the nine divisions that report to the CNO. Both organizations (shown in Figures 3–1 and 3–2) follow traditional organizational models, with nursing as a separate department and most nurses who work in the organization reporting through nursing. Note, however, that some directors, such as the surgical services director, may have additional reporting requirements to other departments and executives, outside of the nursing department and apart from the CNE.

Some medical staff members practicing at a hospital may not be employees of the hospital but instead may be affiliated, voluntary staff. Therefore, they are not part of the direct-line hierarchy in the hospital, indicated on Figure 3–1 as a dotted line. In other cases, physician employees (hospitalists and physician practices) may be hospital employees and report to an organizational executive, shown in Figure 3–2 as a solid line reporting relationship. Figure 3–3 shows the organizational chart of a large government-owned hospital in which physicians are employees of the hospital and directly accountable to the CEO. Regardless of reporting relationships, a hospital cannot function without medical staff any more than it can function without nursing staff. There are established relationships between the medical staff and the employees of the organization.

Most hospitals have a medical board, which has responsibility for the quality of medical care in the organization. Both The Joint Commission and state regulations require that this be a

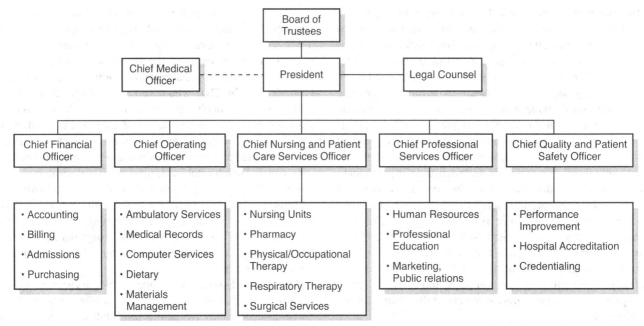

FIGURE 3–1. Organization chart for a moderate-sized community hospital.

formal relationship, but the nature of the relationship varies, depending on whether or not the physicians are organizational employees or affiliates of the organization.

Figure 3–4 shows the organizational chart for a home health agency. Although the chart shows a solid line from staff to patient care manager, this does not necessarily reflect how staff are paid. They may be paid on a per-visit basis but still report directly to a patient care manager.

The most complex health care organizational structures are found in integrated delivery systems. Integrated delivery systems are organizational networks of providers that offer coordinated care across a continuum of health care services and settings.[5] Integrated delivery systems often include a variety of HCOs with various levels of formal relationships. Figure 3–5 shows the organizational chart of a simple integrated health system that owns HCOs, including a physician–nurse practitioner ambulatory care center. Within these systems, hospitals usually have the most complex organizational structure. Also, hospitals and other organizations in an integrated system usually have their own CNE, and there may be a corporate-level chief nurse that has either a direct or an indirect reporting relationship with other system CNEs.

Integrated delivery systems may or may not be affiliated with a managed care organization (MCO). Some MCOs own facilities (e.g., hospitals), professional practices (e.g., multi-specialty group practices), and other services (e.g., laboratories). Other MCOs own only the insurance and management components

and contract for all health provider services with a single system, an integrated system, or multiple systems.

As health care evolves to become more patient-centered, the conceptualization of care as an integrated, seamless, delivery system is likely to become more obvious in our organizational structures. As acknowledged by the IOM, patient-centered care "establishes a partnership among practitioners, patients, and their families . . . to ensure that decisions respect patients' wants, needs, and preferences and that patients have the education and support they need to make decisions and participate in their own care."[6] Under such an approach, care would be focused on the patient's perspective, structured to be more accessible and convenient for the patient and family, and flexible enough to accommodate patient and family needs and preferences.

Attributes of such a patient-centered system would promote: access to care; patient engagement in care; clinical information systems that support high-quality care, practice-based learning, and quality improvement; coordination of care; care delivery via an integrated care team; feedback from patients about their care; and the public availability of information about care.[7] Unfortunately, our health care system still has a way to go. A 2010 report by the Agency for Healthcare Research and Quality identified the following deficiencies in patient-centered care in the United States: barriers in patient–provider and family–provider communication (including communications in the delivery of care to children, older adults, and non–English-speaking

[5]Enthoven, A.C. 2009. Integrated delivery systems: The cure for fragmentation. *Am J Manage Care* 15(10):S284-S290. Retrieved at http://www.ajmc.com/publications/supplement/2009/A264_09dec_HlthPolicyCvrOne/A264_09dec_EnthovenS284to290.

[6]Institute of Medicine 2001. *Envisioning the National Health Care Quality Report.* Washington, DC: National Academies Press.

[7]Retrieved July 26, 2011, at http://www.commonwealthfund.org/Content/Publications/In-the-Literature/2005/Oct/A-2020-Vision-of-Patient-Centered-Primary-Care.aspx.

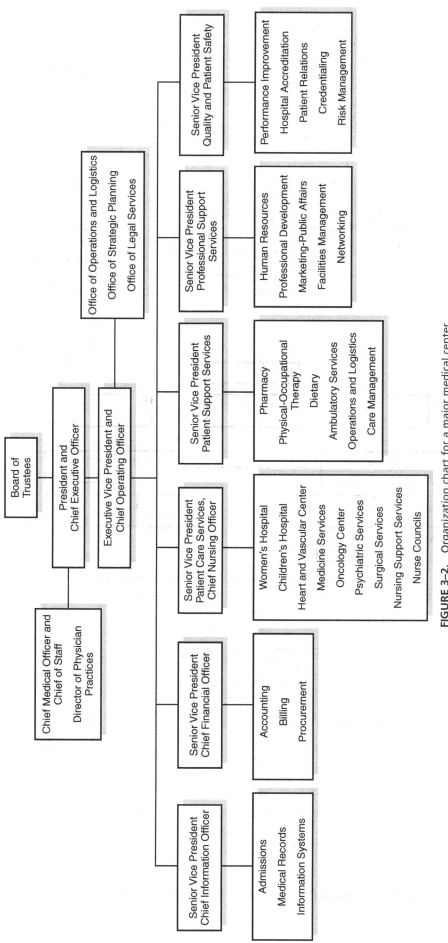

FIGURE 3–2. Organization chart for a major medical center.

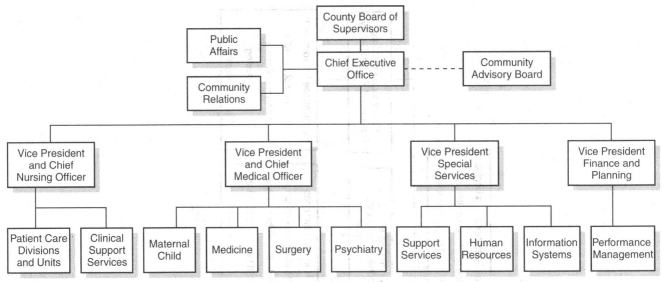

FIGURE 3–3. Organization chart for a government-owned hospital.

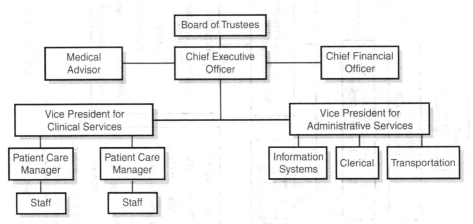

FIGURE 3–4. Organization chart for a (not-for-profit) home health agency.

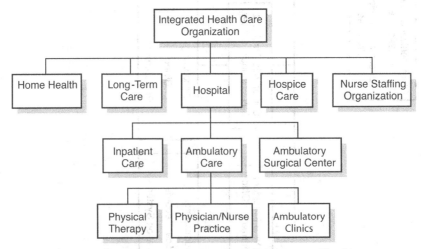

FIGURE 3–5. Organization chart for a (not-for-profit) integrated health care system.

individuals); difficulty reading and understanding prescription medications; difficulty understanding care instructions; challenges navigating the care system; and lack of involvement in care decision making.[8] As integrated and other health systems evolve, the emphasis on becoming more patient-centered must focus on improvements in these very basic aspects of care delivery.

Informal Lines of Authority

The organizational charts shown previously focus primarily on the formal relationships. Informal relationships are not part of the official authority structure of the organization. As such, they come and go, often with the individuals in specific positions. Informal relationships develop gradually over time. Although they have no official standing, they often become an accepted part of the way an organization operates.

Most texts of organizational theory point out that informal lines of authority are often as important, if not more important, as the formal lines of authority. Informal lines of authority are based on the history of the organization, the key players in the organization, and resources controlled by the various players. Depending on the specific history in any particular HCO, the CNE may have more or less authority and responsibility than the organizational chart indicates. This could develop over time with a CNE who happens to have particularly strong personality. The gains of one occupant of a position may even carry over to the successor. So may the losses.

In some organizations, individual key players may have other relationships that are not included on the organizational chart but are widely known. For example, the CNE may be married to an influential physician. This personal relationship allows each of them to have access to information that he or she might not normally have. These two players may then form a coalition to influence certain decisions.

In other cases, key employees may have connections with people important to the hospital. The director of volunteers may be the brother of the major employer in town, which pays for the care of employees who use the hospital. In some organizations, key players share a common history: They went to school together; they both worked together at another hospital; they are members of the same professional organization; they socialize together or attend the same place of worship; or they may be connected through a social networking site. Each of these connections has implications for the sharing of information and support that occurs in the process of running a hospital. The world of social networking has made possible connections and communications that were unimaginable even a decade ago.

A third source of informal authority is control of resources. A common maxim is "He who controls information controls the organization." Financial information is an example of information that may not be freely shared in or among organizations. Another resource is employees. The nursing department is usually the largest hospital department in terms of

employees and therefore has the potential to give the department and the CNE the ability to influence certain decisions and interactions.

The number of employees may not be as influential as bottom-line results. Nursing, although traditionally seen as a cost center rather than a profit center, is becoming increasingly recognized for its impact on the bottom line. Because organizational reimbursement has become more dependent on the prevention of adverse events and hospital-acquired conditions (HACs), the role that nursing plays in profits has become more obvious to organizational leaders. Despite this recognition, the widespread transition of nursing from a cost center to a profit center has not been fully achieved. Nursing must generally work to keep its expenses within budgeted expectations, but certain types of activities in other departments may give them recognition as a profit center. The profit such departments generate may be used as a bargaining chip when organizational resource allocation decisions are made. This means that some managers may exercise greater influence than others. In some cases, managers may bypass the formal lines of authority and jump over one or more levels in the organization, using their power to gain resources to achieve their goals.

Other elements also serve to reinforce informal lines of authority. Physicians admit patients to the hospital. Patients represent revenue. Therefore, physicians have power. The implicit (and sometimes explicit) threat to refer their patients elsewhere allows the medical board to have significant impact in decisions.

Often informal relationships are worked out in hospitals to exchange services. For example, the nurse manager on 3 North may make sure that when the mother of the supervisor of housekeeping is a patient in the hospital, she receives special attention. When 3 North needs extra housekeeping help, the housekeeping department may be more responsive. This "quid pro quo" behavior is common in HCOs and may be used in formal and informal relationships.

Centralized versus Decentralized Organizations

Historically, HCOs have tended to be centralized and bureaucratic. As they became more complex and employed more specialized workers, they became centralized to manage people, budgets, and organizational processes. In such a centralized system, planning, control, and decision-making authority resided with a few managers at the top levels in the organizational hierarchy, generally far from the point of service. The primary advantage of a centralized system is clarity about who makes decisions. The primary disadvantage is frustration by front-line managers and staff because they lack the ability to participate in decision making. A centralized system also requires a top-level executive who is highly knowledgeable about point-of-service processes, yet as HCOs have become increasingly complex, this has become increasingly difficult.

There has been a growing trend toward decentralization in HCOs. In a decentralized HCO, planning, control, and authority for decision making occur much lower down in the organizational hierarchy, much closer to the point of service, and by greater numbers of managers. For example, a 600-bed hospital

---

[8]AHRQ. *2010 National Healthcare Quality & Disparities Report.* Retrieved July 26, 2011, at http://www.ahrq.gov/qual/nhdr10/Chap5.htm.

may be divided into four 150-bed "mini-hospitals" in which authority for decision making resides with the managers.

Nurse councils developed in many shared-governance models are also examples of decentralization. A common councilor model used in many nursing departments is shown in Figure 3–6. At the center of the model is an Executive Council that functions as a steering committee, to which all other councils report and bring issues for decision making. This council may be chaired by the president of the nursing staff (i.e., an elected senior staff member) or the CNE. The four surrounding councils generally make decisions that affect nursing practice in the areas of professional practice, quality, education (or professional development), and research. These four councils are usually chaired by staff nurses and have representatives from all nursing units or patient care divisions. Nursing units often have committees focused in these same four areas that report and bring related issues to the councils for decision making. This approach is a way to give staff nurses a voice in departmental decision making and, when appropriate, a voice in organizational decision making as decisions are spread outside the nursing department to inform organizational policymaking. Figure 3–7 illustrates how such a structure has been applied in practice at a large integrated health system. Note that this system has interpreted the councilor structure just described in a slightly different manner. This reflects the nature of organizations and the fact that organizations operationalize structures in a way that expresses their unique focus and beliefs. Their structure consists of system-wide committees composed of members from all across the health system who work to fulfill the mission and goals of the organization.

In a classic book, Tom Peters suggests that management should be limited to no more than five layers, and he prefers no more than three.[9] He argues for increased authority and responsibility for unit managers, including greater spending authority.

Decentralization enhances the development of unit-based managers, puts authority for making decisions with the people who have the current information, allows management by exception rather than by rule, and allows a quick response to both client need and environmental change. Decentralization also means that unit-based managers encourage staff involvement in decision making and actively engage them in the process. This is particularly important when financial resources are at stake.

For an organization to grow and thrive, it must continually develop its management staff. Decentralization permits the organization to foster management skills and identify successful managers who can be promoted within the organization. A second advantage of decentralization is that the best information needed to make decisions often resides at the unit level

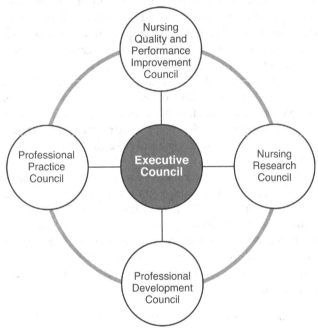

FIGURE 3–6.   Nurse shared governance model.

---

[9]Peters T. 1987. *Thriving on Chaos.* New York: Alfred A. Knopf, p. 359.

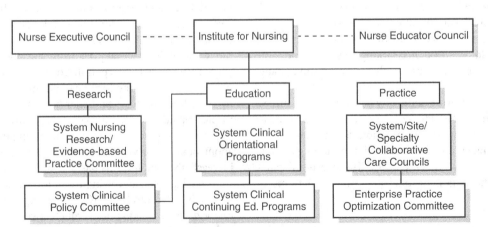

FIGURE 3–7.   Institute for Nursing, a division of the Center for Learning and Innovation, North Shore-Long Island Jewish Health System. Relationships Across the Care Continuum. (Permission to use was obtained from North Shore-Long Island Jewish Health System.)

or in positions closest to the point of care delivery. Unit managers are in constant contact with clients and staff. They know and understand the human, financial, and other needs of these groups better than a manager or executive sitting in a central office.

A third advantage of decentralization is the ability to decentralize exceptions to rules. Although large bureaucratic organizations need policies and rules, exceptions are inevitably necessary. Decentralization allows exceptions to be made at the unit level when appropriate. A good example of this is the ability of nurse managers and other staff to access other organizational resources to bring on additional staff when patient care needs are unmet.

Finally, timeliness is enhanced in a decentralized organization. Centralized organizations take a great amount of time to make decisions as information moves up and then back down through the organizational hierarchy. In a decentralized organization, decisions can be made in a more timely and efficient manner.

Although there is a trend toward decentralization, it does have disadvantages. Decentralization requires that top management relinquish some degree of planning, control, and authority for decision making to managers at lower levels in the organization. This is often very difficult to do. Not only are the right leaders and managers needed for decentralization to be successful, but organizational information and performance systems are needed to support decentralized decision making. To a great extent the degree of decentralization rests on the confidence top management has in the management team throughout the hospital, and on the quality of the performance measurement system in place.

Other problems exist as well. HCOs function in a regulated environment. This environment requires accountability for a myriad of details. External regulators place requirements on everything from how supplies should be stored to what to tell a patient before discharge. In decentralized hospitals, a system for ensuring regulatory compliance may be the greatest challenge.

Communication is a critical factor in a decentralized system. Because more decentralized decisions are made, there must be a working communication system so that top management is informed of decisions in a timely fashion. It is likely that unit-based managers and top managers will have conflicting goals; therefore, communication throughout the organizational hierarchy is essential. For example, the unit-based nurse manager often has a goal of providing high-quality, cost-effective care with the least stress to the staff. Although this goal is consistent with top management, the cost of providing care is often of higher priority to top administration than it may be to the nurse manager. However, nurse managers, and nurses in general, are becoming increasingly fluent in the language of finance and understanding of nursing's impact on the bottom line. This knowledge gives them increasing awareness of the unit's financial goals and concerns. Communication systems that provide accurate and timely financial information are therefore needed to foster communication between nurses and unit managers and between unit managers and top

administrators on matters such as setting, monitoring, and achieving unit, departmental, and organizational financial goals.

Inevitably, managers and executives at all levels of decentralized organizations will make mistakes. Nurse managers at the unit level are no exception; they are human. The organization must tolerate some mistakes and have in place a system to assist managers to learn from, rather than be punished for, exercising reasonable judgments that later turn out to be mistakes. This is consistent with the philosophy of a "just culture," which is a prevalent aspect of patient safety in many HCOs today. This approach focuses on ". . . identifying and addressing systems issues that lead individuals to engage in unsafe behaviors, while maintaining individual accountability by establishing zero tolerance for reckless behavior."[10] Thus, a financial error made by a well-intended manager should be used as a learning and growth opportunity; otherwise, managers may operate in an environment of fear in which innovation is stifled.

To successfully achieve decentralization requires a commitment from the organization for education. This requires that top management provide the necessary education to train its existing managers and to recruit new managers with the appropriate level of education. Unit managers in many HCOs have a baccalaureate degree and a few years of experience, yet many nurse managers may have an associate degree plus experience. The expectations for management roles, however, generally are commensurate with those of someone with graduate education. This is particularly apparent with regard to financial decision making. Budgeting concepts are not commonly taught in undergraduate nursing programs, yet often these undergraduates become the nurse manager of a unit in a few years after graduation. For decentralization to work, there must be a commitment from the organization to ensure that unit-based managers have the appropriate management skills, including knowledge of financial management.

A decentralized environment requires that nurse managers and executives be knowledgeable about budgeting processes and conversant in financial language. The CNE must be informed on organizational finances and financial statements, the nursing department's budget, the resources and needs of other departments, and resource allocation decisions that impact the organizational budget. The nurse manager must understand their unit budgets, how they are derived, how their resources are allocated, how their unit contributes to the nursing departmental and organizational budgets, and the implications of unit spending that reach beyond their unit. This necessitates a close working relationship between nurse managers and the finance department. "Working in silos" is no longer an option for nursing and financial leaders. As one nurse leader put it, "We need to make collaboration between nursing and finance not only an obvious thing but a necessary thing to do."[11]

---

[10]Retrieved July 26, 2011, at http://psnet.ahrq.gov/primer.aspx?primerID=5.
[11]Pamela Thompson, quoted in Clarke R. 2006. Finance and nursing: the business of caring. *Healthc Financ Manage* 60(1):50-56.

✳ THE ROLE OF THE CHIEF FINANCIAL OFFICER AND OTHER FINANCIAL MANAGERS

The CFO is in charge of all of the financial functions of the organization. The financial resources of cash and investments and their sources—loans, contributions, and retained profits—are the domain of the finance function. The generation of accounting information for external reports is the function of financial accounting. The generation of accounting information for use by the organization's own managers is the function of managerial accounting. Financial managers must also consider the organization's internal control system. The CFO is responsible for all of these functions.

The Finance Function

All organizations, whether in the health care industry or not, must manage their financial resources. These resources include *cash, marketable investments,* and *accounts receivable.* Finance is also responsible for managing the sources of these resources, such as notes and accounts payable, loans, and payroll. The finance function includes making and maintaining relationships with banks and other sources of funds for the organization.

Cash must be managed. This includes safeguarding it against misappropriation, ensuring that cash resources are handled efficiently, and ensuring that the organization has sufficient cash for its needs. In the finance function, financial managers consider the timing of cash inflows and outflows from the organization. If it becomes apparent that there will be insufficient cash at times to meet the organization's needs, arrangements must be made to get additional cash. This may require arranging for loans, pushing harder on fund-raising efforts, or in a for-profit organization, selling more shares of its stock.

Finance also actively works to maximize the benefit of *accounts receivable.* Accounts receivable are amounts owed to the organization for the services it has provided. These amounts might be owed by individuals, insurance companies, or the government. Careful management is required to ensure that the organization collects all possible receivables in a timely manner. Eventually, some receivables will prove uncollectible. All large organizations have bad debts. Active management, however, can minimize bad debts. Active management can also result in receivables being collected as quickly as possible. The sooner receivables are collected, the sooner the money is in the organization's bank accounts earning interest for it.

When money is collected for patient care services provided, it is either immediately spent or invested. Part of the finance function is to make decisions regarding appropriate *investments.* It requires care to determine how to invest the money to earn a high return for the organization while safeguarding the money so that the risk from any investment is minimal. HCOs do not want to miss the chance to earn high returns on available cash, nor can they afford to lose their investment by taking excessive risks.

Finance officers also manage cash indirectly by managing the payment of the organization's *obligations.* In some cases, to keep cash invested (earning a return for the organization), the finance managers will defer payment of obligations for a period of time. A choice may be made to pay the telephone bill a month late. This choice must be balanced against the possible negative consequences of the action. The phone bill must not be paid so late that telephone service is discontinued; supply bills must not be paid so late that suppliers stop providing needed clinical supplies to the organization.

If it becomes apparent that there will be insufficient cash to meet obligations—even with borrowing, fund raising, and management of receivables and payables—finance officers will raise the possibility of cost-cutting throughout the organization. Such cost-cutting cannot be authorized without the approval of the CEO. However, because the CFO is not directly above the department managers in the chart of organization, decisions requiring cost-cutting must be made by the CEO and COO. Ultimately, the CEO is responsible to the board. If the organization becomes bankrupt because of insufficient cash to pay obligations as due, the CEO is responsible. If quality of patient care declines because of cost-cutting aimed at saving cash, the CEO is responsible. If the organization loses reimbursements because of adverse events, the CEO is responsible. As a result, the CEO will at times approve requests by the CFO to take actions that affect the departments providing care.

More often, the CEO will push to find other financing alternatives that do not affect care. Although most nurse managers and executives become aware of efforts to cut costs to reduce cash expenses, they are not usually aware of other efforts. Negotiations with banks to increase the amount they will lend or with suppliers requesting that they allow deferred payments are often kept within the finance department. In most organizations, a wide variety of approaches will be assessed and attempted before cost cutting that might affect patient care is implemented.

In the final analysis, however, the finance department can ensure the long-run existence of the organization only if total spending is kept to a level that can be met by total receipts. Because even borrowing money requires cash payments (at least interest), the finance department's efforts to control the organization's sources and uses of money will ultimately have an effect on the operations of the clinical and administrative departments.

The Financial Accounting Function

The financial accounting function of the organization's finance department is different from the finance function. Financial accounting has nothing to do with the decisions of whether to borrow money and, if so, how much and from where. Nor does it concern the efficient management of cash resources, accounts receivable, investments, or obligations of the organization. It is concerned with collecting information about the finances of the organization and translating that information into a form that can be reported to interested individuals outside the organization.

Many individuals are interested in the finances of HCOs. They include government regulators and payers; stockholders, in the case of for-profit organizations; and possible donors, suppliers, and lenders. A great deal of effort by the finance department is consumed by the various reporting requirements of different outside users. The reports generated by the financial management function also provide valuable information to managers within the organization.

The Managerial Accounting Function

Of particular interest to nurse managers and executives is the managerial accounting function of the financial managers of the organization. This function relates to providing financial information that can be specifically used to better manage the organization. Financial managers often request financial information from nurse managers and executives. However, managerial accounting should be a two-way street and should be a give-and-take process. Nurse managers and executives need to learn how to get useful managerial accounting information from financial managers. Understanding the role of managerial accounting should help in that regard.

The first key objective of managerial accounting is to aid in the general management role of planning. Planning is an essential role of management. The organization carries out much of its planning via the budgeting process. The financial managers are responsible for putting together an overall financial plan for the organization that achieves certain goals. Those goals may include growth, expansion of services, or just financial stability. From the perspective of the financial manager, the plans of all the departments must be aggregated to generate a plan for the organization that is workable.

Managerial accounting is also concerned with the role of management in the area of control. To implement a plan, there must be a variety of control reports that managers use. These reports can ensure that suppliers get paid only for items actually delivered and that employees get paid only for an appropriate number of hours or days. The reports may focus on the spending of each department and each area of each department. From the perspective of the finance department, enough information is generated for control to allow the top management team to have the information it desires.

Other managers in the organization, however, have the right to request information in a form that is useful for their control needs. Nurse managers and executives should place demands on accounting to provide information that is both timely and useful. Information does not make decisions; managers do. But managers cannot take actions to control spending if they do not have information about what spending is occurring. Therefore, there should be a demand for all of the information that is needed and for that information to be in a usable format.

Note that there is emphasis on the usability of data. It is not simply an issue of there being too little information. Certainly, receiving too little information leaves managers without the ability to make informed decisions; however, too much information may obscure the relevant data needed to make an appropriate decision. Requiring collection of too much information also interferes with or impedes other responsibilities of line managers and their staff. Line managers must work with the finance department to specify what information is needed and what presentation would be most useful.

One of the most critical problems of management in HCOs is that too often finance tells line managers what information the line managers need and the format in which it will be provided. There is a terrible lack of communication in most organizations. Line managers do not get the information they need, and finance staff members feel abused because the information they provide is not used. For example, there may be times when nurse managers need specific patient care–related information such as patient flow, nurse assignment, and staffing by day of the week, week of the month, or quarter to address specific budget variances. At other times, they may need vacancy, turnover, and cost data to build a case for developing a unit-focused retention plan or to support the provision of a particular type of patient-centered services, such as interpreter services.[12] Thus, there should be ongoing meetings between finance staff and line managers to discuss whether the information generated by staff meets the needs of the line managers and, if not, how the information can be made more useful.

Internal Control Function

Internal control refers to the processes and systems that ensure that the decisions made in the organization are appropriate and receive appropriate authorization. This requires a system of accounting and administrative controls. According to noted accounting authorities,

> *Accounting control comprises the methods and procedures that are mainly concerned with the authorization of transactions, the safeguarding of assets, and the accuracy of accounting records. Good accounting controls help increase efficiency; they help decrease waste, unintentional errors, and fraud.*
>
> *Administrative control comprises the plan of organization (for example, the formal organization chart concerning who reports to whom) and all methods and procedures that help management planning and control of operations. Examples are departmental budgeting procedures and performance reports.[13]*

It is extremely important that HCOs not waste any of their resources. Accounting controls must be in place to minimize the chances of theft or of errors that will detract from the organization's resources. Fraud and embezzlement must be prevented to the greatest extent possible. Therefore, there must be a system of checks and balances that prevents the possibility of one person's withdrawing significant sums of money and misappropriating them. Generally, two signatures are needed for the disbursement of cash so that there is less chance of theft.

Organizations can help minimize risks by following a few general rules:

- Hire qualified, reliable people. As Collins[14] says, get the right people on the bus.
- Create a separation of functions that prevents the disbursement of cash based on authorization by one individual. For example, the same manager should not authorize purchases and verify receipt or pay the supplier.

[12]Esposito-Herr MB, Persinger KD, Reiger MS, Hunt S. 2009. Partnering for better performance: The nursing-finance alliance. *Am Nurse Today* 4(4). Retrieved at http://www.americannursetoday.com/article.aspx?id=2546&fid=2446.

[13]Horngren C, Foster G. 1987. *Cost Accounting—A Managerial Emphasis*, 6th edition. Englewood Cliffs, NJ: Prentice-Hall, p. 910.

[14]Collins J. 2001. *Good to Great: Why Some Companies Make the Leap . . . and Others Don't*. New York: Harper Business.

- Require authorization before disbursement of resources.
- Require documentation of all financial transactions.
- Establish formal procedures.
- Create physical protection, such as safes and locks.
- Enforce vacation and rotation-of-duties policies that ensure that more than one person carries out each task related to money each year.
- Bond employees (i.e., purchase insurance policies to protect the organization against theft by employees).
- Provide for an independent check of financial transactions.

No organization can ever guarantee that it will not lose financial resources. However, it is the role of the financial managers of the organization to establish controls that minimize the possibility of such losses.

✳ THE ROLE OF THE CHIEF NURSE EXECUTIVE IN FINANCIAL MANAGEMENT

In identifying the knowledge and skills required for nurse managers and executives, Mark et al.[15] differentiate two levels. They describe the nurse *executive* as the senior nurse responsible for managing nursing in the entire organization and the nurse *manager* as responsible for an area or program within the organization. The American Nurses Association (ANA) "Scope and Standards for Nurse Administrators"[16] and the American Organization of Nurse Executives (AONE)[17] also define two levels of nurse administrator, consistent with those proposed by Mark et al.

This section discusses the role of the CNE in the financial management of the organization and of the nursing division. Financial management includes management of the financial resources of the organization. This includes not only cash and obligations but ultimately the expenses incurred by the organization and the revenue it generates. In almost all HCOs, the CNE has the authority and responsibility for the expenses incurred by the nursing department. In some HCOs, the CNE also has responsibility for generation of revenues.

Responsibility for expenses means that the CNE is the person who is ultimately answerable for all expenses incurred by the department. The CNE is directly involved in the negotiation process that establishes the level of resources that will be available for the department, and he or she is accountable for any spending above or below the planned level.

Responsibility is starting to extend to revenues as well. Few hospitals hold the CNE accountable for revenues. However, many other types of organizations, such as home health agencies, assign the CNE the authority and responsibility for both expenses incurred and revenues generated.

For example, home health agencies are reimbursed on a per-visit basis. The manager sets appropriate standards for visits per nurse and charges per visit and authorizes other expenses.

In addition to their responsibility for nursing, many hospital CNEs, often those with the title "vice president" or "senior vice president for patient services," are responsible for non-nursing departments. These often include the emergency department and the operating room and sometimes departments such as social work or other professional services. The CNE is frequently responsible for both expense and revenue in those departments. In many home health agencies, the CNE is responsible for all services provided by the agency. In many organizations, the CNE is responsible for new product development, such as an outreach program to elderly adults or development of ambulatory surgery.

As a member of the senior management team, the CNE must have the financial skills of equivalent senior managers. The CNE should have a thorough grounding in applied economics, be familiar with basic accounting principles, and have the skills to analyze financial statements. In addition to these basic skills, the CNE must be highly competent in cost management. To do this, the CNE must understand how to determine the cost of nursing services. To effectively manage costs, it is necessary for the CNE to be effective at strategic planning and controlling operating results.

As a member of the senior management team, the CNE must understand the management of the financial resources of the organization. This includes working-capital management and sources of financial resources. All but the smallest HCOs have financial officers. CNEs need not be financial officers; however, they must understand financial management enough to ask the right questions, comprehend the answers, and participate in senior management decisions about financial management.

✳ THE ROLE OF MIDLEVEL AND FIRST-LINE NURSE MANAGERS IN FINANCIAL MANAGEMENT

The authority and responsibility of midlevel nurse managers (e.g., clinical director of nursing, patient care manager) vary widely from one HCO to another. In small nursing agencies, the midlevel nurse manager is responsible for costs and revenue. The manager of eight nurses in a home health agency may be responsible not only for personnel and related expenses but also for the amount of revenue generated by the staff. In most hospitals, however, midlevel nurse managers are responsible only for direct expenses in their area.

The level of decentralization will determine the knowledge and skills needed by midlevel and first-line nurse managers. It is clear that midlevel and first-line nurse managers require budgeting skills. Although these managers do not require all the knowledge and skills of the CNE, they should be familiar with most of the concepts that are discussed in this book.

In preparation for writing this book, we interviewed a number of CNEs and midlevel and first-line managers. Those we spoke with differentiated the depth of knowledge required

---

[15]Mark B, Turner J, Englebardt S. 1990. Knowledge and skills for nurse administrators. *Nurs Health Care* 11(1):185-189.

[16]American Nurses Association. 2009. *Scope and Standards for Nurse Administrators,* 3rd edition. Washington, DC. Retrieved at http://www.nursebooks.org.

[17]American Organization of Nurse Executives. Competencies for AONE's Certification as Nurse Manager and Leader (CNML) and Certification in Nurse Executive Practice (CENP) are available at http://www.aone.org/aone/certification/about.html.

among levels of nurse managers more than they differentiated among content areas. Most of those we spoke with agreed that in addition to budgeting, midlevel managers must have basic knowledge about applied economics and the financing of health care. In addition, they should understand cost management, including the basic principles of determining the cost of nursing care. Midlevel managers should also have skills in both strategic planning and forecasting. Most of those we interviewed believed that midlevel and first-line managers needed skills in inventory control at the level for which they were responsible, and they may need skills in managing other short- or long-term financial resources and reading financial statements. All agreed that the level of skills required depends on the type of organization and level of decentralization of the organization. For example, whereas many midlevel managers should have skills in securing grants for demonstration projects, research, or ongoing financial needs, most midlevel managers would not need to understand corporate stock issuance or bond ratings.

To competently manage the unit or program, nurse managers need financial skills for planning, control, and decision making. Using forecasting skills, they can estimate services to be delivered in the future and likely labor and supplies needed to provide the services (or evaluate the forecasts provided by other parts of the organization). With this information and solid budgeting skills, they can prepare a budget and, more important, interpret the variance reports either created by themselves or supplied centrally.

Transition from Staff Nurse to Nurse Manager

At some point in their careers, experienced staff nurses find themselves making a decision about whether to advance to a clinical or administrative role. Those who advance in a clinical role, such as moving to a higher level on a clinical ladder or into a patient educator role, may have some need for financial knowledge, but the management of financial resources is not likely a primary aspect of their role. Nurses who move into an administrative role may go straight from the staff nurse to nurse manager role or from an assistant manager to manager role with little or no financial experience or training. Nurses at higher levels on an organization's career ladder may also take on some unit-level financial responsibilities. In fact, it is common for expert clinicians to be recruited into nurse manager roles. The idea is that good clinicians are likely to make good managers.

The reality is that this line of thinking does not always translate to the real world. Without formal or informal training in financial management (and other aspects of management), the clinician turned nurse manager may find her- or himself in a precarious position and actually at a disadvantage in managing the unit. That is not to say that there are no successful nurse managers who have become so without formal financial management training. Rather, the nurse manager who comes into the role without training has to invest a great deal to learn the role and understand financial processes to succeed.

The requirements for certification set forth by the American Nurses Credentialing Center (ANCC), which are based on ANA

standards,[18] recognize that educational qualifications vary by type of nurse administrator certification. The Nurse Executive-Board Certified (NE-BC) targets midlevel managers and includes nurse managers. This level of certification requires a bachelor's or higher degree in nursing and certain levels of experience in the position. The Nurse Executive-Advanced Board Certified (NEA-BC) targets nurses in executive roles and requires a master's or higher degree in nursing or a bachelor's degree in nursing and a master's in another field plus a certain level of experience in an executive-level position. The AONE's educational requirements for certification also vary by level of administrator: Certification as Nurse Manager and Leader (CNML) requires a bachelor's degree in nursing, a bachelor's degree in another field, or a diploma or associate degree in nursing plus certain levels of experience. Certification in Executive Nursing Practice (CENP) requires a master's degree (in nursing or outside of nursing with one degree in nursing) or a bachelor's degree in nursing plus certain levels of experience.[19] Both ANCC and AONE certification require differing levels of financial management.

The roles of today's nurse managers and executives have become increasingly demanding and have greatly expanded as the health care environment has evolved in complexity.[20] Nurse administrators at all levels have taken on greater responsibilities in HCOs, all at a time when there have been declining numbers of nurses who possess the qualifications to fit the responsibilities of their role.[21] Recommendations in the professional literature have called for nurse managers and executives to possess financial, operational, and data utilization skills to develop and defend complex budgets, monitor performance outcomes, gather and use data and facts to develop positions, understand financial statements, advocate for staff, and engage in strategic planning.[22]

In reality, most nurse managers and executives have had a modest amount of formal education in these areas, yet knowledge of financial and operational management is critical if nurse managers and executives are to formulate appropriate solutions to unit and organizational problems and make a positive contribution to the outcomes for the organization as a whole.[23] In fact, a survey of nurse leaders reported that 95% cited graduate education as the ideal preparation for nurse leaders—with the administrative or management specialization in a master's degree in nursing being the top choice, followed by the PhD, dual MSN and MBA, and either MSN or MBA.[24,25]

---

[18]American Nurses Association, *Op. cit.*

[19]American Organization of Nurse Executives, *Op. cit.*

[20]Kleinman C. 2003. Leadership roles, competencies, and education: How prepared are our nurse managers? *J Nurs Admin* 33(9):451-455.

[21]Parsons M, Stonestreet J. 2003. Factors that contribute to NM retention. *Nurs Econ* 21(3):120-126.

[22]See, for example, Oroviogoicoechea C. 1996. The clinical NM: A literature review. *J Adv Nurs* 24:1273-1280; Sovie M. 1994. A key role in clinical outcomes. *Nurs Manage* 25(3):30-34; and Urden L, Rogers S. 2000. Out in front: A new title reflects NMs' changing scope of accountability. *Nurs Manage* 31(7):27-30.

[23]Schmidt D. 1999. Financial and operational skills for NMs. *Nurs Admin Q* 23(4):16-28.

[24]Scoble K, Russell G. 2003. Vision 2020, part I: Profile of the future nurse leader. *J Nurs Admin* 33(6):324-330.

[25]Russell G, Scoble K. 2003. Vision 2020, part 2: Educational preparation for the future nurse manager. *J Nurs Admin* 33(7/8):404-409.

The bottom line is that nurse managers and executives need formal and informal training to be effective in their role. Formal training can take the form of in-house financial management classes offered through the hospital's finance department or a course taken through continuing education. Formal training also can be enrollment in an academic course for credit or enrollment in a degree-granting program in nursing administration, business administration, or health care administration—as is the case with many of you who are reading this book! Courses and degrees can also be obtained through distance education or through online coursework.

Informal training is also critical. This kind of training generally takes the form of mentoring by other nurse managers and executives, and hopefully mentoring by a financial manager or financial staff member. Through formal and informal on-the-job training, new nurse managers can gain a better understanding of how to read a balance sheet and how unit decisions impact organizational performance and vice versa. Over time and through experience, nurse managers are able to apply the skills they learn and gain a better understanding of why certain decisions and actions may or may not be successful. Although training is essential, there is nothing like the actual application of financial principles and "real life" experiences to make it stick.

✳ THE ROLE OF STAFF NURSES IN FINANCIAL MANAGEMENT

Although staff nurses focus primarily on patient care, their knowledge of finances is no less important. In fact, the idea that staff nurses do not need an understanding of finances is absurd in today's complex health care environment. Some schools of nursing may teach some level of financial content to undergraduate nursing students, but the truth of the matter is that those of us who teach nurses have not done a very good job socializing nursing students to the importance of financial knowledge. In turn, nursing students do not come to value the importance of that knowledge.

When nursing students graduate and enter HCOs, they are gradually (if not immediately) faced with clinical care issues that relate to financing, such as getting the necessary patient care supplies and equipment, calling in back-up help, and deciding how much time to spend with their patients to educate them about their diseases. These things may not happen on their first day on the job, but they will happen eventually. At that point, nurses may seek financial information from others, seek out formal or informal training to better understand the operational challenges of patient care delivery in today's financially conscious HCOs, or become so frustrated that they leave the organization or nursing altogether.

Staff nurses have an incredible potential to influence organizational financing, given that they are the most constant presence at the point of care.[26] However, they may be so focused on the day-to-day aspects of delivering care that they do not see how their daily actions in providing patient care influence costs. It is therefore the nurse manager's role to introduce the idea in staff meetings and other forums, brainstorm how staff nurses contribute to the financial aspects of the organization, and make them aware of their role in the financial health of the organization (after all, the organization's financial health is important to their employment!).[27] This has never been more important than now, when the role of nursing in the prevention of adverse events and HACs and their impact on the financial well-being of HCOs is being recognized both in and outside of nursing. As Caroselli[28] acknowledged, "Staff who are aware of and use information about the relationship between their clinical behavior and cost savings could make a major impact on the financial health of their units." Their involvement at unit, departmental, and organizational levels can help nurse managers identify new ways of delivering care and creative strategies for addressing costly processes that bring about efficiencies and more effective delivery of care.

✳ INTERACTIONS BETWEEN FISCAL AND NURSE MANAGERS

Nurse managers have lateral relationships with fiscal managers. As the CNEs in many organizations become part of the top management team, nurse managers become peers of the fiscal officers. At all levels of the organization, however, nurse managers generally have no formal authority to require information or services. Although the CEO may require that fiscal managers provide information to nurse managers, the format may not be presented in a way that is useful to nurse managers. However, to acquire needed and useful information, a collegial relationship between nursing and finance is essential.

Relationships between fiscal departments and nursing are strained in some organizations. Many fiscal officers continue to believe that nurse managers do not need a substantial amount of financial management information. People in the fiscal department may feel threatened when nurse managers ask questions. One CNE told us that when she pointed out systematic inaccuracies in the data she was receiving from the fiscal department, the CFO became hostile. The CNE eventually was fired, in part because she was raising questions that were discomforting. Nurses, on the other hand, believe that financial managers cannot possibly understand aspects of patient care and that they certainly do not share concerns about providing the highest quality of care possible.

These views are changing in many HCOs. Today's health care environment requires that this kind of bickering be deemed unacceptable by leaders at the highest organizational levels. It is certainly not productive, but more importantly, it may contribute to a negative organizational culture. In fact, it is absolutely essential that the interests of nursing and fiscal managers become aligned. Clarke[29] emphasizes that the relationship between

---

[26]Caroselli C. 1996. Economic awareness of nurses: Relationship to budgetary control. *Nurs Econ* 14(5):292-298.

[27]Bradley D, Cornett E, DeLetter M. 1998. Cost reduction: What a staff nurse can do. *Nurs Econ* 16(5):273-276.

[28]Caroselli, *Op. cit.*, p. 292.

[29]Clarke R. 2006. Finance and nursing: The business of caring. *Health Financ Manage* 60(1):50-56.

nurse managers and financial managers must improve because the alignment of quality and costs necessitates a closer relationship between nurse and financial managers. For example, to comply with patient safety standards, the nurse manager needs to communicate to the financial manager why perhaps more time-consuming (and expensive) procedures must be undertaken or why certain patient safety equipment must be included in the budget. Also, the emergence of pay for performance and transparency in public reporting means that hospitals and financial units must be concerned about how care is delivered and communicated to the public.

Building these relationships requires reaching out and breaking down communication barriers between nursing and finance to understand each other's perspective. Nurses need to provide financial managers with clear explanations about clinical processes and language. Financial managers need to help nurse managers learn how to conduct a business analysis for investing in new equipment, staff, programs and services as well as for analyzing the pros and cons of making these investments. This kind of exchange should be apparent at all levels of nursing and finance, and it is important for the CNE and CFO to model these behaviors.[30]

A substantial amount of team building, informal communication, and networking is necessary for nurse managers and fiscal departments to generate and use financial information that is useful for the organization. It is up to both nursing and finance to work cooperatively. Nursing has to take responsibility for investing in and building the nursing–finance relationship even if it takes a while before dividends are received. One example is to invite finance staff to attend nursing council and other committee meetings, as well as to attend staff meetings to explain financial issues or to help address patient care delivery issues that impact or are related to the budget. Another example is for the nurse manager or executive to invite finance personnel to collaborate on projects that may involve the use of financial resources. Establishing a good working relationship with the people who work in finance is well worth the investment.

❋ RESPONSIBILITY ACCOUNTING

The previous sections have focused on the role of financial managers, the role of nurse managers, and their interactions. There has been a presumption that all managers attempt to carry out their activities to the best of their abilities and in the best interests of the organization. The organization, however, needs a way to assess the performance of its managers. That is the role of responsibility accounting. *Responsibility accounting* is an attempt to measure financial outcomes and to assign those outcomes to the individual or department responsible for them so that performance can be assessed.

It is important to note that the performance of a manager is not necessarily the same as the performance of a unit or department. The distinction is primarily concerned with the issue of ability to control outcomes. The philosophy of responsibility

accounting is that managers should be held accountable for things that they can control and should not be held accountable for things that are beyond their control. Therefore, there should always be an attempt to evaluate a unit's or department's performance separately from its manager.

For instance, top management may be concerned that the cost of providing care exceeded expectations because an unexpected shortage of nurses resulted in the use of additional overtime and high-cost agency nurses. In that case, the performance of the nursing units will likely be below expectations. On the other hand, the unit managers should be evaluated on how well they managed the situation. In light of the shortage of nurses, did they make economical choices about when to use overtime, when to hire agency nurses, when to leave a position unfilled for a shift, and when to close beds?

Nurses should always bear this principle in mind, in their interactions both within the nursing department and between the nursing department and the remainder of the organization. Managers and executives should be held accountable only for the things they can control. Without implementation of such a philosophy, managers and executives develop a pervasive negative attitude. When they are considered to have failed because of causes beyond their control, they lose all incentive to attempt to be efficient in the use of resources that are within their control. Why work hard when you will fail no matter what you do? The nurse manager or executive should always evaluate whether the individual or the position held has control over the duties for which he or she is being held accountable.

Managers and executives must also believe that they will be evaluated in a fair manner. In essence, they must trust that the system will generate a fair evaluation of their performance. The performance evaluation of managers and executives in most HCOs focuses on the use of responsibility centers.

Responsibility Centers

A *responsibility center* is a part of the organization, such as a department or a unit, for which a manager is assigned responsibility. There are three general categories of responsibility centers: cost, revenue, and profit.

A *cost center* has responsibility only for the control of expenses. Most nursing units in hospitals are cost centers. This makes sense given the basic concept of responsibility equal to control. The typical first-line nurse manager cannot exercise any control over revenues. This manager does not generate patients, nor is that position responsible for the prices charged to patients. Therefore, it is logical to hold that individual accountable only for expenses.

Units that are solely revenue centers are rare. That would imply that they can control revenues but have no control over expenses. Usually marketing departments are considered *revenue centers* because the organization wants to see specifically how much revenue the marketing effort is generating.

The most common alternative to a unit that is a cost center is a *profit center*. A profit center is responsible for both revenues and costs. Therefore, it is both a cost center and a revenue center. It is responsible for the expenses it incurs as well as the revenues it generates. Most hospital operating rooms are profit

―――――――――

[30]*Ibid.*

centers. In some hospitals, patient care units are now considered profit centers. Many nurses working in ambulatory settings are responsible for managing profit centers. However, health care terminology differs from that used in most industries. The health care industry, traditionally not for profit, prefers to avoid use of the term *profit* and therefore to avoid use of the term *profit center*. It has become the practice in HCOs to use the term *revenue center* to refer to all responsibility units that are both revenue centers and cost centers.

One weakness of hospital management has been its perception of the results of cost centers and revenue centers. Resources have often been more tightly constrained for cost centers than for revenue centers because at the end of a year cost centers show a large balance of expense without any counterbalancing revenue. Revenue centers, on the other hand, show revenue and expense. Many revenue centers show profits. Those profits have been used as a justification for more liberal allocation of resources to those departments. Similarly, managers of revenue centers have been perceived at times as being better managers. This has worked unfairly against nursing departments, which have been considered cost centers.

That approach tends to be somewhat irrational. Expenses are not inherently bad and do not indicate poor management. Patient care cannot be provided without incurring expenses, and there would be no revenue at all without incurring the expenses of departments such as nursing. On the other hand, the existence of profits does not necessarily indicate good management. Evaluations of managers should be based on a standard of comparison. That standard is generally the budget. Both cost and revenue centers should be evaluated against the budgeted amount to assess the performance of the manager.

Even this approach is somewhat simplistic. The budget is based on an expectation of what will happen. If patient volume increases, expectations need to be adjusted. More patients result in more revenues but more expenses as well. Managers must be evaluated in comparison with the budget after it has been adjusted for patient volume and, if possible, patient acuity. The ultimate goal is to evaluate the contribution of the manager apart from factors that are outside the manager's control. That is the only way that managers will perceive that the organizational structure is fair. Fairness is a necessary perception to get the maximum effort from managers.

Today, it is critically important for nurse managers and staff to recognize that adverse events and HACs attributed to patient care units may impact their performance evaluations in the future. The possible link between adverse events and performance requires a frank and open discussion regarding how this sensitive information is tracked and disclosed. It is important for both managers and staff to see and understand the consequences of the care they deliver.

❋ INCENTIVES AND MOTIVATION

The issue of fairness in the evaluation of managers raises the question of goals and attitudes. Organizations are made up of people as much as they are made up of buildings and equipment, if not more so. Individuals, however, have their own

interests as persons as well as employees. It is possible that their own interests will conflict with those of the organization that employs them. In that case, it is vital to attempt to achieve goal congruence. *Goal congruence* simply means that the wants and desires of the organization and of its employees are consistent. Organizations develop a set of incentives for their employees. The goal of those incentives is to encourage employees to work toward achieving the organization's goals.

Large organizations tend to have many layers of management. Each manager in each layer must work constantly to achieve the goals of the organization to have the most effective results. However, there is reason to believe that in many organizations, managers may have reason not to work in the best interests of the organization; what is in the best interests of the organization may not be in the best interests of the individual manager.

Most nurses entered the profession because of a desire to help and to serve people. They did not expect to get rich. Nevertheless, an individual manager may want a big salary, a large office with fancy furniture, and a large staff. The organization would prefer that the manager work for a low salary in a small office with old furniture and minimal staff. Individuals are not bad because they prefer more money and more perquisites. The organization is not bad because it wants to conserve its resources. Yet there must be some meeting of the minds or there will be a constant tension between the wishes of the individuals and the wishes of the organization.

Goal congruence is the meeting of the minds. It is achieved in most cases through a system of incentives. The organization must put forth a system of incentives that makes it worthwhile for the individual to do what is in the best interests of the organization. First-line nurse managers must find a way to provide incentives to the nursing staff. Midlevel nurse managers must find incentives for first-line nurse managers. Associate directors of nursing must find incentives for midlevel managers. CNEs must find incentives for the associate executives and directors of nursing.

Incentives can be provided in a variety of ways. Some organizations use bonuses; others use merit pay increases. Another approach is to provide managers with a letter from their supervisor discussing budget performance. Often simple, explicit recognition of a manager's hard work to achieve the organization's goals is a sufficient motivating tool to gain the benefits of goal congruence. The question of incentives and motivation is discussed further in Chapter 16.

❋ POWER AND POLITICS

Power, authority, and influence have no standard definitions. Hampton et al.[31] have noted that "influence is the process by which one person follows another's advice, suggestion, or order; power is a personal or positional attribute that enables one to influence; and authority is only one of several bases of power—one granted to an influencer-manager by higher

---

[31]Hampton D, Summer C, Webber R. 1987. *Organizational Behavior and the Practice of Management.* Glenview, IL: Scott, Foresman & Company, p. 150.

organizational officials.[22] These authors suggest that power can take many forms:

- Coercive power is based on fear of punishment.
- Reward power is based on hope for reward.
- Legitimate power is based on the belief that the influence has formal authority.
- Referent power is based on charismatic leader traits.
- Expert power is based on the leader's special expertise.
- Representative power is based on the democratic delegation of power to a leader.
- Information power is based on the leader's access to information, both within and outside of the organization.

It is postulated that referent, expert, and informational forms of power are most important for managers of professionals. That is, the managers of professionals will be most effective in influencing others if they are charismatic leaders and are seen as experts by others.[32] In today's HCOs, where information and the ability to link information are at the forefront of transforming care delivery, access to information, knowledge of where it resides, and an understanding of how to acquire and manage it are essential to individual and organizational success.[33]

Access to information and resources in HCOs can serve as a base for power development. Because HCOs are often large and complex, it is difficult to have all the information required to make many decisions. Thus, those who control the information are in a position to be powerful and to influence decision making.

Control of financial information by "administration" and the power associated with it has been seen by many as a reason for the low level of nurses' influence in the organization. Although cynics might argue that this control has been intentional, others argue that many nurses have not sought this information. As nurses understand financial management and gain access to and develop financial information, their ability to influence decision making may improve.

✳ NETWORKING

Because managers and executives are often dependent on others over whom they have no authority, the use of power is critical to the effective manager. Effective managers develop relationships with people in the organization on whom they depend for information and with whom they build coalitions to influence the goals and resource allocation of the organization.

Networking was the buzz word of the 1990s. "I'm going to a networking event" and "I'm networking at lunch today" were heard in HCOs. Today, networks have become so important that social networks in and outside of organizations are studied and recognized as critically important in organizational performance. Networks have been described as horizontal as well as vertical. For most managers, lateral relationships are often more important than vertical relationships in achieving goals.

For example, for the unit manager in a hospital, resources required from dietary and housekeeping are critical to running the unit. Typically, the nurse manager has no direct authority over the housekeepers and dietary aides who perform activities on the unit. Nurse managers must therefore rely on their lateral supervisors, peers, and subordinates to effectively achieve the unit's goals.

Numerous articles have appeared in the nursing literature about networking—what it is, how to do it—and blessing it as a strategy. It is also argued that trade is the basis of networking. Managers trade information and services. They trade the ability to get things done. Effective managers work on building relationships with others so that when they need something (e.g., information, services), they can get it. This occurs both within and outside the organization. Social networking with colleagues via professional and social websites puts a tremendous amount of information readily at nurse managers' and executives' fingertips.

✳ IMPLICATIONS FOR NURSE MANAGERS AND EXECUTIVES

Control of information about revenues, expenses, and operations is the key to financial control. In organizations in which this information is not shared, control is not possible. A second factor is responsibility and authority for revenues in addition to the responsibility for expenses. Efforts on the part of both fiscal managers and nurse managers and executives to share information and cooperate are necessary for successfully managing an organization.

Also, nurse managers and executives should be aware of the critical role they play in engaging staff nurses in the financial management of organizational resources. Over time, the daily actions of staff nurses can have a dramatic impact on the organization's financial bottom line. Focusing on solving point-of-care problems will make nurses' work more efficient and productive and will eliminate waste and potentially costly adverse events and HACs.[34] These occurrences have serious implications for organizations because they can result in nonpayment for care. It is the unit-level nurse manager's role to involve staff and seek their input and together develop strategies for addressing issues of financial concern.

Finally, nurse managers and executives at all levels are playing increasingly important roles in the management of financial resources in HCOs. To do so, they need the requisite knowledge and skills that come from both formal and informal training. This is of critical importance when staff nurses make the transition to nurse manager and executive roles. It is therefore incumbent upon organizational leaders to make a variety of opportunities available to nurse managers and executives so that they develop these new skills and become adept in their roles.

---

[32]*Ibid.*
[33]Yukl, GA. 2011. *Leadership in Organizations*, 7th edition. Upper Saddle River, NJ: Prentice Hall.

[34]Tucker AL 2004. The impact of operational failures on hospital nurses and their patients. *J Oper Manage* 22:151-169.

✳ KEY CONCEPTS

Management's role   Most essential elements are planning, control, and decision making.

Board of trustees or board of directors   Governing body that has the ultimate responsibility for the decisions made by the organization. The board sets the overall direction and adopts goals and objectives for the organization. The CEO reports to the board and is responsible for managing the organization.

Managerial hierarchy   Structure that establishes the authority and responsibility of different individuals within the organization. The board is at the top, with the CEO reporting to the board. The COO reports to the CEO. The CFO and the CNE may report to either the CEO or the COO, depending on the specific organization. The COO, CFO, and CNE each have a number of managers who report directly to them.

Line and staff functions   Line function is the element of running an HCO that is related directly to the provision of patient care. Nurse managers are considered line managers. In contrast, the staff function concerns providing auxiliary assistance or service to the line managers and their departments. Finance officers are staff managers.

Lines of authority   Formal lines of authority may be either direct (full authority), such as in the case of the associate director of nursing reporting to the CNE, or indirect (limited authority), such as the director of dietary reporting to the chief of the medical staff. Informal lines of authority carry no official authority but may have a substantial de facto impact.

Chief financial officer (CFO)   Individual in charge of all of the financial functions of the organization. These include those related to the sources and investment of the organization's financial resources, the generation of accounting information for making external reports, and the generation of accounting information for use by line managers. It also includes the function of internal control.

Chief nurse executive (CNE)   Individual in charge of all of the nursing functions in the organization. This primarily includes all nursing care provided to clients. Other responsibilities include managing the human and financial resources of the nursing department to achieve the health care mission of the department.

Midlevel nurse manager   Responsible for nursing functions on more than one nursing unit or area. This includes all nursing care provided to clients. Other responsibilities include managing the human resources for the manager's area of responsibility. Responsibilities usually include financial management.

First-line manager   Responsible for one patient care unit, area, or group of nursing staff. This includes all nursing care provided to clients. Other responsibilities may include some financial management.

Responsibility accounting   An accounting approach that attempts to measure financial outcomes and assign those outcomes to the individual or department responsible for them. The performance of a manager is not necessarily the same as the performance of a unit or department. Managers should be held accountable only for things they can control.

Responsibility center   Part of the organization, such as a department or a unit, for which a manager is assigned responsibility. HCO responsibility centers are generally divided into cost centers and revenue centers.

Networking   Effective managers and executives develop relationships with people in the organization on whom they depend for information and with whom they build coalitions to influence the goals and resource allocation of the organization. The relationships are often made informally through a shared history (e.g., attending school together) or through a shared professional experience (e.g., participation in professional association activities). Trade is often the basis of networking. A person with information or services, such as financial information, may trade that information for something such as a prompt reply when a request is made. Relationships outside of the organization—via professional and social networking opportunities—enable nurse managers and executives to gain a broader understanding of issues that impact their practice.

Nurse councils   Components of a shared governance structure that aim to give staff nurses a voice in decision making. Common councils are nursing practice, quality of care, education (or professional development) and research councils; an executive council provides a central function to coordinate, facilitate, and integrate the activities of all other councils.

✳ SUGGESTED READINGS

Aiken L, Clarke S, Sloane D: Hospital restructuring: does it adversely affect care and outcomes? *J Nurs Admin* 30(10):457–465, 2000.

Aiken L, Clarke S, Sloane D, et al: Nurses' reports on hospital care in five countries, *Health Aff* 20(3):43–53, 2001.

American Nurses Association: *Scope and standards for nurse administrators,* ed 3, Washington, DC, 2009, ANA. Available at www.nursebooks.org.

Arnold L, Drenkard K, Ela S, et al: Strategic positioning for nursing excellence in health systems: insights from chief nursing executives, *Nurs Admin Q* 30(1):11–20, 2006.

Bradley D, Cornett E, DeLetter M: Cost reduction: what a staff nurse can do, *Nurs Econ* 16(5):273–276, 1998.

Caroselli C: Economic awareness of nurses: relationship to budgetary control, *Nurs Econ* 14(5):292–298, 1996.

Clarke R: Finance and nursing: the business of caring, *Healthc Financ Manage* 60(1):50–56, 2006.

Collins J: *Good to great: why some companies make the leap . . . and others don't,* New York, 2001, Harper Business.

Daft RL: *Organization theory and design,* ed 10, Mason, OH, 2010, Thompson South-Western.

Dreisbach A: A structured approach to expert financial management: a financial development plan for nurse managers, *Nurs Econ* 12(3):131–139, 1994.

Enthoven AC: Integrated delivery systems: the cure for fragmentation, *Am J Manage Care* 15(10):S284–S290, 2009. Available at www.ajmc.com/publications/supplement/2009/A264_09dec_HlthPolicyCvrOne/A264_09dec_Enthoven S284to290.

Esposito-Herr MB, Persinger KD, Reiger MS, Hunt S: Partnering for better performance: the nursing-finance alliance, *Am Nurse Today* 4(4), 2009. Available at www.americannursetoday.com/article.aspx?id=2546&fid=2446.

Evan K, Aubry K, Hawkins M, et al: Whole systems shared governance: a model for the integrated health system, *J Nurs Admin* 25(5):18–27, 1995.

Finkler S: Responsibility centers, *Hosp Cost Manage Account* 3(9):1, 1991.

Gelinas L, Manthey M: The impact of organizational redesign on nurse executive leadership, *J Nurs Admin* 27(10):35–42, 1997.

Hampton D, Summer C, Webber R: *Organizational behavior and the practice of management,* Glenview, IL, 1987, Scott, Foresman, & Company.

Horngren C, Foster G: *Cost accounting—a managerial emphasis,* ed 6, Englewood Cliffs, NJ, 1987, Prentice-Hall.

Institute of Medicine: *Envisioning the National Health Care Quality Report,* Washington, DC, 2001, National Academies Press.

Institute of Medicine: *The future of nursing: leading change, advancing health,* Washington, DC, 2011, National Academies Press.

Jones K: The ins and outs of financial management: an introduction, *Semin Nurse Manag* 1(1):4, 1993.

Kleinman C: Leadership roles, competencies, and education: how prepared are our nurse managers? *J Nurs Admin* 33(9):451–455, 2003.

MacDonald G: Shared governance—a unit based concept, *Axone* 17(1):3–5, 1995.

Mark B, Turner J, Englebardt S: Knowledge and skills for nurse administrators, *Nurs Health Care* 11(1):185–189, 1990.

Oroviogoicoechea C: The clinical NM: a literature review, *J Adv Nurs* 24:1273–1280, 1996.

Page A, editor, Institute of Medicine Committee on the Work Environment for Nurses and Patient Safety, Board on Health Care Services: *Keeping patients safe: transforming the work environment of nurses,* Washington, DC, 2004, National Academies Press.

Parsons M, Stonestreet J: Factors that contribute to NM retention, *Nurs Econ* 21(3):120–126, 2003.

Peters T: *Thriving on chaos,* New York, 1987, Alfred A. Knopf, p 359.

Prince S: Shared governance, sharing power and opportunity, *J Nurs Admin* 27(3):28–35, 1997.

Russell G, Scoble K: Vision 2020, part 2: educational preparation for the future nurse manager, *J Nurs Admin* 33(7/8):404–409, 2003.

Schmidt D: Financial and operational skills for NMs, *Nurs Admin Q* 23(4):16–28, 1999.

Scoble K, Russell G: Vision 2020, part 1: profile of the future nurse leader, *J Nurs Admin* 33(6):324–330, 2003.

Sovie M: A key role in clinical outcomes, *Nurs Manage* 25(3):30–34, 1994.

Sovie M, Jawad A: Hospital restructuring and its impact on outcomes, *J Nurs Admin* 31(12):588–600, 2001.

Tucker A, Edmondson A: Managing routine exceptions: a model of nurse problem solving behavior, *Adv Health Care Manag* 3:87–113, 2002.

Tucker AL: The impact of operational failures on hospital nurses and their patients, *J Oper Manage* 22:151–169, 2004.

Tucker AL, Edmondson AC: Why hospitals don't learn from failures: organizational and psychological dynamics that inhibit system change, *Calif Manage Rev* 45(2):55–72, 2003.

Tucker AL, Nembahard IM, Edmondson AC: Implementing new practices: an empirical study of organizational learning in hospital intensive care units, *Manage Sci* 53(6):894–907, 2007.

Tucker AL, Singer SJ, Hayes JE, Falwell A: Front-line staff perspectives on opportunities for improving the safety and efficiency of hospital work systems, *Health Serv Res* 43(5):1807–1829, 2008.

Urden L, Rogers S: Out in front: a new title reflects NMs' changing scope of accountability, *Nurs Manage* 31(7):27-30, 2000.

Yukl, GA: *Leadership in organizations,* ed 7, Upper Saddle River, NJ, 2011, Prentice Hall.

Zachry B, Gilbert R, Gragg M: Director of nursing finance: controlling health care costs, *Nurse Manag* 26(11):49–53, 1995.

4

Key Issues in Applied Economics

CHAPTER GOALS

The goals of this chapter are to:

- Introduce applied economics and discuss the notion of scarce resources
- Define economic goods and services and the role of utility in determining the demand for goods and services
- Explain the law of supply and demand and the functioning of free markets
- Define the concept of elasticity of demand
- Define and explain economies of scale

- Consider the role of incentives in economic behavior
- Discuss market efficiency and market failure
- Distinguish between redistribution of resources to improve economic efficiency and redistribution for improved equity
- Explain the economic view of the market for nurses and periodic nursing shortages
- Discuss the implications of economics for nurse managers and executives

❋ INTRODUCTION

Economics is the study of how scarce resources are allocated among their possible uses. In the case of health care, economic principles are demonstrated on a daily basis, both to society as a whole and to health care organizations (HCOs). Costly new drugs, treatments, and technologies strain the capacity of individuals, employers, insurers, and society to pay the costs of health care.

Recently, we have observed a number of important changes that impact health care. For example, many employers have eliminated or restricted employee health coverage or benefits. Insurance companies have raised premiums, deductibles, and co-pays. Both of these changes have placed a greater burden of health care costs on individuals. In turn, many people have dropped health insurance coverage because of its cost. Malpractice insurance for health providers has become more costly, forcing some providers to modify their practice, raise prices, or become employees themselves. HCOs have experienced an increase in the number of uninsured patients and reduced reimbursements from insurers. As a result, they have looked for ways to find efficiencies in care delivery, one of which is changing the workload of nurses or the mix of employees deployed to provide care. The passage of the Affordable Care Act (ACA) (discussed in Chapter 2) also represents an attempt to address some of the existing "failures" in our insurance system and in the market for health care. All of these changes relate in some way to the economic principles discussed in this chapter.

Economics also tells us that maintaining and improving the quality of health services costs an ever-increasing amount, even if the care is provided in a totally efficient manner. Cost concerns and resistance by payers to increasing health care costs have reduced payments to health care providers and forced health care managers to make difficult choices in the spending of limited resources.

The bottom line is that Americans have been consuming both more care and more expensive care. The increased cost of providing that care affects us all, whether we are health care consumers, HCO executives or health care professionals. How are the pressures to increase spending reconciled with the constraints imposed by government and payers to control spending? Fundamentally, that is a question of applied economics, the topic of this chapter. As a management or policy tool, economics helps individuals, organizations, and society make optimal use of their limited resources.

The tools of economics are developed from a structure built upon analysis of the behavior of individuals and organizations. This chapter discusses how the law of supply and demand governs a free market. The specific prices charged for products are based on the cost of producing the product. Another important pricing factor is how strongly consumers react to changes in prices. These concepts are discussed in this chapter. Next, the chapter focuses on the role of incentives. Individual (and at times organizational) behavior is often reactive. Therefore, it is possible for an organization, the government, or other payers to generate desired behaviors by creating appropriate incentives.

After the discussion of incentives, the chapter concentrates on issues of market efficiency in the provision of health care services. The basic notions of market efficiency and of redistribution of society's scarce resources are discussed, and a variety of issues related to the failure of the free market are explored. The chapter concludes with a discussion of how economists might view the reasons for periodic nursing shortages and the implications of applied economics for nurse managers and executives.

✳ FUNDAMENTAL CONCEPTS OF ECONOMICS

Economics is the study of the allocation of scarce resources among alternative possible uses. Included in such study are the actions and behaviors of patients, health insurance companies, providers of health care services, and the government. Given the limited nature of resources, efficient use of resources is desired. By studying behavior, economists are able to attempt to ensure that resources are used in an optimal manner.

Economic Goods

Consumers purchase *goods* or *services* provided by suppliers. These goods or services are referred to as *economic goods.* Goods and services are any items that consumers wish to acquire or use. Such goods and services provide a benefit to consumers. Consumers generally acquire goods and services through exchange. Although it is possible to *barter* or exchange some goods or services for other goods or services, most exchanges are facilitated by the use of money. Each good or service has a monetary price.

Consumers have a combination of wealth and income available to make purchases. *Wealth* is the value of all of the resources the consumer currently owns. *Income* is the increase in wealth, or the amount of additional resources the consumer gains over a period of time. Additional dollars of income may come either from working or from profits on investments. The wealth and income of all consumers are limited. No one can afford to buy everything. Therefore, consumers make choices about the things they purchase.

Utility

When consumers purchase goods and services, they gain a benefit from them. The benefit may be physical. For example, without food and water, the individual would die. There is a clear physical benefit from acquiring enough food and water to survive. Other benefits are psychological. Chocolate may be perceived by some to be a pleasurable food. It is not required for subsistence, but it may well be desired. Economists refer to the physical and psychological benefit one receives from goods or services as the *utility* of those items. The more benefit received, the greater the utility.

Utility helps determine how much an individual would be willing to pay to acquire a good or service. Suppose that the price of water is 10 cents a glass. Water is needed for survival, so its utility to the consumer may well exceed 10 cents by a substantial amount. If the utility exceeds the price, the consumer will buy the water at the 10-cent price.

Suppose that the price of chocolate is $5 per bar. One person may not be wild about chocolate. Given the limitation of that person's total wealth and income, a chocolate bar may have utility that makes the chocolate's value only 50 cents. That person would not buy the bar for $5. Other people may get such a large psychological benefit from chocolate that they would be willing to pay up to $10 (or more!) a bar. Some people would buy chocolate for $5. Not everyone receives the same utility from a specific good or service. In other words, the value of different goods and services is different to different people.

The more income an individual has, the more he or she can buy. However, income can also take a non-dollar form. Each year individuals receive a dollar salary from their job, and they also gain some leisure time. That leisure time is itself a form of income. Leisure represents an economic good; it can be consumed. Or, similar to other economic goods, leisure time can be exchanged. A nurse may choose (in some cases) to work more overtime to make more money. In that case, the nurse has decided that there is something that can be purchased with the extra money earned that is worth more than the extra hours are worth as leisure time. The additional utility of the extra dollars exceeds the utility of the leisure time.

It is assumed that rational individuals will act in order to maximize their total utility. To maximize total utility, a mix of goods must be consumed so that the last unit of each type of item consumed yields the same marginal utility per dollar spent. This accomplishes the purchase of a set of goods and services that, in aggregate, provides the most benefit.

Marginal Utility

As an individual makes purchases, actions are taken as if the *marginal utility* (or *marginal benefit*) of each additional purchase is evaluated. The marginal benefit represents the additional benefit or utility gained from a purchase of one more unit of a particular item. A person may have a high marginal utility for one glass of water. However, a second glass of water is not worth quite so much. The twentieth glass of water on a given day may not have much additional utility at all.

How much water is the individual likely to consume? The consumer will select a set of goods and services so that the last unit of each yields the same marginal benefit per dollar spent. By doing this, total utility will be maximized. Any other combination of goods and services would mean that some money was spent on items that provided less utility per dollar than could have been obtained from another item.

Not all individuals have the same marginal utility values. If we were evaluating chocolate, some individuals would value the first piece more highly than others would. The same is true for the second, tenth, and hundredth pieces. This is true for any good. However, by aggregating information about the marginal benefit or utility for all individuals, we can develop information about the overall demand for the good or service.

Marginal Cost

Economists call the price paid for a good or service the *marginal cost.* This tells what it costs the consumer to purchase one more unit of an item. As a result of the argument just presented about utility, economists conclude that any consumer can maximize utility by setting the marginal benefit of purchases equal to the marginal cost. That is, the individual purchases units of each good or service until the marginal benefit of another unit is just equal to the marginal cost.

This is also a useful concept for suppliers. They will make a profit when the price they charge exceeds the cost of making the good or providing the service. Therefore, we would not expect to see a service sold at less than the marginal cost of the resources needed to produce it. Pricing based on marginal costs is discussed further in Chapter 9.

Savings

What if the consumer has made a series of purchases but feels that the benefit from an additional purchase of any item is not worth the price charged even though there is still some money left over? In that case, the individual receives more benefit from saving money than from spending it. Many individuals reach a point where the utility of saving money exceeds the utility of additional expenditures. What benefits can be realized from saving money? Several examples of the benefits individuals have from saving as opposed to direct consumption are protection against future unemployment, creation of a pool of money for a future vacation or retirement, and accumulation of money for a child's college education.

❊ SUPPLY AND DEMAND

Free Enterprise

Economics is governed by the law of supply and demand. *Supply* is the amount of a good or service that all suppliers in aggregate would like to provide for any given price. *Demand* is the amount of a good or service that consumers would be willing to acquire at any given price. The U.S. economy is based on a system of free enterprise, or capitalism. In such a system, any individual can choose whether to invest wealth or capital in a business venture. That venture provides goods and services to the public. Workers can choose whether to work for that venture at the wages offered. Consumers can choose whether to buy the products of the venture at the seller's price. The central theme of the system is freedom of choice.

In theory, such a system would also result in optimal use of society's scarce resources. Supply and demand are automatically equated by a process known as the *market mechanism*. Suppose that there are consumers who would like to purchase a product and suppliers who would like to sell that product. That represents the basis for there to be a *market* for that product. A *free market* (the basis for the capitalistic system) is simply a situation in which sellers are free to charge whatever price they like for their product and buyers are free to purchase or not purchase at the price sellers are charging. Exchange may take place if the buyers and the sellers reach a mutually agreeable price.

In a free market system, suppliers compete with each other for the inputs—labor, materials, and capital—and to sell their outputs. Competition may take a number of forms. One hospital might compete for nurses by offering better working conditions or higher wages. Another might offer more holidays and vacations. One hospital might compete for patients by emphasizing quality of care. Another might stress the convenience of using its facilities. Throughout the economy, the most widely used basis of competition is price. Higher wages are paid to attract employees, and lower prices are charged to attract customers.

In practice, free market conditions do not always exist, and unregulated competition does not always result in optimal use of society's scarce resources. If prices are not set by the results of active competition but by an individual seller or buyer or by a regulator such as the government, the market is not a free market. Buyers may still have the option of buying at the stated price. But sellers are not free to set whatever price they choose. Market failure and regulatory intervention are discussed at greater length later in this chapter.

An Example of Supply and Demand

For simplicity, consider a health care product for which there is clearly a free market: toothpaste. This preventive health care item fits all of the various requirements for a free market. It is widely available, there are a number of competitors, and consumers have a fair degree of choice in whether to make a purchase. Suppose that the suppliers of toothpaste were to charge $10 per tube. At a price that high, many companies would be willing to supply toothpaste because there would be substantial profits. However, few people would want toothpaste so badly that they would be willing to pay the price. Some people would, but not many. Suppliers would be trying to sell more toothpaste than people are willing to buy.

Suppose that there is a total demand for 100 tubes of toothpaste at the $10 price, but there are 10 suppliers who would each like to sell 100 tubes. Obviously, they cannot each sell 100 tubes. They could each sell 10 tubes, but at that low volume, the costs of setting up for production would be so high that it would not be worthwhile. *Equilibrium* is a situation in which the quantity of a good or service offered at the stated price is the same as the quantity that buyers want to purchase at that price. Equilibrium is a stable situation. Buyers and sellers are in agreement, and prices fluctuate little, if at all. If supply and demand are not equal at a given price, the market is in *disequilibrium*. When disequilibrium exists, as in this toothpaste example, there is pressure to either raise or lower the price until equilibrium is achieved.

One supplier will no doubt cut its price in an effort to corner the market. Other suppliers will follow suit or choose not to produce that product.[1] Eventually, in a fully functioning free

---

[1] Note that if a supplier does not match the lower price other suppliers offer, no one will buy from that supplier in a fully functioning free market. Why pay more for exactly the same item? Examples of multiple prices do exist, however. For instance, convenience stores charge higher prices but do not go out of business. This is because the products offered are not identical—that is, the consumer pays for the toothpaste plus the "convenience" of making the purchase at a small nearby store instead of having to get into his or her car and travel all the way to the supermarket and back.

market, a point is reached where the quantity buyers demand at a given price is the same as the supply at that price.

The amount of any item that a consumer wants depends on the price of that item. However, it depends on other factors as well. The utility of water is much higher if water is the only liquid available than it would be if the consumer also had a choice of milk or juice. Such other items are examples of *substitutes*—goods and services that meet the same need. If the price of water increases and the price of milk or juice is less, the demand for these drinks will increase—that is, the consumer drinks more of them because they are cheaper than water. A related concept is that of *complements*. A complement is a good or service that is consumed along with another, such that if the price of one decreases (or increases), the demand for both increases (or decreases). An example is ice cream and chocolate syrup—if the price of ice cream decreases, the demand for both ice cream and chocolate syrup will increase (assuming, of course, a constant supply of both).

The demand of an individual for a specific good or service is also determined in light of the amount of wealth and income a consumer has and the specific preferences of the individual. The aggregate demand for a good or service depends on how these factors affect all consumers.

Suppose the price offered by toothpaste suppliers drops to $6. At that lower price, more people are willing to buy toothpaste. Assume the quantity demanded at that price is 420 tubes. The suppliers lowered the price in an effort to compete for the original demand for 100 tubes. At the lower price, the number of tubes demanded has increased. On the other hand, at a price of $6, the profits per tube are not as great. Some suppliers will leave the industry. At that lower price, suppliers want to sell only 600 tubes, not 1,000. But offering 600 tubes at that price is still greater than the 420 tubes demanded at that price. The market is not yet in equilibrium.

Price will fall further. At a price of $5, buyers want to buy 500 tubes, and sellers want to offer 500 tubes. The demand and the supply are now the same, and they are in equilibrium. It is possible to draw a graph that estimates how many tubes of toothpaste would be demanded by consumers for any given price. The *demand curve (D)* indicates the quantity of toothpaste (horizontal axis) that would be desired by consumers for any given price (vertical axis). Similarly, the *supply curve (S)* indicates the quantity that would be offered by suppliers at any given price. Figure 4–1 presents both the demand and supply curves on one graph. Equilibrium is achieved when the demand and supply curves intersect. Only at that point is there a price that generates exactly the same amount of demand and supply. What is the total dollar size of the toothpaste industry? In equilibrium, a total of 500 tubes are sold at $5 per tube. Therefore, by multiplying the quantity times the price, we find that the industry generates $2,500 of charges or revenue.

Note that there is some unfilled demand even at equilibrium. The demand curve continues to a volume of 900 tubes. That means that consumers could use 900 tubes. But what is the price at 900 tubes? It is zero. The demand would be that high only if the product was offered for free.

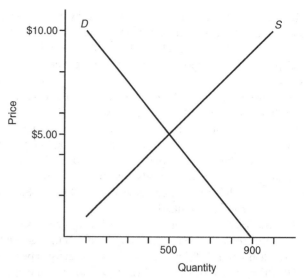

FIGURE 4–1. Supply and demand for toothpaste.

✳ ELASTICITY OF DEMAND

In the toothpaste example, the quantity demanded rose steadily as the price fell. It is a general assumption of economics that demand and price are *inversely* related. That is, as price goes down, the quantity demanded rises; as price rises, the quantity demanded declines. However, an open question is how much more will be demanded as the price declines. Suppliers find this question very interesting. Are profits likely to rise more if prices are raised or lowered? How responsive is a change in demand to a change in price?

The obvious solution is to look at the supply and demand curves and determine how much would be demanded at any given price. However, the specific demand curve for each product, such as that seen in Figure 4–1, is not generally known. Economists draw such diagrams as an analytical tool to study what would happen if a certain pattern of demand existed. Measurement of demand is much more difficult to accomplish. Generally, demand curves are estimated based on a combination of available evidence and suppositions or assumptions.

On the basis of such estimates, economists attempt to determine whether demand is elastic or inelastic. *Elastic* demand is a situation in which an increase or decrease in price results in a proportionately greater change in demand. *Inelastic* demand is a situation in which a decrease in price results in a proportionately smaller decrease in demand. The *elasticity* of a particular good or service reflects the responsiveness of demand for a good or service, or the percent change in demand, relative to a percent change in price.

Suppose that a product's price is cut by 10%. If the increase in demand is more than 10%, the demand is said to be elastic. The more the quantity demanded increases, the more elastic the demand is. Similarly, if the price of the product is increased by 10% and the quantity demanded falls by more than 10%, the demand is considered elastic.

If the quantity demanded were to rise by very little in response to a decline in price, it would hardly be worthwhile for the supplier to cut the price. All customers would get the lower price, but the supplier would get very few new customers. On the other hand, if demand were very elastic, a small price cut would result in a large number of additional customers. In that case, the price cut might be worthwhile.

Certain types of health care services have generally been considered inelastic. When consumers are sick, they want medical care. They tend to be not very sensitive to the price. For example, if a consumer needs a visiting nurse to come to the house, the difference in charge between $80 and $88 may not affect demand substantially.

Suppose that a for-profit home health agency wishes to increase its profits. Currently, the average cost to the agency to provide each visit is $78, and the average price charged per visit is $80. The agency provides 1,000 visits per month and makes a profit of $2,000 per month ($80 price less $78 cost equals a profit of $2 per visit, times 1,000 visits, equals a profit of $2,000).

What would happen if the price were raised by 10%, to $88? If the demand is inelastic, the number of visits might fall by only 5%. In that case, the agency would only have 950 visits (a 5% decrease in volume), but the price for each one would be $88 (a 10% rise in price). The profit of $10 per visit ($88 price less $78 cost) for 950 visits would be far greater than the profit of $2 per visit for 1,000 visits.

On the other hand, suppose a competing visiting nurse association charges only $80 for a similar service. In that case, the demand for the for-profit agency's services might be highly elastic. The 10% price increase could result in a 90% decrease in the quantity demanded. The profit of $10 per visit on 100 visits would not be as high as the profit of $2 per visit on 1,000 visits. Elasticity of demand depends not only on how essential the good or service is but also on the existence of competition in the marketplace.

✳ ECONOMIES OF SCALE

A critical concept in health economics is *economies of scale*. Many decisions nurse managers and executives make require knowledge of the cost per patient. However, that cost is not constant. The cost per patient varies because of economies of scale. Economies of scale refer to changes in the cost per patient as the number of patients changes. Having more patients is referred to as a *larger scale of operations*.

All organizations tend to have some costs that are *fixed* and some that are *variable*. Fixed costs stay the same as the volume of patients increases or decreases. For example, rent on a nursing home building remains the same regardless of whether the nursing home is 50%, 75%, or 100% full. Variable costs increase as the number of patients increases. When one considers all the costs of providing care, the cost per patient decreases as the number of patients increases because there are more patients to share the fixed costs.

Increasing Returns to Scale

Suppose that the fixed costs for a nursing home include rent, heat, and the salary of the administrator, for a total of $200,000 per month. Variable costs include nursing staff, medications, and dietary, for a total of $140 per patient day. If there are 2,000 patient days a month, the cost per patient day is $240, as follows:

Total Fixed Cost	$200,000
Total Variable Cost: $140/day × 2,000 patient days	280,000
Total Cost	$480,000
Divided by Total Patient Days	÷ 2,000
Total Cost per Patient Day	$ 240

However, what if there were 4,000 patient days a month? The fixed cost would still be $200,000. The total variable cost would be $560,000. The total cost would be $760,000, and the cost per patient day would now be only $190:

Total Fixed Cost	$200,000
Total Variable Cost: $140/day × 4,000 patient days	560,000
Total Cost	$760,000
Divided by Total Patient Days	÷ 4,000
Total Cost per Patient Day	$ 190

The cost per patient day has declined as a result of economies of scale, sometimes referred to as *increasing returns to scale*. The importance of this notion is that large volumes make it less costly to treat each patient because of the sharing of fixed costs by the larger number of patients. At some point, however, this trend often reverses.

Decreasing Returns to Scale

At extremely large volumes, *decreasing returns to scale* occur. Decreasing returns refer to the fact that at very large volumes, the cost per patient tends to increase. There are several reasons for this. For one thing, when full capacity is reached (e.g., all beds are full), fixed costs rise. It may be necessary to add a new facility. Another problem is that at very large size, it becomes more expensive for an organization to acquire resources. There may not be any nurses available to staff the extra volume, and this may drive up the costs of labor.

The implication of this is that there is a least cost volume for any organization. At that volume, all economies of scale have been realized, but decreasing returns to scale have not yet set in (Figure 4–2). Cost C represents the least cost per patient. That cost occurs at a volume (i.e., quantity) of Q patients.

✳ ECONOMICS AND INCENTIVES

In the earlier hypothetical toothpaste example, each consumer or supplier acted in his or her own best interest. Suppliers decided whether they wanted to provide a product at different prices, and consumers decided whether they wanted to buy the product at various prices. The decision of each consumer or supplier individually was aggregated to derive a total demand curve and a total supply curve. The assumption that individuals (and suppliers) act in their own best interests is central to economics, and it leads in turn to an important lesson about incentives.

Whenever an action is taken, whether by government, an organization, a supplier, or an individual, the action that is taken may affect other individuals or organizations. Much as in

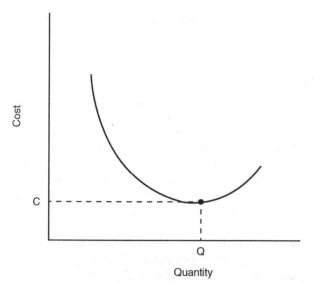

FIGURE 4–2. Economies of scale.

physics, for every action there is a corresponding reaction. Managers and policymakers must be aware that the actions they take may give individuals and organizations incentives to behave in a certain way.

For instance, many health care insurance companies use deductibles, coinsurance, and co-payments. A deductible is a portion of health care cost that the individual must pay before insurance covers any of that individual's costs. Coinsurance is a percentage of each health care bill that the individual must pay out of pocket. A co-payment is a specific amount, such as $20, that a patient must pay per physician visit. Why are these used? The rationale is that if insurance fully covers all costs, the consumer will use (or overuse) health care services for many little problems that do not need medical attention. By making individuals bear some of the cost, they have a personal financial incentive to be more judicious in the use of health services. The lower the cost to the consumer, the greater the demand, as evidenced by demand curves.

The issue of incentives is a concept of economics that has wide applications. Should your employer offer bonuses? One reason to do so is to give individuals an incentive to work harder in the interests of the organization. The bonus provides individuals with more resources. Those resources can be used for consumption or for savings to result in greater total utility.

Consider another example. Should hospitals be paid on a cost reimbursement basis? For many years, that is how Medicare paid hospitals. It was determined, however, that this gave hospitals an incentive to have high costs. Therefore, the cost reimbursement system was replaced by the Diagnosis Related Groups (DRG) system. The DRG system does not reimburse the hospital for its costs; rather, it pays a fixed amount based on the type of patient regardless of length of stay or cost.[2]

---

[2]For patients who have unusually long lengths of stay, there is supplemental payment. However, that payment is kept low so that hospitals do not have an incentive to extend patient stays.

The expectation was that DRGs would give hospitals an incentive to shorten lengths of stay and decrease costs.

✴ MARKET EFFICIENCY

One can view the health services field as having three key economic questions:

1. How much?
2. How?
3. For whom?

How much health services are to be provided? How are they to be produced? And who will receive them? The first two questions relate to efficiency of production; the third relates to distribution of society's scarce resources. The efficiency of the market is judged by how well it responds to these three questions.

In the case of a fully functioning free market, the three questions would solve themselves. *How much* production would depend on the supply and demand curves. Finding the equilibrium price and quantity would determine how much.

The *how* would also be solved at equilibrium. The supplier that is most efficient at the task would be able to offer the service at the lowest cost. As price declines until supply and demand intersect, the less efficient producers will drop out of the competition. When equilibrium is achieved, it means that the existing suppliers must be using efficient techniques or they would have been forced out of business. This means that *technical efficiency* has been achieved. Technical efficiency means that the services are produced using the minimum possible amount of resources for the quantity and quality of output achieved.

For whom is also solved by equilibrium. Any potential buyers who are able and willing to pay the equilibrium price or more will receive the goods or services. Anyone who can or will only pay less than that price will not receive the goods or services. This represents *distributional efficiency*. The market efficiently distributes goods based on the utility of the various consumers.

However, market efficiency does not address the issue of equity or fairness. Is the free market outcome fair for those who are poor? The question of fairness raises the issue of redistribution of resources.

✴ REDISTRIBUTION OF RESOURCES

Government and management tend to have different objectives. The management of an organization may desire to determine how to best provide patient treatment. It uses economics to find the least costly ways to provide a particular level or type of care. This is technical efficiency. The government is interested in distributional efficiency and equity—or could society be made better off by redistribution of resources? These are difficult issues that reflect differences in the objectives and values of business and government; however, reconciling these differences requires an understanding of related economic principles.

Collective Action

Resource redistribution is more than simply taking resources from the rich to help the poor. It is based on a much wider notion of welfare than the use of welfare payments to the poor. The government taxes everyone so that it can have public sewer systems, police, and fire protection. It would be too expensive for any one individual to buy his or her own police department or fire department. The government acts as a central collection organization, taking contributions (taxes) from each individual and putting them all together to be able to do what any one person cannot, such as having fire and police protection. There is little disagreement that such protection is needed and worthwhile.

This is an example of distributional efficiency through government collective action. The government optimizes the result through its redistribution of resources, making everyone better off than they would be without the intervention.

Equity Improvement

A more controversial aspect of resource redistribution concerns taxing one group of individuals to provide a benefit to another group. For example, taxes paid by the working class tend to support Medicare payments made for the elderly population. This makes some individuals better off but others worse off.

Should such redistribution of resources from current workers to the elderly population take place? That is a value judgment, not an economic calculation. In the fire and police department examples, collective action makes everyone better off. Attempts to improve societal equity often improve the utility of some people at the expense of others. How much redistribution should take place? Again, that is a value judgment. Society must make those value decisions. Then economics can focus on whether the money is being used efficiently to achieve society's goals.

✳ MARKET FAILURE

Except for issues of collective action or equity improvement requiring resource redistribution, the free market is generally assumed to be an efficient mechanism. Left to its own devices, it should always find equilibrium between supply and demand. However, it is often contended that the marketplace for health care services is not perfectly efficient. There is a condition referred to as a *market failure*. Market failure means that the market does not function fully and freely. This results in an inability to reach supply and demand equilibrium without intervention. The government often steps in to try to correct market failure.

Market failure can result from a number of different factors. Sometimes government intervention itself is responsible for the failure. Another factor is lack of full information on the part of consumers. Yet another is failure of consumer actions to fully account for the market price because consumers are not directly responsible for full payment of their health care service consumption. Market failure can be caused by lack of full competition, as occurs if either sellers or buyers have monopoly power. Finally, failure can occur when the actions of individuals or organizations do not result in optimal output because their actions do not consider externalities that they generate. All of these factors are discussed here. It should be noted that there may be situations in which there is "no market" to fail. Such may be the case in some local, very rural, or remote areas where there are no providers to deliver care and

thus no competition among providers. Despite this possibility, the larger market for health care services is the focus of our discussion here.

Government Intervention

The free market does not generally result in satisfying all demand. It only results in providing products to consumers who are able and willing to pay a price high enough to make it worthwhile for producers to supply a product. In the health care marketplace, society has generally agreed that at least some elements of health care should be provided to individuals who cannot afford to pay for their care. This represents an equity redistribution of resources based on a value judgment by society.

In redistributing resources, an attempt should be made to avoid creating market distortions. The consequences of redistribution should be analyzed carefully. Consider, for example, that society does ensure that an individual in terrible pain from an abscessed tooth who appears at an emergency department receives care for that tooth, for free if necessary. This is accomplished either through government payment for the services or through legislation mandating that the care be offered whether the patient can afford to pay the charge or not.

Suppose that a member of Congress argues that the nation is spending $4,000 for emergency care for poor individuals with tooth abscesses that could have been saved had those individuals had toothpaste. In our earlier example, we noted that at equilibrium, 500 tubes of toothpaste are purchased at $5 a tube. However, if toothpaste were free, 900 tubes would have been consumed. There is an unmet demand of 400 tubes because of the $5 price. The member of Congress might note that this unmet need is the result of people being too poor to spend their meager resources on toothpaste. At $5 a tube, it would cost the government only $2,000 to buy 400 tubes of toothpaste. This is half as much as is being spent on avoidable emergency care. Therefore, it would be both cheaper and more socially responsible and morally correct to distribute toothpaste and prevent those abscesses. Is that a correct economic analysis?

What happens if the government acts as a buyer for the health care service, be it toothpaste or emergency abscess care? Will the supply curve change? No. The suppliers have calculated their costs, and the curve indicates how much supply they will offer at any given price. What about the demand curve? If the government says it will buy care for poor people, the amount of care demanded at any specific price has changed. To ensure that everyone has toothpaste, 900 tubes must be purchased. The supply curve in Figure 4–3 indicates that the price at which that volume will be available is $9 per tube.

What are the implications of this government decision? First, society must raise taxes by enough to cover the cost of toothpaste provided to those who did not buy it at the market price of $5. Because the free market equilibrium was 500 tubes, the government must buy 400 tubes. At what price? Assuming the government pays the market price, it would have to pay $9 per tube.

However, the government has also introduced another change. At the higher price of $9 per tube, the original demand

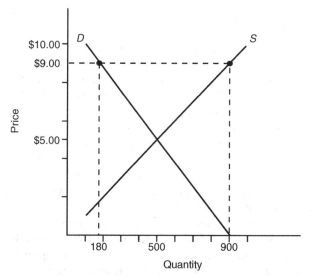

FIGURE 4–3. Supply and demand for toothpaste with government intervention.

is less than 500 tubes. It is only 180 tubes (see Figure 4–3). There are a number of people who were able to buy the toothpaste at a price of $5 but who are unwilling or unable to pay $9 for it. The government policy, however, will ensure that they get the toothpaste by buying it for them. Thus, in the new equilibrium, 180 tubes of toothpaste are bought by consumers at a price of $9 per tube, and 720 tubes are bought by the government at a price of $9 per tube.

Prices have nearly doubled as a result of government intervention. The number of people providing their own care has fallen from 500 to 180. The 180 are each paying nearly twice as much as they had before. In addition, there will be a tax of $6,480 to pay for the 720 tubes at $9 per tube. This compares with the $4,000 tax that was paid to take care of abscesses. It turns out that the new policy of toothpaste instead of abscesses is substantially more expensive, not less expensive as had been proposed.

What is the total size of the toothpaste industry? There are 900 tubes sold at $9 per tube for a total charge of $8,100. Earlier there had been 500 tubes sold for $5 each for a total of $2,500. The good intentions of the government to provide direct care to avoid tooth abscesses has caused the number of tubes sold to nearly double and the revenues of the industry to more than triple. Is it any surprise that health care costs rose dramatically after the introduction of Medicare and Medicaid?

What will be the impact of the 2010 ACA on health care costs? The Centers for Medicare and Medicaid Services estimates that the government will be paying for 50% of all health care costs by 2020, up from 44% in 2010.[3] This will result from more people's having access to care and also from rising costs per unit of care (i.e., similar to producers' supplying more tubes

of toothpaste at a higher price per tube supplied when the government becomes a purchaser). Total health care spending is expected to increase from $2.6 trillion in 2010 to $4.6 trillion in 2020, nearly doubling in 10 years, with per capita spending rising from $8,327 in 2010 to $13,708 in 2020. This projected outcome should not be surprising given an understanding of basic economics. When 30 million more individuals become covered by health insurance, the total costs of providing care rise dramatically.

Does this mean that it was a mistake to create the Medicare and Medicaid programs or to pass the ACA? No. Perhaps society should be willing to spend substantial additional amounts of money to avoid the tooth abscesses, diseases, morbidity, and mortality associated with a large number of individuals without health insurance. Economics is a science, not a political party. Economics is essential because it allows us to analyze the impact of a policy.

Economists would argue that it is inappropriate to adopt a new policy, such as government payment for toothpaste or the ACA, without considering the likely economic implications of that policy action. In other words, an economic evaluation provides an important piece of evidence for decision making. After the costs of an action are known, economics does *not* make recommendations for or against the policy.

Lack of Full Information

A critical factor causing widespread market failure in health care is that consumers typically have far less information than the sellers. This lack of information makes it difficult for buyers to make a rational, informed decision.

Consider an extreme hypothetical example. A consumer has a cough, and the doctor examines him. The doctor concludes that there is a 99.9% chance that the patient simply has a cold. If the patient has a cold, the cough will probably go away in a week or so. After 2 weeks, perhaps 5% of patients will still have a cough.

If the cough does not go away, the doctor could then order an x-ray to determine if the patient has some more serious condition, such as tuberculosis or lung cancer. Assume that a more serious condition occurs in 1 in 1,000 cases.

What if the doctor, who happens to own an x-ray machine in his office, prescribes a chest x-ray for each person with a cough? The doctor has a personal incentive to do this because a profit can be earned on each of 1,000 x-rays. Waiting 2 weeks and then prescribing an x-ray for the 5% who are still coughing will result in only 50 x-rays. In either case, the doctor diagnoses the serious condition. However, in one way he can earn far more money.

Assume that no patient will incur a significant detriment by waiting the 2 weeks for the x-ray. When the physician recommends an x-ray, the patient is usually not an informed buyer. The physician recommends that the x-ray be taken to rule out any serious problem. The unknowing patients agree to the x-ray.

Had the patients been fully informed that they could save their money, wait 2 weeks, and then come back in 2 weeks if they were still coughing, with no risk, many might opt to do so.

[3]Keehan SP, Sisko AM, Truffler CJ, et al. 2011. National health spending projections through 2020: Economic recovery and reform drive faster spending growth. *Health Aff* 30(8):1594-1605. Retrieved July 30, 2011, at http://content.healthaffairs.org/content/early/2011/07/27/hlthaff.2011.0662.abstract.

The lack of complete information takes away an important element of choice from the patient. Even though the Internet enables patients to have far more information today than they have had in the past, health care providers still possess more specific knowledge of health care diseases, processes, and outcomes than patients.

This type of market failure can be corrected by a system of regulations. For example, the government could dictate when it is appropriate to prescribe a chest x-ray. This has occurred to some degree through the development and use of evidence-based practice guidelines by health care provider groups and the implementation of recommendations made by the U.S. Preventive Services Task Force. This latter group is composed of nonfederal providers who come together to review scientific evidence for preventive care and treatments and to make broad recommendations for care delivery. However, the government has provided such restrictive regulations only reluctantly. The health services community has argued, successfully to a great extent, that the potential risk to the health of patients from extremely high regulation outweighs the economic benefits of reductions in inappropriate utilization.

Lack of Direct Patient Payment

The failure of the market to be efficient because of a lack of information is exacerbated by the fact that many patients have Medicare, Medicaid, Blue Cross, or some other insurance plan that will pay part or all of the cost of the x-ray. The high cost of health care services has induced many individuals to acquire health insurance. Health insurance represents a pooling of resources.

On the surface, insurance is clearly a good thing. Rather than some people being lucky and healthy and having little if any cost and others being unlucky and ill and having costs that wipe out their life savings, everyone pays a set insurance premium, such as $8,000 per year. However, there are problems with insurance. After individuals have purchased insurance, there is little incentive for them not to consume great amounts of health care services.

The impact of insurance is similar to the example in which the government purchased toothpaste. When individuals are fully insured (assuming neither deductible nor co-payment), the price to them for health care services drops to zero. In that case, their demand is based on a price of zero. Market failure results in suboptimal use of resources. Health resources are consumed until their marginal utility is nearly zero because of the zero cost. This drives up the total costs of providing health care services.

Monopoly Power

Market failure is often associated with lack of full competition. The basic foundations of free markets assume that there are a large number of buyers and a large number of suppliers for any good or service. If there is only one seller, that seller is referred to as a *monopoly*. Sometimes there are natural monopolies when it makes sense to have only one supplier. Many public utilities fall into that category. Duplication of power plants and power lines would be technically wasteful. In such cases,

government regulates prices to prevent the supplier from charging an excessive amount.

In small communities, hospitals may effectively be natural monopolies. It is too costly to build more than one hospital for the community. In that case, the hospital has the potential to charge substantially more than a hospital in a city with 10 hospitals. In the latter case, an individual wanting elective surgery could shop around for a hospital offering a reasonable price.

Another element of market failure in health care is that consumers often use the health care facilities and organizations used by their physicians. Rather than having to compete directly for patients, hospitals, nursing homes, and home care agencies need only compete for physician referrals. When the physician makes a recommendation, the patient is often locked in even if other suppliers are available that are preferable or cost less. When it comes to the patient's health, especially if there is any chance of death or permanent disability, each health care provider is viewed as unique. For example, if the patient hears that a surgeon is good, the patient will be reluctant to shop around for another surgeon who is cheaper or who operates at a less expensive hospital. Thus, monopoly power sometimes exists for health care providers even in the absence of single supplier monopolies.

If there is monopoly power, the price may not be driven down to a normal equilibrium level. The monopoly might find that more profits can be made at a higher price. Figure 4–4 considers this situation. Equilibrium is at the intersection of the supply and demand curves, with price P1 and quantity Q1. However, what if the monopoly charges price P2? Consumers will only purchase quantity Q2 at that higher price. However, the price is so high that the monopoly may make more profit selling less volume at a high price than by selling a higher volume at the equilibrium price. This is a result of the relatively inelastic demand for health care services. Increases in price may not lower the quantity demanded substantially. With competition, prices would fall to the equilibrium level; without competition, it pays for the provider to keep the price above equilibrium.

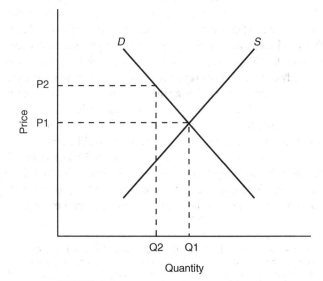

FIGURE 4–4. Example of monopoly power.

The government has traditionally tried to regulate public utility monopoly prices by fixing them at level P1. At that level, consumers purchase Q1 quantity of services, and a free market outcome is achieved through intervention.

To the extent that the government pays health care providers directly for Medicare and Medicaid, the government is involved directly in setting the prices it is willing to pay. However, full regulation of health care pricing has not yet taken place, as it has in the case of public utilities. That means that many health care providers may have the ability to set artificially high prices to generate excessive profits.

Monopsony Power

At the same time, however, insurance companies, and employers are starting to exercise the power of large buyers. Blue Cross exercised such power for many years. Just as it is possible to have a monopoly where there is only one seller, it is possible for there to be just one buyer. If there is only one buyer, it is called *monopsony*.

In recent years, there has been a great proliferation of HMOs and *preferred provider organizations* (PPOs) (see Chapter 2). Insurance companies or employers direct their members or employees to use certain providers of health care in exchange for lower prices. In effect, the insurance companies are behaving as monopsonists. They control the buying of health care services for their populations. That provides them with market power to help them gain a better purchase price for the services.

Just as a supplier with monopoly power can dictate the price at which it sells a good or service, a monopsonist can dictate the price it pays to buy a good or service. For instance, suppose that the only employer for nurses in a geographic area is the local hospital. That hospital would be a monopsony.

The monopsony buyer pays low wages, which reduces the amount of supply. Fewer nurses are willing to work at such low wages. However, the savings from the lower wage offsets the financial losses from the inability to hire more staff. This may result in less care being provided. It is conceivable that part of the reason nursing shortages are frequently observed is that health care providers maintain an artificially low wage level for nurses because of their exercise of monopsony power.

Government-Induced Inefficiency

Another problem that can contribute to market failure is the potential lack of incentives on the part of HCOs to minimize the costs of production. The government is often the cause of this technical inefficiency, because many government programs pay HCOs their costs for providing care to specific groups of patients.

Without economic analysis, it might seem prudent for the government to reimburse an organization for its costs. It should save money because the government will not have to pay for any profit. However, it provides a perverse incentive. It encourages organizations to keep costs high. Why work hard to control costs if you will be paid whatever you spend? There is no reward for low cost. History has shown that schemes that reimburse costs are not good tools for restraining the growth

of health care costs. This rationale provided the basis for moving from a cost-based reimbursement system to a prospective reimbursement system (i.e., one that paid providers a predetermined price for services rather than paying them whatever costs they incurred) and now to a pay-for-performance (or value-based) system, which gives organizations incentives to also improve the quality of services provided (discussed in Chapter 2).

Externalities

A last principal cause of market failure is the existence of *externalities*. Externalities exist when an action by an individual or organization has secondary effects on others that are not taken into account. For example, if a factory pollutes the skies, it may have found the cheapest way to produce its product, but as a side effect, its pollution hurts people. Externalities may present additional costs or benefits to those affected. If a person goes to a hospital and is cured of a contagious disease, it benefits all those who might have caught the disease from that person. If external costs and benefits are not taken into account, a nonoptimal amount of output may be produced. There could be too much pollution or too little health care. This represents a market failure. A mechanism is needed to correct the output level. In the case of pollution, the factory can be fined for polluting to make it realize the full costs of the pollution, including its negative external effect on others. This can cause it to reduce its output of pollution. In the case of health care, the government can tax all individuals for the positive external benefits they receive and use the money collected to pay subsidies for health care.

In fact, the government does take that approach frequently. The government role is essential because of its ability to take collective action. As in the case of police and fire protection, the government can use collective action to benefit society.

❋ THE MARKET FOR NURSES

A problem that has plagued the health care industry periodically for decades is a shortage of nurses, sometimes followed by a surplus. These shortages have come and gone, with at least some shortages being noted in every decade since World War II. A critical issue is determination of whether nursing shortages occur because of market failure or whether the market is in fact functioning normally. The answer has serious ramifications for what the government should do to alleviate nursing shortages when they occur.

It is often argued that the primary cause of most nursing shortages is not a decreasing supply but an increasing demand. The number of nurses needed increases more rapidly than the supply. The result of an increase in demand with supply unchanged is a shift of the demand curve from D to D′ in Figure 4–5A. The new equilibrium, B, has a substantially higher wage than the original equilibrium, A. This higher wage entices more individuals to become educated as nurses. With higher wages, the profession is relatively more attractive than it was at the lower wage. After a number of years, this results in an increased supply of nurses. Figure 4–5B shows the eventual shift in the supply curve as newly trained nurses enter the work

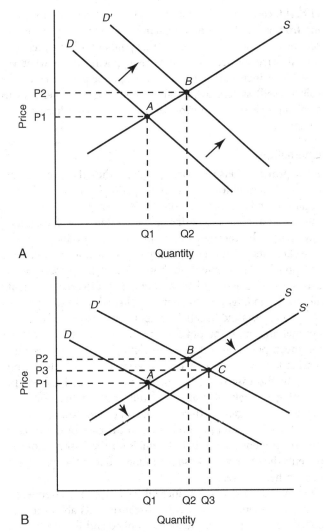

A

B

FIGURE 4–5. **A,** Increase in demand for nurses. **B,** Increase in supply of nurses.

gradually seeking the level at which enough nurses will be available to meet the demand. If demand is continuing to rise during this period, it is difficult for supply to catch up.

The problem is made more complicated by the fact that other industries are also trying to attract qualified labor. An economic analysis of labor in one industry is incomplete if it fails to consider possible increases in demand and wages in other industries.

Therefore, the observed shortages of nurses could be the result of lack of information about the price at which sufficient individuals will be enticed into the industry. Or it could be the result of a moving target. Increasing demand plus wage increases in other industries could create a situation in which prices are rising to attract more nurses but simply not fast enough to eliminate the shortage. Both of these arguments revolve around the lag in time between when prospective future nurses realize that higher wages are available, enroll in nursing school, and graduate or the lag in time required to recruit nurses through other means.

On the other hand, if this were the case, there should be great increases in the numbers of students in nursing schools. It would be easy enough for the health care industry to consider whether wages are high enough by examining whether more students are applying to nursing schools and continuing to raise wages until applications start to rise. If that is not the case, one might argue that the larger employers of nurses are acting in a monopsonist fashion, artificially keeping wages low and enduring a shortage of nurses in exchange for avoiding a higher total payroll cost. Regardless, one must keep in mind that determining whether or not a nursing shortage exists is not just a matter of perceptions in the market. The economic definition of a labor shortage is the condition in which wages rise faster than average during a period of time. Economists must actually look back over time to determine whether or not nursing wages have increased faster than average over a period. This is the only way to know for sure that an economic shortage of nurses has occurred.

There has been considerable debate about whether nurses and advanced practice nurses, in particular, are substitutes or complements to physician care. On the one hand, nurse practitioners who provide the same level and quality of primary care as their physician counterparts at a lower price could be considered substitutes for physicians. A recent integrative review suggests that advanced practice nurses provide at least the same level of care, and perhaps better, than their physician counterparts.[4] In some areas, the wages of nurse practitioners may be less than the wages of physicians; in that case, one could expect there to be increased demand for nurse practitioner services.[5] Increased demand for nurse practitioner services has occurred to some degree but has probably been constrained by the nature and structure of the health care market.

[4]Newhouse RP, Stanik-Hutt J, White KM, et al. 2011. Advanced practice nurse outcomes 1990-2008: A systematic review. *Nurs Econ* 29(5):1-21.

[5]Physician residents may be even less expensive than nurse practitioners in some urban areas, and in this case, the demand for their services may be higher than the demand for nurse practitioners.

force. The new supply, S′, removes the pressure for salaries to increase (faster than the general level of wages in society). A new equilibrium exists at point C.

Note that the equilibrium at C has a lower wage than that at point B. Wages, however, often do not adjust downward. Instead, a period of time may occur during which wages rise extremely slowly, if at all. The higher supply removes the pressure on employers to raise wages.

In fact, more nurses, Q3 compared with Q2, are available. If the price stays at P2, an even greater number of nurses will be available. Consider where the P2 price would intersect with the S′ curve. It is at a quantity substantially higher than Q2 or Q3.

This analysis assumes that everyone has reasonably complete information. It is not likely, however, that employers know how much salaries must rise to reach equilibrium. Therefore, they raise salaries, but not enough, and then wait for more nurses to enter the market (i.e., through nursing school graduations, international nurse migration, or the return of unemployed nurses to work). After a period of time, if the supply of nurses has not risen sufficiently, wages will again rise,

That may change with the implementation of the ACA. On the other hand, few would argue that nurses and nurse practitioners are complements to physician care, such that when the demand for physician services increases, so, too, would the demand for nurses and nurse practitioners.

❋ IMPLICATIONS FOR NURSE MANAGERS AND EXECUTIVES

Accounting and finance are a subset of applied economics. We live in a society whose entire financial structure is built around a system of economics. That economic system permeates all institutions and organizations. It dictates the allocation of society's scarce resources.

The health care system, however, is largely an example of the failure of the economic system. Lack of information, monopoly power, and a variety of other factors cause the laws of supply and demand to fail to achieve normal free market equilibrium level. These failures lead to the need for government to help achieve efficient economic resource allocation.

Externalities and the power of collective behavior hold a special role in health care because of the value to everyone of living in a society that is basically healthy. This means that there is a further need for government intervention.

Compounding the need for a government role even further is the fact that most members of society believe that some degree of resource redistribution is essential for equity as well as for efficiency. This can allow the poorest members of society to be guaranteed at least a minimum level of health care services.

Within this complicated economic environment are nurses who want to know why their organizations do not provide more resources to their departments, why salaries cannot be raised to levels that compensate them more adequately for their skills and the challenges of their jobs, and why everyone is not guaranteed the highest level of care.

The answers to these questions are complex. However, an understanding of the basic law of supply and demand and the inherent limited nature of all resources is a starting point in answering these questions. The complications of market failure further explain why health care is one of the most highly regulated industries and why health care is sometimes viewed as best provided by a not-for-profit organization with a mission of providing care rather than a mission of maximizing profits.

As readers go through the remaining chapters of this book, the laws of supply and demand and the scarcity of resources should be kept in mind. The importance of incentives in understanding the likely behavior of individuals should be considered, as should the efficiency generated by economies of scale. The elements of economics are fundamental to the realm of financial management issues faced by nurse managers and executives.

❋ KEY CONCEPTS

Economics   Study of how scarce resources are allocated among their possible uses. As a management or policy tool, economics is used to ensure that individuals, organizations, and society make optimal use of their limited resources.

Economic goods   Goods or services acquired by consumers that provide physical or psychological benefit. Goods or services are generally acquired through an exchange process.

Utility   Benefit gained by consumers from either consuming or saving resources. Marginal utility is the additional utility gained from consuming one more unit of a particular good or service. Total utility is maximized by purchasing a set of goods and services such that the marginal utility or marginal benefit is the same for each item.

Supply and demand   Supply is the amount of a good or service that all suppliers in aggregate provide at any given price. Demand is the amount of the good or service that consumers are willing to acquire at any given price. At the equilibrium price, the quantity offered and the quantity demanded are identical.

Free enterprise, capitalism, or market economy   System in which each individual can choose whether to invest wealth or capital in a business venture; workers can choose whether to work for that venture at the wages offered, and consumers can choose whether to buy the products of the venture at the requested price.

Elasticity of demand   Degree to which demand increases in response to a price decrease or decreases in response to a price increase. In general, the demand for health services is considered highly inelastic.

Economies of scale   Cost of providing a good or service falls as quantity increases because fixed costs are shared by the larger volume. However, eventually, large volume may lead to decreasing returns to scale because of capacity constraints or shortages of labor or supplies.

Incentives   Economics assumes that individuals and organizations act in their own best interests. Incentives such as health insurance deductibles are used to make it be in the individual's interest to act in a desired manner. They are often used by management to result in an improved use of an organization's scarce resources or by government to improve the use of society's scarce resources.

Market efficiency   In a fully functioning free market economy, resources are optimally allocated and used as a result of the supply-and-demand mechanism.

Redistribution of resources   Even in a relatively efficient market, some government redistribution of resources can provide collective action that makes everyone better off, such as the provision of police and fire protection. Economic analysis can determine which redistributions can make everyone better off and no one worse off. Other redistributions of resources are done to improve equity. They may make some individuals better off and some worse off. Such redistribution requires an equity value judgment. Economics cannot determine a "correct" level of redistribution.

Market failure   Situation in which the free market does not operate efficiently. Market failure may be the result of:

Government intervention   The role of the government in guaranteeing basic medical care to all individuals creates a distortion in the normal equilibrium, the effects of which should be minimized to the extent possible.

Lack of full information   There is a tremendous gap between the knowledge of the patient and the health care provider concerning what services are needed and how important they are. This lack of information prevents consumers from making rational, informed decisions.

Lack of direct patient payment   The existence of health insurance allows individuals to consume more services than they would if they had to directly pay the full cost of the services.

Monopoly or monopsony power   Organizations with monopoly or monopsony power can sometimes make excess profits by maintaining prices of final products at a level higher than equilibrium and the prices of inputs below equilibrium.

Government-induced inefficiency   Decreases in technical efficiency may occur as a result of government reimbursement to health care providers based on the cost of care provided.

Externalities   An action by an individual or organization may have secondary effects on others that are not taken into account. These side effects may present additional costs or benefits to those affected.

✳ SUGGESTED READINGS

Blair R, Harrison J: *Monopsony: antitrust law and economics*, Princeton, NJ, 1993, Princeton University Press.

Cleverley W, Cleverley J, Song P: *Essentials of health care finance*, ed 7, Sudbury, MA, 2011, Jones & Bartlett.

Clewer A, Perkins D: *Economics for health care management*, Upper Saddle River, NJ, 1998, Prentice Hall.

Feldstein P: *Health care economics*, ed 7, Clifton Park, NY, 2011, Thomson Delmar Learning.

Folland S, Goodman A, Stano M: *The economics of health and health care*, ed 6, Upper Saddle River, NJ, 2009, Prentice Hall.

Frech H III: *Competition and monopoly in medical care*, Washington, DC, 2007, AEI Press.

Getzen T: *Health economics and financing*, ed 4, New York, 2010, John Wiley & Sons.

Herzlinger R: *Market-driven health care: who wins, who loses in the transformation of america's largest service industry*, Reading, MA, 1999, Addison-Wesley.

Jacobs P, Rapoport J: *The economics of health and medical care*, Boston, 2003, Jones & Bartlett.

Keehan SP, Sisko AM, Truffler CJ, et al: National health spending projections through 2020: economic recovery and reform drive faster spending growth, *Health Aff* 30(8):1594–1605, 2011.

Newhouse RP, Stanik-Hutt J, White KM, et al: Advanced practice nurse outcomes 1990–2008: a systematic review, *Nurs Econ* 29(5):1–21, 2011.

Phelps C: *Health economics*, ed 4, Reading, MA, 2009, Addison-Wesley.

Quality, Costs, and Financing

CHAPTER GOALS

The goals of this chapter are to:

- Define *quality* and how it is measured
- Discuss value in health care and the impetus for integrating quality, cost, and financing
- Describe the use of report cards in health care
- Examine the role of Magnet and Baldridge designations in shaping hospital quality

- Examine the intricate relationships among costs, quality of care, and health care financing
- Describe incentives in our financing system that support or deter quality
- Introduce the concept of a business case for quality

✻ INTRODUCTION

In the late 1990s and early 2000s, several reports raised concerns about the quality of health care and highlighted the complex relationships among the quality, costs, and financing of health care. The most notable are the Institute of Medicine (IOM) reports, *To Err Is Human: Building a Safer Healthcare System*[1] and *Crossing the Quality Chasm*.[2] *To Err Is Human* estimated that between 44,000 and 98,000 hospital deaths per year were caused by preventable errors in health care. The authors contrasted this loss of life in health care with the loss of life in the airline industry by noting:

The likelihood of dying per domestic jet flight is estimated to be one in eight million.[3] Statistically, an average passenger would have to fly around the clock for more than 438 years before being involved in a fatal crash.

Compared with health care, data from the *To Err Is Human* report suggested that the likelihood of dying from preventable hospital errors is approximately 1 in every 350 to 770 hospital admissions (based on approximately 34 million hospital admissions in 1997). This report noted that even though the

health care system is less safe than other industries and the risk of dying in the health care system is much greater than dying in an airline crash, the public has made few demands to improve the health care system. Why? Perhaps because society views safety problems in health care as provider deficiencies versus systems deficiencies. Yet the costs of health care system deficiencies are great, estimated to range from $17 billion[4] to as much as $29 billion per year.[5]

Crossing the Quality Chasm provided solutions for overcoming the enormous barriers in the health care system that obstruct quality initiatives. This report identified sources of overuse, underuse, and misuse of our health care system, which, in turn, contribute to costs by increasing direct, indirect, and opportunity costs.[6] The authors determined that care in the U.S. health care system should be:

- Safe (avoiding injury to patients)
- Effective (providing care based on scientific knowledge while minimizing the overuse, underuse, or misuse of care)
- Patient-centered (being respectful, responsive, and considerate of patient preferences, needs, and values)
- Timely (minimizing delays and wait times)

---

[1] Kohn L, Corrigan J, Donaldson M. 2000. *To Err Is Human: Building a Safer Healthcare System*. Committee on Quality of Health Care in America, Institute of Medicine. Washington, DC: National Academies Press.

[2] Committee on Quality of Health Care in America, Institute of Medicine. 2001. *Crossing the Quality Chasm*. Washington, DC: National Academies Press.

[3] Source cited: Federal Aviation Administration, Office of System Safety. 1999. *Aviation Safety Reporting System (ASRS) Database*.

[4] Van Den Bos J, Rustagi K, Gray T, et al. 2011. The $17.1 billion problem: The annual cost of measurable medical errors. *Health Aff* 30(4):596-603.

[5] Committee on Quality of Health Care in America, Institute of Medicine, *Op. cit.*, 2001.

[6] Schuster M, McGlynn E, Pham C, et al. 2001. The quality of health care in the United States: A review of articles since 1987. In *Crossing the Quality Chasm*. Committee on Quality of Health Care in America, Institute of Medicine. Washington, DC: National Academies Press.

■ Efficient (avoiding waste)
■ Equitable (providing care that does not vary based on race, gender, geography, or socioeconomic status)

Although these six aims, by themselves, are not revolutionary, the impact of all six aims collectively on health care delivery has been. These two reports have spurred the patient safety movement in health care and countless reports, manuscripts, and studies; almost all of the quality initiatives under way in health care organizations (HCOs) cite these IOM reports as their impetus.

Another IOM report, *Preventing Medication Errors*, suggests that medication errors are even more commonplace in HCOs than one might expect. This report estimated that, on average, a hospital patient runs the risk of being exposed to "more than one medication error each day."[7] Overall, approximately 1.5 million preventable adverse drug events are estimated to occur every year. The report also determined that based on a conservative estimate of 400,000 adverse drug events per year in hospitals, the cost of medication errors would be approximately $3.5 billion.

Why have these reports drawn so much attention? Interestingly, they exposed what many health care professionals have known for a long time: the U.S. health care system does not live up to its potential.[8] This is especially striking—and concerning—when one considers that *the United States spends more on health care than any other country in the world.* Would we—as individual citizens—pay for services that did not live up to our expectations? Would we continue to purchase goods and services time and again that are not a good value? Probably not, unless there were no other options. But that is what makes health care unique: We might switch providers or insurers, but we cannot switch health care systems unless we move to another country.

So that leaves us faced with changing and improving our system to better meet the needs of our society. Assessments of progress in improving the health care system since the IOM reports that made quality and patient safety everyday concerns suggest that a great deal more work is needed before our health care system is safe.[9] A report by the nonprofit Consumers Union (publisher of *Consumer Reports*) estimated that 10 years after *To Err Is Human*, errors accounted for over 100,000 preventable deaths in hospitals per year, largely because of slow progress implementing computerized systems to prevent medication errors in hospitals, slow action by the U.S. Food and Drug Administration (FDA) to address confusion in medication labeling, the lack of transparency in error accountability

and reporting systems, poor national coordination in tracking and reporting errors, and a lack of evidence on health providers' competencies in patient safety practices.[10]

This chapter explores the intricate relationships among health care quality, costs, and financing. We begin with a general discussion and definition of quality and how it is measured and then move to a discussion of the impetus for integrating quality, costs, and financing.[11] We then discuss the emergence of report cards to grade health care providers and the role of quality recognition programs in the health care quality movement. Relationships among health care costs, quality, and financing are explored to highlight the incentives and disincentives in our health care financing system and to address concerns about the *value* of health care. We also discuss issues related to access because these will become more important as future changes in the health system occur. We conclude the chapter by discussing the development of a business case for quality, variations in practice, and short- and long-term costs.

✳ WHAT IS QUALITY, AND HOW IS IT MEASURED?

What is quality? In our society, we've all heard advertising slogans such as "Quality is Job 1." In reality, that slogan is misleading because it does not account for how quality is defined and measured or the costs required for desired levels of quality.

Traditionally, quality was assumed to be an intrinsic part of health care, often without question. The responsibility for quality was concentrated at the top of most HCOs, and the focus was on adhering to certain criteria and standards and ensuring that they were met.[12] These so-called quality assurance programs were often punitive and focused on identifying and punishing individuals who committed errors or failed to adhere to standards.

Today, however, there is a widely held belief that quality in health care is far from what it should be. This belief has fueled changes in how quality is addressed in HCOs. In many HCOs, the responsibility for quality is dispersed throughout the organization, and there has been a shift from focusing on quality assurance to the safety of the systems within which quality is determined, namely how to prevent errors, build safer processes, create a nonpunitive environment or "just culture," address errors that do occur, and continuously improve quality. The intent is that quality efforts should be customer-focused. Today, data bases are commonly developed, maintained, and analyzed in HCOs

[7]Aspden P, Wolcott J, Bootman J, Cronenwett LR. 2007. *Preventing Medication Errors. Committee on Identifying and Preventing Medication Errors, Institute of Medicine.* Washington, DC: National Academies Press.

[8]Berwick D, Joshi M. 2005. Healthcare quality and the patient. In Ransom S, Joshi M, Nash D, editors. *The Health Care Quality Book: Vision, Strategy and Tools.* Chicago: Health Administration Press, pp. 3-24.

[9]See, the following references: Clancy C. 2009. Ten years after "To Err Is Human." *Am J Med Qual* 24(6):252-528; Leape L, Berwick D. 2005. Five years after To Err Is Human: What have we learned? *JAMA* 293(19):2384-2390; and Wachter R. 2004. The end of the beginning: Patient safety five years after "To Err Is Human." *Health Aff* W4:534-545.

[10]Consumers Union. 2009. *To Err Is Human—To Delay Is Deadly: Ten Years Later, a Million Lives Lost, Billions of Dollars Wasted.* Retrieved at http://www.safepatientproject.org/safepatientproject.org/pdf/safepatientproject.org-ToDelayIsDeadly.pdf.

[11]Costs are defined in Chapter 6 as expenses associated with providing care. Financing, discussed in Chapter 2, reflects the ways and means by which health care is paid.

[12]Schiff G, Rucker T. 2001. Beyond structure-process-outcome: Donabedian's seven pillars and eleven buttresses of quality. *Jt Comm J Qual Improv* 27(3):169-174.

using sophisticated statistical tools and processes. The results of these analyses are, in turn, used to develop future quality improvement efforts, such that quality is a never-ending process. Although some HCOs have stronger quality programs and perhaps better outcomes than others, all must have some commitment to quality to survive in today's competitive and complex environment.

The IOM[13] provided the following definition of quality, which is generally accepted in health care:

. . . the degree to which health care services for individuals and populations increase the likelihood of desired health outcomes and are consistent with current professional knowledge.

This definition acknowledges several important points.[14] First, quality is not a static concept but rather a matter of degree. Second, quality increases the *likelihood* of beneficial outcomes but does not necessarily preclude poor outcomes despite even the provision of ideal care. Third, quality is based on the application of the best and most current professional knowledge available. And finally, quality is a very complex dimension that requires the consideration of a broad range of issues to ensure its attainment. Even under the best of conditions, quality may be elusive.

Avedis Donabedian, widely held to be the "father of quality assurance" and of the quality movement in health care,[15] was an outspoken proponent of systems change to improve health care quality. Donabedian acknowledged that defining quality depends on perspective. For example, patients likely define quality differently than clinicians do, and patients and clinicians likely define quality differently than society at large.[16] Donabedian also acknowledged that the definition of quality involves a valuation of benefits, monetary costs, and potential harms in health care, yet the quantification of benefits, costs, and harms is difficult to ascertain and may change over time.

In a seminal article,[17] Donabedian defined quality as a function of structures, processes, and outcomes of care. Measuring quality, in turn, requires an examination of system attributes that represent the structures, processes, and outcomes of care. He described structural aspects of quality as resources used in the provision of care (e.g., physicians, nurses, and other care providers; organizational characteristics), process aspects of quality as the activities involved in providing care (e.g., the model of care delivery used and organizational policies and procedures), and outcomes as the consequences of care (e.g., condition-specific results of care

and patient satisfaction).[18] Donabedian also identified seven pillars or attributes of quality[19]:

- Efficacy: the ability of care to improve health
- Effectiveness: the degree to which attainable health improvements are realized
- Efficiency: the ability to obtain the greatest health improvement at the lowest cost
- Optimality: the most advantageous balancing of costs and benefits
- Acceptability: conformity to patient preferences regarding accessibility, the patient–practitioner relationship, the amenities, the effects of care, and the cost of care
- Legitimacy: conformity to social preferences concerning all of the above
- Equity: fairness in the distribution of care and its effects on health.

The Nursing Role Effectiveness Model, derived from Donabedian's structure–process–outcome framework, has been conceptualized as an approach for measuring and improving quality in nursing.[20] In keeping with Donabedian's approach, this model recognizes that structural and process components affect patient outcomes. Doran and Pringle[21] identified the following as examples of variables that comprise these three components:

- Structure
  - Patients: age, gender, education, type and severity of illness, comorbid conditions
  - Nurses: education, experience
  - Organizational: staffing, staffing mix, workload, and work environment
- Process
  - Nurses' independent role, including patient education and the implementation of nursing interventions
  - Medical care–related role, including medically directed or prescribed care, and the expanded scope of nursing clinical practice
  - Interdependent role: team communication, coordination of care, discharge planning, and case or care management
- Nurse-sensitive outcomes
  - Functional status, self-care, symptom control (including pain management), patient safety and adverse occurrences, and patient satisfaction with care

This model has been tested and validated[22] for its usefulness in capturing nurses' contributions to quality of care in acute

[13]Institute of Medicine, Lohr K, editor. 1990. *Medicare: A Strategy for Quality Assurance.* Washington, DC: National Academies Press, p. 44.

[14]*Ibid.*

[15]Best M, Neuhauser D. 2004. Avedis Donabedian: Father of quality assurance and poet, *BMJ* 13:472-473.

[16]Donabedian A. 1982. *Explorations in Quality Assessment and Monitoring, Volume I. The Definition of Quality and Approaches to Its Assessment.* Ann Arbor, MI: Health Administration Press.

[17]Donabedian A. 1966. Evaluating the quality of medical care. *Milbank Mem Fund Q* 44(3 suppl):166-206.

[18]Donabedian A. 1982. *Explorations in Quality Assessment and Monitoring, Volume II. The Criteria and Standards of Care.* Ann Arbor, MI: Health Administration Press.

[19]For those who would like to know more about these pillars, see Donabedian A. 1990. The seven pillars of quality. *Arch Pathol Lab Med* 114:1115-1118.

[20]Irvine D, Sidani S, McGillis Hall L. 1998. Finding value in nursing care: A framework for quality improvement and clinical evaluation. *Nurs Econ* 16(3):110-131; Irvine D, Sidani S, McGillis Hall L. 1998. Linking outcomes to nurses' roles in health care. *Nurs Econ* 16(2):58-64, 87; Doran D, Pringle D. 2011. Patient outcomes as an accountability. In Doran D, editor. *Nursing-Sensitive Outcomes: State of the Science*, 2nd edition. Toronto: Jones & Bartlett.

[21]Doran and Pringle, *Op. cit.*, 2010, pp. 1-23.

[22]Doran D, Sidani S, Keatings M, Doidge D. 2002. An empirical test of the Nursing Role Effectiveness Model. *J Adv Nurs* 38:29-39.

care. Although further work is needed to understand and measure the coordinating function of nurses, this model aids in understanding nursing's role in the delivery of quality care.

Mitchell and colleagues[23,24] also derived a dynamic model to guide research examining nursing contributions to quality of care from Donabedian's structure–process–outcome framework. This model reflects reciprocal relationships among the health care system within which care is provided, the interventions used, client characteristics, and the outcomes of care. The model emphasizes the need for analysis at the levels of individual, group, community, and population.[25]

The use of Donabedian's structure–process–outcome framework by researchers, scholars, and practitioners as a basis for research and theory development suggests that it is compelling in its ability to capture important aspects of quality in health care. However, even Donabedian's framework does not specify how quality should be measured in each and every case. Lohr[26] emphasized that process and outcome measures should be used to assess quality because emphasizing only one aspect of quality could be misleading. She also pointed out that quality measures should be based on explicit clinical criteria and that quality measures should be adjusted for case mix, patient severity of illness, and patient comorbid conditions.

✳ THE IMPETUS FOR INTEGRATING QUALITY, COST, AND FINANCING

In an ideal world, high-quality care would be a basic characteristic of the health care system. In some cases, it is. However, the reality of our health care system is that

> [u]nfortunately, we have a system with incentives around dollars, not around results that are indicative of quality. Quality cannot drive the system until there are incentives for quality. . . . Those who manage the system have not been convinced of the need to realign incentives at all levels so that quality comes first.[27]

This sentiment is echoed in the IOM's *Crossing the Quality Chasm* report, which called for a greater understanding of how financial and other incentives relate to quality. In some cases, reimbursements to providers are now being based on the outcomes associated with care provided. This is known as *pay for performance* or *value-based purchasing* (see Chapters 2 and 9), but this reimbursement system is still evolving. We know very little about how this system works and whether it will be sustainable over the long run. Anyone who works in the health care system also knows that we have a very long way to go before financial incentives are truly aligned to reward quality.

The impetus for today's focus on quality comes from a variety of public and private sources. The federal government has been a major player in the quality debate in health care. The Advisory Commission on Consumer Protection and Quality in the Health Care Industry (known as the Quality Commission), established by Executive Order in 1996, was created to "advise the President [Clinton] on changes occurring in the health care system and, where appropriate, to make recommendations on how best to promote and ensure consumer protection and quality health care."[28] The Quality Commission delivered "A Consumer Bill of Rights and Responsibilities," which was endorsed by the president, and a final report, "Quality First: Better Health Care for All Americans," which made the following recommendations[29]:

- Provide strong leadership and clear aims for improvement in the health care system
- Advance quality measurement and reporting
- Create public–private partnerships to provide leadership in improving health care quality
- Encourage actions by group purchasers that support and promote quality
- Strengthen the hand of consumers by providing accurate, timely, and useful information
- Focus on the quality of care provided to vulnerable populations
- Promote accountability in the system by adhering to the Patient's Bill of Rights, providing adequate and appropriate oversight, and adhering to quality standards
- Reduce errors and increase safety in health care
- Foster evidence-based practice and innovation
- Adapt HCOs for change that promotes quality
- Engage the health care workforce in quality initiative
- Invest in information systems

The extent to which the Quality Commission's recommendations have been put into place is debatable. Nonetheless, this group's work brought several important quality issues to the forefront and informed quality initiatives that have followed.

More recent federal initiatives are discussed elsewhere in this book (e.g., Chapters 2 and 9), such as the implementation of the Centers for Medicare and Medicaid Services (CMS) pay-for-performance system and the Hospital Quality Initiative. These initiatives are a major step forward in aligning payment with quality incentives, and because CMS is such a prominent player in our health care financing system and exerts such great control in shaping U.S. health care, other major insurers have and will continue to follow suit. These initiatives bundle fees for hospitals and their physician affiliates if they meet certain quality standards in the provision of services for specific, complex procedures, such as heart surgery and hip and knee replacement surgery.

[23]Mitchell P, Ferketich S, Jennings B. 1998. Quality health outcomes model. *Image J Nurs Sch* 30(1):43-47.

[24]Mitchell P, Lang N. 2004. Framing the problem of measuring and improving healthcare quality: has the quality health outcomes model been useful? *Med Care* 42(2 suppl):II-4-I-11.

[25]*Ibid.*

[26]Lohr K. 1997. How do we measure quality? *Health Aff* 16(3):22-25.

[27]Hungate R. 2001. Reflecting on Donabedian. *Health Aff* 20(3):295.

[28]President's Advisory Commission on Consumer Protection and Quality in the Health Care Industry. Retrieved July 31, 2011, at http://www.hcqualitycommission.gov/about.html.

[29]President's Advisory Commission on Consumer Protection and Quality in the Health Care Industry. Retrieved July 31, 2011, at http://www.hcqualitycommission.gov/final.

Today, the Patient Protection and Affordable Care Act (ACA) described in Chapter 2 represents the government's most sweeping attempt to reform the health care system in 45 years. This legislation aims to improve the health of society by increasing access to care via expanded health care coverage to uninsured individuals and improve the health care system by aligning quality metrics with payment mechanisms. For example, this legislation will reduce payments to hospitals for preventable hospital readmissions and for hospital-acquired conditions. Although U.S. hospitals have been focused on improving quality in these key areas, other such efforts are needed to bring about the comprehensive improvements needed in the system.

Another focus on quality comes from the IOM, a nonprofit organization and subsidiary of the National Academy of Sciences that "serves as an advisor to the nation to improve health" and "provides independent, objective, evidence-based advice to policymakers, health professionals, the private sector, and the public."[30] Three important IOM quality reports have already been mentioned in this chapter, which speaks to the significance of these reports. However, there are other IOM reports that pertain to improving the quality of care in the United States and are particularly relevant for nursing. For example, a 1996 IOM report, "Nursing Staffing in Hospitals and Nursing Homes," noted the following:

> . . . [T]here is a serious paucity of recent research on the definitive aspects of structural measures, such as staffing ratios, on the quality of patient care in terms of patient outcomes when controlling for all other likely explanatory or confounding variables.[31]

This 1996 IOM report laid the foundation for the IOM's 2004 report, "Keeping Patients Safe: Transforming the Work Environment of Nurses."[32] This 2004 report linked the nursing work environment with patient safety and outlined a number of recommendations for improving the work environment. These recommendations were far-reaching and largely aimed at the organizations where nurses work, but they also called on the federal government, private organizations, nursing organizations, labor organizations, and policymakers to take actions to improve the work environment for nurses and ultimately improve quality and patient safety.

These reports led to publications in the popular press and numerous research efforts that have helped to inform quality of care efforts, particularly as they pertain to nursing. The most recent IOM initiative relevant to nursing is its partnership with the Robert Wood Johnson Foundation to produce the 2011 report, *The Future of Nursing: Leading Change, Advancing Health.*

As discussed in Chapter 2, this report put forth a series of key messages and recommendations focused on nursing practice, education, interdisciplinary partnerships, and workforce planning. This initiative has been instrumental in coalescing efforts to position nurses as key players in improving the quality and safety of health care in the United States and worldwide.

Other initiatives have also influenced the push toward quality. The Joint Commission, an independent, not-for-profit organization that accredits U.S. hospitals, long-term care facilities, and other HCOs, has as its mission "to continuously improve health care for the public, in collaboration with other stakeholders, by evaluating HCOs and inspiring them to excel in providing safe and effective care of the highest quality and value."[33] In 2002, The Joint Commission introduced its first set of National Patient Safety Goals. Beginning in 2003, hospitals undergoing accreditation by The Joint Commission had to document and demonstrate organizational initiatives that were consistent with these goals. These goals and their associated requirements change annually and are aimed at improving the quality and safety of patient care in HCOs. Because The Joint Commission accredits about 19,000 HCOs and programs in the United States, these goals and requirements are extremely influential in shaping quality and patient safety initiatives nationwide.

Another influential step taken by The Joint Commission was a series of roundtables held on nurse staffing that resulted in a 2002 publication, *Health Care at the Crossroads: Strategies for Addressing the Evolving Nursing Crisis.*[34] This report linked a shortage of nurses with potential quality and patient safety risks and recommended a series of efforts needed to change the nursing practice environment and nursing education and advancement. The report assigned responsibility for meeting those changes to a variety of groups, ranging from The Joint Commission itself to professional organizations, the federal government, and organizations that employ nurses. The report addressed specific financial incentives that are needed to promote quality, improve the nursing work environment, and change nursing education:

> *Make new federal monies available for health care organizations to invest in nursing services. Condition continued receipt of these monies on achievement of quantifiable, evidence-based, and standardized nursing sensitive goals. Align private payer and federal reimbursement incentives to reward effective nurse staffing.*[35]

The Joint Commission subsequently established a Nursing Advisory Council in May 2003 to address the recommendations contained in this report, and this Council remains active today.[36] In recommendations to the Robert Wood Johnson–IOM *Future*

---

[30]Institute of Medicine. Retrieved July 31, 2011, at http://www.iom.edu.

[31]Wunderlich G, Sloan F, Davis C. 1996. *Nursing Staff in Hospitals and Nursing Homes: Is It Adequate?* Committee on the Adequacy of Nurse Staffing in Hospitals and Nursing Homes. Washington DC: National Academies Press, p. 9.

[32]Page A. 2004. *Keeping Patients Safe: Transforming the Work Environment of Nurses.* Committee on the Work Environment for Nurses and Patient Safety. Washington DC: National Academies Press.

[33]The Joint Commission. *About The Joint Commission.* Retrieved July 31, 2011, at http://www.jointcommission.org/about_us/about_the_joint_commission_main.aspx

[34]The Joint Commission. Retrieved July 31, 2011, at http://www.jointcommission.org/assets/1/18/health_care_at_the_crossroads.pdf.

[35]*Ibid,* p. 7.

[36]See, for example, these facts about the Council, retrieved July 31, 2011, at http://www.jointcommission.org/assets/1/18/Nursing_Advisory_Council1.PDF

of Nursing initiative, The Joint Commission highlighted the need for continued efforts to build a culture of quality and safety by expanding leadership opportunities for nurses, redesign nursing education by preparing clinically and culturally competent nurses, and support the study of quality and safety improvements by increasing research funding.[37]

Another influential organization on the health care quality front is the Institute for Healthcare Improvement (IHI), a not-for-profit organization founded in 1991. The IHI's mission is to:

> *. . . improve the lives of patients, the health of communities, and the joy of the health care workforce by focusing on an ambitious set of goals adapted from the IOM's six improvement aims for the health care system—care that is safe, effective, patient-centered, timely, efficient, and equitable. We call this the* **"NO NEEDLESS LIST":** **No** *Needless Deaths;* **No** *Needless Pain or Suffering;* **No** *Helplessness in Those Served or Serving;* **No** *Unwanted Waiting;* **No** *Waste;* **No** *One Left Out.*[38]

An extremely persuasive initiative of the IHI was the "100,000 Lives Campaign." This nationwide initiative began in January 2005 with the goal of saving 100,000 lives in U.S. hospitals over the 18-month period that followed. The IHI proposed that lives would be saved if organizations implemented the following six initiatives[39]:

- Address emerging patient needs at the first signs of patient decline by implementing rapid response teams, an interdisciplinary group of clinicians (including nurses) trained to treat urgent patient needs.
- Prevent unnecessary patient deaths through the use of reliable, evidence-based care for patients with myocardial infarction.
- Prevent adverse drug events by using systems to reconcile differences in patient medication.
- Prevent central line infections by using a series of evidence-based steps in caring for patients with central lines (these steps are called the "Central Line Bundle").
- Prevent surgical site infections by using appropriate and reliable perioperative care.
- Prevent ventilator-associated pneumonia by using a series of evidence-based steps in caring for ventilator patients (these steps are known as the "Ventilator Bundle").

By June 2006, more than 3,000 organizations were voluntarily participating—and investing—in these initiatives, which helped the IHI exceed its original goal of saving 100,000 lives. The IHI subsequently implemented the "5 Million Lives Campaign," launched in December 2006 to address medically induced injuries in health care. This campaign added six additional interventions (high-alert medications, surgical complications, pressure ulcers, methicillin-resistant *Staphylococcus aureus* infections, readmissions for congestive heart failure patients, and providing governing boards with the latest information to accelerate organizational change) to the original set of six. At the close of the 5 Million Lives Campaign in December 2008, more than 4,000 hospitals had voluntarily participated in the initiative and invested considerably in the implementation of these initiatives. However, whether the IHI reached its goal of saving 5 million lives by the end of the campaign is still unknown.[40]

Two other groups have been prominent in bringing about the recent focus on quality in health care, and particularly the focus on quality standards. The National Quality Forum (NQF), a private, not-for-profit organization of members, has the "three-part mission to improve American healthcare by: building consensus on national priorities and goals for performance improvement and working in partnership to achieve them; endorsing national consensus standards for measuring and publicly reporting on performance; and promoting" the attainment of national goals through education and outreach programs."[41] Using a well-established process for reaching consensus among stakeholders,[42] the NQF has endorsed more than 600 consensus standards since its inception.

In 2004, the NQF endorsed a set of performance measures for nursing: the National Voluntary Consensus Standards for Nursing-Sensitive Care.[43] These standards were developed to guide hospitals and other HCOs on a set of common measures that could be used to assess and improve nursing care and patient care quality. Exhibit 5–1 identifies the initial 15 NQF standards for nursing-sensitive care.[44] In a routine "maintenance " review for continued relevancy, eight of the initial 15 nursing sensitive standards were recommended to the NQF Board of Directors for ratification in 2009 (noted in Exhibit 5-1).[45] The Joint Commission also developed an implementation guide for 12 of the original 15 NQF-endorsed measures (also shown in Exhibit 5-1).[46] This action reflects just how

---

[37]See The Joint Commission's testimony to the Robert Wood Johnson Foundation Initiative on the Future of Nursing, at the Institute of Medicine, February 23, 2010, at http://www.jointcommission.org/assets/1/18/RWJ_Future_of_Nursing.pdf.

[38]Institute for Healthcare Improvement. Retrieved July 31, 2011, at http://www.ihi.org/about/Documents/IntroductiontoIHIBrochureDec10.pdf.

[39]Retrieved July 31, 2011 and adapted from http://www.ihi.org/offerings/Initiatives/PastStrategicInitiatives/5MillionLivesCampaign/Documents/Overview%20of%20the%20100K%20Campaign.pdf.

[40]More information on the IHI's "5 Million Lives Campaign" is available at http://www.ihi.org/offerings/Initiatives/PastStrategicInitiatives/5MillionLivesCampaign/Pages/default.aspx.

[41]The National Quality Forum. Retrieved July 31, 2011, at http://www.qualityforum.org/About_NQF/About_NQF.aspx.

[42]The National Quality Forum's Consensus Development Process. Retrieved July 31, 2011, at http://www.qualityforum.org/Measuring_Performance/Consensus_Development_Process.aspx.

[43]National Quality Forum. 2004. *National Voluntary Consensus Standards for Nursing-Sensitive Care: An Initial Performance Measure Set. A Consensus Report.* Washington DC: National Quality Forum. Available at http://www.qualityforum.org/Projects/n-r/Nursing-Sensitive_Care_Initial_Measures/Nursing_Sensitive_Care__Initial_Measures.aspx.

[44]For more details on the measurement of these standards, see the consensus report cited at the above.

[45]Retrieved July 31, 2011, at http://www.qualityforum.org/Projects/n-r/Nursing-Sensitive_Care_Measure_Maintenance/Nursing_Sensitive_Care_-_Measure_Maintenance.aspx.

[46]Retrieved July 31, 2011, at http://www.jointcommission.org/national_quality_forum_nqf_endorsed_nursing-sensitive_care_performance_measures/

❊ **EXHIBIT 5–1** *National Quality Forum–Endorsed National Voluntary Consensus Standards for Nursing-Sensitive Care*

Patient-Centered Outcome Measures	Nursing-Centered Intervention Measures	System-Centered Measures
Death among surgical inpatients with treatable serious complications (failure to rescue)*	Smoking cessation counseling for heart failure[†]	Skill mix of RN, LVN/LPN, UAP, and contracted nurse care hours*[‡]
Pressure ulcer prevalence*[‡]	Smoking cessation counseling for AMI[†]	Nursing care HPPD*[‡]
Falls prevalence*[‡]	Smoking cessation counseling for pneumonia[†]	Scores on the Practice Environment Scale—Nursing Work Index*[‡]
Falls with injury*[‡]		Voluntary turnover for RNs, APNs, LVNs/LPNs, UAPs*[‡]
Restraint prevalence*[‡]		
Urinary catheter–associated UTI for ICU patients*		
CLABSI rate for ICU and high-risk nursery patients*		
VAP for ICU and high-risk nursery patients*		

AMI, Acute myocardial infarction; CLABSI, Central line-associated bloodstream infection; HPPD, Hours per patient day; ICU, intensive care unit; UTI, urinary tract infection ; VAP, Ventilator-associated pneumonia.

*12 NQF Nursing Sensitive Measures included in The Joint Commission's *Nursing Sensitive Care Implementation Guide*, 2009. Retrieved August 1, 2011, at http://www.jointcommission.org/assets/1/6/NSC%20Manual.pdf.

[†]NQF Nursing Sensitive Measure that was submitted to the NQF Board of Directors for Ratification as "Do Not Endorse" by the Consensus Standards Approval Committee. Retrieved August 1, 2011, at http://www.qualityforum.org/About_NQF/CSAC/Decisions/2009/nursingmaintenance.aspx.

[‡]8 Nursing Sensitive Measures recommended for endorsement by the Consensus Standards Approval Committee to the NQF Board of Directors for Ratification. Retrieved August 1, 2011, at http://www.qualityforum.org/About_NQF/CSAC/Decisions/2009/nursingmaintenance.aspx.

Based on information retrieved July 31, 2011, from: http://www.qualityforum.org/Projects/n-r/Nursing-Sensitive_Care_Initial_Measures/Nursing_Sensitive_Care__Initial_Measures.aspx; http://www.qualityforum.org/Projects/n-r/Nursing-Sensitive_Care_Measure_Maintenance/Nursing_Sensitive_Care_-_Measure_Maintenance.aspx; and http://www.jointcommission.org/assets/1/6/NSC%20Manual.pdf.

important these measures have been in shaping organizational quality improvement efforts and research pertaining to the quality of nursing care for some time to come.

The Leapfrog Group, launched officially in 2000, "is a voluntary program aimed at mobilizing employer purchasing power to alert America's health industry that big leaps in health care safety, quality and customer value will be recognized and rewarded."[47] The Leapfrog Group is composed of large Fortune 500 corporations and public agencies that have large numbers of employees for which they must purchase health insurance. These large companies, in many cases, make health insurance available to employees as well as their dependents and organizational retirees. The Leapfrog Group identified four "leaps" or evidence-based practices that, if adopted by HCOs, would improve health care quality[48]: computerized physician order entry (CPOE), evidence-based hospital referrals, intensive care unit (ICU) staffing by physicians experienced in critical care medicine, and organizational progress in attaining safe practices determined by the Leapfrog Safe Practices Score (derived from the NQF's list of Safe Practices). Leapfrog determined that if all hospitals implemented three of these four leaps, it would save up to $12 billion and more than 57,000 lives per year.[49]

Given that this organization is composed of some of the largest public and private organizations to purchase health care, the importance of this group cannot be overestimated.

The Leapfrog Group's Hospital Recognition Program, a pay-for-performance, value-based purchasing program, rewards hospitals based on quality, resource use, and value in the aforementioned areas plus in caring for patients with certain common acute conditions (acute myocardial infarction, pneumonia, newborn deliveries), certain health care–acquired conditions (i.e., pressure ulcer incidence rates, hospital injury rates, central line–associated bloodstream infection rates), and the implementation of policies regarding never-events, and NQF-endorsed safe practices.[50] Hospitals participate in an annual survey to report performance in these areas, and the information provided is benchmarked against Leapfrog's national performance set. Recognition is based on a hospital's "value" score, derived from a hospital's performance on certain quality measures (65% of value score) and resource use (35% of value score).[51] Hospitals that excel in these areas may be recognized by receipt of bonuses, increased reimbursement rates, increased public recognition, and increased market share. In 2011, Leapfrog included the achievement of Magnet Recognition® in its annual survey, which represents recognition of the growing importance of this award in the market.

Although the organizations and initiatives just discussed are not meant to be exhaustive, these and other efforts have converged to spur the focus on quality in health care today.

[47]The Leapfrog Group. *About Us*. Retrieved July 31, 2011, at http://www.leapfroggroup.org/about_us.

[48]The Leapfrog Group. *Fact Sheet*. Retrieved August 8, 2006, at http://www.leapfroggroup.org/about_us/leapfrog-factsheet.

[49]Retrieved July 31, 2011, at http://www.leapfroggroup.org/media/file/FactSheet_LeapfrogGroup.pdf.

[50]The Leapfrog Hospital Recognition Program. Retrieved July 31, 2011, at http://www.leapfroggroup.org/media/file/2009LHRPFactSheet.pdf. See also http://www.leapfroggroup.org/media/file/LHRP_2010scoringmethodology.pdf.

[51]Retrieved July 31, 2011, at http://www.leapfroggroup.org/for_hospitals/fh-incentives_and_rewards/hosp_rewards_prog/4751817/4752142.

Many of these efforts have focused on reducing variations in quality at the provider level by standardizing processes, including the use of checklists, protocols, and standard operating procedures. In many respects, these efforts to standardize and make practice safer are long overdue. Although standardization may help to reduce variations in practice, there are concerns about the bureaucratization, depersonalization, and deprofessionalization that could result.[52] Mick and Mark[53] recommended that serious consideration be given to the type and extent of standardization enforced and to the benefits and costs of standardization.

Efforts have also focused on improving patients' involvement in their care by correcting the information imbalance that has traditionally existed in health care. That is, providers have in-depth knowledge about health care that is actually delivered and the care that should be delivered simply because they are trained in the provision of health care. Consumers, on the other hand, generally lack this in-depth knowledge and often rely on health care providers and other sources (including the Internet) to gather information. Because consumers rely on health care information from a variety of sources, there is a concern about the quality of information they receive. One mechanism for correcting the information imbalance between providers and consumers is the use of quality report cards aimed at equipping consumers with greater knowledge of provider performance and improving consumer choice.

Quality Reporting

The use of "report cards" has increased during the past decade as a way to grade and compare health care providers on measures of quality and performance. Report cards are typically based on available information about provider processes and outcomes, and these report cards are developed using either consumer surveys or audits. They are often constructed from data gathered on large national surveys of health care quality, such as the Health Plan Employer Data and Information Set (HEDIS) and the Consumer Assessments of Health Plans Survey (CAHPS). The intent of report cards is to (1) provide individuals, payers, and other decision makers with information upon which to base choices about providers and locations for receiving health care services and (2) stimulate quality improvements among providers.[54]

There are several public report cards, such as the one developed by the National Committee for Quality Assurance (NCQA). The NCQA is a private, not-for-profit organization dedicated to improving the quality of health care. Its vision is "to transform health care quality through measurement,

transparency and accountability."[55] This organization makes information on health plans available for individuals and families to use in decision making about health plans and insurance. Reports for health plans are constructed using HEDIS, a standardized set of performance measures developed by the NCQA, to determine how plans perform in key areas: quality of care, access to care, and member satisfaction with the health plan and physicians.[56] The NCQA also accredits health plans and HCOs based on quality of care measures and services provided[57] and provides access for its customers to the interactive tool, *Quality Compass*, that uses publicly reported NCQA data to determine a relative resource use quality index. This tool gives purchasers a way to select health plans, conduct a competitor analysis, and examine quality improvement and benchmarking plan performance.[58]

Other health care report cards include The Joint Commission's Quality Check and the Hospital Compare (discussed in Chapter 2 as part of the pay-for-performance discussion). Quality Check[59] is a Web-based tool that allows consumers to compare the quality of care at HCOs accredited by The Joint Commission. Hospital Compare, developed by CMS,[60] is another Web-based tool that provides information to consumers about hospital performance on quality improvement measures and allows them to compare process outcomes at different hospitals. There are also other types of report cards, such as those sponsored by individual states, The Leapfrog Group, and proprietary health care report cards such as *Health Grades* that provide competitive information across health care settings. *Consumer Reports* also offers a variety of resources for consumers to use in making decisions about health care and services, including an interactive tool that provides a state-by-state evaluation of physicians and hospitals,[61] a guide for selecting a long-term care facility,[62] and information about hospital safety based on surveys from both patients and nurses.[63] Finally, *U.S. News & World Report* ranks hospitals and specialty hospitals annually based on organizational reputation, mortality, and other factors, including patient-to-nurse ratios and Magnet Recognition®.[64]

[52]Mick S, Mark B. 2005. The contribution of organizational theory to nursing health services research. *Nurs Outlook* 53(6):317-323.

[53]*Ibid.*

[54]RAND. 2002. *Research Highlights: Report Cards for Health Care.* Retrieved September 3, 2006, at http://www.rand.org/pubs/research_briefs/RB4544/index1.html.

[55]National Committee for Quality Assurance. *About NCQA.* Retrieved August 8, 2006, at http://www.ncqa.org/tabid/65/Default.aspx.

[56]National Committee for Quality Assurance. Retrieved August 8, 2006, at http://www.ncqa.org/tabid/187/Default.aspx.

[57]For more details on NCQA's report cards, please see NCQA Report Cards, retrieved at http://www.ncqa.org/tabid/60/Default.aspx.

[58]Retrieved July 31, 2011, at http://www.ncqa.org/tabid/177/Default.aspx.

[59]Retrieved July 31, 2011, at http://www.qualitycheck.org/consumer/searchQCR.aspx.

[60]Retrieved July 31, 2011, at http://www.hospitalcompare.hhs.gov/hospital-search.aspx?AspxAutoDetectCookieSupport=1.

[61]Retrieved July 31, 2011, http://www.consumerreports.org/health/doctors-hospitals/doctors-and-hospitals.htm.

[62]Retrieved July 31, 2011, at http://www.consumerreports.org/health/doctors-hospitals/nursing-home-guide/0608_nursing-home-guide.htm.

[63]Patients beware: 731 nurses reveal what to watch out for in the hospital. *Consumer Reports.* Retrieved July 31, 2011, at http://www.consumerreports.org/health/doctors-hospitals/hospitals/overview/hospitals-and-nurses-ov.htm.

[64]Retrieved July 31, 2011, at http://static.usnews.com/documents/health/best-hospitals-methodology.pdf?s_cid=related-links:TOP.

The American Nurses Association's (ANA) "Nursing Care Report Card for Acute Care"[65] was developed to assess the contribution of nursing care to health care quality.[66] The following nursing care-specific indicators were developed[67-69]:

- Structural aspects of care: mix of registered nurses (RNs), licensed practical nurses (LPNs), and other nursing personnel; total nursing care hours per patient day
- Processes of care: skin integrity; nurse satisfaction
- Care outcomes: nosocomial infection rate; patient injury rate; patient satisfaction with nursing care, pain management, and educational information

On the basis of evaluations of these indicators, the ANA has reported that an inverse relationship exists between the number of licensed nursing hours per acuity-adjusted day and patient length of stay, and an inverse relationship also exists between likelihood of adverse patient events (e.g., postoperative infections, pressure ulcers, urinary tract infections) and a "richer" staff mix that included more RNs.[70] Although there were problems associated with the use of the ANA's report card indicators in the early stages of development,[71] many of these problems have been or are being addressed.[72]

The ANA's report card evolved into the National Database of Nursing Quality Indicators (NDNQIs),[73] an initiative that gathers unit-level nurse-sensitive data from U.S. hospitals. Hospitals pay an annual fee based on the number of beds (reported fees range from $1,800 for hospitals with fewer than 25 beds to $8,400 for hospitals with more than 500 beds in 2011) to participate in the NDNQI.[74] Although this is a proprietary database that belongs to the ANA, participating organizations receive unit-level reports for their organization quarterly. At the time of this writing, more than 1,400 hospitals across the United States were members of the NDNQI and in turn part of the ANA's quality reporting effort.[75]

Despite the potential of quality report cards, there are ongoing questions about the reliability and validity of report card indicators, the standardization of their use, and the availability of data.[76] In general, however, the use of report cards raises more fundamental questions: Do they achieve their intended purpose (i.e., do patients and purchasers use them to make cost and quality decisions)? Do they encourage HCOs to improve quality and patient outcomes? Do they instead simply encourage HCOs to meet certain standards to increase payments?

Using the results of several studies, the RAND Corporation determined that report cards have had little influence on consumer decision making and changing physician behavior, yet health provider organizations have been responsive in making improvements based on the results of these report cards.[77] In fact, improvements have been noted in diabetes care, women's health screening, childhood immunizations, smoking cessation, and management of heart disease. This finding is supported by other researchers,[78] who have suggested that the public reporting of quality information stimulates an increased emphasis on quality improvement initiatives in organizations where quality performance was low and in turn add value when quality objectives are achieved.

Some of the reasons offered in the RAND report for consumers' lack of report card use are that the information is not presented in an appealing and understandable format, the information is not relevant to their situations, the abundance of information is overwhelming, help is needed to make sense of the information, information is not always readily available (i.e., consumers do not have it when they need it, or even if it is available, they do not have time to seek the information and review it when they need it), and consumers are uncertain about the trustworthiness of the data.[79] The report goes on to say that the use of report cards could be increased if information were provided and communicated in a more organized manner, if targeted educational initiatives were provided for consumers, and if more systematic usability testing of public report cards were conducted to determine the most useful formats.

Another study suggested that hospitals and other providers have been more willing to embrace quality reporting efforts because they are linked to payment.[80] The study authors found that because these report cards are tied to payment and because hospitals tend to receive payment from multiple sources, hospitals may participate in multiple and varied reporting programs, each

[65]American Nurses Association. 1995. *Nursing Care Report Card for Acute Care*. Washington, DC: American Nurses Association.

[66]Moore K, Lynn M, McMillen B, Evans S. 1999. Implementation of the ANA Report Card. *J Nurs Adm* 29(6):48-54.

[67]American Nurses Association. 1997. *Implementing Nursing's Report Card: A Study of RN Staffing, Length of Stay, and Patient Outcomes*. Washington, DC: American Nurses Association.

[68]Jennings B, Loan L, DePaul D, et al. 2001. Lessons learned while collecting ANA indicator data. *J Nurs Adm* 31(3):121-129.

[69]McGillis Hall L. 2002. Report cards: Relevance for nursing and patient safety. *Int Counc Nurses* 49:168-177.

[70]Rowell P. 2001. Lessons learned while collecting ANA indicator data: The American Nurses Association responds. *J Nurs Adm* 31(3):130-131.

[71]Jennings B, et al., *Op. cit.*, 2001.

[72]Rowell P, *Op. cit.* See also Montalvo I. (September 30, 2007). The National Database of Nursing Quality Indicators™ (NDNQI®) *OJIN* 12(3), Manuscript 2; and Clarke SP, Donaldson NE. 2008. Nurse staffing and patient care quality and safety. In *Patient Safety and Quality: An Evidence-Based Handbook for Nurses*. Rockville, MD: Agency for Healthcare Research and Quality. Retrieved at http://www.ncbi.nlm.nih.gov/books/NBK2676/.

[73]For more information, please visit http://www.nursingquality.org/Default.aspx.

[74]Retrieved July 31, 2011, at https://www.nursingquality.org/BecomeA Participant.aspx.

[75]Retrieved July 31, 2011, at http://www.nursingworld.org/MainMenu Categories/ThePracticeofProfessionalNursing/PatientSafetyQuality/Publications/Hospital-Profiles.aspx.

[76]McGillis Hall, *Op. cit.*, 2002.

[77]RAND Corporation. 2006. *Research Brief. Document number RB-9053-2*. Retrieved July 31, 2011, at http://www.rand.org/pubs/research_briefs/RB9053-2.html.

[78]Hibbard J, Stockard J, Tusler M. 2003. Does publicizing hospital performance stimulate quality improvement efforts? *Health Aff* 22(2):84-95. See also http://www.cfah.org/hbns/preparedpatient/Prepared-Patient-Vol1-Issue11.cfm and What can we say about the impact of public reporting? Inconsistent execution yields variable results. *Ann Intern Med* 148:160-161.

[79]RAND Corporation, *Op. cit.*, 2006.

[80]Pham H, Coughlan J, O'Malley A. 2006. The impact of quality-reporting programs on hospital operations. *Health Aff* 25(5):1412-1422.

with a different focus.[81] Also, whereas quality reporting programs that were perceived as necessary (e.g., CMS and The Joint Commission) tended to provide incentives that "pushed" the organization to improve quality, other programs such as the IHI, state quality improvement organizations, and professional organizations that offered tools and resources to the organizations to change practices, provided incentives that "pulled" the organization to improve care processes. This study also reported that despite the increase in quality improvement resources that comes with participation in these report card programs, the resources available for quality measurement and improvement remain inadequate. Most frequently cited as lacking were information technology systems to support quality improvement efforts. The authors recommended that policy efforts be directed toward coordinating quality reporting programs to avoid duplication and to standardize data collection across programs as well as to support and encourage improvements in information technology systems.[82]

Balanced Scorecards

Another type of report card used by organizations is the balanced scorecard.[83] Balanced scorecards are used internally for strategic management purposes and as a way to examine performance. Typically, performance is monitored in four areas[84]:

- Customer perspective
- Financial perspective
- Internal processes (including human resources)
- Learning and growth

Within these four areas, organizations identify and examine their performance on a key set of measures selected based on the importance to the organization. Information obtained from this self-evaluation is typically shared within the organization to improve processes, but it may be used as the framework for reporting to boards of directors and even the public, if desired. Balanced scorecards are valuable to organizations because they allow organizations to look inward to determine the degree to which they have met their strategic objectives.

In HCOs, balanced scorecards provide the vehicle by which organizations can integrate and disseminate clinical, operational, and financial data to inform decision making.[85] The Clinical Value Compass uses a similar approach for improving and disseminating information about clinical care throughout the HCO. In this case, patient care processes and outcomes are assessed based on specific clinical, functional, cost, and patient satisfaction outcomes.[86]

The Magnet Movement

Kramer and Schmalenberg[87] present a historical overview of the quality movement in nursing based on Magnet hospitals. Magnet hospitals are organizations that are recognized as providing excellent, high-quality nursing care while attracting and retaining nurses. The Magnet hospital concept was originally conceived to address concerns about recurring nursing shortages, specifically, to identify and examine HCOs that were particularly good at recruiting and retaining nurses and in turn delivering high-quality care. The original Magnet hospital study, conducted in 1982 and 1983, was grounded in the structure–process–outcome framework of Donabedian. The early research on Magnet hospitals reported that both nurse satisfaction and retention were related to nurses' ability to deliver quality care. Magnet hospitals of the time were claimed to be analogous to Peters and Waterman's "Best Run" companies, described in their now classic book *In Search of Excellence*.[88]

The Magnet Hospital concept has evolved over time, with the launch of the Magnet Recognition® Program and the development of its "14 forces of magnetism" in the early 1990s. The first hospital received Magnet designation in 1994. Today, the American Nurses Credentialing Center's (ANCC) Magnet Recognition Program offers certification to hospitals that meet its standards. At the time of this writing, almost 400 hospitals have been designated as Magnet facilities.[89]

To receive the Magnet certification, hospitals are assessed based on the degree to which they excel in five key areas:

- Transformational Leadership
- Structural Empowerment
- Exemplary Professional Practice
- New Knowledge, Innovations, and Improvements
- Empirical Quality Outcomes

These five areas were derived from the original "14 forces of magnetism" to streamline the Magnet application process and the documentation required.[90] Linkages between the original forces of magnetism and the new model components are shown in Table 5-1.

Hospitals are required to make application to ANCC to be considered for recognition, and to pay various required fees, which include an application fee (estimated at $3,900), an appraisal fee (based on the number of licensed acute care beds, ranging from $13,750 for 100 beds or fewer to $57,850 up to 950 beds plus $65 per additional bed or $27,850 for an independent outpatient care center), a document review fee ($2,500 for the team leader plus $2,000 for each team member), and a site visit fee ($1,850 per appraiser per day).[91] Each

[81]*Ibid.*

[82]*Ibid.*

[83]McGillis Hall, *Op. cit.*, 2002.

[84]See the classic work of Robert Kaplan and David Norton cited at the end of this chapter for more details on the balanced scorecard.

[85]See, for example, Oliveira J. 2001. The balanced scorecard: An integrative approach to performance evaluation. *Healthc Financ Manage* 55(5):42-46; and Zelman WN, Pink GH, Matthias CB. 2003. Use of the balanced scorecard in health care. *J Health Care Finance* 29(4):1-16.

[86]Nelson E, Mohr J, Batalden P, Plume S. 1996. Improving health care, part 1: The clinical value compass. *Jt Comm J Qual Improv* 22(4):243-258.

[87]Kramer M, Schmalenberg C. 2005. Best quality patient care: A historical perspective on magnet hospitals. *Nurs Adm Q* 29(3):275-287.

[88]Peters RJ, Waterman RH. 1982. *In search of excellence*. New York: Harper Row.

[89]Retrieved July 31, 2011, at http://www.nursecredentialing.org/Magnet/FindaMagnetFacility.aspx.

[90]Retrieved July 31, 2011, at http://www.nursecredentialing.org/Magnet/ProgramOverview/New-Magnet-Model.aspx.

[91]Retrieved July 31, 2011, at http://www.nursecredentialing.org/Magnet ScheduleFees.aspx.

✳ **TABLE 5–1** *A Comparison of the Original and New Magnet Approaches*

	Original Magnet Approach: 14 Forces of Magnetism	Reflected in . . .	New Magnet Approach: 5 Model Components
1	Quality of Nursing Leadership	⇒	Transformational Leadership
2	Organizational Structure	⇒	Structural Empowerment
3	Management Style	⇒	Transformational Leadership
4	Personnel Policies & Programs	⇒	Structural Empowerment
5	Professional Models of Care	⇒	Exemplary Professional Practice
6	Quality of Care	⇒	Empirical Quality Outcomes
7	Quality Improvement	⇒	New Knowledge, Innovations, Improvements
8	Consultation & Resources	⇒	Exemplary Professional Practice
9	Autonomy	⇒	Exemplary Professional Practice
10	Community & Health Care Organization	⇒	Structural Empowerment
11	Nurses as Teachers	⇒	Exemplary Professional Practice
12	Image of Nursing	⇒	Structural Empowerment
13	Interdisciplinary Relationships	⇒	Exemplary Professional Practice
14	Professional Development	⇒	Structural Empowerment

Based on information obtained from American Nurses Credentialing Center, Magnet Recognition Program Model® http://www.nursecredentialing.org/Magnet/NewMagnet/Model.aspx; and Overview of ANCC Magnet Recognition Program® (2008), http://www.nursecredentialing.org/Magnet/NewMagnetModel.aspx. Accessed April 7, 2012.

facility prepares an application describing the structures and processes that reflect sources of evidence for the model components and associated empirical outcomes. During a site visit, the facility receives an in-depth review of documentation provided with its application and undergoes a rigorous onsite assessment by a minimum of two expert appraisers to verify and expand on information provided. The Magnet Model and supporting documentation serve as the basis for the onsite visit that lasts usually a minimum of 2 days. Public comments are also sought by ANCC for organizations undergoing assessment as part of their evaluation to verify information provided in the application and observations made during the site visit.[92]

Research has shown that patients cared for at Magnet facilities may have better outcomes. For example, one of the earliest outcomes studies reported that patient mortality was lower in Magnet hospitals,[93] and subsequent studies have reported that patient satisfaction is higher[94] and falls are lower[95] in Magnet versus non-Magnet hospitals. Nurses also perceived a more supportive work environment, higher job satisfaction, and lower levels of burnout in Magnet hospitals.[96] However, recent studies have reported that there were no differences between Magnet and non-Magnet hospitals in nurses' perceptions of working conditions, and that, in some cases, the outcomes achieved in non-Magnet hospitals may be as good or better than those of Magnet hospitals[97] It is also unclear whether the public truly appreciates Magnet Recognition® and what it represents or whether they use this information to make decisions about where to receive care. Although Magnet facilities may have a good reputation within their communities and in turn may enjoy patient loyalty because of that reputation, Magnet facilities may not necessarily derive direct financial benefits from their recognition as a Magnet hospital. This may change, however, as influential purchasing groups such as Leapfrog (described earlier) consider Magnet Recognition® in their approaches for making value-based purchasing decisions, and as influential rating groups, such as *U.S. News & World Reports*, include Magnet Recognition® in their methodologies for ranking hospitals.

Based on a program developed by the Texas Nurses Association to recognize small and rural hospitals, the ANCC rolled out its Pathway to Excellence® program in 2007. The Pathway program is more broadly focused on all types of organizations, including long-term care organizations.[98] Organizations awarded this recognition must reflect a work environment that fosters nursing excellence and support 12 standards, including control

[92]Retrieved July 31, 2011, at http://www.nursecredentialing.org/Functional Category/FAQ/DEO-FAQ.aspx. See also eligibility requirements for individual organizations applying for Magnet status at http://www.nursecredentialing.org/OrgEligibilityRequirements.aspx and health care systems applying for Magnet status at http://www.nursecredentialing.org/SysEligibilityRequirements.aspx.

[93]Aiken L, Smith H, Lake E. 1994. Lower Medicare mortality among a set of hospitals known for good nursing care. *Med Care* 32:771-787.

[94]See Aiken L, Sloane D, Lake E. 1997. Satisfaction with inpatient acquired immunodeficiency syndrome care: A national comparison of dedicated and scattered-bed units. *Med Care* 35(9):948-962; and Aiken L, Sloane D, Lake E, et al. 1999. Organization and outcomes of inpatient AIDS care. *Med Care* 37(8):760-772.

[95]Lake ET, Shang J, Klaus S, Dunton NE. 2010. Patient falls: Association with hospital Magnet status and nursing unit staffing. *Res Nurs Health* 33(5): 413-425.

[96]Laschinger HKS, Shamian J, Thomson D. 2001. Impact of Magnet hospital characteristics on nurses' perceptions of trust, burnout, quality of care, and work satisfaction. *Nurs Econ* 19(5):209-219.

[97]See Trinkoff AM, Johantgen, M, Storr CL, et al. 2010. A comparison of working conditions among nurses in Magnet® and Non-Magnet® Hospitals. *J Nurs Adm* 40(7/8):309-315; and Goode CJ, Blegen MA, Park SH, et al. 2011. Comparison of patient outcomes in Magnet® and non-Magnet® hospitals. *J Nurs Adm* 41(12), 517-523.

[98]Retrieved July 31, 2011, at http://www.nursecredentialing.org/Pathway/AboutPathway.aspx.

over practice, and a work environment and systems in place that support quality and safe nursing care. The application fee for this program is $700, which is considerably less than the Magnet program fee. Other fees are also required, including a document submission fee (ranging from as low as about $6,000 for smaller acute care or long-term care facilities to more than $22,000 for larger ones and between $8,000 and $15,000 for ambulatory or independent outpatient facilities), a clarification fee (if additional document reviews are needed), and an annual review fee of $250.[99] Pathway recognition may be sought by organizations that do not desire (or cannot afford) to apply for Magnet Recognition® or as the first step for organizations before they apply for Magnet Recognition®. At the time of this writing, about 70 organizations in 16 states had been recognized as Pathway organizations.[100]

Chief executive officers (CEOs) and other hospital leaders have begun to appreciate the importance of Magnet Recognition® and Pathway Excellence® designation, especially in competitive markets where there may be other Magnet or Pathway facilities nearby. Chief nurse executives (CNEs) are expected to be knowledgeable of the process needed to achieve these recognitions, and many are recruited to HCOs based on their experiences leading Magnet or Pathway initiatives.

Magnet designation represents a significant investment for HCOs, yet that investment is purported to be offset by lower nurse recruitment and turnover costs.[101] Drenkard contends that a return on investment (ROI) can be estimated to illustrate the benefits of Magnet Recognition® and used to evaluate long-run financial gains. These returns come in the cost savings achieved through increased staff nurse retention and lower burnout; decreased vacancy and turnover costs; decreased agency use; decreased staff injuries; and increased patient, nurse, and quality outcomes. Drawing on the literature, Drenkard estimated the overall cost savings for a 500-bed hospital to be around $2.3 million.[102] However, beyond the direct costs associated with the Magnet program is the investment to change the nursing and organizational culture from one that focuses exclusively on costs to one that strives to balance costs and quality by way of the magnet components.[103] There is a need for research to document the costs and benefits associated with Magnet Recognition® and each of its components and to determine whether the benefits of obtaining Magnet status outweigh the costs of doing so. Until such research is available, organizations must review the literature; weigh the costs and benefits of acquiring and maintaining Magnet

Recognition®; and calculate their own ROI based on their philosophy of care delivery, belief in the program, and commitment to quality nursing care.

The Baldridge Award

A national award that recognizes quality and excellence in the business sector is the Malcolm Baldridge National Quality Award. This award, named after Secretary of Commerce Malcolm Baldridge, was established by Congress in 1987. The Baldridge Award is a prestigious award that is made by the president of the United States to recognize organizations that excel in seven areas[104]:

- Leadership
- Strategic planning
- Customer focus
- Measurement, analysis, and knowledge management
- Workforce focus
- Operations focus
- Results

The award is not given for specific products or services but rather for quality performance. Up to three awards may be given each year in the following categories: manufacturing, service, small business, education, health care, and nonprofit.[105] Responsibility for program oversight is within the U.S. Department of Commerce, and the program is managed by an agency within it, the National Institute of Standards and Technology (NIST).

To be considered for this award, organizations must submit an application documenting excellence in the seven areas just listed, pay a series of fees,[106] and undergo a rigorous organizational analysis and assessment by a Board of Examiners. The Board of Examiners is composed of a minimum of eight quality experts. Public and private organizations are eligible to apply for this award. Many well-known U.S. organizations have received this award, such as Nestlé, Honeywell, AT&T, Motorola, and Boeing, as well as some that are not as widely recognized, such as Pal's Sudden Service, Texas Nameplate Co., Inc., and the Chugach School District. At the time of this writing, 12 HCOs had received the Baldridge Award.

Obviously, HCOs can set a goal of applying and receiving recognition from both Baldridge and Magnet®. In fact, some of the Baldridge Award winners in health care are Magnet hospitals. However, because of the time and expense associated with both programs, HCOs may be faced with choosing to invest in one program over the other. According to studies conducted by the NIST, the Government Accounting Office, and others,

[99]Retrieved July 31, 2011, at http://www.nursecredentialing.org/Pathway/PathwayFees.aspx.

[100]Retrieved July 31, 2011, at http://www.nursecredentialing.org/Pathway/DesignationOrganizations.aspx.

[101]Brady-Schwartz D. 2005. Further evidence on the Magnet Recognition Program: Implications for nursing leaders. *J Nurs Adm* 35(9):397-403.

[102]Drenkard K. 2010. The business case for Magnet. *J Nurs Adm* 40(6): 263-271.

[103]McClure M, Hinshaw A. 2002. *Magnet Hospitals Revisited: Attraction and Retention of Professional Nurses.* Washington, DC: American Nurses Publishing. See also Russell J. 2010. Journey to Magnet™: Cost vs. benefits. *Nursing Econ* 28(5):340-342.

[104]Retrieved July 31, 2011, at http://www.nist.gov/baldrige/publications/criteria.cfm.

[105]Retrieved July 31, 2011, at http://www.nist.gov/baldrige/about/baldrige_faqs.cfm.

[106]Organizations may be required to pay all or some of the following fees: an eligibility fee of $150; an application fee ranging from $1,250 for some educational programs, $3,500 for small businesses, and as much as $7000 for large organizations; a supplemental fee is required for the site visit; and a $1,250 processing fee is required for applications submitted on a computer disk. For more information see specific to health care, see http://www.nist.gov/baldrige/enter/health_care.cfm (retrieved July 31, 2011).

"investing in quality principles and performance excellence pays off in increased productivity, satisfied employees and customers, and improved profitability—both for customers and investors."[107] Does either of these awards ensure the best possible quality 100% of the time? Not necessarily.

The decision to invest in pursuing Magnet designation or the Baldridge Award depends on the strategic goals of the organization at any point in time. Baldridge acknowledges that its criteria are consistent with those of the Magnet Recognition® Program, The Joint Commission Accreditation, and IHI initiatives.

✳ RELATIONSHIPS AMONG HEALTH CARE QUALITY, COSTS, AND FINANCING

The relationship among health care quality, costs, and financing is very complex, and although these aspects of care delivery are linked in some formal ways, they are indelibly linked in many informal ways. Although the definition of quality and in turn its presence or absence may depend on perspective, costs are incurred regardless. Moreover, although our financing system is moving toward pay for performance, not all payments are based on quality. In some cases, payment may be made to providers based on their performance on certain outcomes, but meeting certain thresholds on certain outcomes does not mean that high-quality care is necessarily provided.

A few definitions are important to clarify when discussing health care quality, costs, and financing. *Value,* defined broadly, is the relationship between costs and quality[108]:

Value = Quality/Cost

The relationship between cost and quality is illustrated in Figure 5-1. Moving from low costs or expenditures to higher costs, quality increases. Some argue that efforts to increase quality may reach a point where increased expenditures result

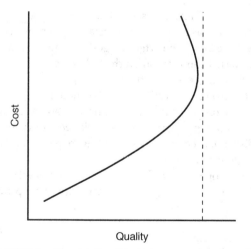

FIGURE 5–1. The relationship between cost and quality.

in no further increases in quality—and may actually lead to a reduction in quality. In other words, putting ever-increasing amounts of money into quality improvement efforts may not always achieve the outcomes intended. This point can be illustrated using an example from research. Blegen and colleagues examined the relationship between nurse staffing and patient outcomes.[109] They reported that as the proportion of RN staffing increased, rates of adverse outcomes decreased—up to a point. When RN proportion increased above 87%, adverse outcomes also increased. To bring this back to costs, this finding suggests that simply spending more and more money to increase RN staffing levels alone and beyond certain levels may not improve quality. The same general relationship may hold as shown in Figure 5-1. An important question that must be asked is how we can increase quality without simply increasing costs. Porter and Teisberg argue that high quality may actually cost *less*.[110]

One way to achieve quality and lower costs is by focusing on *efficiency,* or the "mix of health care resource inputs that produce optimal quantity and quality of health and health care outputs."[111] Put another way, efficiency is the relationship between inputs and outputs[112]:

Efficiency = Output/Input

Inputs are generally taken to be direct costs (e.g., labor, capital, equipment), but they also can be in the form of indirect costs, such as staff time required to engage in certain processes. Efficiency is generally concerned with eliminating unnecessary procedures, waste in the system, and administrative costs.[113] If we can do more with less or even accomplish the same result with less input, efficiency increases.

Another way to achieve quality and lower costs is by focusing on *effectiveness,* or the degree to which outcomes or results are achieved as intended. In health care, effectiveness means that a treatment, service, or technology provides a benefit to recipients under *usual* or natural circumstances.[114] Effectiveness in health care also implies the appropriate use of knowledge and evidence to achieve a desired outcome while considering patients' values.[115]

The relationship among quality, costs, and financing is muddied by the fact that the persons or groups that receive care generally want the highest quality care possible regardless of cost and certainly without full knowledge of costs. Because

[109]Blegen MA, Goode CJ, Reed, L. 1998. Nurse staffing and patient outcomes. *Nurs Res* 47(1):43-50.

[110]Porter ME, Teisberg EO. 2006. *Redefining Health Care: Creating Value-Based Competition on Results.* Cambridge, MA: Harvard Business Review Press.

[111]Committee on Redesigning Health Insurance Performance Measures, Payment, and Performance Improvement Programs. 2006. *Performance Measurement: Accelerating Improvement.* Institute of Medicine. Washington, DC: National Academies Press.

[112]Palmer S, Torgerson D. 1999. Economics notes: Definitions of efficiency. *BMJ* 318(7191):1136.

[113]Committee on Quality of Health Care in America, *Op. cit.,* p. 52.

[114]Retrieved September 11, 2006, at http://www.nlm.nih.gov/nichsr/ihcm/01whatis/whatis08.html#Effectiveness. Effectiveness is distinguished from efficacy in that efficacy implies that a benefit is achieved under ideal or controlled conditions.

[115]Committee on Quality of Health Care in America, *Op. cit.,* pp. 47-48.

[107]*Ibid.*

[108]Folland S, Goodman A, Stano M. 2009. *The Economics of Health and Health Care,* 6th edition. Upper Saddle River, NJ: Prentice-Hall.

the person or groups receiving care do not know the actual costs of care, they are unable to determine whether the care they receive is a good value or to determine the level of care that they are willing to purchase. Enthoven[116] argues that knowledge of quality, product features, and prices or costs is needed to discern value and to make purchasing decisions in health care. Making purchasing decisions in health care without knowledge of quality and costs is like taking a best guess or even rolling the dice.

Unfortunately, this approach to decision making in health care is all too common. There is a great deal of "medical guesswork" that goes into health care decision making, and the health care industry at large still knows very little about the treatments that really work and why.[117] This lack of knowledge affects the information that gets passed on to patients and patients' ability to determine the value of care they will receive.

The other complicating factor is that in our financing system, a third party (i.e., not the person giving or receiving the care but another entity) generally makes decisions about the type and amount of care that will be purchased for those who receive care. This third party (i.e., the payer or insurer) also has some say in the price of the care that is provided. Thus, payers have some level of knowledge of costs and quality, and they in turn make decisions for those who will receive care. Insurers determine who receives care and the type of care they receive, and they select plans that will deliver the care for the price negotiated. Payers also manage patient enrollment into plans and the risks associated with the care patients receive and create price-elastic demand by forcing providers to reduce prices in order to increase revenues.[118] It is the payer that estimates value, not the person receiving care, and the payer may well have a stronger interest in low costs than in high quality. Thus, choices about the quality and costs of health care are filtered through the payer.

The IOM *Crossing the Quality Chasm*[119] report identified several sources of costs associated with quality. There are the obvious costs of measuring, monitoring, and maintaining a quality improvement program in HCOs and all of the training and prevention planning that goes with the process. There are also short- and long-term investments that must be incurred to ensure the integrity and maintenance of a quality program. However, some costs are often "unseen," such as those incurred when a service is not delivered (i.e., underuse of care), when services are delivered but not needed (i.e., overuse), or when services are delivered inappropriately (misuse). Other examples include the redundancy in patient testing and the duplication of services that often occurs in health care, simply for the convenience of providers or to protect them from litigation. The lack of information-sharing among providers adds costs, delays care, and puts the burden of undergoing sometimes uncomfortable and painful procedures on patients unnecessarily. Costs are also associated with poor quality—that is, organizations may be willing to incur the costs of "redoing" a process if needed but unwilling to incur the upfront costs to deliver a service the right way in the first place. Finally, psychological costs are associated with poor quality, such as frustrated staff, loss of professional integrity, turnover, dissatisfied patients, errors, and a bad reputation.

Research at Dartmouth has shown that both costs and quality vary by geographic region and the practices within them. For example, some regions within the United States spend much less on health care than others but achieve better patient outcomes. Dartmouth researchers determined that health care spending could be reduced by as much as 20% to 30% (and maybe more) if higher-spending regions adopted similar care delivery practices and achieved the same level of quality as certain low-spending regions.[120]

An important question to ask is what structural changes in the U.S. health care delivery and financing system would allow us to purchase more quality with the dollars we currently spend? A follow-up question is if structural changes can be made, how would we go about making such changes? Although there is general agreement that system changes are needed to provide incentives that promote quality, there are differing perspectives on the specific changes needed to increase our purchasing power. For example, in 2011 the U.S. Department of Health and Human Services adopted recommendations from the IOM regarding coverage of all contraceptive methods as a preventive benefit free of co-payment responsibility.[121] Some might contend that this preventive benefit will save society money over time, but others might argue that removing the need for any deductible or co-payment will result in overconsumption of these services, resulting in a net increase in costs.

Porter and Teisberg[122] argue that mistargeted competition in health care has impeded the satisfactory performance of the U.S. health care system. They suggest that our health care system has based competition on the following:
- The wrong level (i.e., the insurer)
- The wrong objective (i.e., cost reduction)
- The wrong form (i.e., competition among plans; competition among providers to be included in plans based on discounts; competition about who pays: the plan, the provider, or the patient)
- The wrong level in the market (i.e., local level)
- The wrong strategies and structure (i.e., providing a broad or shallow range of services)

---

[116]Enthoven A. 1993. The history and principles of managed competition. *Health Aff* 12(suppl):27-43.

[117]Carey J. May 29, 2006. Medical guesswork. *Bus Wk* 3983:72-79.

[118]*Ibid.*

[119]Committee on Quality of Health Care in America, *Op. cit.,* 2001.

[120]Retrieved July 31, 2011, at http://www.dartmouthatlas.org/keyissues/issue.aspx?con=1338.

[121]See http://www.hhs.gov/news/press/2011pres/08/20110801b.html (retrieved August 4, 2011).

[122]Porter M, Teisberg E. 2004. Redefining competition in health care. *Harv Bus Rev* 82(6):65-76. See also Porter ME, Teisberg EO. 2006. *Redefining Health Care: Creating Value-Based Competition on Results.* Cambridge, MA: Harvard Business Review Press.

- The wrong information (i.e., information is not available to all, and the best available information is not always known or used by providers)
- The wrong incentives for payers (i.e., payers benefit by enrolling healthy individuals or charging premiums, coinsurance, and co-payment rates or denying coverage to those who are sick)
- The wrong incentives for providers (i.e., providers are rewarded financially if they minimize patient referrals, spend less time with patients, discharge patients quickly, and readmit patients only if necessary, yet the fear of malpractice often encourages overtreatment).

The authors propose instead that competition should focus on prevention; creating and improving value in the system; developing deep levels of expertise; creating regional or national markets; providing information to consumers and payers about providers, treatments, and alternatives; providing incentives so that payers help enrollees find the best care value; simplifying administrative and billing processes; and encouraging providers to develop areas of excellence and expertise, measure and enhance quality and efficiency, and set up systems to eliminate mistakes and improve standards. The ACA addresses some of these issues (e.g., prevention, focusing on value-based purchasing, simplifying administrative processes, addressing mistakes), and other resources have been put into place outside of this effort (e.g., hospital report cards and websites for comparing providers), but the degree to which these objectives will be achieved—or not—is merely speculation at this point.

Enthoven and Tollen[123] provide a counterargument that suggests competition should be focused at the level of systems of care versus the individual level of provider as advocated by Porter and Teisberg. Enthoven and Tollen define *systems of care* as integrated delivery systems, or large, multi-specialty group practices networked with hospitals, laboratories, pharmacies, and other essential facilities and services supported by per-capita prepayment (see Chapter 2 for a more detailed description of managed care and per-member payment). They acknowledge that consumers should have a choice of integrated delivery systems. They also argue that to align provider incentives with patients' interests, systems of care must have the following characteristics: risk-adjusted prepayment to reward providers for keeping patients healthy; use of appropriate, evidence-based care; coordination of care across the care continuum (i.e., from home, to hospital, to home care); comprehensive patient records for the sharing of information; and incorporated strategies to improve efficiency.

An important issue in the discussion of health care costs, quality, and financing is *access*. The ANA has long held that issues pertaining cost, quality, and access represent the cornerstone of its agenda.[124] A classic definition of access to care is the "fit" between the client and the health care system regarding the availability of care, the adaptability of care to patients' needs (and of patient to the system), the affordability of care, and the acceptability of care.[125] Many individuals do not have access for all of these reasons. However, over the past 2 decades, the primary reason, unfortunately, pertains to costs. Insurance coverage, often considered a proxy for access, is now lacking for some 50 million people in the United States.[126] In a recent report, the United States was last among seven countries (Australia, Canada, Germany, the Netherlands, New Zealand, the United Kingdom, and the United States) on dimensions of access to care, costs, and safety and ranked sixth on overall quality.[127] As discussed in Chapter 2, the United States spends almost double the per-capita spending of all other countries, yet many people in the United States do not have access to care. The authors of a recent report attribute the United States' poor ranking to a lack of universal health coverage, which is available in the other six countries. Also, Americans with health problems reported the greatest difficulty accessing care.[128] This lack of access to needed care affects the overall health of our society and contributes to a revolving door system in which patients receive care in overburdened emergency departments, public health system, or free clinics. In essence, the lack of access to care may add more costs back into a costly system. These issues will be even more important in the coming years as the ACA is put into place. Will resources continue to flow to hospitals? Will procedures with questionable effectiveness still be recommended and reimbursed? Only time will tell how these issues are addressed in the changes that lie ahead.

Given the sources of impetus for examining quality and integrating quality, costs, and financing cited earlier, there is little argument that changes are needed to address quality, costs, and financing issues. The bigger concern is how health care providers can best achieve quality efficiently and effectively. Although Porter and Teisberg and Enthoven and Tollen offer differing perspectives on structural systems changes needed to better integrate quality, costs, and financing, others suggest that a business case can be made for investing in quality.

A Business Case for Quality

A business case is simply a position on whether or not an investment should be made in a project or initiative based on a systematic evaluation of the worth or value of the project or initiative. A business case involves the calculation of costs and benefits, rates of return on investments, break-even points, and other financial indices.[129] The development and interpretation of a business case will depend on perspective.

[123]Enthoven A, Tollen L. 2005. Competition in health care: It takes systems to pursue quality and efficiency. *Health Aff (Millwood)* W5-420-W5-433.

[124]Retrieved July 31, 2011, at http://nursingworld.org/FunctionalMenu Categories/AboutANA/WhatWeDo/Reports/AgendafortheFuture.aspx.

[125]Penchansky R, Thomas WJ. 1981. The concept of access: Definition and relationship to consumer satisfaction. *Med Care* 19(2):127-140.

[126]Retrieved July 31, 2011, at http://www.kff.org/uninsured/upload/7451-06. pdf.

[127]Retrieved July 31, 2011, at http://www.commonwealthfund.org/~/media/ Files/Publications/Fund%20Report/2010/Jun/1400_Davis_Mirror_Mirror_on_ the_wall_2010.pdf.

[128]*Ibid.*

[129]Jones C. 2005. The costs of nursing turnover, part 2: Application of the Nursing Turnover Cost Calculation Methodology. *J Nurs Adm* 35(1):41-49.

Consideration must be given to the entity (or entities) required to make investments and the entity (or entities) to which the returns accrue. That is, do investments and returns accrue to the organizational provider? The clinicians? The purchaser? The employer? Society? Some combination thereof? An important aspect of the business case is that the returns do not necessarily accrue to the entity making the investment. Another important point is that returns may not accrue during the timeframe expected.

Leatherman and colleagues[130] examined whether improved quality provides a return on investment as well as the kinds of HCOs that realized a financial benefit. They examined improvements in chronic disease management, patient safety, waste reduction, prevention, and approaches to value-based purchasing by estimating the financial and clinical implications of quality in four specific cases: the management of high-cost pharmaceuticals, diabetes management, smoking cessation, and employer-based wellness programs.

The results of their study were inconclusive but enlightening. For example, the high-cost pharmaceutical programs they examined had a favorable financial impact on patients and society but an unfavorable financial impact on the care provider and mixed returns for the purchaser. The diabetes management program had an unfavorable financial impact on the care provider but a favorable financial impact on the purchaser, the patient, and society. The smoking cessation program had an unfavorable financial impact on the care provider and a neutral and unknown impact on the purchaser but a favorable impact on the patient and society. Finally, the wellness program had a favorable impact on the care provider, the purchaser, the patients, and society.

Interestingly, the authors made several observations worth noting. First, there is a failure in our system of financing to pay for quality, yet the system is willing to pay for system defects. For example, some aspects of the diabetes care management and smoking cessation programs could not be billed to anyone, yet these care management services were essential to the provision of the service. Also, payers incurred costs long after patients' problems developed. To overcome this problem, Leatherman and colleagues recommended that the government and other purchasers consider care management activities as essential, versus optional, services.

Second, they noted that consumers are unable to distinguish quality. To overcome this problem, they recommended that patients demand defect reports; that clinicians and organizations publicly report performance and defect problems; and that the government and payers release hospital-specific mortality data, educate the public on optional models of care delivery, and pay differentially for higher cost patients.

Third, they noted that returns may not accrue immediately and are often displaced far into the future. They recommend that the government and payers address this problem by offering capitated population-based payment, unifying Medicare Parts A and B (see Chapter 2 for a discussion of capitated payment and Medicare), paying for case management, providing disincentives for changing caregivers, and investing in prevention and chronic care programs.

Fourth, they emphasized the disconnect between consumers and payers and suggested that consumers pay for the care they prefer within a set of options. They also recommended that the government and payers encourage innovations in care (e.g., chronic care management) and experiment with paying for nontraditional care delivery methods (e.g., e-mail consultation). Finally, they noted that there is uneven access to information among clinicians, making the implementation of evidence-based practice challenging. They recommended that consumers become savvy in acquiring science-based protocols to discuss with their clinicians, that providers adopt electronic patient records and other mechanisms of decision support, and that the government and payers support the development of an information infrastructure and use their paying power to enforce the use of evidence-based practice.

This analysis tells us that there is much more we need to know to determine a business case for quality in all instances. For example, in another study (discussed in more detail in Chapter 9), Needleman and colleagues[131] examined three nurse staffing scenarios and reported that there is an "unequivocal" business case for increasing nurse staffing under one of the three scenarios they examined (i.e., raising the proportion of RN staffing without changing the number of total licensed hours of care provided), but the business case was less clear among the other choices.

Attempts to develop a business case for quality represent an important step toward better understanding the cost and financing implications of quality and for evaluating investment decisions based on differing levels of inputs and outputs. By doing so, patients, payers, and providers can use this information to trade off the costs they are willing to incur for varying levels of quality. Reiter and colleagues urge HCOs to adopt the business case approach to more clearly delineate the costs and investments of quality-enhancing interventions and to encourage the uptake of known, successful, and evidence-based quality improvements.[132] These authors provide a checklist that can be used to assess organizational readiness for developing a business case for quality improvement initiatives. This approach can also help to identify the actions and policies that are needed to better align our system of rewards and incentives to provide more value for patients, providers, and society.

✳ IMPLICATIONS FOR NURSE MANAGERS AND EXECUTIVES

Quality is a complex issue that can be difficult to define and measure. However, an understanding of the concept and its relationship to cost and financing issues is critically important

---

[130]Leatherman S, Berwick D, Iles D, et al. 2003. The business case for quality: Case studies and an analysis. *Health Aff* 22(2):17-30.

[131]Needleman J, Buerhaus P, Stewart M, et al. 2006. Nurse staffing in hospitals: Is there a business case for quality? *Health Aff* 25(1):204-211.

[132]Reiter KL, Kilpatrick KE, Greene SB, et al. 2007. How to develop a business case for quality. *Int J Qual Health Care* 19(1):50-55.

for nurse managers and executives. The momentum to place quality in the forefront of health care has been building over the past 2 decades. Unfortunately, we have only scratched the surface in understanding the financial incentives needed to affect quality initiatives and truly making headway in improving the quality of health care.

Report cards are a mechanism for publicly reporting quality information to patients and purchasers. The idea behind making quality information publicly available to patients and purchasers is that they will use the information to make decisions about providers, where and how care will be received or provided, and the value of the care they can expect to receive. Although report cards may be an important incentive that encourages HCOs to initiate quality improvement efforts, the use of public report cards has not been widely adopted by consumers. This may be partly because patients go where their physicians practice or affiliate and often cannot exercise a great deal of choice in where they receive care. Studies also indicate that the information contained in report cards is not presented in a useful and understandable format for consumers, is not readily available, is not relevant to their situations, and is not necessarily trusted by consumers.

Despite the availability of report cards, consumers in the United States still do not receive the health care they need. A RAND report suggests that adults across the United States receive only about half of the care that they should receive, and that "all adults in the United States are at risk for receiving poor health care," regardless of where they live; why they seek care; where and from whom they receive care; or their race, gender, or financial status.[133] This may be partly because of individuals' lack of access to health care coverage, which in turn may limit their ability to pay for the care they receive. Thus, many complex issues in our system need to be addressed before report cards or any other tools can help to close the gap between what should be done and what is done in health care.

Balanced scorecards allow organizations to look inwardly to evaluate themselves in the areas of financial performance, customer perceptions and satisfaction, internal processes (generally administrative processes), and the ability to learn and grow. They also allow organizations to determine the degree to which they have met their strategic objectives. They hold promise for HCOs in that they integrate clinical, operational, and financial data, and this information can be shared more broadly within the organization to inform decision making.

Both the Magnet Recognition® Program and the Baldridge Award are intended to recognize excellence and quality. HCOs have to weigh the costs and benefits of pursuing these specific quality recognition awards and rely on their organizational objectives in making strategic decisions to pursue them. Regardless of whether a specific recognition is being sought, nurse managers and executives are intimately involved in the "journey" to achieve quality.

Numerous issues in nursing pertain to the quality, cost, and financing of health care. Better care processes can be devised by adopting quality measurement and improvement techniques and through the appropriate use of technology in delivering care. Quality involves not only the end results— patient outcomes and organizational performance—but also a focus on structures and processes that support care delivery. Investing in quality often requires changing the culture, or the accepted way of doing things, on work units and within organizations. This is no small feat, and changing the culture may take years to accomplish. To effectively achieve this kind of deep-level change, nurse managers are called upon to engage front-line staff. Nurse managers must work with staff to build buy-in by involving staff in the process of change as well as by listening and acting on staff needs and concerns.

Patient satisfaction, an outcome often associated with quality, is correlated with nurse satisfaction (discussed in greater detail in Chapters 10 and 13).[134] Newman and Maylor[135] attempt to link patient and nurse satisfaction in their "nurse satisfaction, quality of care, and patient satisfaction chain." In this model, the authors argue that nurses' satisfaction with their job and the work environment may be an antecedent to nurses' ability to actually meet quality of care expectations and patient satisfaction. This approach implies that efforts to improve quality, particularly patient satisfaction, must consider nurses' satisfaction and the work environment. It is therefore incumbent upon nurse managers to appreciate these relationships and to recognize the importance of involving staff in quality initiatives.

Nurse managers and executives must also be aware of the "bigger picture" of quality within and outside of their organizations. They should become involved in organizational strategic planning efforts during which decisions would be made about, for example, pursuing Baldridge, Magnet, or any other type of quality recognition. Nurse managers have important information that can be used to guide these decisions, such as firsthand knowledge of quality performance issues at the point of care delivery, nursing performance outcomes that contribute to quality, and nursing quality issues within the context of the overall organization.

The relationship among quality of care, costs, and health care financing is intricate and complicated. Incentives within our financing system both support or deter quality. The ACA puts forth different incentives that will change the way health care is delivered, change current practices in caring for certain types of patients, and change the ways in which health care is financed. It is up to the nurse manager to be aware of these issues and to minimize the impact of disincentives on quality of care to the extent possible.

---

[133]RAND Corporation. 2006. Research Highlights: The first national report card on quality of health care in America. Retrieved July 31, 2011, at http://www.rand.org/pubs/research_briefs/RB9053-2.html.

[134]Kessler D, Mylod D. 2011. Does patient satisfaction affect patient loyalty? *Int J Health Care Qual,* 24(4):266-273.

[135]Newman K, Maylor U. 2002. Empirical evidence for "the nurse satisfaction, quality of care, and patient satisfaction chain." *Int J Health Care Qual* 15(20):80-88.

Nursing has a long-standing focus on the moral and ethical responsibility to provide the best and highest quality of care for patients. Often, however, nurse managers are faced with budget constraints, staff shortages, and budget-cutting initiatives that put them in a position in which they may be asked to compromise their moral and ethical beliefs. For example, new equipment upgrades are being made almost constantly, and with each upgrade, there is usually some improvement in the product. When is the appropriate time to replace a piece of equipment with the latest version? Another tough position for nurse managers is the justification of staffing increases. What appropriate financial arguments can be used to justify increased staffing requests? If faced with both of these problems at the same time, how does the nurse manager make resource allocation decisions? There are no easy answers to these questions, and finding the answers often involves issues that are ethical in nature. These decisions also require that careful consideration be given to whether the investment is worth the cost or whether the investment is properly timed. The costs of nurse staffing may be minor compared with the denial of payment to organizations for adverse events and hospital-acquired conditions. When faced with such dilemmas, nurse managers may be called upon to build a strong argument—or a business case—using financial and other performance data to assess whether investments in certain quality initiatives should be made.

Achieving quality in HCOs requires an investment. The development of a business case allows managers to illustrate whether, how, and when efforts to invest in quality will pay off. Unfortunately, without building a business case, the expected payoff may not be known, and the derivation of benefits may not occur until far into the future. Also, although some returns may accrue to the organization, others may instead accrue to patients or society. When minimal direct financial returns accrue to the organization, decisions will need to be made about whether an investment is appropriate or whether the payoff to society will result in goodwill toward the organization that makes the investment worthwhile.

It is therefore of paramount importance that nurse managers collaborate with their financial colleagues to understand the process of building a business case, to develop their case, and to have a voice in determining how the business case will be interpreted. Although a business case can be used to justify certain investments in quality, nurse managers need other information to make trade-offs between the costs and quality of care, such as that obtained from the use of quality measures and benchmarking (discussed in Chapter 18).

McCloskey[136] recommends that costs and quality be viewed simultaneously. That is, when there are concerns about containing costs and cost-cutting options are being considered, nurse managers should ask, "Containing cost—at what risk to quality? " On the other hand, when the concerns are about quality and investing in quality initiatives, nurse managers should ask, "Quality—but at what cost?"

Several evidence-based interventions are known to improve patient outcomes and quality of care and decrease costs. The Olds Nurse-Family Partnership is a nonprofit organization that has been supported primarily by public and private funding. This model, developed by Dr. David Olds, was envisioned using nurse home visits to help young, often poor, mothers take better care of themselves and their babies.[137] This model now provides assistance to more than 20,000 mothers and their children in more than 20 states.[138] The Transitional Care Model, developed by Dr. Dorothy Brooten[139] and first tested as a way to provide high-quality, low-cost, early discharge care to very low birth weight babies and their families, used advanced practice nurses to transition babies and families from hospital to home care. The model assessed quality by examining patient outcomes, costs, and patient satisfaction. This model has been tested in different patient populations—from infants to elderly adults[140]—and, in all cases, this model has demonstrated lower costs and improved patient outcomes. More recently, Dr. Mary Naylor has applied the model in several studies of elderly adults[141] and home care,[142] and the model is now being tested in CMS demonstration projects.

Nursing is a large and integral component of health care and can contribute in innovative ways to the future of health care delivery. Given the importance of nurses' role, variations in care that relate to nursing have implications for nurse managers. Variations in care may affect quality based on patient outcomes, and they may affect costs if there is overuse, underuse, or misuse of care. To adequately address variations in care, nurse managers should advocate the use of current research and evidence-based practice to inform the development of standards of care and to ensure that nursing care and practice are based on the best available knowledge and research. Nurse managers must also have a strong understanding and appreciation of nursing's impact on the quality and costs of patient care and to articulate this understanding to organizational leaders and staff. Their insights can contribute to the development of a more comprehensive approach for improving the quality and safety of care in HCOs and in turn the costs incurred and financing available to the organization.

[136]McCloskey J. 1995. Breaking the cycle. *J Prof Nurs* 11(2):67.

[137]Retrieved July 31, 2011, at http://www.rwjf.org/files/publications/other/DavidOldsSpecialReport0606.pdf.

[138]*Ibid.*

[139]Brooten D, Kumar S, Brown L, et al. 1986. A randomized clinical trial: Early discharge and nurse followup of very low birthweight infants. *N Engl J Med* 315:934-939. (Reprinted in Rinke LT, editor. 1987. *Outcome Measures in Home Care.* New York: National League for Nursing, pp. 95-108.)

[140]See Brooten, Naylor MD, York R, et al. 2002. Lessons learned from testing the Quality Cost Model of Advanced Practice Nurse Transitional Care. *J Nurs Scholarsh* 34(4):369-375.

[141]Naylor M, Brooten D, Campbell RL, et al. 2004. Transitional care of older adults hospitalized with heart failure: A randomized, controlled trial. *J Am Geriatr Assoc* 52(5):675-684.

[142]Naylor MD 2006. Transitional care: A critical dimension of the home healthcare quality agenda. *J Healthc Qual* 28(1):48-54.

✳ KEY CONCEPTS

Quality "The degree to which health care services for individuals and populations increase the likelihood of desired health outcomes and are consistent with current professional knowledge."[143] Donabedian defined quality as a function of structures, processes, and outcomes of health care and recognized that measurement of quality requires an examination of system attributes that pertain to structures, processes, and outcomes of care.[144]

Structure Resources used in the provision of care, such as physicians, nurses, and other care providers, and organizational characteristics.[145]

Process Activities involved in providing care, such as models of care delivery, and organizational policies and procedures.[146]

Outcomes Consequences or results of care, such as condition-specific results of care, and patient satisfaction.[147]

Report card Quality reporting strategy that grades health care providers on measures of quality and performance to provide individuals, payers, and other decision makers with information upon which to base health care decisions.[148]

Balanced scorecard An internal organizational report card used by organizations for strategic management purposes to examine performance. Typically, performance is monitored in four areas: customer perspective, financial perspective, internal processes (including human resources), and learning and growth.[149]

Value The relationship between costs and quality, which can be expressed as follows[150]:

$$Value = Quality/Cost$$

Efficiency "Mix of health care resource inputs that produce optimal quantity and quality of health and health care outputs."[151] Inputs can be direct costs (e.g., labor, capital, equipment) and indirect costs (e.g., time). Efficiency can be expressed as follows[152]:

$$Efficiency = Output/Input$$

Effectiveness Degree to which outcomes or results are achieved as intended. Effectiveness also means that a treatment, service, or technology provides a benefit to recipients under usual or natural circumstances.[153] Effectiveness implies the appropriate use of knowledge and evidence to achieve a desired outcome while considering patients' values.[154]

Business case Position on whether or not an investment should be made in a project or initiative based on a systematic evaluation of the worth or value of the project or initiative. Involves the calculation of rates of return on investments, break-even points, costs and benefits, and other financial indices.[155]

Cost Amount spent to acquire or maintain a good or service.

Access to care The availability of care that is appropriate and adaptable to patients' health needs, acceptable to the patient, and affordable.

Price Amount charged for a particular service.

[143]Institute of Medicine, Lohr K, editor. 1990. *Medicare: A Strategy for Quality Assurance*. Washington, DC: National Academies Press, p. 44.
[144]Donabedian A, *Op. cit.*, 1966.
[145]Donabedian A, *Op. cit.*, 1982.
[146]*Ibid.*
[147]*Ibid.*
[148]RAND, *Op. cit.*, 2002.
[149]Oliveira J, *Op. cit.*, 2001.
[150]Folland S, *Op. cit.*, 2009.
[151]Committee on Redesigning Health Insurance Performance Measures, Payment, and Performance Improvement Programs, *Op. cit.*
[152]Palmer and Torgerson, *Op. cit.*, 1999.
[153]Retrieved September 11, 2006, at http://www.nlm.nih.gov/nichsr/ihcm/hsrckey.html.
[154]Committee on Quality of Health Care in America, *Op. cit.*, pp. 47-48.
[155]Jones, *Op. cit.*, 2005.

✳ SUGGESTED READINGS

Aiken L, Sloane D, Lake E: Satisfaction with inpatient acquired immunodeficiency syndrome care: a national comparison of dedicated and scattered-bed units, *Med Care* 35(9):948–962, 1997.

Aiken L, Sloane D, Lake E, et al: Organization and outcomes of inpatient AIDS care, *Med Care* 37(8):760–772, 1999.

Aiken L, Smith H, Lake E: Lower Medicare mortality among a set of hospitals known for good nursing care, *Med Care* 32:771–787, 1994.

American Nurses Association: *Implementing nursing's report card: a study of RN staffing, length of stay, and patient outcomes*, Washington, DC, 1997, American Nurses Association.

American Nurses Association: *Nursing care report card for acute care*, Washington, DC, 1995, American Nurses Association.

Berens M: Nursing mistakes kill, injure thousands, *Chicago Tribune* Sept 10, 2000. Available at www.chicagotribune.com/news/specials/chi-000910nursing1,1,2682439.story?ctrack=1&cset=true. Accessed November 26, 2006.

Berwick D, Joshi M: Healthcare quality and the patient. In Ransom S, Joshi M, Nash D, editors: *The health care quality book: vision, strategy and tools*, Chicago, 2005, Health Administration Press, pp 3–24.

Best M, Neuhauser D: Avedis Donabedian: father of quality assurance and poet, *BMJ* 13:472–473, 2004.

Blegen MA, Goode CJ, Reed L: Nurse staffing and patient outcomes, *Nurs Res* 47(1), 43–50, 1998.

Brady-Schwartz D: Further evidence on the Magnet Recognition Program: implications for nursing leaders, *J Nurs Adm* 35(9):397–403, 2005.

Brooten D, Kumar S, Brown L, et al: A randomized clinical trial: early discharge and nurse followup of very low birthweight infants, *N Engl J Med* 315:934–939, 1986. (Reprinted from Rinke LT, editor: *Outcome measures in home care*, New York, 1987, National League for Nursing, pp 95–108.)

Brooten D, Naylor MD, York R, et al: Lessons learned from testing the Quality Cost Model of Advanced Practice Nurse Transitional Care, *J Nurs Scholarsh* 34(4):369–375, 2002.

Carey J: Medical guesswork, *Bus Wk* 3983: 72–79, 2006.

Clancy C: Ten years after "To Err Is Human," *Am J Med Qual* 24(6):252–528, 2009.

Consumers Union: *To err is human—to delay is deadly: ten years later, a million lives lost, billions of dollars wasted*, 2009. Available at www.safepatientproject.org/safepatientproject.org/pdf/safepatientproject.org-ToDelayIsDeadly.pdf.

Donabedian A: Evaluating the quality of medical care, *Milbank Mem Fund Q* 44(Suppl 3):166–206, 1966.

Donabedian A: *Explorations in quality assessment and monitoring, volume I. The definition of quality and approaches to its assessment*, Ann Arbor, MI, 1982, Health Administration Press.

Donabedian A: *Explorations in quality assessment and monitoring, volume II. The criteria and standards of care*, Ann Arbor, MI, 1982, Health Administration Press.

Donabedian A: The seven pillars of quality, *Arch Pathol Lab Med* 114:1115–1118, 1990.

Doran D: *Nursing-sensitive outcomes: state of the science*, ed 2, Toronto, 2010, Jones and Bartlett Publishers.

Doran D, Sidani S, Keatings M, Doidge D: An empirical test of the Nursing Role Effectiveness Model, *J Adv Nurs* 38:29–39, 2002.

Drenkard K: The business case for Magnet, *J Nurs Adm* 40(6):263–271, 2010.

Drenkard KN: Sustaining Magnet: keeping the forces alive, *Nurs Adm Q* 29(3):214–222, 2005. Available at http://nursingworld.org/ancc/magnet/forms/StudentManual.pdf.

Enthoven A: The history and principles of managed competition, *Health Aff* 12(Suppl):27–43, 1993.

Enthoven A, Tollen L: Competition in health care: it takes systems to pursue quality and efficiency, *Health Aff (Millwood)*: w5-420–w5-433, 2005.

Folland S, Goodman A, Stano M: *The economics of health and health care*, ed 6, Upper Saddle River, NJ, 2009, Prentice-Hall.

Goode CJ, Blegen MA, Park SH, et al: Comparison of patient outcomes in Magnet® and non-Magnet hospitals, *J Nurs Adm* 41(12):517–523, 2011.

Hibbard J, Stockard J, Tusler M: Does publicizing hospital performance stimulate quality improvement efforts? *Health Aff* 22(2):84–95, 2003.

Hungate R: Reflecting on Donabedian, *Health Aff* 20(3):295, 2001.

Institute for Healthcare Improvement: *The breakthrough series: IHI's collaborative model for achieving breakthrough improvement*, 2003. Available at http://www.ihi.org/NR/rdonlyres/3F1925B7-6C47-48ED-AA83-C85D-BABB664D/0/TheBreakthroughSeriespaper.pdf.

Institute of Medicine, Lohr K, editor: *Medicare: a strategy for quality assurance*, Washington, DC, 1990, National Academies Press, p 44.

Institute of Medicine Committee on Identifying and Preventing Medication Errors, Aspden P, Wolcott J, et al, editors: *Preventing medication errors*, Washington, DC, 2007, National Academies Press.

Institute of Medicine Committee on Quality of Health Care in America: *Crossing the quality chasm*, Washington, DC, 2001, National Academies Press.

Institute of Medicine Committee on Quality of Health Care in America, Kohn L, Corrigan J, Donaldson M, editors: *To err is human: building a safer healthcare system*, Washington, DC, 2000, National Academies Press.

Institute of Medicine Committee on Redesigning Health Insurance Performance Measures, Payment, and Performance Improvement Programs: *Performance measurement: accelerating improvement*, Washington, DC, 2006, National Academies Press.

Irvine D, Sidani S, McGillis Hall L: Finding value in nursing care: a framework for quality improvement and clinical evaluation, *Nurs Econ* 16(3):110–131, 1998.

Irvine D, Sidani S, McGillis Hall L: Linking outcomes to nurses' roles in health care, *Nurs Econ* 16(2):58–64, 87, 1998.

Jennings B, Loan L, DePaul D, et al: Lessons learned while collecting ANA indicator data, *J Nurs Adm* 31(3):121–129, 2001.

Jones C: The costs of nursing turnover, part 2: application of the nursing turnover cost calculation methodology, *J Nurs Adm* 35(1):41–49, 2005.

Kaplan R, Norton D: How to implement a new strategy without disrupting your organization, *Harv Bus Rev* 84(3):100–109, 2006.

Kaplan R, Norton D: Putting the balanced scorecard to work, *Harv Bus Rev* 71(5):134, 1993.

Kaplan R, Norton D: The balanced scorecard: measures that drive performance, *Harv Bus Rev* 70(1):71–79, 1992.

Kaplan R, Norton D: Transforming the balanced score-card from performance measurement to strategic management: part I, *Account Horiz* 15(1):87–104, 2001.

Kaplan R, Norton D: Transforming the balanced score-card from performance measurement to strategic management: part II, *Account Horiz* 15(2):147–160, 2001.

Kaplan R, Norton D: Using the balanced scorecard as a strategic management system, *Harv Bus Rev* 74(1):75–85, 1996.

Kessler D, Mylod D: Does patient satisfaction affect patient loyalty? *Int J Health Care Qual*, 24(4):266–273, 2011.

Kramer M, Schmalenberg C: Best quality patient care: a historical perspective on magnet hospitals, *Nurs Adm Q* 29(3):275–287, 2005.

Lake ET, Shang J, Klaus S, Dunton NE: Patient falls: association with hospital Magnet status and nursing unit staffing, *Res Nurs Health* 33(5):413–425, 2010.

Laschinger HKS, Shamian J, Thomson D: Impact of Magnet hospital characteristics on nurses' perceptions of trust, burnout, quality of care, and work satisfaction, *Nurs Econ* 19(5):209–219, 2001.

Leape L, Berwick D: Five years after To Err Is Human: what have we learned? *JAMA* 293(19):2384–2390, 2005.

Leatherman S, Berwick D, Iles D, et al: The business case for quality: case studies and an analysis, *Health Aff* 22(2):17–30, 2003.

Lohr K: How do we measure quality? *Health Aff* 16(3):22–25, 1997.

McCloskey J: Breaking the cycle, *J Prof Nurs* 11(2):67, 1995.

McClure M, Hinshaw A: *Magnet hospitals revisited: attraction and retention of professional nurses*, Washington, DC, 2002, American Nurses Publishing.

McGillis Hall L: Report cards: relevance for nursing and patient safety, *Int Counc Nurs* 49:168–177, 2002.

Mick S, Mark B: The contribution of organizational theory to nursing health services research, *Nurs Outlook* 53(6):317–323, 2005.

Mitchell P, Ferketich S, Jennings B: Quality health outcomes model, *Image J Nurs Sch* 30(1):43–47, 1998.

Mitchell P, Lang N: Framing the problem of measuring and improving healthcare quality: has the quality health outcomes model been useful? *Med Care* 42(2 suppl):II-4-I-11, 2004.

Moore K, Lynn M, McMillen B, Evans S: Implementation of the ANA report card, *J Nurs Adm* 29(6):48–54, 1999.

National Quality Forum: *National voluntary consensus standards for nursing-sensitive care: an initial performance measure set. A consensus report* (website). Washington, DC, 2004, National Quality Forum. www.qualityforum.org/pdf/nursing-quality/txNCFINALpublic.pdf. Accessed November 26, 2006.

Naylor M, Brooten D, Campbell RL, et al: Transitional care of older adults hospitalized with heart failure: a randomized, controlled trial. *J Am Geriatr Assoc* 52(5):675–684, 2004.

Naylor MD: Transitional care: a critical dimension of the home healthcare quality agenda, *J Healthc Qual* 28(1):48–54, 2006.

Needleman J, Buerhaus P, Stewart M, et al: Nurse staffing in hospitals: is there a business case for quality? *Health Aff* 25(1):204–211, 2006.

Nelson E, Mohr J, Batalden P, Plume S: Improving health care, part 1: the clinical value compass, *Jt Comm J Qual Improv* 22(4):243–258, 1996.

Newman K, Maylor U: Empirical evidence for "the nurse satisfaction, quality of care, and patient satisfaction chain," *Int J Health Care Qual* 15(20):80–88, 2002.

Oliveira J: The balanced scorecard: an integrative approach to performance evaluation, *Healthc Financ Manage* 55(5):42–46, 2001.

Page A, Committee on the Work Environment for Nurses and Patient Safety: *Keeping patients safe: transforming the work environment of nurses,* Washington, DC, 2004, National Academies Press.

Palmer S, Torgerson D: Economics notes: definitions of efficiency, *Br Med J* 318(7191):1136, 1999.

Penchansky R, Thomas WJ: The concept of access: definition and relationship to consumer satisfaction, *Med Care* 19(2):127–140, 1981.

Pham H, Coughlan J, O'Malley A: The impact of quality-reporting programs on hospital operations, *Health Aff* 25(5):1412–1422, 2006.

Porter M, Teisberg E: Redefining competition in health care, *Harv Bus Rev* 82(6):65–76, 2004.

Porter ME, Teisberg EO: *Redefining health care: creating value-based competition on results*, Cambridge, MA, 2006, Harvard Business Review Press.

President's Advisory Commission on Consumer Protection and Quality in the Health Care Industry: (website). www.hcqualitycommission.gov/about.html. Accessed August 8, 2006.

RAND: *Research highlights: report cards for health care* (website), 2002. www.rand.org/pubs/research_briefs/RB4544/index1.html. Accessed September 3, 2006.

RAND Corporation: *Research highlights: the first national report card on quality of health care in America* (website), 2006. www.rand.org/pubs/research_briefs/RB9053-2/index1.html. Accessed September 3, 2006.

Reiter KL, Kilpatrick KE, Greene SB, et al: How to develop a business case for quality, *Int J Qual Health Care* 19(1):50–55, 2007.

Rowell P: Lessons learned while collecting ANA indicator data: the American Nurses Association responds, *J Nurs Adm* 31(3):130–131, 2001.

Russell J: Journey to Magnet™: cost vs. benefits, *Nursing Econ* 28(5):340–342, 2010.

Schiff G, Rucker T: Beyond structure-process-outcome: Donabedian's seven pillars and eleven buttresses of quality, *Jt Comm J Qual Improv* 27(3): 169–174, 2001.

Schuster M, McGlynn E, Pham C, et al: The quality of health care in the United States: a review of articles since 1987. In Institute of Medicine Committee on Quality of Health Care in America, editor: *Crossing the quality chasm,* Washington, DC, 2001, National Academies Press.

Trinkoff AM, Johantgen, M, Storr CL, et al: A comparison of working conditions among nurses in Magnet® and Non-Magnet® hospitals, *J Nurs Adm* 40(7/8):309–315, 2010.

Van Den Bos J, Rustagi K, Gray T, et al: The $17.1 billion problem: the annual cost of measurable medical errors, *Health Aff* 30(4):596–603, 2011.

Wachter R: The end of the beginning: patient safety five years after "To Err Is Human," *Health Aff* W4:534–545, 2004.

Wunderlich G, Sloan F, Davis C, Committee on the Adequacy of Nurse Staffing in Hospitals and Nursing Homes: *Nursing staff in hospitals and nursing homes: is it adequate?* Washington, DC, 1996, National Academies Press, p 9.

Zelman WN, Pink GH, Matthias CB: Use of the balanced scorecard in health care, *J Health Care Finance* 29(4):1–16, 2003.

✳ FINANCIAL ACCOUNTING

Financial accounting is the area of financial management that focuses on how well the organization is doing from a financial perspective. Chapter 6 presents the basic principles of accounting, along with related terminology, and addresses the compilation of accounting information into financial reports that can be used by the organization's managers and other interested individuals to manage operating units and aid in making resource allocation decisions. Chapter 7 explains the techniques commonly used to analyze and interpret the financial condition of an organization and the financial results of its activities.

Accounting Principles

CHAPTER GOALS

The goals of this chapter are to:

- Explain why accounting is important to health care organizations
- Describe the basic framework of accounting, including the fundamental equation of accounting
- Introduce the balance sheet and the statement of operations
- Define a wide range of common accounting terminology

- Explain the process of recording accounting information and then summarizing and reporting that information
- Introduce and define the most common and important generally accepted accounting principles
- Describe the use of fund accounting in not-for-profit health care organizations
- Discuss the implications of financial accounting for nurse managers and executives

❋ INTRODUCTION

Accounting is a system that lets us keep "account" of things. Health care organizations (HCOs) have formalized accounting systems that track the financial well-being and financial success of the organization. The organization may or may not exist in order to make profits. Even if the organization is a for-profit organization, profits may not be its only goal. The primary goal of the organization may be to provide health care services. Nevertheless, the financial well-being and financial success of the organization are critical because the organization must be financially viable to meet its goals related to providing care.

Unless satisfactory financial results are achieved, at best, the organization will not be able to acquire the latest technologies or expand services; at worst, it will not be able to pay its bills. In the worst-case scenario, the organization will possibly cease providing any care at all.

Therefore, a critical job of financial managers is to compile a set of financial reports, officially called *financial statements* but often referred to simply as "the financials." The goal of these financials is to convey information about the organization's financial condition and the financial results of its activities. This information can be used by banks to decide whether to lend money to the organization, by philanthropists to determine whether to donate money, and by suppliers to decide whether to extend credit. They can also be used by the organization's managers to decide whether the organization's financial results are satisfactory and how they could be improved.

The information contained in these reports can help nurse managers and executives know whether the organization has sufficient resources to provide larger raises, add staff, or agree to capital expenditure requests or whether the organization will need to substantially cut expenses just to avoid going out of business. Power is often said to reside with those who possess information. Certainly, an ability to understand and interpret the financial results of the organization is critical to ensuring that nursing receives an appropriate share of available organizational resources. Thus, the study of financial accounting and financial statements is not just an "academic" exercise but one that provides nurse managers and executives with the tools necessary for critically analyzing the financial status of the organization.

Every time an employee is paid, a bill is issued to a patient, or a supply item is purchased, a financial event or transaction has occurred. All organizations have a great number of financial transactions. Even a small nursing practice has hundreds or thousands of events each year that have a financial impact. A small home health care agency likely has tens of thousands of such events during the year, and a large medical center may have tens of millions of such events. The job of accounting is to develop a system that can record each of the many events that have financial implications, summarize them, and report them in a manner that is useful to managers and other interested individuals.

This task is accomplished via the techniques of *financial accounting*. Financial accounting is a system that records each financial event as it occurs, summarizes all of the events, and provides reports that indicate the impact of these events on the financial status of the organization. Accounting is not a science. It is based on a generally accepted set of conventions, rules, and terminology.

This chapter begins with an explanation of the basic framework upon which modern accounting rests. Then it introduces the central financial statements:

- Statement of financial position (or balance sheet)
- Statement of operations (or income statement)
- Statement of changes in net assets (or changes in equity)
- Statement of cash flows

Understanding these financial statements is difficult if for no other reason than that the accounting terminology they use is generally new to readers. Thus, a section on terminology is provided in this chapter.

The chapter then discusses how financial information is recorded and reported by HCOs. Such reporting often follows a set of rules that in the United States are referred to as *generally accepted accounting principles* (GAAP). Furthermore, there are some specialized GAAP that health care providers must follow. Several of the most important of these principles are discussed in this chapter. Outside of the United States, more than 120 countries follow a set of accounting rules that are called *International Financial Reporting Standards* (IFRS). IFRS are similar to GAAP in many respects, but there are some differences. There is currently a movement to adopt IFRS in the United States, and this could happen sometime later in this decade.

The chapter concludes with a brief discussion of accounting's implications for nurse managers and executives.

✳ THE BASIC FRAMEWORK OF ACCOUNTING

Accounting systems are established based on one widely accepted *axiom*. This axiom is the basic equation of accounting:

$$\text{Assets} = \text{Liabilities} + \text{Owners' Equity}$$

Assets are valuable resources that are owned by the organization. They may be either physical (having substance and form, e.g., a table or building) or intangible (e.g., the reputation the organization has gained for providing high-quality health care services). *Liabilities* are legal financial obligations the organization has to outsiders. Essentially, they represent money that the organization owes to someone. These liabilities represent claims against some of the organization's assets. *Owners' equity* represents the portion of an organization's assets that belong to its owners.

The left-hand side of the equation represents all of the valuable resources of the organization. The right-hand side of the equation indicates who owns all of those resources. Note that the owners' equity is a residual amount. When one subtracts the claims of outsiders from the total of the organization's assets, whatever is left belongs to the organization or its owners. Because the owners' equity is a residual value, which rises and falls in response to changes in the assets and liabilities, the equation will always remain in balance. The owners' equity balance will be whatever it must be for the

equation to be in balance. That forms the basis for all bookkeeping or accounting.

If the organization is a for-profit business, the owners may be sole proprietors (just one owner of the business), partners, or stockholders, depending on whether the organization is legally established as a proprietorship, partnership, or corporation, respectively. The owners' equity belongs to the owners of the organization. In the case of a not-for-profit organization, there is no owner per se. The organization exists for the good of the community at large. No individuals are entitled to benefit from any profits that might be generated by the organization. In not-for-profit organizations, the owners' equity is referred to as the *net assets*. When accountants use the term *net*, it generally refers to an amount after something has been subtracted. Note that the fundamental equation of accounting can be transformed as follows:

$$\text{Assets} = \text{Liabilities} + \text{Owners' Equity}$$
$$\text{Assets} - \text{Liabilities} = \text{Owners' Equity}$$

And for not-for-profit organizations use, the term *owners' equity* is replaced with *net assets,* so the equation becomes:

$$\text{Assets} - \text{Liabilities} = \text{Net Assets}$$

Here it becomes a bit easier to see where the term *net assets* originates. If you take assets and subtract liabilities, the amount left over is the net assets because that is the portion of assets not required for the payment of liabilities.

✳ THE KEY FINANCIAL STATEMENTS

Four key statements are central to reporting on the financial results and financial condition of an organization. They are the *statement of financial position* (often called the balance sheet), the *operating statement* (sometimes referred to as the income statement), the *statement of changes in net assets* (or statement of changes in equity), and the *statement of cash flows*. The first two are discussed here and the remaining two in Chapter 7.

The Statement of Financial Position

The most essential of the organization's financial reports is a document officially called the statement of financial position. It is usually called the balance sheet. The role of the balance sheet is to indicate what the organization owns and owes at a specific point in time.

The balance sheet summarizes the fundamental equation of accounting. The assets are shown on the left side (or top) of the statement. The liabilities and owners' equity are shown on the right side (or bottom) of the statement. A balance sheet for the hypothetical ABC Health Care not-for-profit organization appears in Table 6–1. Because the balance sheet is based on the fundamental equation of accounting, the total of the assets must always be equal to the total of liabilities plus owners' equity. The left and right sides of the balance sheet must have the same total and therefore be in balance.

We will discuss the specific parts of the balance sheet shown in Table 6–1 later in this chapter. Additional sample balance sheets for a for-profit nursing home, a not-for-profit home

❋ **TABLE 6–1**

ABC Health Care
Statement of Financial Position
as of June 30, 2012
(000s Omitted)

Assets		Liabilities and Net Assets	
Current Assets		**Current Liabilities**	
Cash	$ 150	Wages payable	$ 1,123
Marketable securities	220	Accounts payable	2,430
Accounts receivable, *net* of $436	2,319	Notes payable	500
allowance for bad debts		Deferred revenue	300
Inventory	832	Taxes payable	145
Prepaid assets	46	Total current liabilities	$ 4,498
Total current assets	$ 3,567		
Fixed Assets		**Long-Term Liabilities**	
Property, plant, and equipment	$43,470	Mortgage payable	$ 3,560
Less accumulated depreciation	17,356	Bonds payable	20,000
Net property, plant, and equipment	$26,114	Total long-term liabilities	$23,560
Sinking fund	1,737		
Investments	341	**Net Assets**	
Goodwill	3,231	Unrestricted	$ 5,412
Total fixed assets	$31,423	Temporarily restricted	520
		Permanently restricted	1,000
		Total net assets	$ 6,932
Total Assets	**$ 34,990**	**Total Liabilities and Net Assets**	**$ 34,990**

health agency, and a not-for-profit ambulatory clinic may be found in the Appendix to Chapter 7.

The Operating Statement

When services are provided to patients, a charge is generally made. The monies that the organization is legally entitled to collect in exchange for the services that have been provided are called *revenues*. The costs of providing services are *expenses*. The revenues less the expenses represent the profit or loss of the organization.

Most organizations in industries other than health care refer to a statement that compares revenues to expenses as an *income statement*. This is because revenue less expense is defined as *net income* or *profit* of the organization. However, in the health care industry, the statement that provides information about revenues and expenses is referred to as the *operating statement* or *statement of operations*. This helps the reader understand that profits may not be the primary goal of the organization. But we still need to understand the results of the organization's operations that relate to generating revenues and incurring expenses.

This book uses the term *not-for-profit* rather than the common term *nonprofit*. The term *nonprofit* implies that the organization does not make a profit. That is not a correct inference. A key goal of for-profit companies is to earn a profit. In not-for-profit organizations, profit is not the primary goal, but it is acceptable and even desirable for the organization to make a profit. Literally, such organizations are NOT in business FOR

the purpose of making a PROFIT. So *not-for-profit* is a more descriptive term, and it is widely used by financial managers. Not-for-profit organizations are exempt from a variety of taxes and are sometimes referred to as tax-exempt organizations.

Whether an organization is for-profit or not-for-profit, profits *are* a necessary element for several reasons. First, to fulfill their mission, many HCOs must adopt new, expensive technologies as they become available. Profits earned on current patient services help to pay for the adoption of new technology tomorrow. Second, many HCOs want to expand both the range of services they offer and the number of people served. Such expansion requires the reinvestment of profits. Third, the effect of inflation is to constantly increase the cost of replacing buildings and equipment as they wear out. Some profits must be earned to allow for accumulation of enough money to pay for replacement of facilities at higher prices than they originally cost. Finally, some profits are needed as a margin of safety to protect against an unexpected emergency.

Therefore, not-for-profit HCOs do not exist for the purpose of making a profit, but making a profit does not represent improper behavior. Rather, it is indicative of an organization that will remain healthy enough to continue to provide services to its community.

An operating statement for the hypothetical ABC Health Care appears in Table 6–2. Additional sample operating statements for a for-profit nursing home, a not-for-profit home health agency, and a not-for-profit ambulatory clinic may be found in the Appendix to Chapter 7.

✳ **TABLE 6–2**

ABC Health Care
Statement of Operations
for the Fiscal Year Ending June 30, 2012
(000s Omitted)

Revenues	
Patient revenues	$18,230
Other operating revenues	1,919
Total	$20,149
Expenses	
Wages for clinical services	$10,325
Patient care supplies and food	934
Housekeeping services	654
Operation and maintenance of plant	1,221
Administrative services	2,343
Depreciation and amortization	1,433
Bad debt expense	436
Interest	2,333
Total	$19,679
Operating Income	$ 470

✳ ACCOUNTING TERMINOLOGY

Accounting is often referred to as the language of business. Numerous accounting terms have become part of the everyday vocabulary of running an organization. Given the background you now have in the basic framework of accounting and the balance sheet and statement of operations, we can turn our attention to introducing the most common terms.

Assets

Some of the most common terms related to assets include the following:

- Liquid assets
- Current assets
- Cash equivalents
- Marketable securities
- Liquidate
- Accounts receivable
- Allowance for uncollectible accounts or allowance for bad debts
- Inventory
- Prepaid assets
- Fixed assets
- Depreciate
- Depreciation
- Accumulated depreciation
- Sinking fund
- Goodwill
- Intangible
- Amortization

All of these terms are discussed in this section. (They are listed above in the order in which they will be discussed.) Consider Table 6–1. One of the first things to note about the balance sheet is the remark "000s Omitted" in the heading of

the statement. This means that all numbers are shown in thousands. For example, the Cash entry of $150 in Table 6–1 is really $150,000. There are several reasons numbers in financial statements are commonly shown this way. One reason is that the financial statement is less cumbersome to read if numbers are shown in thousands. For some very large organizations, such as some hospitals, numbers are shown in hundreds of thousands or millions. More importantly, financial statements are not as accurate as most people assume. Most accounting systems have many clerical errors. To eliminate all the errors would be extremely costly. Therefore, financial statements should be thought of as being reasonably, but not precisely, accurate. Showing the numbers in thousands, hundred thousands, or even millions helps to convey that the numbers are not exact to the penny or even to the nearest hundred dollars. So, if $150,354.28 is shown as $150, it takes the focus off the exact amount of $150,354.28, which might not be precisely correct.

The balance sheet presents the organization's assets in order of liquidity from the most liquid to the least liquid. *Liquid assets* are cash or other assets that can be converted quickly to cash to pay the liabilities of the organization. Buildings and equipment are examples of illiquid assets (having little liquidity). Organizations that have a great amount of cash and other liquid assets are in a relatively safer position than those that are "illiquid." The most liquid assets are placed near the top of the balance sheet to give them prominence. This is done because one primary purpose of financial statements is to convey the financial stability of the organization—its ability to continue in business.

The first section on the asset side of the balance sheet is *current assets*. These are the resources that are cash, can be converted to cash within 1 year, or will be used up within 1 year. Current assets are often referred to as short-term or near-term assets. Current assets are more liquid than assets that are not current.

Within the current assets category, the first asset listed is cash. Cash includes not only money on hand but also *cash equivalents,* such as savings and checking accounts and short-term certificates of deposit. The next item is *marketable securities.* This includes investments in stocks and bonds. Similar investments are also included on the balance sheet under the heading of long-term asset investments. *Long-term assets* are assets that will not be used up or converted to cash within 1 year. The primary difference between marketable securities and long-term investments is intent. If management intends to sell, or *liquidate,* the stocks or bonds within 1 year of the balance sheet date, they are marketable securities. If the intent is to hold those securities for more than 1 year, they are long-term investments.

The next current asset listed after marketable securities is *accounts receivable.* These are amounts owed to the organization by purchasers of the organization's goods or services. Often a transaction occurs "on account." This means that payment is not made immediately. Instead, an account is opened that tracks the transaction until payment is made. For the provider of the service, the unpaid amount is referred to as an *account receivable*. For the purchaser of the service, there is a mirror image, referred to as an *account payable*.

Accounts receivable are shown on the balance sheet at their "net" value. This refers to the fact that HCOs often have bad debts; that is, there are some patients for whom payment is never received even though the patients were expected to be able to pay for the care. Although the health care provider may not know who will not pay, an estimate must be made, and the amount of receivables shown on the balance sheet should be only the net amount that the organization estimates it will receive. If the gross amount of receivables outstanding were shown on the balance sheet, there would be an overestimate of the value of that asset. Therefore, there is established an *allowance for uncollectible accounts,* sometimes called an *allowance for bad debts* or an *allowance for doubtful accounts*. In Table 6–1, the total accounts receivable are $2,755,000, but when we subtract an estimated uncollectible portion of receivables equal to $436,000, the net accounts receivable are shown as $2,319,000.

Inventory is the next item listed in current assets. This represents the various supplies that will be used to provide goods or services. If a home health agency sells walkers and wheelchairs to its clients, it may keep a stock of them on hand. A hospital might need a wide variety of medical supplies such as sutures. Those supply items that are purchased and then used in providing services are not considered expenses as soon as they are purchased; rather, they become a valuable resource, inventory, which becomes an expense only as it is used up.

The last item shown in current assets in Table 6–1 is *prepaid assets*. This represents assets that have been paid for and have not yet been used but will be used within 1 year. This includes items such as fire insurance premiums or rent paid in advance. These items are not expected to be converted back into cash, but they will be used up within 1 year, so they are considered current assets.

Fixed assets are listed on the balance sheet after current assets. Fixed assets consist primarily of property, plant, and equipment. This refers to the land, buildings, and pieces of equipment owned by the organization. Land is expected to last forever. However, buildings and equipment physically wear out with the passage of time. From an accounting perspective, they are said to *depreciate,* or decline in value or productive capability.

Suppose that a building costs $40 million when it is new, and it is expected to last 40 years. Rather than showing the entire cost of the building as an expense in the year it is purchased, accountants require that the cost be spread out over the expected useful lifetime of the building. The allocation of the $40 million cost over 40 years is referred to as *depreciation*. The amount of the original cost allocated as an expense each year is the depreciation expense for that year. The total amount of depreciation that has been taken over the years the organization has owned the asset is referred to as the *accumulated depreciation*.

For instance, if the organization is taking depreciation expense of $1 million per year on the $40 million building and it has owned the building for 10 years, the accumulated depreciation is $10 million and the net value of the building is $30 million. The financial statements will disclose the original cost, the accumulated depreciation, and the net value. Note, however, that financial statements do not list each building and each piece of equipment. Instead, all similar items are combined and shown as one summary amount. In Table 6-1, the property, plant, and equipment line represents the buildings owned by the organization, the land, and all pieces of equipment.

During the years that buildings and equipment get old, the organization tries to charge enough for its services to be able to collect an adequate amount of money to replace these assets when they have exhausted their useful life. However, sometimes the organization spends that money for current activities rather than saving it to replace long-term assets. To ensure adequate accumulation of resources for future major investments in buildings and equipment, the organization will sometimes establish a *sinking fund*. This is simply a segregated group of investments that can be used only for a specified purpose, generally replacement of plant and equipment or repayment of a loan taken to purchase that building and equipment.

The only asset on the example balance sheet that has not yet been discussed is *goodwill*. This is an *intangible* asset. It represents a measure of the value of the organization that goes beyond its specific physical assets. This includes good relationships with suppliers, a favorable reputation for high-quality care, and other similar values that are not easily quantified. Although most organizations have goodwill, usually they do not show it or any other intangible assets on their financial statements. This is because accountants have trouble measuring the true value of an organization's goodwill.

The only time that intangible assets appear on a financial statement is when the organization has purchased the intangible asset from someone else. Generally, this occurs when one organization acquires another organization and has paid more than the value of that organization's specific tangible assets. In that case, accountants assume that the excess paid must have been a payment for the general goodwill of the organization. Otherwise, rather than buying the second organization, the buyer would have simply purchased similar tangible assets. Therefore, the excess paid is shown as goodwill.

The term depreciation is only used for identifiable physical assets. The equivalent of depreciation for intangible items is referred to as *amortization*. Amortize means to spread out or allocate. The cost of the intangible asset is spread out or allocated as an expense over the expected useful lifetime of the asset. Amortization is recorded for a wide variety of intangibles, such as copyrights and patents, but is not done for goodwill. Goodwill is considered to continue at the same level for an indefinite period unless subsequent information indicates that its value has clearly been impaired.

Liabilities and Owners' Equity

The terms to be discussed in this section include the following:
- Current liabilities
- Long-term liabilities
- Wages payable
- Accounts payable

- Notes payable
- Taxes payable
- Federal Insurance Contributions Act (FICA)
- Deferred revenues
- Mortgage payable
- Bonds payable
- Permanently restricted net assets
- Temporarily restricted net assets
- Unrestricted net assets
- Stockholders' equity
- Par value
- Retained earnings

Liabilities are divided on the balance sheet into *current liabilities* and *long-term liabilities*. Current liabilities are obligations that are expected to be paid within 1 year. Long-term liabilities are obligations that are not expected to be paid within the coming year.

Current liabilities in Table 6–1 include wages payable, accounts payable, notes payable, deferred revenue, and taxes payable. *Wages payable* simply represent amounts that are owed to employees. *Accounts payable* generally represent amounts owed to suppliers (e.g., pharmaceutical or medical supply companies). *Notes payable* represent obligations to repay a loan. Depending on when the loan must be repaid, some notes payable are long-term liabilities. *Taxes payable* represent taxes owed to a local, state, or federal government. For-profit organizations must pay real estate, sales, and income taxes. Not-for-profit organizations are generally exempt from those taxes. However, even if an organization is not-for-profit, it will likely have some tax obligations. These usually relate to payroll deductions for employee income taxes and Social Security taxes (i.e., *FICA*) as well as unemployment and workers' compensation taxes.

Deferred revenues are somewhat more complex. These represent payments that the organization has received in advance of providing its services. For example, suppose that under an arrangement with an employer in the area, your organization will provide primary care to that employer's employees. The employer makes quarterly payments in advance. The payment at the end of this year covers care to be provided in the first 3 months of next year. The money has been received, but the organization has not yet delivered any care. This money received will represent revenue in the future, but that recognition is deferred until the services have been provided. Until then, this deferred revenue is treated as a liability because the organization is liable to repay the money it received if it does not keep its part of the bargain and provide the agreed-upon care.

Table 6–1 indicates two types of long-term liability: *mortgage payable* and *bonds payable*. A mortgage payable represents a loan secured by a specific asset. Mortgage payments, including interest and a portion of the liability balance, are generally made monthly. If the organization defaults on its required payments, the lender can take the asset and sell it to recover the balance of the loan.

A bond payable represents a formal borrowing arrangement in which a security, called a bond, represents the debt. The security is legally transferable. For instance, one person lends money to a hospital and receives the bond. The individual can sell that bond to another person. The hospital is then obligated to repay the money borrowed to the new owner of the bond. Often, interest on bonds is paid only twice a year (semiannually), and the principal amount borrowed is not repaid at all until the maturity or termination date of the bond. Bondholders typically are general creditors. Their loan to the organization is secured by all the assets of the organization rather than by a specific asset. When insufficient cash is available to make payments due to creditors, the organization may be forced into bankruptcy. Creditors with loans secured by specific assets get paid from the proceeds of the sale of those specific assets before general creditors get paid anything.

The last section on the balance sheet is net assets or owners' equity. Note that all of the valuable resources of the organization are on the asset side of the balance sheet. This section just indicates ownership of some of those assets.

There are three parts to the net assets section of the balance sheet of not-for-profit organizations, as seen in Table 6–1. These are *permanently restricted net assets, temporarily restricted net assets,* and *unrestricted net assets.* Permanently restricted net assets result from endowment gifts. Assets that have been given as a permanent endowment gift can never be spent by the organization. The donation is invested, and the income from the investment can be used for operating expenses. Temporarily restricted net assets are the result of gifts that have restrictions on their use. The restrictions relate to a specific use for the donated assets, or a specific time period before the assets can be used. For example, the assets may only be used for a specific research project. All net assets that are neither permanently nor temporarily restricted are unrestricted.

If ABC Health Care were a for-profit (or proprietary) organization, the balance sheet's assets and liabilities would appear the same as they do in Table 6–1. However, the owners' equity section of the right side of the balance sheet would be different. For-profit organizations would typically have "*Stockholders' Equity*" as the main owners' equity heading, instead of "Net Assets." A typical owners' equity section for a for-profit organization might appear as follows:

Stockholders' Equity

Common Stock at Par Value	$ 100
Additional Paid-in Capital	900
Retained Earnings	5,932
Total Stockholders' Equity	$6,932

For-profit corporations sell shares of ownership in the organization. By doing so, the corporation acquires money it needs to operate a business, and the individuals receive shares of stock that represent ownership of the company. In many cases, corporations have issued stock that has a stated, or *par,* value. Par value is a technical legal concept that protects the stockholders from being sued for the debts of the corporation. Generally, as long as an investor pays more than the par value to buy stock from a corporation, creditors can sue the corporation for money owed to them, but they cannot sue the individual stockholders.

This means that stockholders have limited liability. They can never lose more than the amount they paid to purchase the stock. In contrast, sole proprietors and partners are liable for all of the debts of an organization that they own.

For example, a new nurse practitioner company might issue 1,000 shares of $1 par value stock at $10 per share. The corporation would receive $10,000 in cash (i.e., 1,000 shares × $10 issue price per share = $10,000). The stock would show up in the Stockholders' Equity section of the balance sheet as Common Stock at Par Value of $1,000 (i.e., 1,000 × $1 par value = $1,000) and Additional Paid-in Capital of $9,000. The additional paid-in capital is simply the difference between the par value of the stock issued and the actual amount that the organization received for the stock it issued.

The *retained earnings* line in the Stockholders' Equity section represents the amount of profits that have been earned by the organization over the years that have not been distributed to the owners in the form of a dividend. Often organizations retain profits and use them for expansion of services offered. However, retained earnings do not represent cash but rather reflect a claim on ownership of a portion of the assets that appear on the left side of the balance sheet.

Revenues and Expenses

Table 6–2 presents an operating statement for discussion. The terms to be discussed based on this statement include the following:

- Revenues
- Net patient revenues
- Operating revenues
- Contractual allowances
- Wage, patient care supply, depreciation, administrative, and other operating expenses
- Bad debts
- Charity care

The operating statement starts with *net patient revenues* and other *operating revenues* (e.g., gift shop or cafeteria sales).[1] Net patient revenue represents the amount that the organization is legally entitled to collect. This is usually less than the amount

the organization charges for its services. In many cases, governments (Medicare and Medicaid) and insurers (including health maintenance organizations [HMOs]) pay a rate lower than the health care provider charges. These discounts are referred to as *contractual allowances.* Accounting rules require that patient revenues be shown after discounts have been deducted. The amount of contractual allowances does not have to be shown on financial statements.

Expenses are subtracted from revenues on the operating statement. Expenses are the costs related to generating the revenues of the organization. These include *wages, patient care supplies, depreciation, administrative costs,* and a wide variety of other types of costs.

The amounts charged that the provider is legally entitled to collect are included as *revenues.* Then the portion of that amount that the organization is not able to collect is subtracted as a *bad debt* expense. This contrasts with the accounting treatment for contractual allowances and charity care. The organization is not entitled to collect contractual allowances, so those amounts are never included in net patient revenues. Therefore, they do not have to be subtracted as bad debts. Similarly, *charity care* is not included in revenues because the organization never expects to collect payments for charity care in the first place. So charity care is also not subtracted as a bad debt expense. However, the costs of providing charity care are included with the other expenses on the operating statement.

✳ THE RECORDING AND REPORTING PROCESS

How does one develop financial statements? The financials are based on recording each individual event that has a financial impact on the organization, aggregating that information, and finally developing a summarized report.

Journal Entries

When a financial event occurs, it is recorded in a *journal.* The journal is called the book of original entry because it is the first place that the accounting system recognizes the event. When the event is recorded, it is called a *journal entry.* The journal provides a complete chronological financial history of the organization. Each journal entry must leave the fundamental equation of accounting in balance. For example, if we buy supplies, the asset "supplies" increases on the left side of the equation. Also, if we have not paid for the supplies, the liability, "accounts payable," increases on the right side of the equation. This leaves the equation in balance.

As a technical way to minimize arithmetic errors, accountants use *debits* and *credits* (abbreviated *Dr.* and *Cr.* based on the Latin roots of the words). A debit is simply an increase in an item on the left side of the fundamental equation of accounting. A credit is simply an increase in an item on the right side of the equation. Decreases are the opposite: A decrease in an asset is a credit and a decrease in a liability is a debit. The bookkeeping rule—debits must equal credits—is a way to help ensure that as we record journal entries, the fundamental equation is always kept in balance. Managers who are not financial managers do not have to ever get involved in debits and credits. If financial managers use those terms, one

---

[1]Until the late 1990s, the first line on an operating statement of a HCO was gross patient revenues. Gross revenues are the charges for all service care provided. However, in most cases, HCOs receive less than 100% of their charges. Some patients are too poor to pay the full charge (resulting in charity care), some patients just never pay their bill (resulting in bad debts), and some payers receive discounted prices (contractual allowances). Therefore, the operating statement at one time would start with gross charges on the first line, and then amounts for contractual allowances, bad debts, and charity care would be subtracted. This approach is no longer permitted under GAAP as put forth by the authoritative accounting body, the Financial Accounting Standards Board.

Consider a car dealership that negotiates the price at which each car is sold. Would the auto dealer report revenue as the total of the actual amounts that all the cars were sold for or the total of the sticker (list) prices? Clearly, the sales are the sum of the negotiated prices, not the artificially high list prices shown on the car stickers. The old health care approach was comparable to showing the total of the sticker prices of the cars rather than the total of the agreed-upon prices. As the discounts allowed in health care became larger and larger, the gross charge became less and less of a relevant measure of the true revenues of the organization.

should simply ask them to explain which account balances have increased and which have decreased.[2]

Ledgers

Although the journal provides a complete and permanent financial chronological history, it is somewhat cumbersome to use. If one wanted to know how much cash the organization had, one would have to go back to each journal entry, see whether it changed the cash balance, and sum all the journal entries that had an impact on cash. To simplify this process, accounting uses a set of *ledgers*.

A ledger is referred to as a *book of accounts*. Each page in the book represents a different item that we would like to keep track of or keep "account" of. When the journal entry is recorded, each item in the journal entry is *posted* to a ledger account. Posting means to copy over or transfer the item. Thus, if a patient pays $100 that had been owed for 2 months, the journal entry would show cash going up and accounts receivable going down. In addition to recording that journal entry, the accountant would also add $100 to the cash ledger account (to show an increase in cash) and deduct $100 from the accounts receivable ledger account (to show a decrease in the amount that our customers still owe us). At any point in time, if we would like to know how much cash we have, we do not have to go through all the individual journal entries; instead, we can simply go to the ledger and look at the current balance in the cash account.

In today's computerized environment, almost all organizations maintain their accounting records using computer software systems. Such systems simplify the process of recording journal entries and keeping ledgers up to date. So a ledger book generally does not have actual pages for each account but rather is a set of electronic files.

Reporting Information

When journals and ledgers are maintained, it is a straightforward process to report the financial results of the organization. At the end of an accounting period, the accumulated balance in each ledger account is reported on the appropriate financial statement.

Asset and liability accounts are used to prepare a balance sheet. Revenue and expense accounts are used to prepare an operating statement. The excess of revenues over expenses (called the *net income* or the *increase in net assets*) represents a profit that is retained in the organization. It causes the net assets at the beginning of the year to increase to its level at the end of the year.

The organization can generally choose a financial or *fiscal* year-end date that is convenient. *Fiscal years* do not have to coincide with the calendar year. In some states, there is a regulation that mandates a particular year end. Unless that is the case, most organizations choose to end their fiscal year when they are at a relatively slow time in their operations, so that the extra bookkeeping needed at year end does not impose an unnecessarily great burden. Thus, if things ease off over the summer, June 30 might be chosen for the end of the fiscal year.

The use of ledger account balances to create financial statements allows a tremendous number of financial events to be summarized. The financial statements in turn convey to the user information about the organization's financial position and the financial results of its activities.

❋ GENERALLY ACCEPTED ACCOUNTING PRINCIPLES

Accounting is a set of rules, not a clear-cut science. These rules are generally followed by both *internal* and *external accountants*. Each organization employs its own in-house accountants who keep track of financial information throughout the year as it occurs. These accountants are referred to as *internal accountants*. There are also accountants who work for separate certified public accounting companies. These accountants are referred to as *external accountants* or *external auditors*. Many organizations hire certified public accountants (CPAs) to *audit* or examine their financial records once a year.

A CPA is someone who has been licensed by the state. Licensing as a CPA indicates a level of expertise in accounting and auditing. *Auditing* is a function that examines the accuracy and completeness of financial records. In an audit by a CPA, the financial records of the organization are examined to discover significant errors, evaluate the organization's accounting system, and determine whether financial statements have been prepared in accordance with GAAP.

Generally accepted accounting principles are rules established by the Financial Accounting Standards Board (FASB). CPAs are required to indicate whether an audited set of financial statements is in compliance with GAAP. Many HCOs are required to have financial statements that have been audited by a CPA; therefore, the use of GAAP is common in the health care industry. A few of the most common and important GAAP discussed here include the following:

- Entity concept
- Going-concern concept
- Matching principle and cash versus accrual accounting
- Cost principle
- Objective evidence
- Materiality
- Consistency
- Full disclosure

---

[2]The use of debits and credits is complicated by the fact that each organization looks at the world from its own viewpoint. For instance, if a long-term care (LTC) facility receives a debit memo from the bank, it reduces its cash on deposit at the bank. However, cash or bank deposits are assets, and we have said that debits represent asset increases or liability decreases. How can we understand why a bank debit memo would reduce your bank deposit asset? You would think a debit would increase your bank balance. The seeming paradox is caused by the fact that the bank looks at the world from its own perspective. When you have money on deposit in a bank, the bank owes that money to you. On your records, you have a bank deposit asset. But on the bank's records, it has a liability to repay the money you put on deposit. When the bank issues a debit memo (let's say they are charging the LTC facility for printing new checks), they are saying they owe the LTC facility less money. They are taking money out of its account to pay for the check printing. The bank's liability to repay the LTC facility has decreased. When a liability decreases, the result is a debit. However, that is from the bank's perspective. From the LTC facility's perspective, its bank deposit asset has decreased, and that transaction is recorded on the records of the LTC facility as a credit. Think about your own use of a debit card. When you buy something with your debit card, the bank records a debit to your account on its books because it owes you less money, so its liability to you went down. But from your perspective, you would record a credit to your bank account because the balance in that asset account dropped.

The Entity Concept

The *entity* is the person or organization that is the focus of attention. A large medical center that includes a hospital, nursing school, medical school, and long-term care facility is an entity. Accounting records may be kept for that entity as a whole. However, the hospital, nursing school, medical school, and long-term care facility that make up the medical center are each entities as well. Financial records could be maintained separately for each of these subentities. When financial statements are prepared, it is important to identify the specific entity to which the statements relate.

All accounting transactions must take the perspective of the entity for which the financial statements report. For example, suppose that we are interested in learning about the finances of the nursing school. Suppose further that the nursing school purchased some supplies from the hospital but has not paid for them. On the financial records of the nursing school entity, there would be an account payable to indicate the obligation to pay for the supplies. On the records of the hospital entity, there would be an account receivable because it has not yet been paid for the supplies it provided.

Going Concern

The second critical GAAP is that of the *going concern*. There is a presumption when accounting records are prepared that the entity is going to continue in business into the future. If there is a strong possibility that the entity is going to go out of business, that possibility must be disclosed by the organization's auditor. The reason for this stems from the fact that assets may be valuable to an ongoing organization but have much less value if the organization goes out of business.

The Matching Principle and Cash versus Accrual Accounting

The simplest way to record revenues and expenses is on a *cash basis*. When cash is received, revenue is recorded. When cash is paid, expense is recorded. This easy approach does not necessarily give a fair picture of what has happened to the organization in any given fiscal year. Suppose that we provide care near the end of the year to a patient who immediately pays the organization. However, our staff will not be paid their biweekly salary until the second day of the next year. The profit for the year will be overstated because it does not reflect all the costs of providing the care.

To avoid such results that do not truly reflect how well the organization did in a given year, accountants rely on the *matching principle*, which gives rise to *accrual accounting*. The matching principle requires that organizations record expenses in the same year as the revenues they help to generate. Thus, revenue and related expense are matched. Revenues are recorded in the accounting period that the organization becomes legally entitled to them. Even if the cash is not yet received, the organization accrues (i.e., accumulates or adds) the revenue to other current year revenue to find the total revenue for the year. The cost of resources consumed to generate that revenue is recorded as an expense in the same year as the revenue is recorded, whether we have paid for those resources yet or not.

Accrual accounting helps the organization provide a full picture of current year activities. For example, patient revenue that is not actually collected from insurance companies until the year after the service is provided is considered to be revenue the year we care for the patient. Accrual accounting also gives rise to depreciation, ensuring that part of the cost of a fixed asset is recorded as an expense in each year that the fixed asset is used to generate revenues rather than all in the year the asset is purchased. Accrual accounting is more complicated than cash accounting. However, because it provides a fairer picture of what has occurred in each year, it is required for organizations that prepare their financials in accordance with GAAP.

The Cost Principle

The cost of any resource is the amount that the organization pays to acquire that resource. Assets are generally recorded on the balance sheet at a value equal to their cost.

There are some exceptions to this straightforward concept; for example, depreciation charges off the original cost of some assets over a period of years. Therefore, the net plant (building) and equipment value will appear on the balance sheet at a level lower than the original purchase cost. The reported balance is called the *net book value*. It is net because it represents cost less the accumulated depreciation that has been recorded all the years that the building and equipment have been owned.

The *cost principle*, seemingly innocuous, creates serious problems in the interpretation of balance sheet information because over time, the value of many assets may vary from their original cost. For example, land may rise substantially in value. Nevertheless, it remains on the balance sheet at its cost. This is largely the result of the principle of objective evidence.

Objective Evidence

The principle of *objective evidence* holds that information reported on financial statements should be based on objective, verifiable evidence. This is evidence on which a wide group of different individuals could all be expected to agree.

For example, there could be considerable discussion concerning what a patient monitor is currently worth. Some might argue that it is worth what we paid for it. Others might contend that it is worth what we could sell it for. Another choice is that it is worth the amount we would have to spend if we were to replace it today. Yet another view would be that its value is based on the revenues it allows the organization to generate. Each of these perspectives has some merit; however, most of them are subjective measures.

How much revenue will a hospital generate because it has a particular patient monitor? That is clearly subject to speculation. We cannot know what future revenues will be. How much could we get for the monitor if we were to sell it? Again, this is a speculative question unless we actually sell the monitor, which we have no intention of doing. Accountants wish to avoid speculation because it makes it hard to interpret financial statement information. Was the estimate of value made by an optimist or a pessimist? It is much simpler to use objective, verifiable evidence.

As a result, accountants record the value of most assets at their cost because we can generally get agreement on the exact amount that was paid to acquire an asset. On the up side, the user of the financial statement does not have to worry about the introduction of bias in valuing the asset. On the down side, balance sheet information is often not a good measure of what assets are really worth. In many cases, the assets that appear on financial statements substantially underestimate the value of the assets owned by the organization.

In contrast, however, GAAP require marketable securities to be shown at their fair market value. They are valued at their fair market value because actual transactions in the stock and bond markets provide objective evidence of the value of stocks and bonds at any point in time.

Materiality

The accounting process requires the recording of thousands, millions, and even billions of individual financial transactions. Practice has shown that it is generally impossible to undertake such a task and expect it to be error free. In general, errors occur with any accounting system, and to try to eliminate all errors would be extremely costly. Therefore, accounting systems are designed to try to minimize the number and size of errors.

How many errors of what size are acceptable? To answer that question, accountants rely on the concept of *materiality*. Individual error, or all errors in aggregate, can be tolerated if not material in amount. What amount represents a material error? Is it $5, or $500, or $50,000? The answer to that question depends on a number of factors, such as the size of the organization. Accountants do not have a standard dollar cutoff that can be arbitrarily applied to all organizations; rather, they focus on the likely users of the financial information. An error in a financial report that would cause a user of the financial statement to change a decision is material.

Suppose we expect the organization's financial statements to be used by a bank when it decides whether to lend money to the organization. Assets overstated by a small amount would probably have no effect on the bank's loan decision. If assets are mistakenly overstated by a substantial amount, the bank might lend money to the organization that it would not have loaned if it had known the correct amount of assets. That would be a material misstatement of financial position. Therefore, accountants must decide what amount of money in a given situation is so large that it would likely affect the decisions of users of the financial statement. Then the accountant must attempt to ensure that if any errors of that magnitude occur, they are discovered and corrected before the financial statements are disseminated.

Note that the final financial statements are therefore not expected to be error-free. They are only expected to be free of any material errors.

Consistency

In some instances, organizations are allowed choices among alternative allowable accounting methods. The choice may have an impact on the balance sheet and the operating statement of the organization. In such cases, the organization should be consistent in its choice from year to year. This reflects the principle of *consistency*. To vacillate would confuse users of the financial statement who might be attempting to compare the organization's financial performance from year to year.

Full Disclosure

Financial statements should be a fair representation of the financial position and results of operations of an organization in accordance with GAAP. The principle of *full disclosure* is simply a catchall. This principle requires disclosure of any information that would be needed for the financial statements and accompanying notes, taken as a whole, to present a fair representation of the finances of the organization.

✳ FUND ACCOUNTING

Historically, not-for-profit organizations developed specialized accounting methods to deal with the unusual *fiduciary* nature of the organizations. A fiduciary is someone in a position of trust. The fiduciary of a not-for-profit organization controls assets that belong to the community. For-profit corporations can be expected to be closely monitored by the owners of the organization. Not-for-profit organizations have no owners, and therefore there are fewer "watchdogs" making sure that managers work to carry out the mission of the organization. The response to this problem was to divide authority, preventing any one manager of a not-for-profit organization from having excessive control over the organization and its assets. This divided authority was accomplished by using *fund accounting*.

Fund accounting is a system of separate financial records and controls. Distinct funds are established. Each fund has control over certain portions of the assets of the organization, and each fund has its own separate set of financial records. One could prepare a balance sheet for each fund. Typical HCO funds include the *general operating fund,* which is considered *unrestricted* and can be used for any valid organizational purpose. Other funds are typically *restricted,* and their assets can be used only for their stated purpose. These funds include the *endowment fund* and a variety of *special purpose funds.* Donor restrictions can be removed only by the donor.

Historically, a different manager had control over each fund. This, for example, prevents the chief operating officer, who is in charge of day-to-day operations, from embezzling the endowment fund. It also prevents the commingling of funds (i.e., mixing together in one pot). This assures donors that endowment funds will not be used to pay for current activities or for purposes other than those which the donors intended.

Fund accounting divides the resources available to it into separate categories, called *funds*. The term *fund balance* then results from the idea that when the liabilities of each fund are subtracted from its assets, the remaining amount is the balance owned by the organization, or simply the fund balance. The fund balance represents the net assets for one specific fund.

Over the past half-century the use of separate fiduciaries for each fund has mostly been discontinued. For example, the chief executive officer of most organizations has substantial control over all of the organization's funds. Nevertheless, many not-for-profit HCOs continue to use fund accounting because it helps provide assurance that restricted assets are used for their intended purpose.

Although many not-for-profit HCOs use fund accounting for internal purposes, all funds must be combined when audited financial statements are prepared. It is believed that viewing the results of operations and the financial condition of the organization as a whole allows for a better understanding of the organization.

✳ IMPLICATIONS FOR NURSE MANAGERS AND EXECUTIVES

Basic accounting concepts are critical tools for nurse managers and executives on two levels. First, nurse managers and executives must be able to communicate with financial managers of the organization. Second, accounting provides information that is of critical value to nurse managers and executives as they help to steer the overall direction of the organization.

The need to garner resources for nursing and to work with the organization to control the use of resources requires that nurse managers and executives be able to communicate with financial managers, or at least to some extent, be able to speak their language. Many aspects of basic accounting have become part of the lives of most managers. For example, journal entries are a common bookkeeping element with which most managers are familiar, at least on a mechanical level.

Going beyond that mechanical level and learning about things such as GAAP will allow the nurse manager and executive to comprehend why certain things are done, such as depreciating equipment. It should also serve to put many of the bookkeeping tasks nurse managers and executives perform into their broader context.

Furthermore, nurse managers and executives must look beyond their departments to focus on what the organization as a whole must do to survive and thrive in a difficult economic environment. An understanding of accounting and financial statements is critical to being able to assess the financial position of the organization. That information in turn is needed to be able to participate in an informed manner concerning the critical strategic decisions faced by HCOs.

Chapter 7 takes the nurse manager or executive a step further in developing the capability to understand the organization's financial situation with a discussion of interpretation and analysis of information contained in financial statements.

✳ KEY CONCEPTS

Accounting   System used to track financial events and provide information essential to undertaking the financial well-being and financial success of the organization.

Fundamental equation of accounting   Assets = Liabilities + Net Assets. Assets are the valuable resources owned by the organization; liabilities are amounts the organization owes to outsiders; net assets, or owners' equity, is the portion of the organization's assets owned by the organization or its owners.

Balance sheet or statement of financial position   Financial statement that presents the financial position of the organization at a specific point in time.

Operating or income statement   Financial statement that presents the financial results of the organization's revenue and expense activities for a specific period of time.

Depreciation   Allocation of a portion of the cost of an asset with a multi-year life into each of the years the asset is expected to be used to help generate revenues.

Journal   Book (or computer file) in which the financial events of the organization are recorded in chronological order.

Ledgers   Set of individual accounts. Information from the journal is transferred (posted) to the ledger accounts so that the balance in any account can be easily determined and reported on financial statements.

Generally accepted accounting principles (GAAP)   Set of rules adopted by the accounting profession that facilitates interpretation of financial statements by users outside the organization.

Fund accounting   Accounting system used by many not-for-profit HCOs that establishes a complete distinct set of accounting records for separate groupings of the organization's assets. These groupings consist of a general unrestricted operating fund and a series of restricted funds set aside for specified purposes such as endowment or research projects.

✳ SUGGESTED READINGS

American Institute of Certified Public Accountants: *AICPA audit and accounting guide for health care organizations with conforming changes as of May 1, 1999,* New York, 1999, AICPA.

Finkler S, Ward D, Calabrese T: *Fundamentals of accounting for health care organizations,* ed 2, Sudbury, Mass, 2012, Jones & Bartlett.

Gapenski L, Pink G: *Understanding healthcare financial management,* ed 6, Chicago, 2011, Health Administration Press.

Granof M, Khumawala S: *Government and not-for-profit accounting: concepts and practices,* ed 5, Hoboken, New Jersey, 2011, John Wiley & Sons.

Horngren C, Sundem G, Elliott J, Philbrick D: *Introduction to financial accounting,* ed 10, Upper Saddle River, New Jersey, 2011, Prentice Hall.

Keown A, Martin J, Petty J: *Foundations of finance,* ed 7, Upper Saddle River, New Jersey, 2011, Prentice Hall.

Larkin R, DiTommaso M: *Wiley not-for-profit GAAP 2011, interpretation and application of generally accepted accounting principles,* Hoboken, New Jersey, 2011, John Wiley & Sons.

Nowicki M: *The financial management of hospitals and healthcare organizations,* ed 4, Chicago, 2008, Health Administration Press.

Rittenberg K, Gramling A: *Auditing: a business risk approach,* ed 8, Mason, Ohio, 2012, SouthWestern College Publishing.

Tracey J: *How to read a financial report,* ed 7, Hoboken, New Jersey, 2009, John Wiley & Sons.

Zelman W, McCue M, Glick N: *Financial management of health care organizations: an introduction to fundamental tools, concepts, and applications,* ed 3, Hoboken, New Jersey, 2010, Jossey-Bass.

Analysis of Financial Statement Information

CHAPTER GOALS

The goals of this chapter are to:

- Introduce techniques for the interpretation and analysis of financial statements
- Explain the role and nature of an independent audit and the information available in an audited report
- Introduce and describe the statement of cash flows
- Introduce and describe the statement of changes in net assets
- Discuss the types of information contained in notes that accompany financial statements

- Discuss how to assess the financial performance of an organization, including the use of the statements, notes, and ratio analysis
- Provide definitions of common ratios and examples of ratio analysis
- Distinguish between financial statements and other management reports
- Consider the implications of financial statement analysis for nurse managers and executives

✳ INTRODUCTION

Much of accounting is useful for any manager carrying out the day-to-day activities of an organization. Understanding the general financial status of the organization can help managers to better focus their department's efforts to help the overall organization. In addition, as nurse managers and executives work to gain a more central role in management of the organization as a whole, it becomes important to be able to understand as much as possible about the overall financial well-being of the organization. Nurses want to become part of major decisions, such as whether to add or replace equipment and buildings and the choice of how to finance such expansions. To get involved in broader issues than the management of a unit or department, it is necessary to be able to interpret and analyze information about the financial status of the organization.

Chapter 6 discussed the fundamental concepts of financial accounting. The framework of accounting, terminology of accounting, the balance sheet (statement of financial position), the operating statement, recording and reporting of accounting information, generally accepted accounting principles (GAAP), and fund accounting were all covered. These concepts provide a foundation for understanding the accounting elements of the organization. However, it does not provide the reader with the tools necessary to interpret and analyze the information that the accounting process can make available. Those tools are the subject of this chapter.

One of the most useful financial documents is the annual *audit report*. This report includes key financial statements, notes to the financial statements, and an opinion letter from an independent auditor. The information contained in an audit report provides a solid foundation for gaining an understanding of the historical results and current financial condition of the organization. This chapter begins with a discussion of the independent audit.

An audit report includes the balance sheet and the operating statement (see Chapter 6). It also generally includes a statement of cash flows and a statement of changes in net assets. All of these statements are essential for gaining a full understanding of the finances of the organization, and a discussion of them is included in this chapter.

Generally accepted accounting principles require that an audit report provide full disclosure of relevant items. To comply with that principle, audited financial statements include a set of notes that provide vital information in addition to the data contained in the financial statements themselves. An explanation of the nature and typical contents of the notes follows the discussion of the statement of cash flows and the statement of changes in net assets.

All managers should first carefully read the auditor's opinion letter, the financial statements themselves, and the notes that accompany them to gain a thorough understanding of the organization's finances. In addition, the technique of ratio analysis is widely used to provide additional insights. This chapter focuses on several critical types of ratios.

Not all information that a manager might desire is in the audit report. Additional financial documents, called *management reports,* can be generated to provide managers and other interested parties with a wealth of additional data. The chapter concludes with a discussion of management reports and how they differ from traditional financial statements, followed by a discussion of the implications of this chapter's contents for nurse managers and executives.

✳ THE AUDIT

An audit is an examination of the organization's financial statements and supporting documents. Many individuals and businesses need financial information about the organization. This includes the organization's own managers, as well as philanthropists, banks, bondholders, vendors (i.e., suppliers), and regulatory agencies. Users from outside the organization want to feel certain they can rely on the information contained in the financial statements. For this reason, many, if not most, health care organizations (HCOs) use a certified public accountant (CPA) to perform an independent audit of their financial statements.

There are a number of purposes for an independent audit. The first is to examine the internal controls that the organization has built into its accounting system to minimize arithmetic and other clerical errors and to reduce the chances of embezzlement or fraud. The second is to examine a sample of the organization's accounting records to determine whether it is reasonable to conclude that material errors have not occurred or to find them and allow them to be corrected if they have occurred. The next purpose is to determine whether the financial statements are a fair representation of the financial results of the organization in accordance with GAAP. The credibility of an HCO's accounting information is often supported by the results of an independent audit.

When a CPA firm completes an audit, it issues two letters: a *management letter* and an *opinion letter.* These letters are essentially the end product of what may represent months of detailed investigation.

The management letter is a letter from the CPA to the board of trustees or directors of the organization; its contents are generally not disclosed to the public. This letter discusses the strengths and weaknesses of the internal control system of the organization. Accountants test records on a very limited basis. Accountants cannot be expected to uncover all errors, frauds, or embezzlements in their limited examination. Therefore, it is important for the organization to have a system that limits the opportunity not only for errors but also for theft or fraud. In the management letter, the auditor provides advice on how to strengthen the system. Also noted are apparent weaknesses that would cause the organization's activities to be inefficient, although that is not the main focus of a financial audit.

The opinion letter is also addressed to the board of trustees or directors, but this letter is often presented to interested parties, such as regulators, payers, and potential creditors. All internal managers have a stake in understanding how well their organization is doing. Therefore, all internal managers should make a point of obtaining a copy of the opinion letter and audit report each year. An example of the opinion letter is presented in Exhibit 7–1. The opinion letter in the exhibit notes that financial statements from the years 2012 and 2011 have been audited. The tables in Chapter 6, for simplicity, showed information for only 1 year. However, it is general practice to provide at least 2 years' worth of audited information at a time so that the user can compare the previous year's results with those of the current year.

The standard opinion letter has three paragraphs (although these are sometimes all combined into one paragraph): an opening or introductory paragraph, a scope paragraph, and an opinion paragraph (see Exhibit 7–1). Additional paragraphs are included if unusual circumstances require further explanation.

The opening paragraph describes what the auditor was hired to do. Many CPA firms provide a range of consulting services to HCOs. This paragraph explains to the user that an audit was undertaken and explicitly points out that the HCO's management bears the ultimate responsibility for the contents of the financial statements. Auditors merely examine the statements that are management's representation and ultimate responsibility.

The scope paragraph describes in brief what is done as part of an audit of financial statements. This paragraph explains the type of procedures auditors follow in carrying out an audit, including complying with a set of generally accepted auditing standards.

✳ EXHIBIT 7–1 *Opinion Letter*

Report of The Independent Auditors

To the Directors of ABC Health Care:

We have audited the accompanying statements of financial position of ABC Health Care as of June 30, 2012 and 2011 and the related statements of operations, changes in net assets, and cash flow for the years then ended. These financial statements are the responsibility of the ABC Health Care's management. Our responsibility is to express an opinion on these financial statements based on our audits.

We conducted our audits in accordance with generally accepted auditing standards. Those standards require that we plan and perform the audit to obtain reasonable assurance about whether the financial statements are free of material misstatement. An audit includes examining, on a test basis, evidence supporting the amounts and disclosures in the financial statements. An audit also includes assessing the accounting principles used and significant estimates made by management, as well as evaluating the overall financial statement presentation. We believe that our audits provide a reasonable basis for our opinion.

In our opinion, the financial statements referred to above present fairly, in all material respects, the financial position of ABC Health Care as of June 30, 2012 and 2011, and the results of its operations, changes in net assets, and cash flow for the years then ended in conformity with generally accepted accounting principles.

Steven A. Finkler, CPA

April 20, 2013

The opinion paragraph describes whether the financial statements provide a fair representation of the financial position, results of operations, changes in net assets, and cash flows of the company in the opinion of the auditor. An opinion, such as this one, that says the financial statements "present fairly," indicates that in the opinion of the auditor, exercising due professional care, there is sufficient evidence of conformity to GAAP. This is referred to as a "clean" opinion.

In some cases, the audit opinion letter also includes additional paragraphs containing explanations. This is generally the case if there is significant uncertainty or a material change in the application of GAAP. When extra paragraphs are included or if the auditor does not indicate that, in his or her opinion, the financials are a fair representation, then the user should be alerted to exhibit caution, and the contents of that paragraph or paragraphs should be closely examined.

✳ BALANCE SHEETS AND OPERATING STATEMENTS

Reviewing the auditor's opinion letter is the first step in the analysis of financial statements. Any unusual elements of the letter should be noted for later investigation. The next step is a careful review of the statement of financial position (balance sheet) and the operating statement. These statements were introduced in Chapter 6.

It is important to read through each statement carefully. Are there any numbers that seem out of line (too high or too low)? Are there indications of strength or weakness? Do things seem to be improving or getting worse? These two statements alone are inadequate to gain a full understanding of the organization's finances. However, they provide critical information for starting to gain an overall picture of the organization's financial status.

✳ STATEMENT OF CASH FLOWS

An audited report also includes a statement of cash flows. Recall that GAAP include a principle of matching revenues and related expenses in the same accounting period, the one in which the revenues are legally earned. However, the result of that principle is that the statement of revenues and expenses or operating statement is prepared on an accrual basis. It reports the amount of revenue to which the organization is entitled, not how much it has received in cash.

However, the flow of cash in and out of an organization is also critical. It is important to know the organization's revenue. But bills must be paid with cash. Knowing when cash is received or paid is critical. One must be able to know if there will be enough cash to undertake desired projects or purchase capital equipment and whether the organization has sufficient cash to be financially stable. Therefore, a statement of cash flows is generally required.

The balance sheet tells how much cash the organization has at the end of each accounting period. By comparing this balance from year to year, one can see how much the cash balance has changed. However, that does not explain where the organization gets its cash or how it uses its cash.

The statement of cash flows provides information on where the organization's cash comes from and where the cash goes. This provides a substantially improved sense of what things the organization will have sufficient cash to undertake. Table 7–1 is a simplified example of a statement of cash flows. (Note that parentheses on a financial statement indicate a subtraction or negative number.) Additional sample cash flow statements for a for-profit long-term care (LTC) facility, a not-for-profit home health agency, and a

✳ TABLE 7–1

ABC Health Care
Statement of Cash Flows
for the Fiscal Years Ending June 30, 2012 and 2011
(000s Omitted)

	2012	2011
Cash Flows from Operating Activities		
Collections from patients and third-party payers	$17,825	$16,232
Collections from other operating activities	1,919	1,432
Payments to suppliers	(2,122)	(1,876)
Interest payments	(2,333)	(2,290)
Payments to employees	(14,228)	(12,055)
Net cash from operating activities	$ 1,061	$ 1,443
Cash Flows from Investing Activities		
Earnings from restricted investments	$ 350	$ 350
Increase in sinking fund	(300)	(280)
Net cash from investing activities	$ 50	$ 70
Cash Flows from Financing Activities		
Payments of mortgage principal	$ (2,000)	$ (1,800)
Borrowing from bank	500	0
Net cash used for financing activities	$ (1,500)	$ (1,800)
Net Increase/(Decrease) in Cash	$ (389)	$ (287)
Cash, Beginning of Year	539	826
Cash, End of Year	$ 150	$ 539

not-for-profit ambulatory clinic may be found in the Appendix to this chapter.

For the most recent year, which ended on June 30, 2012, what does this statement tell the manager? The organization's receipts came from patient care and, to a lesser extent, from other operating activities. Cash used for operations went primarily into wages, supplies, and interest. However, note from the statement that cash also comes from and is used for investing and financing activities. For example, $350,000 of cash was generated from earnings on investments.

It is also interesting to note that for hypothetical ABC Health Care, even though there was a positive cash flow of $1,061,000 from operating activities, the cash for the year decreased by $389,000, from a starting balance of $539,000 to an ending balance of $150,000. If cash falls again next year by $389,000, the organization will run out of cash.

In fact, it would appear that the organization did run out of cash during the current year! Note that there was a $500,000 loan from a bank that was taken out during the year (see Cash Flows from Financing Activities in Table 7–1). Why did this happen? In trying to interpret financial statements, the first question to ask is whether operating activities are self-sufficient. Is enough cash being generated from those activities to sustain their cost? In this case, the answer is yes. Even though overall cash is falling, and in fact a loan had to be taken out, there was a positive $1,061,000 cash flow from operations in 2012.

The problem appears to be caused by a $2 million payment of mortgage principal. The cash excess from operations was not enough to offset the large mortgage payment, and therefore additional borrowing was necessary. From the point of view of an internal manager, the next important question is whether a similar payment will be required in the coming years and, if so, whether there will be sufficient cash to cover it.

The balance sheet for ABC Health Care appears in Table 7–2. Looking at the long-term liabilities, you will see that at the current rate of payment, it will take nearly 2 more years to fully pay off the mortgage (i.e., $2 million of principal was paid in 2012, and there is still an outstanding balance of $3,560,000).[1] This is disturbing. It means that if 2013 is about the same as 2012, it will be necessary to borrow another $500,000 from the bank. What if 2013 is worse than 2012?

Trends are extremely important in examining financial information. Is 2013 likely to be better, the same, or worse than 2012? Table 7–3 presents comparative operating statements for ABC Health Care. Note from those statements that the increase in unrestricted net assets (i.e., the organization's profits) fell dramatically from 2011 to 2012 (from $1,197,000 to $470,000). The cash flow statement (see Table 7–1) shows that net cash flows from operating activities fell nearly $400,000 from 2011 to 2012 (from $1,443,000 to $1,061,000).

Does ABC have a cash crisis now? No. It has cash in the bank. Is it facing a cash flow crisis? That may well be the case. Even though the organization has had profits in the past and even though it generates a positive cash flow from its activities, it is rapidly draining its cash resources.

---

[1]This balance sheet is somewhat simplified. In actual practice, the mortgage liability would be split into (1) the portion to be paid within the next year, which would be shown as a current liability under the title of Current Portion of Long-Term Debt, and (2) the portion to be paid more than 1 year into the future.

✳ **TABLE 7–2**

ABC Health Care
Statement of Financial Position
as of June 30, 2012 and 2011
(000s Omitted)

Assets	2012	2011	Liabilities and Net Assets	2012	2011
Current Assets			**Current Liabilities**		
Cash	$ 150	$ 539	Wages payable	$ 1,123	$ 1,018
Marketable securities	220	230	Accounts payable	2,430	2,575
Accounts receivable, *net* of $436			Notes payable	500	0
and $328 allowance for bad debts	2,319	1,722	Deferred revenue	300	0
Inventory	832	342	Taxes payable	145	176
Prepaid assets	46	52	Total current liabilities	$ 4,498	$ 3,769
Total current assets	$ 3,567	$ 2,885			
Fixed Assets			**Long-Term Term Liabilities**		
Property, plant, and equipment	$43,470	$43,470	Mortgage payable	$ 3,560	$ 5,560
Less accumulated depreciation	17,356	16,085	Bonds payable	20,000	20,000
Net property, plant, and equipment	$26,114	$27,385	Total long-term liabilities	$23,560	$25,560
Sinking fund	1,737	1,437			
Investments	341	341	**Net Assets**		
Goodwill	3,231	3,393	Unrestricted	$ 5,412	$ 4,942
Total fixed assets	$31,423	$32,556	Temporarily restricted	520	170
			Permanently restricted	1,000	1,000
			Total net assets	$ 6,932	$ 6,112
Total Assets	$ 34,990	$ 35,441	**Total Liabilities and Net Assets**	$34,990	$35,441

ABC Health Care
Statement of Operations
for the Fiscal Years Ending
June 30, 2012 and 2011
(000s Omitted)

	2012	2011
Revenues		
Patient revenues	$18,230	$17,578
Other operating revenues	1,919	1,432
Total	$20,149	$19,010
Expenses		
Wages for clinical services	$10,325	$ 9,525
Patient care supplies and food	934	802
Housekeeping services	654	589
Operation and maintenance of plant	1,221	1,003
Administrative services	2,343	2,050
Depreciation and amortization	1,433	1,433
Bad debt expense	436	328
Interest	2,333	2,083
Total	$19,679	$17,813
Increase in Unrestricted Net Assets	$ 470	$ 1,197

What response should be taken? That is a difficult question. ABC has a number of options. It could actively work to cut costs. Or it could refinance the mortgaged item, spreading payments further into the future. The ability to do that would largely depend on the likely remaining useful life of the mortgaged property.

Or it could increase the *unsecured* $500,000 loan that had already been taken out. The organization could use its cash flow statement to show a bank, well in advance of a cash crisis, that there is a current need for additional cash. However, that need will only persist for several years until the mortgage is paid off. At that point, the positive cash flow from operating activities can be used to repay the bank. ABC should also be concerned that the $500,000 loan taken out in 2012 is due for payment in 2013. The organization knows that it is due in 2013 because it is listed as a short-term liability on the balance sheet (see Table 7–2). ABC should be working on converting that to a long-term loan that will not need to be repaid until after the mortgage is paid off.

If the organization and its managers face the coming cash crunch in advance, a variety of options are available. However, without a document such as the statement of cash flows to examine and analyze, the organization might think everything is okay. Then one day when the cash runs out and the managers have no understanding of why, the consequences may be far more severe, often leading to employee layoffs (and reduced patient quality of care) or worse. The process of financial analysis allows actions at an early stage when there is time to find the most palatable solution.

Another measure of cash flow that some organizations look at is earnings before interest, taxes, depreciation, and amortization (EBITDA, pronounced eh-BIT-dah). Some experts argue

that EBITDA gives a sense of the cash flow that is under the control of managers. After all, managers may not be involved in the decision to borrow money, so interest may be excluded. Taxes are required by law and therefore are less subject to managerial control. Depreciation and amortization are expenses that recognize that the organization is using up assets, but they do not require current cash payments.

Sometimes EBITDA may be shown on an operating statement. More commonly, it is derived by taking the increase in net assets or the net income of the organization and adding back interest expense, income taxes (if any), depreciation, and amortization.

Extreme caution should be used when dealing with an organization that uses the EBITDA measurement. The measure is often improperly used as a general measure of cash flows from operations. It is incorrect to assume that EBITDA is cash flow that is available for management to use as it deems appropriate. In fact, interest and taxes must be paid using cash. Although depreciation and amortization do not require cash currently, they do indicate that the facilities are aging. Eventually, cash will be needed to replace those facilities if the organization intends to maintain the quality of care it offers.

Sometimes EBITDA is used to justify acquisitions of physician practices or other HCOs. Some managers use it to argue that the organization can afford to borrow money to acquire other organizations. They contend that if EBITDA indicates that there is sufficient cash being generated to pay the interest and principal payments on the debt that would be incurred to buy those organizations, it is safe to make the acquisitions. However, if they anticipate using the entire EBITDA amount to pay interest and principal on new debt, how will they pay the current interest expenses and taxes? And where will the money come from to replace the facilities as they become outdated? Using EBITDA to justify large cash outlays to make acquisitions can have serious negative long-term consequences.

✳ STATEMENT OF CHANGES IN NET ASSETS OR EQUITY

There is a fourth financial statement for HCOs: the statement of changes in net assets or equity (Table 7–4). This statement reconciles the net assets or owners' equity from the end of the previous year to the end of the current year.

This statement is valuable because it shows the changes within each class of net assets: unrestricted, temporarily restricted, and permanently restricted. This financial statement provides the user with information about both temporary and permanent restrictions, investment income restricted for specific purposes, and net assets released from restrictions. Alternatively, the statement for a for-profit organization shows how the issuance of stock increases owners' equity and how the payment of dividends reduces it. Additional sample financial statements reflecting the change in net assets for a for-profit LTC facility, a not-for-profit ambulatory clinic, and a not-for-profit home health agency may be found in the Appendix to this chapter. Note that the changes in net assets do not have to be shown in a separate statement. For the for-profit LTC facility

✳ **TABLE 7–4**

ABC Health Care
Statement of Changes in Net Assets
for the Fiscal Year Ending June 30, 2012
(000s Omitted)

	Net Assets		
	Unrestricted	**Temporarily Restricted**	**Permanently Restricted**
Net assets July 1, 2011	$4,942	$170	$1,000
Increase in unrestricted net assets	$ 470		
Restricted contributions and grants		$ 0	$ 0
Investment income	0	350	0
Net assets released from restrictions	0	0	
Change in net assets	$ 470	$350	$ 0
Net assets June 30, 2012	$5,412	$520	$1,000

in the Appendix, the changes in net assets appear in a combined statement of operations and retained earnings. For the ambulatory clinic, these changes appear in a combined statement of operations and changes in net assets.

✳ **NOTES TO FINANCIAL STATEMENTS**

The purpose of financial statements is to convey information to individuals interested in the financial situation of the organization. However, in most instances, the statements themselves are inadequate to provide complete information. Additional information is conveyed by appending notes to the financial statements. The purpose of these notes is to ensure full disclosure of all relevant information needed for the financial statements to constitute a fair representation of the financial position, results of operations, and cash flows of the organization in accordance with GAAP.

Financial statements without notes may be inadequate for several reasons. In some cases, organizations are allowed a number of choices of how to record and report financial results (e.g., how to report inventory). Two identical hospitals with exactly the same inventory might report a different asset value on the balance sheet and a different operating income, depending on the accounting choice made for reporting inventory. A note must disclose the choice that was made so that the reader can compare financial statements of different organizations on an informed basis.

Sometimes notes are required to disclose particular types of information that do not otherwise appear on the financial statements. For example, financial statements of HCOs must disclose the amount of charity care provided by the organization. This specific information may be of interest to users of the financial statements and in most instances would not be available without the notes that accompany the statements.

On occasion, there is some important fact that the statements simply do not capture. For instance, a pending malpractice suit would have no impact on the financial statements. No payment or loss occurs until the case has been decided. However, a large potential loss may be of significant importance to users of the financial statement. Until the case is concluded, the lawsuit represents a *contingent liability*. There may be liability or there may not; it is contingent on the uncertain outcome of the suit. Disclosure of such a possible loss is made in the notes that accompany the statements.

A typical set of notes begins with a summary of significant accounting policies. This is a general statement covering a wide variety of issues. The entity for which the statements were prepared is described. Other information might include organizational policy with respect to charity care. Exemption from income taxes might be noted. Accounting treatment of donor pledges that have not yet been received in cash may be explained. Many other items of general background information may be contained as well.

Following the summary of accounting policies are a number of notes on specific topics. There is a note about charity and other uncompensated care. Next, the relationship between the organization and third-party payers is often intricate, involving the rights of the third parties to conduct their own audits and revise the amounts due. Such relationships often merit a specific note. The property, plant, and equipment information shown on the balance sheet is often presented in a highly summarized form; more detailed information is provided in a note. Malpractice issues, pension plans, and commitments such as future lease payments represent the most common types of notes. Other notes explain unusual circumstances.

Although the notes are sometimes quite involved and may seem peripheral to some readers, accountants believe that the information they contain is essential. To help convey that fact, each financial statement has a footnote on the same page as the statement, referring readers to the notes that accompany the financial statements.

✳ **RATIO ANALYSIS**

In addition to a review of the financial statements themselves and the notes that accompany them, a third major component of the interpretation of financial statement information is *ratio analysis*. A *ratio* is an examination of the relationship between two numbers. This is accomplished by dividing one number by another. Sometimes the result is multiplied by 100% to convert it into a percentage. A number of examples are provided below. The comparison often yields insights that otherwise would not be gained.

In hospitals and other inpatient facilities, one of the most common ratios is not developed from financial statement information. It is the *occupancy rate*, which is the number of occupied beds divided by the total number of beds, multiplied by 100%. Suppose that a hospital has 150 occupied beds on average. Is that good or bad? Generally, from a financial perspective for reasons related to costs, the more beds occupied, the better. This is discussed in Chapter 8. However, that still does not make clear whether 150 is good or bad. If the hospital has only 160 beds, then the occupancy rate is 94% (150 ÷ 160 × 100%), which is very good. If the hospital has 300 beds, the occupancy rate is only 50% (150 ÷ 300 × 100%), which is not very good. The fact that there are 150 filled beds does not convey valuable information; the ratio of 94% occupancy or 50% occupancy is more informative.

The issue of comparisons is at the root of ratio analysis. Not only is one number compared with another, but ratios are also often compared with each other. A ratio by itself may not clearly be good or bad. Therefore, in ratio analysis, one generally asks the question "Good or bad relative to what?" The easiest comparison is of a ratio with itself for the same organization over time. Suppose that the current occupancy rate is 70%. Knowing that the occupancy rate for the past 3 years has fallen from 90% to 80% to 70% tells us something very different about the organization than knowing that the ratio has risen from 50% to 60% to 70%. In both cases, the occupancy ratio is 70%, but one would draw very different conclusions about the status of the organization after considering the trends over time.

A second type of comparison is that of the ratio for the organization compared with information for the entire industry. For example, Ingenix annually calculates a large number of different financial ratios, such as those shown below, for hospitals all over the country. A hospital can compare its own ratios with those of other hospitals throughout the country or region. Furthermore, with that service, hospitals can compare themselves with others of similar size. Other health care industries, such as LTC facilities, home care agencies, and nursing schools, have their own associations that sometimes generate ratios on an industry-wide basis.

A third focus for comparison should be with a specific similar competitor. Comparing the ratios for an organization with those of another organization just like it can provide a number of important insights about differences. Investigation of those areas can yield important information for improving the functioning of the organization.

Before the specific classes of ratios are discussed, several notes of caution are appropriate. First, one cannot rely on the information from just one or a few ratios. Second, the information that ratios draw from financial statements may be misleading.

Any one ratio is similar to one mosaic tile. One can tell very little about a mosaic from just one tile. A large number of tiles are needed to develop a pattern. It is quite possible for one ratio to cause a user to draw wrong conclusions. What if an HCO is in desperate financial condition? As a result of severe financial losses, the organization sells one of its buildings. Immediately after the building is sold, the organization will have a large amount of cash. Ratios that look at liquid assets will imply that the organization is in an extremely strong financial position. With the building gone, however, losses may become even greater. Only a thorough review can provide information on which to base inferences.

Ratios generally use numbers from the financial statements. This may not yield meaningful results in all cases. For example, GAAP require land and some other assets to be valued at their cost. However, assets are often worth far more than their cost. Therefore, ratios that include land may be misleading to the user. Another problem is that GAAP allow choices of accounting method in some cases. When one prepares a ratio, the information concerning the choice made (which is generally specified in the notes) is lost to some extent. When comparisons are made of ratios from different organizations, it is difficult to take into account the differing accounting choices made by those organizations.

Except for the occupancy rate ratio, the ratios discussed here are from financial statement information. However, as you become familiar with the concept, bear in mind that a ratio is simply a comparison of one number with another. The ratios discussed below are not an exhaustive list; many additional ratios can be conceived and calculated. They may be financial, using information from the financial statements; they may be financial but use information not available on financial statements (perhaps departmental budget information); or they may be nonfinancial, such as the occupancy rate ratio. Managers should attempt to consider relationships that can generate new informative ratios.

The five major classes of financial statement ratios are common size, liquidity, solvency, efficiency, and profitability. Each is discussed next in some detail.

Common Size Ratios

The first type of ratio is the common size ratio. Several typical common size ratios are defined in Exhibit 7–2. The goal of common sizing is to make an organization comparable to other organizations of different sizes. For example, the hypothetical ABC Health Care has $150,000 in cash at the end of June 30, 2012 (see Table 7–2). Is that the right amount of cash? Organizations want to have neither too little cash (potential for inability to pay bills and bankruptcy) nor too much cash (wasted investment opportunities). But how much is appropriate?

Suppose that XYZ Health Care has $300,000 in cash. Does that mean that ABC has too little or that XYZ has too much? Before this question can be answered, the cash balance must be viewed in light of the relative size of each organization. A larger organization would be expected to need more cash for its activities. We are really interested in which organization has *relatively* more cash.

The common size ratio helps by putting everything into perspective based on organizational size. Each asset is divided by total assets to find its ratio as a percentage of total assets. Each liability and net asset category is divided by total liabilities plus net assets (sometimes referred to as "total equities"). Each item on the operating statement is divided by total revenues. Thus,

EXHIBIT 7–2 Some Key Common Size Ratios

$$\text{Cash to Total Assets} = \frac{\text{Cash}}{\text{Total Assets}}$$

$$\text{Accounts Receivable to Total Assets} = \frac{\text{Accounts Receivable}}{\text{Total Assets}}$$

$$\text{Current Assets to Total Assets} = \frac{\text{Current Assets}}{\text{Total Assets}}$$

$$\text{Current Liabilities to Total Equities} = \frac{\text{Current Liabilities}}{\text{Total Equities}}$$

$$\text{Total Expenses to Total Revenues} = \frac{\text{Total Expenses}}{\text{Total Revenues}}$$

$$\text{Operating Income to Total Revenues} = \frac{\text{Operating Income}}{\text{Total Revenues}}$$

cash for ABC is $150,000 compared with total assets of $34,990,000 (cash and total assets values from Table 7–2).

$$\text{Cash to Total Assets} = \frac{\text{Cash}}{\text{Total Assets}}$$

$$\text{Cash to Total Assets 2012} = \frac{\$150,000}{\$34,990,000} \times 100\%$$
$$= 0.4\%$$

Dividing the cash by total assets and multiplying by 100% to convert to a percentage, we find that ABC's cash is four tenths of 1% of its assets. Assume that XYZ has total assets of $15 million. Its $300,000 of cash would then be 2% of total assets. Assume that XYZ's 2% cash to total assets ratio has been fairly stable over the past few years; that is, it was about 2% in the previous several years and the most recent year.

We still do not know if XYZ has too much cash or ABC has too little. However, now the relative portions of assets held in cash are known. This one ratio alerts management to the possibility that cash levels may be too low. This would tend to confirm some of the conclusions drawn from an examination of the cash flows statement. At the end of 2011, ABC's cash of $539,000 was 1.5% of total assets. From 2011 to 2012, the cash to total assets ratio fell from 1.5% to 0.4%. This downward trend over time further confirms the possibility that ABC is dangerously low on cash.

Similarly, a common size ratio can be developed for each class of asset, liability, net asset, revenue, and expense. For example, interest expense of $2,333,000 is 12% of total revenues (see Table 7–3; $2,333,000 ÷ $20,149,000 × 100%) for 2012. For the previous year, interest was 11%. This increase is slight but might reflect the increasing dependence ABC has on borrowed resources. Again, a comparison with XYZ or with the industry, also showing trend information over time, would be useful.

Liquidity Ratios

One key point of any ratio analysis is an attempt to determine whether the organization has sufficient assets that are cash, or will become cash soon, that can be used to pay current liabilities as they come due. The common size cash ratio is one attempt to look at liquidity. In addition, a class of ratios focuses specifically on the question of liquidity. Several common liquidity ratios are defined in Exhibit 7–3.

The most widely used liquidity ratio is the *current ratio*. This compares current assets with current liabilities. Rules of thumb are often dangerous because each industry, and each organization within an industry, has special circumstances. Nevertheless, a rule of thumb of a current ratio of 2.0 has become widely accepted. This implies $2 of current assets for every $1 of current liabilities. The reasoning is that current liabilities generally must be paid within several months. However, current assets may take longer to be converted into cash. For example, inventories must first be consumed in providing patient care to be converted into accounts receivable; then accounts receivable may take several or more months to be collected.

For ABC Health Care, with the information from Table 7–2, the current ratios for 2011 and 2012 were:

$$\text{Current Ratio} = \frac{\text{Current Assets}}{\text{Current Liabilities}}$$

$$\text{Current Ratio 2011} = \frac{\$2,885,000}{\$3,769,000}$$
$$= 0.77$$

$$\text{Current Ratio 2012} = \frac{\$3,567,000}{\$4,498,000}$$
$$= 0.79$$

Over this short period, the ratio was fairly constant. It is often desirable to view ratios over a longer time frame, perhaps 3 to 5 years, to fully observe trends or patterns. Plotting ratios on graphs each year can be particularly helpful. For example, Figure 7–1 shows three possible 5-year comparisons for the current ratio for ABC Health Care. Each one tells a story at a glance.

Figure 7–1A shows an upward trend. Although we might be concerned that the current ratio level is below the rule of thumb of 2.0, at least things seem to be going in the right direction. Figure 7–1B shows no discernible trend. We are below the rule of thumb of 2.0. Things are not getting better, but at least they are not getting worse. In Figure 7–1C, we see a declining

EXHIBIT 7–3 Some Key Liquidity Ratios

$$\text{Current Ratio} = \frac{\text{Current Assets}}{\text{Current Liabilities}}$$

$$\text{Quick Ratio} = \frac{\text{Cash} + \text{Marketable Securities} + \text{Accounts Receivable}}{\text{Current Liabilities}}$$

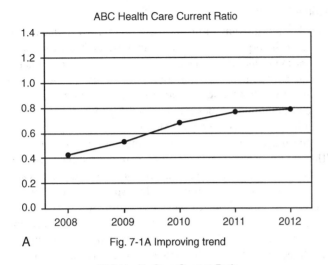

A   Fig. 7-1A Improving trend

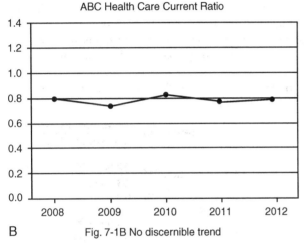

B   Fig. 7-1B No discernible trend

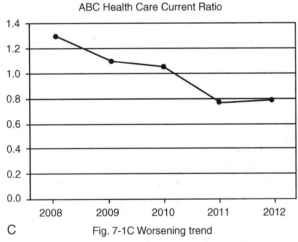

C   Fig. 7-1C Worsening trend

FIGURE 7–1.   Graphs of current ratio over 5 years.

trend. ABC's ratio used to be higher, but it has been falling in recent years. That would not be a good sign for the organization, and managers would need to take action to make sure the fall does not continue.

Another widely used liquidity ratio is the *quick ratio*. This ratio only includes current assets that can be quickly converted

to cash. Recognizing the time it takes before inventory is used to provide care, inventory is excluded from the ratio. The quick ratio therefore divides the total of cash itself, marketable securities, and accounts receivable (which can be used as collateral for a loan if necessary) by current liabilities. For ABC, the quick ratio over the past 2 years, using data from Table 7–2, is:

$$\text{Quick Ratio} = \frac{\text{Cash} + \text{Marketable Securities} + \text{Accounts Receivable}}{\text{Current Liabilities}}$$

$$\text{Quick Ratio 2011} = \frac{\$539,000 + \$230,000 + \$1,722,000}{\$3,769,000}$$
$$= 0.66$$

$$\text{Quick Ratio 2012} = \frac{\$150,000 + \$220,000 + \$2,319,000}{\$4,498,000}$$
$$= 0.60$$

These results are not dramatically different from those of the current ratio. However, there is a falloff in the ratio from 2011 to 2012 that might warrant further attention, especially in light of the other things that have turned up concerning the organization's cash flow. Keep in mind that the major focus of the liquidity ratios is on the ability of the organization to meet its obligations over the coming year.

Solvency Ratios

In contrast, solvency ratios represent an attempt to assess the organization's ability to meet its payment obligations over a longer period of time, such as the next 5 years. Some of these ratios are often referred to as *coverage ratios*. Several common solvency ratios are defined in Exhibit 7–4. These ratios emphasize cash payments that must be made every year to avoid default. Such payments include interest and principal payments on loans.

The *total debt to equity ratio* is a generic ratio looking at long-term solvency. If this ratio is high, creditors are supplying a substantial portion of all resources used by the organization. This in turn makes it more difficult for the organization to borrow further, if it were to become necessary.

For instance, suppose that a for-profit home care agency had $2 million in assets, $1 million in debt, and $1 million in stockholders' equity. The assets might consist of accounts receivable, inventory, buildings, and equipment. Creditors would perceive that there were $2 of assets available to protect every dollar loaned to the organization. Even if the organization fell on hard times, it could sell off assets to pay creditors. In bankruptcy sales, however, buyers know that the seller must sell; therefore, they often pay less than the assets might otherwise be worth.

In this example, even if each asset were sold for only half its balance sheet value, there would be enough money to pay creditors 100% of the amount owed them. That is, if the $2 million in assets were sold for just $1 million, that would generate enough money to pay the $1 million to the creditors, even though it would not leave anything for the owners. But what if there were $1,500,000 of debt and only $500,000 of stockholders' equity?

✳ **EXHIBIT 7–4** *Some Key Solvency Ratios*

$$\text{Total Debt to Equity} = \frac{\text{Current Liabilities} + \text{Long-Term Debt}}{\text{Net Assets}}$$

$$\text{Interest Coverage} = \frac{\text{Cash Flow from Operating Activities} + \text{Interest Expense}}{\text{Interest Expense}}$$

$$\text{Debt Service Coverage} = \frac{\text{Cash Flow from Operating Activities} + \text{Interest Expense}}{\text{Principal Payments} + \text{Interest Expense}}$$

$$\text{Plant Age} = \frac{\text{Accumulated Depreciation}}{\text{Annual Depreciation Expense}}$$

Then each asset would have to be sold for three quarters of its balance sheet stated value, not just for half, for creditors to recover their money. This creates more risk for lenders, because the assets may not all sell for three quarters of their balance sheet value. This means that creditors are less content if the debt to equity ratio rises.

Discontent on the part of creditors may block the ability to borrow, which in turn may generate a cash crisis. Therefore, it is important to monitor and control the debt to equity ratio. Total debt is equivalent to total liabilities. For ABC Health Care:

$$\text{Total Debt to Equity} = \frac{\text{Current Liabilities} + \text{Long-Term Debt}}{\text{Net Assets}}$$

$$\text{Total Debt to Equity 2011} = \frac{\$3,769,000 + \$25,560,000}{\$6,112,000}$$
$$= 4.8$$

$$\text{Total Debt to Equity 2012} = \frac{\$4,498,000 + \$23,560,000}{\$6,932,000}$$
$$= 4.0$$

The rule of thumb commonly used for a debt to equity ratio is 1. That implies total liabilities of $1 for every $1 of net assets. In the health care industry, this ratio is often higher, sometimes going as high as 3. In both 2011 and 2012, the total debt to equity ratio is high for ABC. In 2011, there was almost $5 of debt for each dollar of net assets. However, the trend is good. Although the ratio remains high, it has fallen dramatically. This is a positive sign. It tends to indicate that the problems ABC faces are related to short-term liquidity but not necessarily to long-term solvency. On the other hand, because of the high debt to equity ratio, it may not be possible for ABC to borrow in the short term to solve its short-term cash liquidity problems.

Examination of the *interest coverage ratio*, also called the times-interest earned ratio, provides information about the ability of the organization to meet its current interest payments. Often failure to meet interest payments creates the crisis that results in bankruptcy. The top half, or numerator, of this ratio consists of two parts. First, the cash flow from operations, is taken from the cash flow statement (see Table 7–1).

Next, interest paid (also from Table 7–1) is added to this amount. This is because the amount paid for interest was subtracted from cash flows when we subtracted payments made for our various operating expenses. We want to add the interest to find the cash flow that was available to pay interest before the payment of interest was made.

$$\text{Interest Coverage} = \frac{\text{Cash Flow from Operating Activities} + \text{Interest Expense}}{\text{Interest Expense}}$$

$$\text{Interest Coverage 2011} = \frac{\$1,443,000 + \$2,290,000}{\$2,290,000}$$
$$= 1.6$$

$$\text{Interest Coverage 2012} = \frac{\$1,061,000 + \$2,333,000}{\$2,333,000}$$
$$= 1.5$$

The interest coverage ratio is not particularly encouraging. The cash flow into the organization that is available to pay interest is only enough to pay the interest that was due about 1.5 times over. This means that if for any reason the cash coming into the organization were to fall by an amount equal to half the amount of interest itself, there might be a default.

This indicates a need to closely examine not only interest but also the required principal payments. The numbers for cash flow from operating activities, cash payments for interest, and principal payments can all be found on the statement of cash flows (see Table 7–1). The debt service coverage ratio provides that information:

$$\text{Debt Service Coverage} = \frac{\text{Cash Flow from Operating Activities} + \text{Interest Expense}}{\text{Principal Payments} + \text{Interest Expense}}$$

$$\text{Debt Service Coverage 2011} = \frac{\$1,443,000 + \$2,290,000}{\$1,800,000 + \$2,290,000}$$
$$= 0.91$$

$$\text{Debt Service Coverage 2012} = \frac{\$1,061,000 + \$2,333,000}{\$2,000,000 + \$2,333,000}$$
$$= 0.78$$

The debt service coverage ratio paints a bleak picture for ABC. Apparently, to cover both interest and debt principal payments, the organization spends more money than it brings in. In 2011, the organization's cash fell by nearly $300,000. In 2012, the cash balance fell by nearly $400,000; in addition, the organization borrowed $500,000 from the bank.

This would not appear to be a financially stable position. On the other hand, the large mortgage payments that were made in 2011 and 2012 presumably will continue for only about 2 more years before the mortgage is fully repaid, as noted in the earlier discussion of the cash flow statement. The organization's managers, however, should be taking specific actions to provide the cash that will be needed to make those payments. Also, the $20 million bonds payable must be examined. When is it due? What plans are being made to repay that principal? Even if the payment is not due for 10 years, there should be a plan now for actions that must be taken to ensure that cash will be available to pay the bond liability when it comes due.

Care should be taken in interpreting these ratios, however. Any one ratio gives only a part of the overall picture. For instance, ABC owns investments and marketable securities worth more than $600,000, and these can be used to offset much of the cash shortfall during the coming year, if necessary.

Another focus of solvency ratios is on whether the organization is keeping its plant up to date. Failure to keep facilities up to date often reduces the competitiveness of an organization, worsening the financial problems that caused it to be unable to keep its facilities up to date in the first place.

In the case of ABC Health Care:

$$\text{Plant Age} = \frac{\text{Accumulated Depreciation}}{\text{Annual Depreciation Expense}}$$

$$\text{Plant Age 2011} = \frac{\$16,085,000}{\$1,433,000}$$
$$= 11.2$$

$$\text{Plant Age 2012} = \frac{\$17,356,000}{\$1,433,000}$$
$$= 12.1$$

The accumulated depreciation (from Table 7–2) represents all of the depreciation charged over the years the organization has owned its buildings and equipment. By dividing that total by one year's depreciation (from Table 7–3), one can find approximately how many years the assets have been depreciated. It appears that the buildings and equipment for this organization have aged from about 11 years old on average to about 12 years old on average.

In other words, the plant has aged approximately one full year in the last year. That is cause for concern. It means there has been no significant updating of facilities or addition of equipment in the past year. If substantial amounts of additional buildings or equipment had been purchased, the current depreciation would be higher because there would be depreciation on those new facilities. That in turn would make the ratio lower. The average age of plant would decline or at least rise less rapidly. In light of what is known about the organization's cash situation, this is not surprising. Nor

is it a serious problem unless it is allowed to continue for more than just a few years.

The average age of plant, which uses accumulated depreciation from the balance sheet and depreciation expense from the operating statement, is another ratio that would benefit greatly from some comparison with specific competitors and the industry in general. It would be helpful to know if ABC's facilities are old or new when compared with other organizations' facilities.

Efficiency Ratios

Ratios can be used as an indicator of whether the organization is being run efficiently. This is done on an organization-wide basis. Organizations may have inefficiencies in their operations. The ratio technique will not specifically identify particular inefficiencies; rather, it can provide some overall measures to assess total relative efficiency of the organization. Several common efficiency ratios are defined in Exhibit 7–5. These are often referred to as *asset turnover ratios*.

The efficiency measure that tends to receive the most attention is *days receivable*. This is a measure of how long it takes, on average, to collect receivables. After money has been collected, it can be used to pay the organization's bills or it can invested and earn interest. In contrast, while we are waiting to collect our receivables, they provide no direct benefit to the organization. Therefore, it is generally preferable to keep the average collection period short. The days receivable ratio is often called the *average collection period ratio*.

To calculate days receivable, one first measures the patient revenue per day. This simply requires dividing the total patient revenue by the number of days in the year. If the total accounts receivable is then divided by the patient revenue per day, the result is the number of days worth of patient billings that are tied up in accounts receivable. For ABC,

$$\text{Patient Revenue per Day} = \frac{\text{Patient Revenue}}{365}$$

$$\text{Days Receivable} = \frac{\text{Accounts Receivable}}{\text{Patient Revenue per Day}}$$

$$\text{Patient Revenue Per Day 2011} = \frac{\$17,578,000}{365}$$
$$= \$48,159$$

$$\text{Days Receivable 2011} = \frac{\$1,722,000}{\$48,159} = 35.8$$

$$\text{Patient Revenue Per Day 2012} = \frac{\$18,230,000}{365}$$
$$= \$49,945$$

$$\text{Days Receivable 2012} = \frac{\$2,319,000}{\$49,945} = 46.4$$

In the health care industry, it is common for it to take substantial periods of time before payment is received for some patients. Therefore, the 35.8 average days until collection in

✳ **EXHIBIT 7–5** *Some Key Efficiency Ratios*

$$\text{Patient Revenue Per Day} = \frac{\text{Patient Revenue}}{365}$$

$$\text{Days Receivable} = \frac{\text{Accounts Receivable}}{\text{Patient Revenue Per Day}}$$

$$\text{Revenue to Assets} = \frac{\text{Total Revenue}}{\text{Total Assets}}$$

✳ **EXHIBIT 7–6** *Some Key Profitability Ratios*

$$\text{Operating Margin} = \frac{\text{Operating Income}}{\text{Total Revenue}} \times 100\%$$

$$\text{Profit Margin} = \frac{\text{Change in Net Assets}}{\text{Total Revenue}} \times 100\%$$

$$\text{Return on Net Assets} = \frac{\text{Change in Net Assets}}{\text{Net Assets}} \times 100\%$$

2011 would be considered a fairly good result. And without knowing the 2011 ratio, the 46.4-day result for 2012 would not necessarily be considered bad. However, the trend from 2011 to 2012 is not good. It represents a substantial deterioration.

This may have been caused by slowing of payments by insurance companies or Medicaid and Medicare. Such slowing may be beyond the control of the organization. Or it might be caused by lack of attention to prompt mailing of bills, accurate documentation of bills, or vigorous collection efforts. Such events should be within the organization's control. Ratios are limited. They cannot explain underlying events or causes. However, they are effective for alerting managers to situations that need attention.

Another popular efficiency ratio is *revenue to assets*, often called the *total asset turnover*. This ratio tells how many dollars of revenues have been generated by each dollar invested in assets. It is foolish to waste resources. It does not make sense to use far more assets to provide care than are necessary. If your organization generates $1 of revenue for each dollar of assets invested but other organizations in your field generate $3 of revenue for each dollar of assets, it would seem to imply that your organization is not efficient in the use of its assets. For ABC:

$$\text{Revenue to Assets} = \frac{\text{Total Revenue}}{\text{Total Assets}}$$

$$\text{Revenue to Assets } 2011 = \frac{\$19,010,000}{\$35,441,000} = 0.54$$

$$\text{Revenue to Assets } 2012 = \frac{\$20,149,000}{\$34,990,000} = 0.58$$

Without industry comparisons, these numbers tell relatively little. The increase from 0.54 to 0.58 would seem to be an improvement. However, bear in mind that relatively little, if any, fixed assets were acquired this year. Thus, revenues rose without the addition of assets. However, although this increase makes this ratio look better in the short run, it has other potentially negative long-run consequences. Again, we see that individual ratios cannot be considered by themselves.

Profitability Ratios

The last major class of ratios is profitability ratios. As noted earlier, it is appropriate for not-for-profit organizations to earn a profit. Even if profits are not part of the organizational mission, they are essential to accomplishing that mission. Therefore, it is sensible to focus at least some attention on the success of the organization in earning profits. Several common profitability ratios are defined in Exhibit 7–6.

The first two ratios considered in Exhibit 7–6 are simply common size ratios. However, they focus attention directly on profits. The *operating margin* considers revenues and expenses before unusual gains or losses. That focus keeps attention on the normal day-to-day activities of the organization.

The operating margin specifies what percentage of each dollar of revenues is left as profit before unusual items are considered. The *profit margin* or total margin ratio looks at *all* revenues, expenses, gains, and losses, and it measures what percentage of revenues is left as an excess of revenues over expenses (i.e., net income or change in net assets). Because of inconsistent definition of contributions and investment earnings as operating revenue or non-operating items, it is important to place more weight on the profit margin than on the operating margin when interorganizational comparisons are made. For ABC, there were no unusual gains or losses, so the operating and profit margins are identical. Using data from Table 7–3, they are as follows:

$$\text{Profit Margin} = \frac{\text{Change in Net Assets}}{\text{Total Revenue}} \times 100\%$$

$$\text{Profit Margin } 2011 = \frac{\$1,197,000}{\$19,010,000} \times 100\% = 6.3\%$$

$$\text{Profit Margin } 2012 = \frac{\$470,000}{\$20,149,000} \times 100\% = 2.3\%$$

The profit margin has fallen off considerably. If this represents a trend of declining profitability, it is important. A ratio such as this represents a warning sign that cannot be ignored.

Another important profit measure is the *return on net assets*. Essentially, either the owners (of a for-profit organization) or the community (in the case of a not-for-profit organization) has invested valuable resources in the organization. One can compare the change in net assets with the total net assets to get a measure of the financial return the community is earning from its investment. Remember in looking at these that the change in net assets is essentially the organization's profits for the year, and the net assets are the owners' equity of the organization. In the case of ABC, the ratios are as follows:

$$\text{Return on Net Assets} = \frac{\text{Change in Net Assets}}{\text{Net Assets}} \times 100\%$$

$$\text{Return on Net Assets 2011} = \frac{\$1,197,000}{\$6,112,000} \times 100\% = 19.6\%$$

$$\text{Return on Net Assets 2012} = \frac{\$470,000}{\$6,932,000} \times 100\% = 6.8\%$$

However, this ratio is only a part of the return to the community. The community also receives the benefits related to the health care services provided. One should exercise extreme care in using the return on net assets (also called return on equity) ratio. It does not serve as a full measure of the benefits generated by the use of the assets invested in the organization because it ignores the health benefits to the community.

It is entirely possible to use a wide variety of additional ratios in each of the areas discussed previously or to create other ratios. The essence of ratio analysis is to find two numbers that, when compared, yield some beneficial insight.

✳ MANAGEMENT REPORTS

The financial statements generated by the accounting process are of great potential value to managers of an HCO. However, it should be noted that they are designed primarily with outside users in mind. They focus on reporting the financial history of the organization. By contrast, management reports focus on the future.

The role of management reports is to provide any information that can aid the manager to improve the organization's future results. Unlike financial accounting reports, which are limited by the specific rules of GAAP, management reports need only be useful. GAAP serve a purpose in providing a sound basis of comparability for outsiders to use. An outsider familiar with GAAP can learn much about the organization from financial statements prepared following GAAP. Internal users of information need not be limited by that desire for comparability or by an ability to understand an organization from the outside.

Another problem with GAAP financial statements is that they tend to be highly summarized. There is no detailed information by department. To operate efficiently, organizations assign responsibility to individual unit and department managers. These managers cannot control results without having information specific to their departments. Managers can use department-level information to calculate ratios. Those ratios can then be tracked over time to assess whether there is improvement or deterioration in financial results at the department level.

Therefore, it is not only allowable but also desirable for internal managers to request a wide variety of additional financial information. It is possible to structure any set of reports that contain information that management believes will help in managing the organization better. Every organization will develop its own unique reports. Such reports need not follow GAAP and will not be the same at every organization. Throughout the remainder of this book, a number of different financial reports are discussed that will aid managers in the process of managing efficiently and effectively.

✳ IMPLICATIONS FOR NURSE MANAGERS AND EXECUTIVES

Nurse managers and executives should endeavor to obtain a copy of their organization's financial statements, preferably audited financial statements. There will often be resistance to providing such statements. Ultimately, information represents power, and unfortunately, some individuals do not want to share power. "Why do you need those statements?" they may ask. "Your concern should be with the management of your department." Yet how is it possible to manage a department in isolation from what is happening to the organization as a whole? The sharing of financial information with managers ultimately benefits the entire organization.

Management of a department takes place within the organization. Restrictions are often placed on salary increases or capital acquisitions. Are those restrictions justified? If they are, the financial managers should be pleased to share the financial statements to prove how bad things really are. Doing so is an excellent way to help rally all members of the organization in support of the organization in its financial crisis. On the other hand, if the hard times are really not so hard, managers have the right to know that as well.

It is critical that the chief nursing executive be a part of the organization's top management team. That job should not be focused on running the nursing department but on helping the organization make the correct organization-wide decisions. Understanding the finances of the organization is critical to such decisions.

Even at lower levels of nursing management, it makes little sense to try to manage in a vacuum. All members of the management team can be more effective the better they understand their organization and its finances.

✳ KEY CONCEPTS

Independent audit   Examination of an organization's financial statements and supporting documents by an outside independent auditor. The audit examines the organization's internal controls, searches for material errors, and determines whether the statements have been prepared in accordance with GAAP.

Opinion letter   Letter from a CPA indicating whether the audited financial statements conform to GAAP, in the opinion of the CPA.

Analysis of financial statements   Review of the opinion letter, the balance sheet, the operating statement, the cash flow statement, the statement of changes in net assets, notes to the financial statements, and ratios related to the financial statements.

Statement of cash flows   Financial statement that shows where the organization's cash came from and how it was used over a specific period.

Statement of changes in net assets   Financial statement that summarizes items that affect the organization's unrestricted, temporarily restricted, and permanently restricted net assets.

Notes to the financial statements   Supplementary and explanatory information; a critical element of an overall presentation of the organization's financial information. These notes are required to ensure that adequate and full disclosure of all relevant information, in accordance with GAAP, is made.

Ratios   Comparisons of one number with another to provide some insight or understanding of the finances of the organization that would not be realized from looking at each number individually. Ratios should be compared over time as well as with the industry norms and with those reported by specific competitors.

Common size ratios   Comparisons of financial statement numbers with key numbers on the financial statements to take into account the relative size of the organization.

Liquidity ratios   Comparisons aimed at determining the organization's ability to meet its obligations over the coming year.

Solvency ratios   Comparisons aimed at determining the organization's ability to meet its obligations over the long term.

Efficiency ratios   Comparisons aimed at determining the relative efficiency of the organization's use of its resources.

Profitability ratios   Comparisons aimed at determining the relative profitability of the organization.

Management reports   Any reports other than the four central financial statements, that are prepared to provide managers with information to aid in management of the organization.

✳ SUGGESTED READINGS

American Institute of Certified Public Accountants: *AICPA audit and accounting guide for health care organizations with conforming changes as of May 1, 1999,* New York, 1999, AICPA.

Cleverley W, Cleverley J, Song P: *Essentials of health care finance,* ed 7, Sudbury, Mass, 2011, Jones & Bartlett.

Finkler S, Ward D, Calabrese T: *Fundamentals of accounting for health care organizations,* ed 2, Sudbury, Mass, 2012, Jones & Bartlett.

Gapenski L, Pink G: *Understanding healthcare financial management,* ed 6, Chicago, 2011, Health Administration Press.

Granof M, Khumawala S: *Government and not-for-profit accounting: concepts and practices,* ed 5, Hoboken, New Jersey, 2011, John Wiley & Sons.

Horngren C, Sundem G, Elliott J, Philbrick D: *Introduction to financial accounting,* ed 10, Upper Saddle River, New Jersey, 2011, Prentice Hall.

Ingenix: *2011 almanac of hospital financial and operating indicators,* Eden Prairie, Minn, 2011, Ingenix.

Keown A, Martin J, Petty J: *Foundations of finance,* ed 7, Upper Saddle River, New Jersey, 2011, Prentice Hall.

Larkin R, DiTommaso M: *Wiley not-for-profit GAAP 2011, interpretation and application of generally accepted accounting principles,* Hoboken, New Jersey, 2011, John Wiley & Sons.

Nowicki M: *The financial management of hospitals and healthcare organizations,* ed 4, Chicago, 2008, Health Administration Press.

Rittenberg K, Gramling A: *Auditing: a business risk approach,* ed 8, Mason, Ohio, 2012, SouthWestern College Publishing.

Tracey J: *How to read a financial report,* ed 7, Hoboken, New Jersey, 2009, John Wiley & Sons.

Subramanyam K, Wild J: *Financial statement analysis,* ed 10, Columbus, Ohio, 2009, McGraw-Hill Irwin.

Zelman W, McCue M, Glick N: *Financial management of health care organizations: an introduction to fundamental tools, concepts, and applications,* ed 3, Hoboken, New Jersey, 2010, Jossey-Bass.

Additional Sample Financial Statements

In Chapters 6 and 7, sample financial statements were provided for a not-for-profit organization, ABC Health Care. These examples show the general form of statements for health care organizations (HCOs). In this appendix, sample financial statements are provided for a for-profit long-term care (LTC) facility, a not-for-profit home health agency, and a not-for-profit ambulatory clinic.

Tables 7A–1 through 7A–3 provide sample statements for the Finkler Nursing Home, a for-profit LTC facility. How do these statements differ from those presented in Tables 7–1 through 7–4? Look first at the statement of financial position (balance sheet, Table 7A–1). The asset side of the balance sheet is largely the same for for-profit and for not-for-profit organizations, regardless of the type of organization. There are a few items in the asset section we did not see in Table 7–2. One of these is *assets limited as to use*. There are a variety of reasons why an organization might have assets that are limited. For a LTC facility, it is common for there to be money that the residents have given the facility to hold. Those amounts can be used to pay for the personal needs of the resident (e.g., for a haircut, clothing purchase, gift shop, café, or newspaper). The resident just charges the purchase of such items, and they are paid for by the LTC facility from the resident's account. Even though the LTC facility holds the money, it cannot use that money as it sees fit, so it segregates the funds on the balance sheet. A liability will also appear, showing that the facility owes that money to the residents.

Another asset on Table 7A–1, which we did not see earlier, is *Estimated third-party payer settlements*. Many third party payers—Medicare and Medicaid in particular—audit health care providers to see if they were charged the correct amount. The result of these audits is often an adjustment requiring the provider to return some money to the payer (in which case the provider shows a liability on its balance sheet until it makes the payment) or the payer to pay additional amounts to the provider (in which case there is an asset on the balance sheet until that amount is received). Because these audits are so prevalent, providers are required to make an estimate of the amount that eventually will be received or paid and show it on their balance sheet even if the audit has not yet taken place.

The Finkler Nursing Home in Table 7A–1 also shows a *Deferred tax asset*. Although we often joke about unethical businesses having "two sets of books," that is in fact commonly the case for for-profit organizations. They will have a set of books, or accounting records, that are prepared according to generally accepted accounting principles (GAAP) and another set that follows tax regulations. For instance, the depreciation approach used for reporting to stockholders is different from that required for tax purposes. The result is that an organization may

wind up paying taxes sooner or later than would be expected under GAAP. If the organization defers paying taxes until the future, a deferred tax liability should be recorded. If the organization winds up paying taxes sooner than GAAP would expect, a deferred tax asset should be recorded.

In the owners' equity section of the balance sheet, we see the major difference from a not-for-profit organization. Here we see that instead of Net Assets broken down into unrestricted, temporarily restricted, and permanently restricted net assets, we have Stockholders' Equity divided into *common stock* and *retained earnings*. In this case, the amounts paid for common stock at par and additional paid-in capital are not broken out on separate lines, although sufficient information is provided to segregate those amounts if desired. See Chapter 6 for a discussion of common stock at par and additional paid-in capital.

In Table 7A–2, the operating statement and the statement reflecting changes in equity have been combined into one statement of operations and retained earnings. Also of note in this sample statement: information has been subtotaled to yield EBITDA (earnings before interest, taxes, depreciation, and amortization) information. This is not a required presentation. Generally, for financial statements prepared for external use, the user would have to make some calculations to arrive at the EBITDA amount because at least depreciation and amortization, and more generally interest and taxes as well, are treated as operating expenses and are subtracted to arrive at operating income. Notice that if the net income from this year is combined with the beginning balance for retained earnings, we arrive at the year-end balance for retained earnings.

Contrast Table 7–1 with Table 7A–3. Table 7–1 is a simplified cash flow statement. Table 7A–3 is more typical of how cash flow information is presented in accordance with GAAP. In the two tables, the second and third sections, Cash Flows from Investing Activities and Cash Flows from Financing Activities, are similar. However, the Cash Flows from Operating Activities is much more complex in Table 7A–3. This is called the *indirect method,* and it requires the statement to start with the organization's net income or increase in net assets and to reconcile changes in various operating accounts to determine the cash flows from operations. This is a very technical process and is generally only relevant to financial managers. Nonfinancial managers, however, should be aware that the Net Cash Provided by (or Used for) Operating Activities is a key number on the financials, and they should not let the complexity of the top section of this statement deter them from questioning the adequacy of the Net Cash Provided by Operating Activities.

Tables 7A–4 through 7A–6 provide sample statements for a not-for-profit ambulatory clinic. Table 7A–4 provides a balance

✳ **TABLE 7A–1**

Finkler Nursing Home
Statements of Financial Position
As of

	December 31, 2012	December 31, 2011
Assets		
Current assets:		
Cash and cash equivalents	$ 261,250	$ 354,750
Investments	412,500	
Assets limited as to use	137,500	137,500
Resident receivables, net of allowance for doubtful accounts of $18,425 in 2012 and $14,575 in 2011	445,500	418,000
Estimated third-party payer settlements	195,250	170,500
Interest receivable	19,250	
Supplies	129,250	118,250
Prepaid expenses	8,250	5,500
Deferred tax asset	33,000	38,500
Total current assets	1,641,750	1,243,000
Assets limited as to use, net of current portion	475,750	412,500
Property and equipment		
Land	563,750	563,750
Land improvements	101,750	88,000
Buildings	3,847,250	3,847,250
Furniture, fixtures, and equipment	627,000	519,750
	5,139,750	5,018,750
Less accumulated depreciation	577,500	387,750
Property and equipment, net	4,562,250	4,631,000
Other assets	412,500	349,250
Total Assets	$7,092,250	$6,635,750
Liabilities and Stockholders' Equity		
Current liabilities:		
Current maturities of long-term debt	$ 137,500	$ 137,500
Accounts payable	214,500	143,000
Accrued payroll and other expenses	481,250	517,000
Resident deposits	137,500	123,750
Other current liabilities	203,500	41,250
Total current liabilities	1,174,250	962,500
Deferred tax liability	16,500	38,500
Long-term debt, less current portion	4,675,000	4,812,500
Total Liabilities	5,865,750	5,813,500
Stockholders' Equity		
Common stock, $10 par value, authorized 20,000 shares, issued and outstanding 14,000 shares	192,500	192,500
Retained earnings	1,034,000	629,750
Total Stockholders' Equity	1,226,500	822,250
Total Liabilities and Stockholders' Equity	$7,092,250	$6,635,750

See the notes that accompany the financial statements.

sheet for the Kovner Ambulatory Clinic. This statement is not substantively different from the balance sheet shown in Table 7–2. Note, however, that from the presentation we must presume that the clinic has no net assets that are either temporarily or permanently restricted. Table 7A–5 presents the statement of operations and changes in net assets for the clinic. This is a very similar presentation to that in Table 7A–2, the Finkler Nursing Home statement of operations and retained earnings.

Table 7A–6 shows an alternative form for the cash flow statement. This statement is a mix of Tables 7–1 and 7A–3. This is an acceptable presentation in accordance with GAAP. It

starts out with the approach taken in Table 7–1. Then, at the bottom of the statement, there is a reconciliation that provides the required information that had been presented in the top section of Table 7A–3. Although many people believe the approach used in Tables 7–1 and 7A–6 is easier to understand, Table 7A–3 is the format that is most commonly used by HCOs regardless of whether they are for-profit or not-for-profit organizations.

Tables 7A–7 through 7A–10 provide sample statements for a not-for-profit home health agency. Notice that each type of provider organization will have items on the financial

✳ TABLE 7A–2

Finkler Nursing Home
Statements of Operations and Retained Earnings
For the Years Ended

	December 31, 2012	December 31, 2011
Revenue		
Net resident revenue	$5,948,250	$5,359,750
Interest	49,500	60,500
Other revenue	184,250	19,250
Total Revenue	6,182,000	5,439,500
Expenses		
Salaries and wages	2,664,750	2,527,250
Medical supplies and drugs	1,405,250	1,372,250
Insurance and other expenses	594,000	484,000
Provision for bad debts	253,000	228,250
Expenses before interest, taxes, depreciation and amortization	4,917,000	4,611,750
Earnings before interest, taxes, depreciation, and amortization (EBITDA)	1,265,000	827,750
Interest expense	451,000	473,000
Provision for income taxes	220,000	79,750
Depreciation	189,750	156,750
Net income	404,250	118,250
Retained earnings, beginning of year	629,750	511,500
Retained earnings, end of year	$1,034,000	$ 629,750

See the notes that accompany the financial statements.

✳ TABLE 7A–3

Finkler Nursing Home
Statements of Cash Flows
For the Years Ended

	December 31, 2012	December 31, 2011
Cash Flows from Operating Activities		
Net income	$404,250	$118,250
Adjustments to reconcile net income to cash provided by operations:		
Depreciation	189,750	156,750
Provision for bad debts	253,000	228,250
Loss on sale of property	0	30,250
Change in deferred income taxes	(16,500)	(38,500)
(Increase)/decrease in:		
Resident accounts receivable	(280,500)	(112,750)
Other current assets	(96,250)	(77,000)
Estimated third-party settlements	(24,750)	(27,500)
Increase/(decrease) in:		
Accounts payable and other accrued expenses	35,750	118,250
Deposits from residents	13,750	(13,750)
Other current liabilities	162,250	(30,250)
Net cash provided by operating activities	640,750	352,000
Cash Flows from Investing Activities		
Proceeds from sale of property		5,500
Purchase of investments	(412,500)	0
Purchase of equipment	(121,000)	(217,250)
Purchase of assets, limited as to use	(63,250)	
Net cash used for investing activities	(596,750)	(211,750)
Cash Flows from Financing Activities		
Payment of long-term debt	(137,500)	(137,500)
Net cash provided by (used in) financing activities	(137,500)	(137,500)
Net (decrease)/increase in cash and cash equivalents	(93,500)	2,750
Cash and cash equivalents at beginning of year	354,750	352,000
Cash and cash equivalents at end of year	$261,250	$354,750

See the notes that accompany the financial statements.

✳ TABLE 7A–4

Kovner Ambulatory Clinic
Statements of Financial Position
As of

	December 31, 2012	December 31, 2011
Assets		
Current assets:		
Cash and cash equivalents	$ 130,000	$ 152,000
Receivables for patient care, net of allowance for uncollectible accounts of $30,000 in 2012 and $10,000 in 2011	580,000	556,000
Estimated retroactive adjustments—third party payers	38,000	64,000
Accounts receivable—other	26,000	16,000
Supplies	42,000	36,000
Prepaid expenses and deposits	10,000	18,000
Total current assets	826,000	842,000
Property and equipment, at cost:		
Land	200,000	200,000
Land improvements	644,000	644,000
Buildings	1,364,000	1,364,000
Equipment	2,780,000	2,778,000
	4,988,000	4,986,000
Less accumulated depreciation	434,000	200,000
Property and Equipment, net	4,554,000	4,786,000
Other assets		
Advances receivable	28,000	10,000
Total Assets	$5,408,000	$5,638,000
Liabilities and Net Assets		
Current liabilities:		
Notes payable	$ 276,000	$ 288,000
Accounts payable	104,000	174,000
Accrued payroll and vacation	66,000	44,000
Estimated retroactive adjustments—third-party payers	60,000	48,000
Financing advance from third-party payers	0	2,000
Total current liabilities	506,000	556,000
Net assets—unrestricted	4,902,000	5,082,000
Total Liabilities and Net Assets	$5,408,000	$5,638,000

See the notes that accompany the financial statements.

✳ TABLE 7A–5

Kovner Ambulatory Clinic
Statements of Operations and Changes in Net Assets
For the Years Ended

	December 31, 2012	December 31, 2011
Revenues and gains:		
Net patient service revenue	$1,720,000	$ 714,000
Other	58,000	30,000
Total revenue and gains	1,778,000	744,000
Expenses		
Salaries and wages	970,000	486,000
Medical supplies and drugs	378,000	132,000
Insurance	308,000	196,000
Provision for bad debts	28,000	8,000
Depreciation	234,000	200,000
Interest	40,000	36,000
Total expenses	1,958,000	1,058,000
Operating loss	(180,000)	(314,000)
Net assets, beginning of year	5,082,000	5,396,000
Net assets, end of year	$4,902,000	$5,082,000

See the notes that accompany the financial statements.

✳ TABLE 7A–6

Kovner Ambulatory Clinic
Statements of Cash Flows
For the Years Ended

	December 31, 2012	December 31, 2011
Operating Activities		
Cash received from patients and third-party payers	$1,732,000	$736,000
Cash received from others	42,000	12,000
Interest received	6,000	22,000
Interest paid	(30,000)	(32,000)
Cash paid to employees and suppliers	(1,740,000)	(864,000)
Net cash provided by (used in) operating activities	10,000	(126,000)
Investing Activities		
Purchase of equipment	(2,000)	(8,000)
Advances made to affiliate	(18,000)	(10,000)
Net cash used for investing activities	(20,000)	(18,000)
Financing Activities		
Proceeds from notes payable	0	288,000
Payments on notes payable	(12,000)	0
Net cash provided by (used in) financing activities	(12,000)	288,000
Net increase in cash and cash equivalents	(22,000)	144,000
Cash and cash equivalents at beginning of year	152,000	8,000
Cash and cash equivalents at end of year	$ 130,000	$152,000
Reconciliation of change in net assets to net cash provided by operating activities:		
Change in net assets	($ 180,000)	($314,000)
Adjustments to reconcile change in net assets to cash provided by operations:		
Provision for bad debts	28,000	8,000
Depreciation	234,000	200,000
(Increase)/decrease in:		
Accounts receivable	(24,000)	(38,000)
Other current assets	2,000	(4,000)
Increase/(decrease) in:		
Accounts payable, accrued payroll, and vacation costs	(48,000)	20,000
Other current liabilities	(2,000)	2,000
Net cash provided by operating activities	$ 10,000	($126,000)

See the notes that accompany the financial statements.

statements that are relevant to their industry. For example, note on Table 7A–7, the balance sheet for the Jones Home Health Agency, one of the assets it lists separately is vehicles. If staff members are traveling a lot in company cars, this item may be significant enough in amount to warrant its own asset line on the balance sheet.

Another asset on this balance sheet that we have not seen before is *Deferred financing charges.* When long-term debt is issued, substantial accounting, legal, and underwriting fees are often related to the issuance. We might be tempted to treat them as an expense in the year they are incurred. However, from the perspective of accrual accounting, we will have the benefit of the long-term loan for many years, so we should spread out the cost of issuing the debt, just as we would depreciate a piece of equipment over the years we use it. The costs involved in issuing the debt are said to be *amortized,* or allocated to each of the years when the debt will be outstanding. The portion that has not yet been amortized will be treated as an asset, just as equipment is an asset until it is used up.

✳ TABLE 7A–7

Jones Home Health Agency
Statements of Financial Position
As of

	December 31, 2012	December 31, 2011
Assets		
Current assets:		
Cash and cash equivalents	$ 148,000	$ 82,000
Investments	294,000	274,000
Receivables for patient care, net of allowance for uncollectible accounts of		
$121,000 in 2012 and $60,000 in 2011	1,504,000	952,000
Other receivables	54,000	44,000
Total current assets	2,000,000	1,352,000
Investments	200,000	200,000
Equipment		
Medical and office equipment	112,000	78,000
Vehicles	100,000	74,000
	212,000	152,000
Less accumulated depreciation	(90,000)	(48,000)
Equipment, net	122,000	104,000
Deferred financing charges, net of accumulated amortization of $30,000 in 2012		
and $20,000 in 2011	40,000	50,000
Total Assets	$2,362,000	$1,706,000
Liabilities and Net Assets		
Current liabilities:		
Current portion of long-term debt	$ 26,000	$ 26,000
Accounts payable	80,000	42,000
Accrued payroll and vacation	992,000	704,000
Estimated third-party payer settlements	56,000	62,000
Advances from third-party payers	140,000	132,000
Total current liabilities	1,294,000	966,000
Long-term debt, less current portion	210,000	236,000
Total liabilities	1,504,000	1,202,000
Net Assets		
Unrestricted	660,000	334,000
Temporarily restricted	18,000	10,000
Permanently restricted	180,000	160,000
Total net assets	858,000	504,000
Total Liabilities and Net Assets	$2,362,000	$1,706,000

See the notes that accompany the financial statements.

There is nothing particularly noteworthy about the Jones statement of operations in Table 7A–8. The Jones Home Health Agency has a separate statement of changes in net assets, shown in Table 7A–9. Notice that separate information is provided for unrestricted, temporarily restricted, and permanently restricted net assets. The amounts for the three categories are then summed to find the overall impact of changes on total net assets. The Table 7A–10 statement of cash flows provides the reconciliation approach discussed earlier.

As you look at the financial statements for different types of HCOs—for-profit versus not-for-profit ones, hospital versus LTC facility versus clinic, and so on—you may notice minor

✳ TABLE 7A–8

Jones Home Health Agency
Statements of Operations
For the Years Ended

	December 31, 2012	December 31, 2011
Revenues, gains, and other support:		
Net patient service revenue	$8,084,000	$5,374,000
Contributions	10,000	44,000
Net assets released from restrictions	10,000	0
Other revenue	26,000	12,000
Gains on investments	54,000	64,000
Total revenue, gains, and other support	8,184,000	5,494,000
Expenses		
Salaries and wages	5,428,000	3,670,000
Medical supplies and drugs	2,084,000	1,350,000
Insurance and other expenses	180,000	166,000
Provision for bad debts	92,000	42,000
Depreciation	42,000	30,000
Interest	32,000	38,000
Total expenses	7,858,000	5,296,000
Excess of revenue over expenses and change in unrestricted net assets	$ 326,000	$ 198,000

See the notes that accompany the financial statements.

✳ TABLE 7A–9

Jones Home Health Agency
Statements of Changes in Net Assets
For the Years Ended

	December 31, 2012	December 31, 2011
Unrestricted net assets		
Excess of revenue over expenses	$326,000	$198,000
Increase in unrestricted net assets	326,000	198,000
Temporarily restricted net assets		
Contributions	18,000	10,000
Net assets released from restrictions	(10,000)	0
Increase in temporarily restricted net assets	8,000	10,000
Permanently restricted net assets		
Contributions	20,000	12,000
Increase in permanently restricted net assets	20,000	12,000
Increase in net assets	354,000	220,000
Net assets, beginning of year	504,000	284,000
Net assets, end of year	$858,000	$504,000

See the notes that accompany the financial statements.

✳ TABLE 7A–10

Jones Home Health Agency
Statements of Cash Flows
For the Years Ended

	December 31, 2012	December 31, 2011
Operating Activities		
Cash received from patients and third-party payers	$7,442,000	$5,084,000
Other receipts from operations	44,000	64,000
Cash paid to employees and suppliers	(7,358,000)	(5,082,000)
Interest paid	(22,000)	(28,000)
Nonoperating revenue	46,000	44,000
Net cash provided by operating activities	152,000	82,000
Investing Activities		
Purchase of equipment	(60,000)	(38,000)
Purchase of investments	(20,000)	(30,000)
Net cash used for investing activities	(80,000)	(68,000)
Financing Activities		
Proceeds from contributions restricted for:		
Endowment	20,000	12,000
Other financing activities:		
Payment of long-term debt	(26,000)	0
Net cash provided by (used in) financing activities	(6,000)	12,000
Net increase in cash and cash equivalents	66,000	26,000
Cash and cash equivalents at beginning of year	82,000	56,000
Cash and cash equivalents at end of year	$ 148,000	$ 82,000
Reconciliation of change in net assets to net cash provided by operating activities:		
Change in net assets	$ 354,000	$ 220,000
Adjustments to reconcile change in net assets to cash provided by operations:		
Increase in permanently restricted net assets	(20,000)	(12,000)
Provision for bad debts	92,000	42,000
Depreciation	42,000	30,000
Amortization of deferred financing charges	10,000	10,000
(Increase)/decrease in:		
Accounts receivable	(644,000)	(300,000)
Other receivables	(10,000)	8,000
Increase/(decrease) in:		
Accounts payable, accrued payroll, and vacation costs	326,000	76,000
Estimated third-party settlements	2,000	8,000
Net cash provided by operating activities	$ 152,000	$ 82,000

See the notes that accompany the financial statements.

differences. In fact, even in comparing two for-profit LTC facilities or two not-for-profit clinics, you will see differences. However, keep in mind that the similarities are much more important than the differences. After you have become familiar with the basics of financial statements, you will know enough to understand the parts of each statement. And you should always feel comfortable asking questions about any individual items you do not understand because they do tend to be specific to each organization, and it is reasonable for a manager not to understand a specific item or items on the financials until he or she asks a financial manager about it (them).

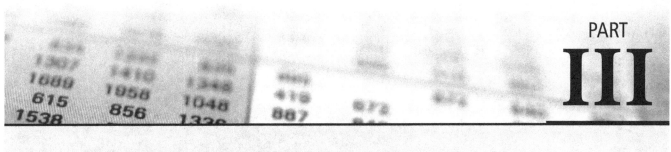

❋ COST ANALYSIS

One of the most critical areas of financial management is analysis and control of costs. Costs represent half of the financial equation. The surplus (profit) or deficit (loss) of an organization each year depends on its revenues and its expenses or costs.

The first chapter in Part III, Chapter 8, deals with basic issues of cost management. The chapter introduces definitions of critical terms and discusses the nature and behavior of costs. The relationship between patient volume and costs is stressed. Techniques are also provided for the prediction or estimation of future costs. Finally, the chapter provides a method to determine when a program or project or service will have sufficient volume to break even, that is, be financially self-sufficient.

Chapter 9 moves from basic cost concepts to the broader issue of cost measurement. There are two primary focuses: One is on how health care organizations (HCOs) collect cost information by cost center and assign that information first to revenue centers and ultimately to patients. The second is on how to cost out nursing services.

The Medicare step-down cost-finding and rate-setting methods are presented and contrasted with more recently developed methods. Attention is also placed on understanding product-line costing. Issues of patient classification systems and staffing are considered. Standard costing techniques are discussed.

Costing out nursing is a topic of much interest to nurses, nurse managers, and executives. As HCOs are increasingly forced to operate in a constrained financial atmosphere, chief executive officers look to nurse managers and executives at all levels to take a greater role in controlling costs. Financial reimbursement for nursing services is also discussed.

Chapter 10 addresses a concern that peaks during periods of nursing shortages but that requires managerial attention regardless of whether there is a current shortage of nurses. That is the issue of measuring the costs of recruiting and retaining staff. Ways to measure those costs and to include them in the budget are discussed.

Nurse managers and executives must have a solid background in costing out nursing to understand the costs of their units and services. The information presented in the chapters in this section will aid them in managing staff and other resources more effectively.

Cost Management

CHAPTER GOALS

The goals of this chapter are to:

- Define basic cost terms
- Explain the underlying behavior of costs and the importance of that behavior for decision making
- Provide tools for cost estimation

- Explain how costs can be adjusted for the impact of inflation
- Provide the tools of break-even analysis

❋ INTRODUCTION

Cost control is a major element of the job for all nurse managers and executives. Basic knowledge of costs and their behavior is central to an understanding of the expenses incurred in the cost centers under a manager's control. The skillful management of costs is an essential element of the financial success of any health care organization (HCO). However, cost management is complicated.

Many cost terms commonly used are not well understood. Direct costs, indirect costs, average costs, fixed costs, variable costs, and marginal costs are concepts that managers use and must understand clearly. This chapter stresses the definitions of these and other key terms.

The relationship of fixed and variable costs is the most fundamental cost concept. The total costs incurred by HCOs depend directly on the interplay between fixed and variable costs. Building on these concepts is the issue of volume. Volume ultimately becomes a critical aspect of almost every successful HCO and of every failing one.

HCOs are not static; rather, they are constantly in a state of flux and change. Services are added; other services are deleted. Some areas of the organization expand; others contract. To a great extent, these changes are dictated by clinical factors, technologies, and the introduction of evidence-based practices. However, every change has an impact on organizational cost. In each case, managers should determine whether the financial impact of a proposed change will be favorable or unfavorable for the organization. Although an unfavorable financial impact may not mean that a service must be deleted, a good manager makes decisions based on as much information as possible. One approach, called *marginal cost analysis,* is critical to generating information for such decisions.

Another important area of cost management is cost estimation. What will costs likely be in the coming year? That question requires careful management attention. This chapter provides several techniques to help in exploring that topic.

The last major topic covered in this chapter is break-even analysis (BEA). BEA addresses the issue of the volume of patients required for a program or service to become financially self-sufficient.

❋ BASIC COST CONCEPTS

The most critical of cost concepts is referred to as *cost behavior.* Cost behavior is the way that costs change in reaction to events within the organization. If patient volume rises by 5%, what do costs do? What if patient volume falls by 5%? How can one predict whether total costs will exceed revenues or remain less than revenues? Which factors are related to stable costs and which to rising costs?

Cost behavior depends on the specific elements of cost in any cost center or organization. A *cost center* is any unit or department in an organization for which a manager is assigned responsibility for costs. Some types of costs are stable, changing little, if at all, even in response to significant changes in patient work load. Other costs are highly changeable, reacting directly to other changes in the organization.

This section of the chapter lays out a framework on which to develop an understanding of how costs behave in HCOs.

Definitions

Cost measurement is more complex than one might expect. When someone asks what something costs, accountants have trouble responding with a direct answer. The reason is that the appropriate measure of cost depends substantially on the intended use for the cost information. Finding out what it cost to treat each patient last year is very different from calculating what it might cost to treat one more patient next year. The cost per patient when 100 patients are treated may be very different from the cost per patient when 500 patients are treated.

To make sense in this complicated area, all managers (nurse managers, executives, and accountants) must rely heavily on a consistent set of definitions. The definitions provided here form the basis of a common language so that when a cost per patient is cited, all managers can interpret that information in the same way and effectively communicate with each other.

Service unit A basic measure of the product or service being produced by the organization, such as discharged patients, patient days, home care visits, emergency department treatments, or hours of surgery.

Cost information is often collected on a *service unit* basis. This is an important concept for managers because they need to know the cost per service unit as it pertains to their area of responsibility and other areas of the organization. Within one HCO, a number of different types of service units may exist. For example, the operating room (OR) may use hours of surgery, but a medical-surgical unit uses patient days.

Direct costs
a. Costs that are incurred within the organizational unit for which the manager has responsibility are referred to as direct costs of the unit.
b. Costs of resources for direct care of patients are referred to as the direct costs of patient care.
Indirect costs
c. Costs that are assigned to an organizational unit from elsewhere in the organization are indirect costs for the unit.
d. Costs within a unit that are not incurred for direct patient care are indirect costs of patient care.

Direct costs are a particularly difficult concept because their definition relates to the object of the analysis. If one were interested in the direct cost of patient care (definition "b") for a specific medical-surgical unit, that cost would not include the cost of the unit manager's time spent on administrative duties or the cost of clerical personnel in the unit. It likewise would not include the cost of a nurse's restocking a supply cart. It would, however, include the cost of clinical supplies used, as well as the cost of nursing time spent with a patient.

From a broader systems perspective, however, all of these costs are direct costs. This perspective applies when one is contrasting all the costs assigned to a unit or department. For the unit as a whole (definition "a" above), all nursing salaries and clerical salaries incurred within the unit are direct costs. Costs assigned to the unit from outside, such as marketing, laundry, or housekeeping, are indirect costs to the unit. Similarly, nursing professional development and education, as well as a portion of the salary of the chief nurse executive (CNE), are indirect costs to a specific unit. However, from the perspective of the nursing department as a whole, rather than that of one unit, the salary of the CNE is a direct cost.

Laundry costs are considered indirect by both the manager for the unit and the CNE for the nursing department. The labor and other costs of the laundry department are clearly incurred neither directly within individual nursing units nor within the nursing department as a whole, even though nursing may control the amount of laundry it uses (definition "c"). But that does not mean that laundry costs are considered indirect costs by everyone. The manager of the laundry department would consider all costs incurred in that department as direct costs. Perspective is critical in the classification of a cost as direct or indirect. From a focus on patient care, indirect costs would include all costs that are not direct patient care costs (definition "d").

Full cost Total of all costs associated with or in an organizational unit or activity. This includes direct and indirect costs.

For example, all of the costs of a hospital would represent its full or total costs. Moving to the department or unit level, it is important to include not only direct costs but also all indirect costs. In this case, full costs include an appropriate share of laundry, administration, billing, engineering, medical records, housekeeping, marketing, and so forth. The question of what is an appropriate share of costs to assign to each cost center is difficult and is addressed in Chapter 9.

Average cost Full cost divided by the volume of service units.

Many questions faced by managers require information on the cost per patient, per treatment, or per patient day. These all represent average costs. Each cost center may use its own service units and calculate its own average cost.

Fixed costs Costs that do not change in total as the volume of service units changes.
Variable costs Costs that vary directly with changes in the volume of service units.

The salaries of the CNE and unit nurse managers do not change day by day as the census changes. Other staff salaries also do not change on a daily basis, such as the unit clerks, assistant nurse managers, schedulers, or staff educators. Therefore, these costs are fixed costs. Supplies that are used for every patient are variable. The more patients, the more supplies used.

The definition of the service unit measure is crucial in defining fixed and variable costs. For example, although most clinical supplies used in a hospital vary with the number of patient days, surgical supplies are more likely to vary with the number of surgical procedures, and clinic supplies will likely vary with the number of clinic visits.

Relevant range Normal range of expected activity for the cost center or organization.

Fixed costs are fixed over the relevant range. Suppose that a 30-bed nursing unit anticipated an average occupancy rate of 75%. It might be reasonable to expect the unit to have an 80% or even 85% occupancy rate. However, a rate of 160% would clearly be beyond the reasonable anticipated rate for that unit. To accommodate such a large number of patients, the hospital would have to add another nursing unit.

Within the normal relevant range, the costs for the salary of the nurse manager would be fixed. However, if occupancy reached 160%, there might well be expansion to two units, with a manager for each. The fixed costs would rise. Fixed costs are fixed only within the relevant range.

Marginal costs Extra costs incurred as a result of providing one more service unit, such as one extra patient day or one more type of service.

Marginal cost information is critical in the decision-making process. Managers are often interested in how costs change when the number of patients cared for changes. If we treat one more patient, how much more money will we have to spend? This differs to some extent from variable costs. What if a piece of equipment is at its capacity? To treat one more patient, we will incur not only variable costs such as supplies but also the fixed costs from purchasing another piece of equipment. Marginal cost would include both variable and fixed costs that change from adding an extra patient or extra group of patients.

Marginal costs are often used to analyze major changes, such as the addition of a whole new service. Suppose that a hospital does not currently provide liver transplantation. Marginal costs focus on what it would take to add the new liver transplantation program to the hospital's range of services.

For example, because no transplants are done currently, it is probable that the hospital would need equipment, supplies, and personnel to provide that service. The supplies represent a variable cost. For each transplant done, the hospital will need additional clinical supplies. However, the equipment represents a fixed cost. After the equipment is purchased, it can be used for many transplants. Because both the supplies and the equipment are needed for the first transplants, both the supplies and equipment costs are marginal costs of adding that service.

If one considers the total costs incurred by an organization before it makes a change and the total costs after it makes the change, the difference in costs represents the marginal costs of that change.

Mixed costs Costs that contain both fixed and variable cost elements.

An example of a mixed cost is electricity. The OR Department uses some electricity every day to light hallways and for other purposes not related to the number of patients. That portion of electric usage is a fixed cost. Much of the electricity used by the department is used in the operating suites. The more surgeries, the more electricity used. Therefore, it has a variable component as well. Similarly, a home health agency would have mixed costs for transportation if it used agency-owned cars. Some costs would be fixed, such as annual maintenance, and some costs, such as gas, would vary with the number of home visits.

Mixed costs create some problems for managers. If the number of service units for a cost center rose by 10%, one would expect fixed costs to stay unchanged. One would expect variable costs to rise by 10%. Mixed costs would be expected to rise but by some amount greater than 0% and less than 10%. Methods are provided later in this chapter for estimating the change in mixed costs resulting from a change in patient volume.

Step-fixed or step-variable cost Costs that are fixed over small ranges of activity that are less than the relevant range.

Nursing units often require a fixed number of nurses on duty for a range of patients. Within that range of patients, the nursing personnel cost remains fixed. However, if the number of patients increases by a large enough number, additional personnel will be needed. That personnel level is then fixed over a new, higher range of activity. The key to step costs is that they are fixed over volume intervals but vary *within* the relevant range.

These concepts are discussed in greater detail throughout this chapter. We will use a variety of examples and graphs to explain cost concepts.

Fixed versus Variable Costs

The total costs of running a department are generally divided into costs that are fixed and costs that are variable. The concepts of fixed and variable costs are often conceptualized with the use of graphs. In the following example, the service unit measure is assumed to be patient days. Figure 8–1 provides an example of fixed costs. Specifically, the graph shows the annual salary for a unit nurse manager for the coming year. The salary is $100,000.[1]

That salary is a fixed cost for the organization. The salary paid to a nurse manager is not dependent on any patient-volume statistic. In Figure 8–1, the vertical axis shows the cost to the institution. As one moves up this axis, costs increase. The horizontal axis shows the number of patient days. The farther to the right one moves, the more patient days the institution has.

Note that the fixed costs appear as a horizontal line. This is because regardless of the volume, the salary for the nurse manager will remain the same. Thus, the cost is the same for 8,000, 10,000, or 12,000 patient days.

Variable costs fluctuate with the volume of service units. Most variable costs are supply costs (e.g. general patient care supplies, linens, dietary stock, and pharmacy supplies). To illustrate how variable costs are determined, suppose that each patient on a 32-bed general medicine unit has his or her

---

[1]Total compensation includes the nurse manager's salary plus benefits. Benefits are an additional percentage on top of base salary and often vary between 25% and 35%, depending on the local market and organizational policies.

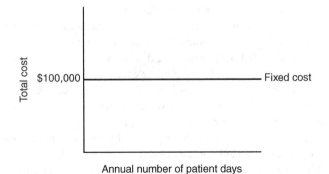

FIGURE 8–1. Fixed costs: cost for a nurse manager.

temperature taken twice a day using either an oral or a tympanic thermometer. However, the unit's practice council recommends that the unit change from taking patients' temperatures with a tympanic device to using an oral device only, with disposable thermometer covers. Based on this policy change, the nurse manager expects that each patient on the unit would use a minimum of two oral thermometer covers per day, but use of disposable covers will vary directly with patient volume. The nurse manager determines that, when purchased from an approved hospital vendor, each thermometer cover costs about $0.05; if two a day are used for each patient, the cost of those items is $0.10 for each patient each day. The more patient days, the more the cost for that disposable item in the total nursing unit budget.

Consider Figure 8–2. This graph plots the cost for disposable thermometer covers as they vary with patient volume. As in Figure 8–1, the vertical axis represents cost, and the horizontal axis represents patient volume. Unlike Figure 8–1, which shows some amount of cost even at a volume of zero, this graph shows zero cost at a volume of zero because with zero patient days, none of this particular supply is used. The total variable cost increases by $0.10 for each extra patient day.

Rather than assume that the unit is filled to capacity every day, the nurse manager could use the average number of patient days to calculate the number of oral thermometer covers needed and consequent costs. The general principle is that the more patient days, the greater the cost for a disposable or any variable cost item in the total nursing unit budget. For instance, in Figure 8–3, dashed lines have been inserted to show the cost when there are 10,000 patient days and the cost when there are 50,000 patient days. As you can see, $1,000 is spent on the disposable item if there are 10,000 patient days and $5,000 if there are 50,000 patient days.

The total of the fixed and variable costs is shown in Figure 8–4. This figure combines the fixed costs from Figure 8–1 with the variable costs from Figure 8–3. Note that in the graph, the total costs start at $100,000, even if volume is

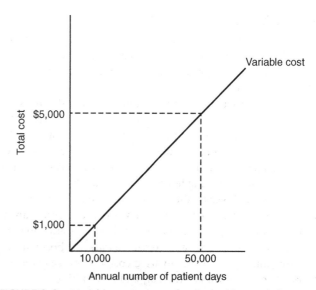

FIGURE 8–3. Variable costs: costs of a disposable supply item at volumes of 10,000 and 50,000 patient days.

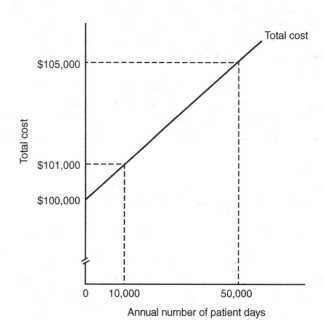

FIGURE 8–4. Total costs for a unit.

zero, because of the fixed cost of the nurse manager's salary. Although this example is used to illustrate a point, the same principle applies for small equipment that is "charged" per patient use or any other purchase that must be determined based on patient volume. Another important issue is that some variable supply costs, such as linens and dietary, are purchased as a contracted service (e.g., the organization "contracts" with a linen service to provide all of the linens used), and others are obtained through negotiated rates with vendors (e.g., the organization negotiates with a vendor to provide certain supplies at an agreed-upon rate). On some contracts, the costs of supplies per unit may actually decrease as volume increases.

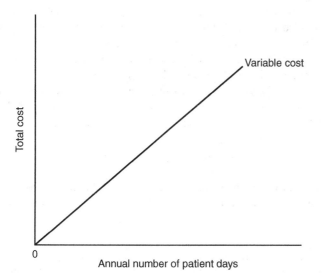

FIGURE 8–2. Variable costs: costs of a disposable supply item.

Cost Graphs and the Relevant Range

One potential problem exists with this type of graphic analysis of fixed and variable costs. That concerns the *relevant range*. The relevant range represents the likely range of activity covered by a budget.

Variable costs increase proportionately over the relevant range. However, it is unlikely that the hospital will pay $0.05 for each disposable thermometer cover at *any* volume level. If purchases increase substantially, the hospital will probably get a price reduction per unit. On the other hand, if purchases decrease substantially, the hospital would possibly have to pay more per unit. However, the variable costs may reasonably be considered to increase proportionately over the relevant range.

As noted earlier, fixed costs are not fixed over any range of activity. If a nursing unit has zero patient days, the hospital will close the unit and not have any fixed cost for a nurse manager. If patient volume rises substantially and exceeds the capacity of the unit, the hospital might need to open a second unit and incur the additional cost of a second nurse manager. The costs, however, are fixed over the relevant range.

Essentially, variable costs do not increase by exactly the same amount per unit over *any* range of volume, and fixed costs do not remain fixed over *any* range of volume. However, for most budgets, volume expectations for the coming year do not assume drastic changes.

When fixed and variable costs are graphed, the relevant range issue is often ignored; costs appear fixed over all ranges of activity in the graph. However, the user of the graph should bear in mind that the graph's information is accurate only within the relevant range.

Many costs are *step-fixed* and vary within the relevant range but not smoothly. They are fixed over intervals shorter than the relevant range. See Figure 8–5 for a graphic representation of step-fixed costs.

For example, staffing patterns may be such that a nursing unit will use several nurses to cover a range of work load (or demand). If that range is exceeded, the unit will have to hire new permanent nursing staff or contract with an outside agency for additional nurses on a short-term basis to staff the unit. Clearly, more patient days or greater average acuity

requires more nursing care hours. However, if the staffing pattern is based on the delivery of about 10.6 hours of nursing time per patient day, the unit would not expect to hire a nurse for an additional 10.6 hours every time the patient-day census increased by one. If the hours were consistently at this level, the nurse manager could use this information to help justify an additional permanent position. It should be noted that the hours per patient day also vary by type of unit. The nursing care hours per patient day on a special care unit are often higher than on a general medical unit.

As long as there is a staffing plan that indicates the number of nurses needed for any volume of patient days, the presence of step costs does not present a major budgeting problem.[2] Generally, because of the use of overtime and agency nurses, a step-fixed pattern of cost is estimated by treating the staffing costs as if they were variable. Although this will not give a precise result, it is usually a reasonable approximation.

The Impact of Volume on Cost per Patient

If a nurse manager were to ask what it costs to treat patients on the unit, accountants would probably answer, "It depends." Costs are not unique numbers that are always the same. The cost to treat a patient depends on several critical factors. One of these is the volume of patients for whom care is being provided. Although other factors may explain the costs to treat patients on a particular unit—namely, acuity, type of patients being cared for on the unit, and the experience or expertise level of staff—our focus here is primarily on volume.

Suppose that a unit has fixed costs of $400,000 and variable costs per patient day of $400. With these hypothetical data, what is the average cost per patient day? If there are 3,000 patient days for the year, the total costs are the fixed cost of $400,000 plus $400 per patient day for each of the 3,000 patient days. The variable costs are $1,200,000 (i.e., $400 per patient day × 3,000 patient days). The total cost is $1,600,000 (i.e., $400,000 fixed cost + $1,200,000 variable cost). The cost per patient is $533 (i.e., $1,600,000 total cost ÷ 3,000 patient days) per patient day.

However, what if there are only 2,500 patient days? Then the variable costs, at $400 per patient day, are $1,000,000, and the total cost is $1,400,000. In this case, the cost per patient day is $560. The cost is higher because there are fewer patients sharing the fixed costs. Each patient day causes the hospital to spend another $400 of variable costs. The $400,000 fixed cost remains the same regardless of the number of patient days. If there are more patient days, each one shares less of the $400,000 fixed cost. If there are fewer patient days, the fixed cost assigned to each rises. Table 8–1 calculates the fixed, variable, total, and average costs per patient at a variety of patient volumes for this scenario.

Figure 8–6 shows the average cost at different patient volumes. The cost declines as the volume of patient days increases

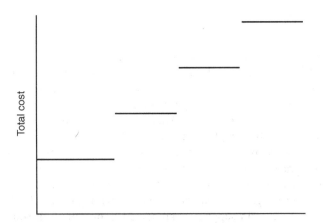

FIGURE 8–5.   Example of step-fixed costs.

Annual number of patient days

Total cost

---

[2]Note that such staffing plans often give the volume of patient days, adjusted for acuity level. See Chapter 13 for a discussion of using acuity for staffing calculations.

✳ **TABLE 8–1** *Fixed, Variable, Total, and Average Costs at Various Patient Volumes*

Volume (A)	Fixed Cost (B)	Variable Cost (C = $400 × A)	Total Cost (D = B + C)	Average Cost (E = D ÷ A)
1	$400,000	$ 400	$ 400,400	$400,400
50	400,000	20,000	420,000	8,400
100	400,000	40,000	440,000	4,400
500	400,000	200,000	600,000	1,200
1,500	400,000	600,000	1,000,000	667
2,500	400,000	1,000,000	1,400,000	560
3,000	400,000	1,200,000	1,600,000	533

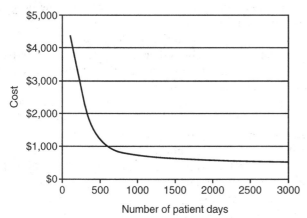

FIGURE 8–6. Average cost per patient day.

because more patients are sharing the fixed costs. In Chapter 4 this result was referred to as *economies of scale*.

Suppose there are only 500 patient days. The total variable costs of $400 per patient day are $200,000, and the total cost is $600,000. The cost per patient day is $1,200, more than double the previous cost per patient results at 2,500 and 3,000 patient days.

In trying to understand costs, it is critical to grasp the concept that because fixed costs do not change in total, the cost per patient or per patient day does change as volume changes. The greater the volume, the greater the number of patients available to share the fixed costs. Because costs depend on volume, there is no unique answer to the question "What is the cost per patient day?" That question can only be answered by giving the cost per patient day assuming a specific volume of patients. The volume of patients is critical.

One implication of this result is that HCOs almost always find higher volume preferable to lower volume. As volume increases, the average cost per patient declines. If prices can be maintained at the original level, the declining cost will result in lower losses or higher profits.

Marginal Cost Analysis

Another costing concern is the issue accountants and economists refer to as *marginal cost analysis*. Decisions to change the volume of a service or to change the specific types of services offered should be based on marginal rather than average costs.

If someone were to ask the nurse manager the cost of treating a particular type of patient, the answer should be, "It depends." The previous section pointed out that cost depends on the number of patients. It also depends on why we want to know. If the question is just one of historical curiosity, the average cost is an adequate response. However, if the information will be used for decision making, that response may well be incorrect.

Suppose the hospital was trying to decide whether to negotiate with an insurer to accept additional patients of the same average acuity and mix as the 2,500 patient days the hospital currently has. The insurer has offered $500 per patient day for 500 patient days. From the earlier calculations, the cost per patient for 500 patient days is $1,200! However, the hospital would not be providing only 500 patient days of care. It already has 2,500 patient days. From the earlier chart, the average cost is $560 per patient day at 2,500 patient days. At 3,000 patient days, the average cost would be $533. Given that information, would it pay to accept the additional patients at a price of only $500?

It definitely would. Why should the hospital accept $500 if the additional patient days will cost at least $533? Actually the additional patient days will not cost at least $533. All of the patients, on average, will cost that amount. The $533 includes a share of both fixed and variable costs. If the unit is going to have at least 2,500 patient days regardless of the insurer negotiation outcome, the fixed costs of $400,000 will be incurred no matter what. The fixed costs will not change if the hospital has the extra 500 patient days.

Decisions such as this one require marginal analysis. The "margin" refers to a change from current conditions. "A patient on the margin" refers to adding one more patient or reducing volume by one patient. Marginal costs are the costs for treating one more patient.

On the *margin* in this case, if the hospital were to take the additional patients, it would have more variable costs but would not have any additional fixed costs (assuming that 3,000 patient days is within the relevant range). Each extra patient causes the hospital to additionally spend only the variable costs of $400 per patient day. That is less than the $500 the insurer has offered to pay. The hospital will be better off by $100 for each additional patient day.

The additional costs incurred for additional patients are often referred to as the *marginal, out-of-pocket,* or *incremental costs*. If fixed costs were to rise because the relevant range was exceeded, those costs would be included appropriately in the incremental costs along with the variable costs. The key element in marginal costing is that the only costs relevant to a decision are those that change as a result of the decision.

The decision may be to add a new service or to close down an existing one. It may be to expand volume (as in the previous example) or to contract volume. In any case, when a decision is being made that involves changing patient load, the essential information to be considered is the revenues and costs that change. Effective managerial decisions require that the manager know the amount by which total costs will increase and the amount by which the total revenues will increase or, alternatively, the amount by which both will decrease. Costs that do not change in total for the organization are not relevant to the decision. Fixed costs generally do not increase when additional patients are added (within the relevant range), and therefore they do not affect marginal costs.

Marginal cost analysis is sometimes referred to as *relevant costing*. The concept of so-called relevant costing is that all decisions should be based only on costs that are relevant to the decision. The simplest way to think about this concept is to consider costs before and after a change. The only relevant costs are those that change as a result of the decision. The approach applies equally to revenues.

In the hospital-insurer example, suppose that before the insurer negotiation, the hospital was receiving $550 for each of its 2,500 patient days. Total revenue ($550 × 2,500) was $1,375,000. Total costs were $1,400,000 (calculated earlier). The hospital was losing $25,000, the amount that the $1,400,000 total costs exceeded the $1,375,000 of revenues. If the insurer business is accepted, the additional revenue would be $500 times 500 patient days, or $250,000. The total costs for 3,000 patient days (calculated earlier) are $1,600,000. The cost increase of going from 2,500 patient days to 3,000 patient days is only $200,000 (i.e., $1,600,000 total cost for 3,000 patient days versus $1,400,000 total cost for 2,500 patient days).

The total costs with the insurer's patients are $1,600,000, and the total revenues are $1,625,000 (i.e., the original $1,375,000 + $250,000 revenue from the insurer). The unit has gone from a loss of $25,000 to a profit of $25,000. The costs have increased by $200,000, and the revenues have increased by $250,000. The amount by which the extra revenues exceed the extra costs for the 500 insurer patients accounts for the turnaround from a loss to a profit. This should not be surprising. The extra revenue per patient day is $500. The cost per additional patient day is $400. The difference between incremental revenue of $500 per patient day and incremental cost of $400 per patient day is a profit of $100 per patient day. This extra profit of $100 for each of the 500 insured patient days accounts for exactly the $50,000 profit from the insurer patients, which turned a $25,000 loss into a $25,000 gain.

If the hospital had used average cost information for its decision, it would have turned away the extra business and lost the chance to turn a $25,000 loss into a $25,000 profit. The $500 per patient day revenue is less than the $533 average per patient day cost. However, the average cost is not relevant for such decisions because it incorrectly assumes that each extra patient day will cause the hospital to have additional variable and fixed costs. The incremental cost is relevant because it considers only the additional revenues and additional costs that the hospital will have as a result of the proposed change.

Relevant Cost Case Study

Assume that a hospital is trying to decide whether to perform liver transplant surgery.[3] The finance department has prepared a financial projection of the expenses for the service, which appears in Table 8–2. Which elements of the table are not relevant costs for the decision?

The first questionable item in the financial projection is the cost of the program supervisor. It is quite possible that one individual will be given the responsibility for the liver transplant program. However, one must question whether a new manager will be hired just for that position or whether the responsibility will be assigned to a manager who would be managing other units or working on various other things in any case. Does the hospital actually spend more for supervisors if it has this program than it would if it did not? If the answer is that no more money is spent on supervision if the program exists than if it does not, the cost is not relevant.

The costs of the staff in the OR during the transplantation are probably relevant. By adding more patients, more nursing staff will be needed. The same is true of the technician. On the other hand, it is not clear that the secretary and the orderly are relevant costs. The manager must assess whether the addition of the program will necessitate having an additional full- or part-time secretary or orderly. If existing staff carry a heavier burden with no staff additions, the costs are not relevant unless additional overtime is incurred. In that case, it would be the overtime cost that was relevant.

Allocation of building overhead is clearly a nonrelevant cost. The building will depreciate in any case. Unless remodeling is done to accommodate the program or unless the organization must acquire additional space, building depreciation should not be considered in making a decision regarding

✳ **TABLE 8–2** *ABC Hospital Liver Transplant Program Financial Projections*

Operating Expenses	
Nurse program supervisor	$ 100,000
OR nurses (RN: circulating, scrub)*	190,000
Technician*	55,000
Orderlies*	40,000
OR receptionist/secretary*	35,000
Benefits*	126,000
Medical supplies*	300,000
Allocation of building depreciation	20,000
Allocation of OR equipment depreciation	40,000
Telephone allocation*	7,500
Office supplies*	5,000
Allocation of malpractice insurance and overhead not included above*	300,000
Medical director fees	150,000
Nursing staff orientation and training costs	15,000
Computers and software	10,000
Fees (Center of Excellence, others)	20,000
Total	$1,413,500

*Expense items assumed to vary directly with the number of operations.
Note: These numbers are hypothetical and do not reflect the true costs related to liver transplantation.

---

[3]This discussion is not intended to be a comprehensive analysis of all the relevant and nonrelevant costs related to liver transplantation. Its purpose is merely to provide readers with some examples of costs that are not relevant to a particular decision.

whether to offer the program. The same is true for equipment depreciation. Assuming that no additional equipment is acquired for the program, depreciation is not a relevant cost. On the other hand, some new equipment will likely be required, and depreciation of any equipment specifically purchased for the program is a relevant cost.

Malpractice insurance is a peculiar item. In some hospitals, it is based on past experience. In other hospitals, it is based on the sum of the riskiness of the patients and services of the hospital. Liver transplantation can be a risky operation. However, patients are aware of the associated risk. An assessment must be made concerning whether this program increases the risk of lawsuits and malpractice findings against the hospital. If so, the malpractice insurance costs will probably increase as a result of the program, and the cost is considered relevant.

Accountants may still argue that a portion of the non-relevant cost items must be assigned to the program so that the full costs of the liver transplantation program will be known. That is, "All costs must be allocated to all activities to be fair, or else why should any costs be allocated to any activities?" Managers would argue that it is preferable not to allocate any costs rather than to allocate costs in such a way as to result in poor managerial decisions. If it is decided not to add the liver program because of costs allocated to it that are not relevant, then the accounting system is a hindrance to the organization's success. The analysis of the new program must allow the manager to know how much *more* cost the organization will have with the program than without the program.

Whether preexisting costs are allocated to the program or not, the important thing to keep in mind is that when decisions are made, relevant costs are the only costs that should be considered.

✳ COST ESTIMATION TECHNIQUES

One of the most difficult parts of financial management is the prediction of costs. This is an essential component of financial management. Budgets contain cost estimates. Trying to predict how much will be spent on each type of expenditure in the coming year presents great problems for both inexperienced and experienced managers. Managers must have ways to estimate such costs.

One approach is to simply look at what happened during the current year and predict next year's cost using the same information, with an increment for inflation. At the other extreme is an approach that says it is desirable to do better next year than this year, so it is appropriate to budget a certain percentage less than was spent this year. In each case, the approach is far too simplistic. A priori, there is no reason to believe that next year will be just like this year, and simply wishing to spend less than the current year will not make it so.

Some sort of clear method is needed that will help predict what will happen next year based on the past. Some way to formally consider why that prediction may not come true is also needed. Finally, if costs are to be reduced below the predicted outcome, there must be a specific plan that the nurse manager believes will accomplish the cost cutback.

This section considers several methods of cost estimation. Not all elements of the budget are simply costs. Items such as the number of patient days must be predicted as well. A discussion of general forecasting is presented in Chapter 21. Here the focus is solely on prediction of costs.

Often historical information about costs incurred can be a great aid in predicting what costs will be in the future. This is especially true in the case of mixed costs, which have both fixed and variable cost elements. Cost estimation techniques look at historical information and compare the change in cost over time with the change in volume over time to isolate fixed and variable costs.

If costs rise as volume rises, what could account for the increase in costs? Fixed costs, by definition, do not change as volume changes. Therefore, any change in cost as volume changes must be attributable to the variable cost. By seeing how much costs change for a change in volume, it is possible to calculate the variable cost per unit. After the variable cost per unit is known, the total variable cost for any volume can be determined by multiplying the variable cost per unit by the volume. Then fixed cost can be determined as well. The difference between the total cost for any volume and the total variable cost for that volume is the fixed cost. The fixed and variable cost information can then be used to estimate costs for the coming year based on a forecast of the volume in the coming year.

There is one critical problem in the flow of logic that allows cost estimation. Changes in cost over time are assumed to be the result only of changes in volume. However, to some extent, changes in cost over time are the result of other changes. One possible type of change is evolving clinical practice. For example, a new technology may require more intravenous solutions than were needed before patients had access to that technology. Other reasons costs may change are because evidence-based practice changes are implemented or because there is a change in the types of medications used to treat certain patient populations. Managers should always adjust any estimates they make for the impact of any changes that they anticipate.

Another problem is inflation. If inflation were a constant percent that was the same each year, one could argue that past inflation could be ignored and inflation would automatically be built into predictions for the future. However, inflation rates tend to fluctuate from year to year. Over a period of years the fluctuations can be substantial. Therefore, to be able to predict fixed and variable costs, the data should be adjusted for the effect of inflation.

Adjusting Costs for Inflation

Suppose that a nurse manager is interested in determining how much the total registered nurse (RN) staff costs of the unit will be for fiscal year 2013.[4] This hypothetical unit is staffed with a

---

[4] A fiscal year may start at any convenient date, not necessarily January 1. For example, fiscal years often begin on July 1 and end on June 30 or begin on October 1 and end on September 30. If fiscal year 2013 begins on July 1, the time period would cover July 1, 2012, through June 30, 2013.

minimum of 10 full-time equivalent (FTE) RNs for any volume up to 9,000 patient days at a certain acuity level. The cost of those 10 FTEs is fixed because the unit will always have at least that cost. As volume increases above 9,000 patient days, additional nursing time will be needed. In 2011, patient days numbered 9,800, and the cost, including fringe benefits, was $666,400. In 2012, the patient days totaled 11,000, and the cost was $792,000. The cost increase of $125,600 was attributable to both the increased volume and inflation.

Most readers are probably familiar with the Consumer Price Index (CPI), the most widely used measure of inflation. The CPI and many other indexes of inflation, such as the hospital market basket index, were developed by or for the federal government. The CPI measures the relative cost of a typical basket of consumer goods. Whatever the basket of goods costs in the base year is considered to be 100% of the cost in that year, or simply 100. The index is revised, and a new base year is established from time to time. If it costs twice as much to buy the same goods in a year subsequent to the base year, the index would be 200% of the base year costs, or simply 200.

The U.S. Department of Commerce's Bureau of the Census annually publishes the *Statistical Abstract of the United States*. Included in that book are "Indexes of Medical Care Prices." There are several quite useful indexes under that heading, including the index of medical care services and the hospital daily room rate index. The CPI is also published online and available for reviewing historical information.

In this example, the nurse manager wants to forecast the variable cost per patient day of nursing labor for 2013 using current dollars as of the end of fiscal year 2012. If information from 2008 through 2012 is used, the nurse manager will have to find the value of an appropriate index in each of those years. The financial managers in most health care institutions can provide nurse managers with appropriate indexes adjusted for labor costs in the specific geographic area. Failing that, most library reference sections can assist with current index information. Assume that an appropriate index has values as follows:

2008	258
2009	287
2010	318
2011	357
2012	395

Suppose also that the following cost and volume information is available:

Year	Patient Days	Cost
2008	8,000	$720,000
2009	8,700	809,100
2010	8,850	862,875
2011	9,800	996,600
2012	11,000	1,188,000

It appears that costs have risen from 2008 to 2010 even though volume is below 9,000 patient days in each of those years. Because the staffing is fixed at 10 FTEs for any volume

below 9,000 patient days, the cost is expected to be about the same in each of those 3 years and to increase only as volume increases above 9,000 patient days, thus requiring more nursing staff. The cost information, however, is not comparable because of the impact of inflation. Even if the number of FTEs did not change, the total cost would rise because of annual pay raises. To make the numbers reasonable for comparison purposes, they must be restated in *constant dollars*, that is, in amounts that have been adjusted for the impact of inflation.

That adjustment can be done by multiplying the cost in any given year by a fraction that represents the current value of the index divided by the value of the index in the year the cost was incurred. This is not a complicated procedure. For example, in 2008, the cost was $720,000. The hypothetical index value is 395 for fiscal year 2012. In 2008, it was 258. Multiplying $720,000 by the fraction 395/258 results in a cost of $1,102,326, which is the 2008 cost adjusted to year 2012 dollars. Now the $1,188,000 spent when there were 11,000 patient days in 2012 can be compared with $1,102,326, the constant-dollar cost of 8,000 patient days in 2008. In a similar fashion, all of the data can be restated in year 2012 dollars, as in Table 8–3.

Inflation accounts for changes in prices. One example of a change in prices is a change in wages. Wage rates are the price an organization pays for labor. Note that adjusted for inflation, there was very little change in costs from 2008 to 2010, the period during which the staffing was fixed, because patient days were less than 9,000. However, the actual dollars spent in those years, before adjusting for inflation, rose from $720,000 to $862,875. Such an increase might at least partly reflect the impact of rising salaries.

These index values are hypothetical. Managers should consult their organization's financial managers for an appropriate inflation index and its actual values for their specific geographic region.

High-Low Cost Estimation

The high-low approach is a relatively simple, quick-and-dirty approach to cost estimation. It is unsophisticated and therefore not terribly accurate, but in many cases, it may be "good enough." It certainly is better than simply taking a guess.

The key to the high-low method is the fact that fixed costs do not change at all in response to changes in volume. The way the method works is to look at the organization's cost for a specific item over a period of approximately 5 years. Costs adjusted for inflation should be used, as described previously.

The use of 5 years is arbitrary. It might be more appropriate to use a longer period, but one would not want to use data from

✳ **TABLE 8–3** *Adjusting Costs for Inflation*

Year	Patient Days	Original Cost		Index Fraction		Adjusted Cost
2008	8,000	$ 720,000	×	395/258	=	$1,102,326
2009	8,700	809,100	×	395/287	=	1,113,570
2010	8,850	862,875	×	395/318	=	1,071,810
2011	9,800	996,600	×	395/357	=	1,102,681
2012	11,000	1,188,000	×	395/395	=	1,188,000

much less than 5 years. Less than 5 years should be used only if there have been substantial changes in the unit that make earlier data no longer relevant. For the period chosen, find the highest volume and the lowest volume and compare the costs at these two volumes.

The amount by which the costs changed from the lowest to highest volume should be compared with the amount by which the volume changed. In the example from the previous section, the highest volume in the last 5 years was 11,000 patient days, and the cost for nursing labor that year for the unit was $1,188,000 in constant dollars. The lowest volume in the last 5 years was 8,000 patient days, and the constant dollar inflation adjusted cost in that year was $1,102,326. In this case, whereas inflation-adjusted costs increased by $85,674, volume increased by 3,000 patient days. If $85,674 is divided by 3,000 patient days, the result is $28.558 per patient day. Although it is certainly likely that nursing labor is a step-fixed cost and therefore will not go up by $28.558 for *each* additional patient day, that volume provides a reasonable measure of the amount of additional nursing services needed per patient day when there are significant changes in volume.

If the variable cost per patient day is $28.558, what is the fixed cost?[5] The yearly total variable cost is first found by multiplying the variable cost per patient day by the number of patient days ($28.558 × 8,000 = $228,464). The total nursing labor cost for 8,000 patient days was $1,102,326 in 2008; if $228,464 is the variable cost, then the remainder, $873,862, represents the fixed cost. Similarly, for 11,000 patient days at $28.558 per patient day, the variable cost is $314,138; given a total cost of $1,188,000 in 2012, the fixed cost would be $873,862. The fixed cost is expected to be the same at either volume level because by definition it is fixed.

This fixed and variable cost information can be used in preparing next year's budget. If 12,000 patient days are expected, costs will be expected to rise by $28.558 × 1,000 patient days, or $28,558. The fixed cost portion will not change. Because this information was calculated using 2012 constant dollars, both the fixed and variable costs will have to be adjusted upward for the expected 2013 salary increases or, more generally, for the expected impact of inflation during the next year.

The high-low method is not accurate because it considers only the experience of 2 years. One or both of the 2 years chosen may have had some unusual circumstance that would skew the costs in that year. A superior prediction is possible if some method is used that takes more experience into account. *Regression analysis* can provide such a prediction.

Regression Analysis

The volume of patient days and the total cost for those days for a number of years can be plotted on a graph. The horizontal axis represents volume, and the vertical axis represents cost.

The result is a scatter diagram. The points on the graph each represent a volume and the cost at that volume. If a line is drawn approximating the points, it can be used for future predictions. By selecting any expected volume on the horizontal axis, it is possible to go vertically up to the line and then from the line move horizontally across to a point on a vertical cost axis. That point represents the prediction of cost. For example, Figure 8–7 shows a scatter diagram with a line drawn approximating the points.

The difficulty in drawing the diagonal line connecting those points is properly placing it so that it will give accurate predictions. Regression analysis is a technique that applies mathematical precision to a scatter diagram. Regression selects the one line that is effectively closest to all the individual points on the scatter diagram and that will therefore best predict cost for the future. This can fairly accurately break down costs into their fixed and variable components.

Simple linear regression analysis can take all available past information into account in estimating the portion of any cost that is fixed and the portion that is variable. The phrase *simple linear regression* refers to several issues. First, it is simple in the sense that there is only one *dependent* variable and one *independent* variable. Cost is the dependent variable being estimated. Cost *depends* on the value of the independent variable.

An independent variable is a *causal* factor. For example, the most significant causal factor for nursing costs might be patient days. The more patient days, the greater the costs for nursing. Patient days *cause* costs to be incurred. For the admissions department of the hospital, it is not patient days but rather the number of patients that is important because admission time is the same for each patient regardless of the ultimate length of stay.

The second part of the phrase *simple linear regression* refers to the presumption that cost behavior can be shown in a linear fashion—that is, using a straight line. For example, what if a

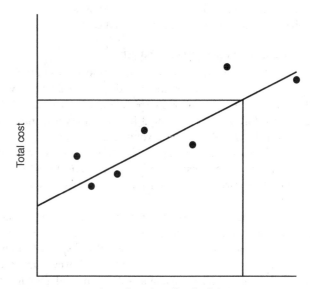

FIGURE 8–7. Predicting costs from a scatter diagram.

---

[5]It is always a good idea to avoid rounding off numbers that will be used in subsequent computations. In this example we are not rounding off $25.558 to $25.56 because it would impact the fixed and variable costs to be calculated using this number.

slightly lower price per disposable supply unit is paid for every increase in volume (e.g., $ 0.75 for one unit, $0.7499 per unit for two units, $0.7498 per unit for three units, and so on)? In that case, Figure 8–2 is not an accurate reflection of how variable costs change. It is necessary to draw a curved line on the graph, but the mathematics involved with curved lines instead of straight lines are far more complicated. Variable costs are generally treated as if they are linear even if that is only an approximation of their true behavior.

Finally, the term *regression* refers to trying to regress, or bring all the points from the scatter diagram as close as possible to the estimated line.

For example, suppose that the CNE desires to make a rough starting prediction for the total cost of all patient care units in a hospital for the coming year. If last year there were 50,000 patient days and this coming year patient days are expected to be 52,000, there is a 4% expected increase in the number of patient days. However, it cannot be assumed that all costs of running the unit will go up by 4%, because some costs, such as the salary of the CNE, are fixed and will not rise in proportion to the number of patient days.

The high-low method is one way to make the prediction, but this method relies on only two data points. Far greater accuracy in breaking out fixed and variable costs is possible if the past years' costs on a very detailed basis are examined, cost item by cost item, to determine which were fixed and which were variable. That is a very time-consuming procedure. Gathering information costs money, and even if the information is gathered, there are always some costs that cannot be separated into fixed and variable components without some estimating method, because they are mixed costs. For example, nonmedical supplies, such as paper, pens, and forms, are needed to some extent regardless of patient volume. On the other hand, the more patients, the more non-medical supplies used.

How can costs be divided into their fixed and variable components and less money spent on gathering information than if each line item from past years is examined? Regression analysis can help to separate these mixed costs.

Mixed Costs and Regression Analysis

Suppose it is known that last year the combined cost of the salary of the nurse manager and the disposable supplies was $105,000 and that the number of patient days was 50,000. This uses the information represented in the graphs presented in Figures 8–1 through 8–3. The volume of patient days is expected to rise to 52,000 next year. Should the $105,000 cost be increased by 4% because volume is increasing by 4%? No. Some costs are fixed. Only variable costs increase as volume increases.

In this scenario, one would expect costs to increase by $200, or $0.10 for each extra patient day, because it is known in this simple example that variable costs for the disposable thermometer covers were $0.10 per patient day. However, in dealing with a more realistic example with many different fixed, variable, and mixed costs, the variable costs per patient day are not necessarily known.

✳ **TABLE 8–4** *Historical Data for Thermometer Cover Costs*

Year	Patient Days	Cost
2003	40,000	$104,100
2004	42,000	104,200
2005	43,000	104,300
2006	44,000	104,400
2007	45,000	104,500
2008	46,000	104,600
2009	47,000	104,700
2010	48,000	104,800
2011	49,000	104,900
2012	50,000	105,000

Suppose that the historical information in Table 8–4 were available (already adjusted for inflation using the indexing technique). If the high-low technique were used to evaluate the fixed and variable costs, there would be a very strange result. The highest cost is $105,000, and the lowest cost is $104,100; thus, costs have risen by $900. At the same time, volume has increased from 40,000 patient days to 50,000, or an increase of 10,000. When $900 is divided by 10,000 patient days, a variable cost of $0.09 per patient day results. Is that an accurate estimate? No, because it is known that the variable cost is $0.10 per patient day. What might be the cause of the discrepancy?

It is possible that 2003 was the first year that a new disposable oral thermometer cover was used. Perhaps many of them were defective and were thrown away, or perhaps some were wasted because of lack of familiarity with using them. In any case, if more than $0.10 per patient day was spent on disposable thermometer covers in the low-volume year, the costs were unduly high in that year. Therefore, the change in cost from 2003 to 2012 looks unrealistically low, and the variable cost measure is unrealistically low.

At the other extreme, had there been unusual waste (perhaps the fault of the nurses but possibly because of quality problems with a large batch of the disposable item) in the most recent, high-cost year, the change in cost would look especially high, and the variable cost per unit would have come out to more than $0.10. As has been stated before, if one relies on just two data points, as the high-low method does, results are subject to the whims of unusual events in either of those years.

In reality, one would not expect to use exactly $0.10 per patient day on disposable supplies in any year. For one reason or another, some patients will have their temperature taken only once on a given day. This might be caused by admission to the hospital late in the day, for instance. On the other hand, patients with a fever will no doubt have their temperature taken more often. A more likely pattern of costs is shown in Table 8–5.

Simply looking at this list does not provide a lot of insight about fixed and variable costs. Figure 8–8 shows a scatter diagram for these data. One can roughly see how costs increase as volume increases. A straight line cannot be drawn through all of the points on this scatter diagram. However, the regression technique uses all of the available information to select a line

※ TABLE 8–5 *More Likely Historical Cost Pattern*

Year	Patient Days	Cost
2003	40,000	$104,100
2004	42,000	104,180
2005	43,000	104,360
2006	44,000	104,380
2007	45,000	104,530
2008	46,000	104,670
2009	47,000	104,690
2010	48,000	104,880
2011	49,000	104,890
2012	50,000	105,000

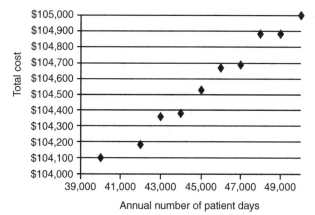

FIGURE 8–8. Scatter diagram of total costs for nursing.

that will provide the best estimate in the absence of any other information.

Regression analysis uses information about the dependent and independent variables in the past to develop an equation for a straight line. As part of that process, it calculates a constant value and a coefficient for the independent variable. If the dependent variable is the cost, the constant represents the fixed cost, and the coefficient of the independent variable represents the variable cost.

Regression analysis is a statistical technique. A detailed discussion of statistics is beyond the scope of this book. However, many mechanical approaches to regression have made it a workable tool used in HCOs. Regression can be performed on many handheld calculators. A wide variety of statistical programs and spreadsheet programs for personal computers also have regression capability.

Turning back to the scatter diagram in Figure 8–8, it is possible to use regression analysis to predict what the costs will be for the nursing unit next year if there are 52,000 patient days. Regression analysis will determine a specific line to plot through this scatter diagram that will give the best possible estimate of fixed and variable costs and therefore allow prediction of the cost next year.

Basically, the process requires several simple steps. First, determine the cost associated with each volume of patient days. For instance, when there were 40,000 patient days, the cost was $104,100. The independent variable, patient days, is often referred to as the X variable because it is plotted on the horizontal axis. The dependent variable, cost, is often referred to as the Y variable because it is plotted on the vertical axis.

Any computer program will require the X values and the Y values for each year. With that information, it is generally only necessary to give a command to compute the regression to complete the process. It is important not to let the extremely quantitative nature of regression theory learned in a statistics course discourage you from attempting to use this tool. In practice, very little mathematics is required of the user. Regression is a tool for better management. The major difficulty in using regression is simply fear of the process.

In the example, regression analysis using the data in Table 8–5 predicts that the fixed cost is $100,226 and the variable cost is $0.0956 per unit. Figure 8–9 shows the resulting line. If extended to the left, it would have its intercept at $100,226, increasing with a slope of 0.0956. These figures are not exactly the expected variable cost of $0.10 per patient day and fixed cost of $100,000 for the salary of the nurse manager. They are, however, better estimates than those the high-low method would give. The high-low approach predicts a fixed cost of $100,000 and variable cost of $0.09 per patient day. Regression analysis is an inexpensive, potentially very useful, and relatively simple way of estimating fixed and variable costs and helping to predict future costs.

For any number of patient days predicted, it is now possible to multiply by 0.0956 and then add $100,226 to get a forecast of future costs. With many computer software programs and packages, the process is made even simpler by requiring only that the forecast volume be entered into the computer along with the historical data. The software will then generate the estimated cost for the coming year automatically based on the forecast volume. Remember, however, that it is necessary to adjust upward the resulting cost for expected increases caused by inflation for the coming year.

Although you will soon find this approach quite simple, it is useful only as a tool to aid you in managing. It should not be allowed to take over the role of your judgment. The mathematical model is quite accurate in predicting the future if nothing has changed. It is your role as a manager to know if there are reasons that costs are likely to change from their past patterns.

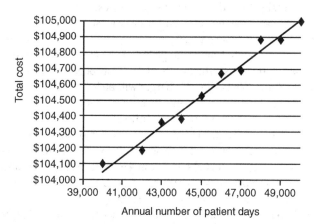

FIGURE 8–9. Simple linear regression of total costs for nursing.

For instance, if you know that 2003 was the first year disposable thermometer covers were used and that there was an awful lot of waste that year, you might want to eliminate that year from the analysis. If you do, your regression results will show fixed costs of $99,997 and variable costs of $0.1005. Recall that the fixed costs were actually $100,000 and the variable costs $0.10. As you can see, the input of judgment into the process can substantially improve the resulting estimates.

When regression analysis is performed, one statistic that is generally provided by the calculator or the computer is R squared (R^2). That value can range from a low of zero to a high of 1.0. If the value is close to zero, it means that the independent variable does not do a very good job of explaining the changes in the dependent variable. An R^2 value of 0.20, for example, might indicate that patient days are not a good predictor of nursing cost. On the other hand, an R^2 of 0.80 would indicate that it is a very good predictor. However, it is possible to become even more exact in estimating costs.

Multiple Regression Analysis

There is a type of regression analysis that is more sophisticated than simple linear regression. It is called *multiple regression* because it allows for use of multiple independent, or causal, variables. The use of simple linear regression can be a substantial aid in estimating future costs because it is so efficient at predicting the fixed cost and the variable cost per unit when there is one major independent variable. Sometimes, however, there are several key variables. For instance, suppose that the nursing costs vary not only with the number of patient days but also with the number of patients. That is most probably the case.

Certainly, the costs vary with the number of patient days. The more patient days, the more temperatures to be taken, pulses to be checked, medications to be administered, and so on. However, for each patient, there are certain costs that vary with the number of patients, not with the number of patient days (e.g., a health history must be recorded, a chart must be set up, a patient care plan must be established, valuables must be stored, orientation must be given, discharge planning and education must be done, and so on). Thus, there may be instances when having fewer patients with a long length of stay will cost less than having more patients with a short length of stay, even if the total patient days are the same. For example, consider 10 patients each staying on a unit 5 days versus 5 patients each staying 10 days. There are 50 patient days in both cases, and the costs of taking vital signs and giving medications are the same. In the 5 patient case, the number (and cost) of admissions, histories, charts, plans, and discharges will be lower. So it is likely that the cost of a nursing unit varies with both the number of patient days and the number of admissions.

Most handheld business calculators cannot perform multiple regression. However, most statistical programs for personal computers can handle this easily, as can Personal Digital Assistants (PDAs), tablet personal computers, and other handheld computerized devices. Instead of simply entering the X and Y values for each year into the calculator or computer, the user enters an X value for the historical information for each of the independent variables as well as the Y value. To predict a future cost, the user provides the computer with, for example, the expected number of patient days and the expected number of patients to predict the expected costs.

Sometimes the multiple regression level of sophistication adds extra work and complexity without substantially changing the results. Recall that when all is said and done, the result is just an estimate; all types of events can happen in the future that will throw off the estimate, no matter how finely tuned it is. It is not necessary to add complexity for its own sake. At times, however, multiple regression can produce information that would not otherwise be available.

For example, more and more attention has been placed on measures of patient acuity, or the level of intensity of required nursing services. It certainly is clear that the amount of nursing services varies not just with the number of patient days but also with the severity of the patients' illnesses. If data about the number of patient days and the average acuity level are used as independent variables, the accuracy of estimated costs might improve substantially.

Another use for multiple regression is in investigatory work with respect to costs. Suppose that there is a strong feeling by the nursing staff that the way a particular physician practices medicine is extremely costly. This is common in the OR, where particular surgeons often exhibit out-of-the-ordinary behavior. The number of operations by a specific physician each year can be used as an independent variable. Costs increasing as a result of more cases by that physician will show up as a positive coefficient for that independent variable. The nurse manager will then have evidence to support the more general feelings of the staff that the physician is an unusually high resource consumer.

Readers of this book are encouraged to pursue the topic of regression analysis further. This should be done on both a conceptual basis, reviewing the underlying principles and theories of regression analysis, and on a practical basis, using a computer software package to perform some regression analyses for financial decision making.

✳ BREAK-EVEN ANALYSIS

Up to this point, the general behavior of costs (fixed versus variable) has been discussed, as well as the techniques for cost estimation (high-low and regression). Attention will now be focused on using cost information for understanding whether a particular unit or service will lose money, make money, or just break even. This technique is useful for the evaluation of both new and continuing projects or services. It is often used in developing a business plan. Business plans are discussed in Chapter 22.

Nurse managers and executives in many instances find it necessary to be able to determine whether a program or service will be profitable. One key to profitability is volume. Prices are often fixed. Average cost, however, is not fixed. As the number of patients rises, the cost per patient falls because of the sharing of fixed costs. One cannot simply compare price and average cost and determine that a program or unit will make a profit or a loss. To determine whether something will be profitable, it is critical to know the volume of patients.

As noted earlier, BEA is a technique to find the specific volume at which a program or service neither makes nor loses money. Forecast information about the likely volume of the service can be compared with break-even volume to predict whether there will be profits or losses.

BEA is based on the following formula:

$$\text{Break-Even Quantity (Q)} = \frac{\text{Fixed Costs (FC)}}{\text{Price (P)} - \text{Variable Cost per Patient (VC)}}$$

or

$$Q = \frac{FC}{P - VC}$$

where Q is the number of patients needed to just break even, FC is the total fixed cost, P is the price for each patient, and VC is the variable cost per patient. At a quantity lower than Q, there will be a loss; at a quantity higher than Q, there will be a profit.

The basis for the formula is the underlying relationship between revenues and expenses.[6] If total revenues are greater than expenses, there is a profit. If total revenues are less than expenses, there is a loss. If revenues are just equal to expenses, there is neither profit nor loss, and the service is said to just break even. Expenses are the sum of total fixed costs and total variable costs.

Example of Break-Even Analysis

Suppose that a new home health agency opens in a rural area.[7] It charges, on average, $50 per visit. The agency has fixed costs of $10,000 and variable costs of $30 per patient visit. If there are no patients at all, there is no revenue, but there are fixed costs of $10,000, and there is a $10,000 loss. If there were 100 patients, there would be $5,000 of revenue ($50 × 100 patients), $10,000 of fixed cost, and $3,000 of variable cost ($30 × 100 patients). Total costs would be $13,000 ($10,000 of fixed cost + $3,000 of variable cost), revenues would be $5,000, and there would be a loss of $8,000.

Each additional patient brings in $50 of revenue but causes the agency to spend only $30 more. The difference between the $50 price and the $30 variable cost—$20—is called the *contribution margin (CM)*. If the CM is positive, it means that each

extra unit of activity makes the organization better off by that amount. The CM from each patient can be used to cover fixed costs; if all fixed costs have been covered, it represents a profit.

In this example, when there are 100 patients, there is $20 of CM for each of the 100 patients, or a total CM of $2,000. Note that the loss with zero patients was $10,000, but it was only $8,000 when there were 100 patients. The loss decreased by $2,000, exactly the amount of the total CM for those 100 patients.

How many visits would the agency need to break even? The answer is 500. If each additional patient generates $20 of CM, then 500 patients would generate $10,000 of CM (500 patients × $20 = $10,000), exactly enough to cover the fixed costs of $10,000. If the agency has 500 patients, it will just break even.

This could have been calculated using the formula

$$Q = \frac{FC}{P - VC}$$

or

$$Q = \frac{\$10,000}{\$50 - \$30} = \frac{\$10,000}{\$20} = 500 \text{ Visits}$$

BEA can also be viewed from a graphic perspective, as shown in Figure 8–10. The total cost line starts at $10,000 because of the fixed costs. The total revenue line starts at zero because there is no revenue if there are zero patients. Where the revenue line and the cost line intersect, they are equal, and the agency just breaks even. Note that with fewer patients than at the break-even point, the cost line is higher than the revenue line, and there will be a loss; with more patients than at the break-even point, the revenue line is higher than the costs, and a profit is made.

Before the introduction of prospective payment systems and Diagnosis Related Groups (DRGs), most break-even analyses in hospitals focused on the number of patient days needed to break even. Hospitals do not get paid for extra patient days under a prospective payment system. Therefore, there is now attention on the total number of patients needed to break even rather than on patient days. BEA can also be performed based

---

[6]The formula may be derived as follows:
1. Profit = Revenues − Costs, or Profit = Revenues − Fixed Costs − Total Variable Costs
2. At the break-even quantity, profit is zero, so: 0 = Revenues (R) − Fixed Costs (FC) − Total Variable Costs (TVC)
3. Moving revenue to the left side of the equation and multiplying the equation by − 1 yields: R = FC + TVC
4. Revenue is the price per unit (P) multiplied by the quantity of units (Q), and total variable costs are the variable costs per unit (VC) multiplied by the quantity of units (Q). Therefore: (P × Q) = FC + (VC × Q)
5. Moving VC to the other side of the equation: (P × Q) − (VC × Q) = FC
6. Factor out Q from the left side of the equation: Q × (P − VC) = FC
7. Divide both sides of the equation by (P − VC) to yield the formula Q = FC/(P − VC)

[7]These data are hypothetical and used for simplicity. They do not reflect the actual cost of a home health visit.

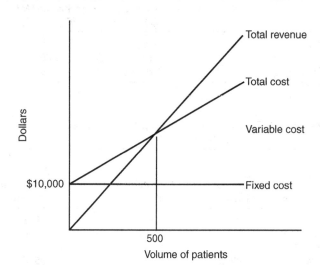

FIGURE 8–10. Break-even analysis.

on the number of surgeries or clinic visits or other appropriate service unit volume measures.

When there are different types of patients, BEA becomes somewhat more complicated. The formula presented at the beginning of this section assumes that there is only one price and one variable cost and therefore one CM. If there are different types of patients with different prices and different variable costs, it is necessary to find a weighted-average CM. That weighted average can be divided into the fixed costs to find the break-even volume for all patients.

For example, suppose that there are three classes of home care visits, referred to here as complex, moderate, and simple. The price for the visits is $80, $50, and $30, and the variable costs for the visits are $55, $30, and $20, respectively. The CM for each type of visit can be calculated by subtracting the variable cost from the price, as shown in Table 8–6.

The crucial piece of information for calculating the break-even point is the relative proportion of each type of visit. Management of the home health agency expects that 20% of all visits are complex, 30% are moderate, and 50% are simple. This information can be used to determine a weighted-average CM. This requires multiplying the individual CM for each type of visit by the percentage of patients that receive that type of visit. The results are added together to get an overall weighted-average CM, as shown in Table 8–7.

This $16 weighted CM represents the average CM for all types of visits. It can be used to calculate the break-even quantity. Assume that fixed costs are $10,000. The break-even quantity of visits is as follows:

$$Q = \frac{FC}{P - VC} = \frac{FC}{CM}$$

or

$$Q = \frac{\$10,000}{\$16} = 625 \text{ Visits}$$

※ **TABLE 8–6** *Contribution Margin by Type of Patient Home Visit*

	Price (A)	Variable Cost (B)	Contribution Margin (C = A − B)
Complex	$80	$55	$25
Moderate	50	30	20
Simple	30	20	10

※ **TABLE 8–7** *Calculation of Weighted Average Contribution Margin*

Visit Type	Percentage of Visits		Contribution Margin		Weighted Average Contribution Margin
Complex	20	×	$25	=	$ 5
Moderate	30	×	20	=	6
Simple	50	×	10	=	5
Total	100				$16

Of the total of 625 visits needed to break even, 20%, or 125, are complex; 30%, or 188, are moderate; and 50%, or 312, are simple.

This method works for three different kinds of patients. What if there are more than three kinds? The same weighted-average approach that can be used to find the break-even volume when there are three different types of patients can be used even if there are hundreds of different types of patients, as is the case with the prospective payment system example.

What if there is more than one price for each type of visit? Medicaid pays one price, Medicare another, private insurers another, and self-pay patients yet another. This still can work within the same framework as has been presented. It will be necessary to calculate a weighted-average CM, treating each payer for each type of visit as a separate group. For example, if Medicaid pays $40 per visit regardless of the type of visit and the other payment rates are the same as indicated earlier, the CM by type of visit by payer will be as shown in Table 8–8.

If it is possible to anticipate the percentage of each type of visit, a weighted-average CM can be estimated. Assume that 10% of all visits are Medicaid complex visits and 10% are other complex visits. Assume that 20% of all visits are Medicaid moderate visits and 10% are other moderate visits. Assume that 30% of all visits are Medicaid simple visits and that 20% are other simple visits. The weighted-average CM will be as shown in Table 8–9.

The break-even volume can then be calculated as follows:

$$Q = \frac{FC}{P - VC} = \frac{FC}{CM}$$

or

$$Q = \frac{\$10,000}{\$13} = 769 \text{ Visits}$$

The number of visits of any type can be determined by multiplying the 769 break-even volume times the percentage of visits in any given class. For example, because 30% of the visits are Medicaid simple, 30% of 769, or 231, Medicaid simple visits can be expected at the break-even level.

Some managed care organizations (MCOs) pay home care agencies on a case basis rather than a visit basis. With some patients paid on a case basis and others on a visit basis, these calculations become complex.

※ **TABLE 8–8** *Contribution Margin by Type of Patient Home Visit and by Payer*

Visit Type	Price (A)	Variable Cost (B)	Contribution Margin (C = A − B)
Complex Medicaid	$40	$55	($15)
Complex other	80	55	25
Moderate Medicaid	40	30	10
Moderate other	50	30	20
Simple Medicaid	40	20	20
Simple other	30	20	10

✳ **TABLE 8–9** *Calculation of Weighted-Average Contribution Margin with Multiple Payers*

Visit Type	Percentage of Visits		Contribution Margin		Weighted-Average Contribution Margin
Complex Medicaid	10	×	($ 15)	=	($ 1.50)
Complex other	10	×	25	=	2.50
Moderate Medicaid	20	×	10	=	2.00
Moderate other	10	×	20	=	2.00
Simple Medicaid	30	×	20	=	6.00
Simple other	20	×	10	=	2.00
Total	100				$13.00

Using Break-Even Analysis for Decision Making

If a particular service is expected to have a volume of activity well in excess of the break-even point, managers have a clear-cut decision to start or continue the service. If the volume is too low to break even, several options exist.

One approach is to lower the volume needed to break even. There are three ways to reduce the required break-even level. One approach is to lower the fixed costs. In some cases, it might be possible to do that. Another alternative is to increase prices. Price increases will increase the CM per patient. This strategy will also have the effect of lowering the break-even point. However, price increases might reduce the expected volume. In that case, the price increases will defeat their purpose. Also, prices are sometimes regulated and beyond the control of the organization. Finally, one can try to reduce the variable cost per unit. This might be accomplished by increased efforts toward improved efficiency.

If it is not feasible to change fixed costs, price, or variable costs, an organization can try to attract more patients so that volume will rise above the break-even point. In the example presented, what type of visits would be desirable? The most desirable type of visit is a non-Medicaid complex visit. That visit yields a CM of $25. The least desirable is a Medicaid complex visit. The CM is negative. For each additional Medicaid complex visit, the agency loses money. In this particular example, the most attractive visit brings the highest revenue. However, the focus should not be on revenue. If the highest-revenue visit also has extremely high variable costs, that visit might not be as attractive as one with lower revenue and much lower variable costs. The attractiveness of additional visits is determined by how much CM they provide to the organization.

Break Even and Capitation

As managed care has become more and more prevalent, many negotiated contracts call for capitated payments. In such an arrangement, the MCO pays the health care provider a set amount for each member for each month. This is called the per member per month (PMPM) payment. Under capitation, an increase in the amount of services provided to patients will not cause revenues to increase at all. On the other hand, an increase in the number of members will increase revenues.

Suppose that an MCO offered to pay a home health agency $1 PMPM to provide all home care services for all of its members. Over the course of a year, revenue would be $12 per member ($1 PMPM × 12 months = $12). Assume that the agency's variable costs are $30 per visit. Furthermore, the agency will have increased fixed costs of $10,000 if it takes the MCO members. How many members will the MCO need to have for the home health agency to break even on the contract?

We can use BEA to calculate the break-even number of members. The fixed costs are $10,000. The variable costs are $30 per visit. The price is $12 per member per year. However, we do not have enough information to calculate the break-even point because we know only the variable cost per visit. We need to know the variable cost per member per year. To find the break-even volume of members, it is necessary to predict the utilization levels—that is, how many home visits each member will have.

Most individuals will not need any visits in a typical year. Suppose that the average person consumes 0.3 visits in a given year. The variable cost for 0.3 visits per year is $9 (the $30 variable cost per visit multiplied by 0.3 visits per year). That $9 represents the variable cost per member per year. We can now calculate the break-even point as follows:

$$Q = \frac{FC}{P - VC}$$

$$Q = \frac{\$10,000}{\$12 - \$9} = 3,333 \text{ Members}$$

Both the price and the variable costs in the calculation are per member per year. The quantity calculated represents the number of members needed to break even. If the MCO guarantees 5,000 members, the agency will likely make a profit. If there are only 2,000 members, it will lose money.

What if the agency has other fixed costs as well? Are they needed for the calculation? No. The determination of whether the MCO contract is profitable depends only on the marginal costs of the contract. Fixed costs that exist whether the agency contracts with the MCO or not are not relevant to the decision or the calculation. What if the MCO contract did not cause fixed costs to rise at all? Then the contract would be profitable for the agency as long as the revenue per member per year exceeded the variable cost per member per year.

Break-Even Analysis Cautions

A few words of caution are advisable when working with BEA. First, after a break-even point has been calculated, one must decide whether it is likely that volume will actually be achieved. That requires a volume forecast (see Chapter 21). To the extent that the forecast of volume is incorrect, the decision to go ahead with a new service may turn out to be a bad one even if the BEA is perfect.

Another potential problem is that BEA assumes that prices and costs are constant. If it can be reasonably expected that prices will fall over time, a higher volume will be needed to keep a service viable unless variable or fixed costs fall as well. On the other hand, if prices are expected to rise faster than costs, a marginal service today may become profitable over time even without an increase in volume.

Another consideration is that there is an assumption that the mix of patients will stay constant. Suppose that in the earlier example, over time, there are more and more Medicaid complex visits. The CM for such visits is negative. If the demographics of the population are such that a shift in mix in that direction is likely, the results of the BEA require close scrutiny. Will there be enough of those visits to shift a profitable service over to a loss?

As with all budgeting tools, judgment is essential. The nurse manager or executive must examine the assumptions of any modeling technique through experience, insight, and thought and consider the reasonableness of the results. If a result does not seem to make sense, often that is because it does not! However, BEA is a tool that can help give a manager a firm starting point in understanding whether a project or service is likely to be financially viable.

✳ IMPLICATIONS FOR NURSE MANAGERS AND EXECUTIVES

Assessing costs is complex. In general, costs do not increase in direct proportion with volume. The implications of this fact are that if money is lost on a particular program, the solution may be to increase patient volume for that program. More patients do not necessarily mean greater losses. It is possible that volume increases can turn a loss into a profit. Understanding how that can happen requires an understanding of cost behavior. Some costs are fixed; others are variable. The result of that basic nature of costs is that the cost per patient will decline with increasing volume. The greater the number of patients who share the fixed costs, the lower the average cost per patient. Costing is further complicated by the fact that additional patients do not cause costs to increase by the average cost per patient. Decisions that are in the organization's best interests often require marginal cost analysis.

An important part of the budgeting process is the prediction of costs. Estimated costs can be based on historical cost information. Some estimation relies on using the historical information to isolate variable costs from fixed costs. To make such calculations, it is first necessary to convert historical cost information into common or constant dollars. This requires *indexation* of costs for the impact of inflation. Indexation is a process that adjusts a dollar value for the impact of inflation over a period of time by using a *price index,* such as the CPI. A price index is a tool that indicates year-to-year changes in prices. Through the use of indexed historical costs, the results of the cost estimation process will be in constant dollars. In preparing next year's budget, the cost estimate has to be adjusted upward by the anticipated inflation rate over the next year.

After constant-dollar information is available, costs can be estimated using the high-low method, simple linear regression, or multiple regression analysis. Being able to estimate fixed and variable costs is a potentially valuable tool. To apply the results, however, projections of the estimated number of patients, patient days, acuity level, and so forth are needed. Chapter 21 focuses on the process of forecasting such data.

BEA is a tool that allows one to focus specifically on the quantity of patients needed for a program, project, or service to be financially viable. Its foundations are in fixed and variable costs. At low volumes of patients, the average cost may surpass the revenue per patient. As the number of patients increases, the cost per patient falls, because fixed costs are shared by more patients. Eventually, the cost per patient falls below the revenue. BEA allows the manager to determine what the break-even quantity is so that a reasonable decision can be made about the likely financial viability of a program, project, or service.

From the perspectives of nurse managers and executives, the topics of this chapter have critical implications. At the most basic level, falling volume will mean rising cost per patient. In such cases, it is likely that a revenue crisis will exist, and actions to restrain costs should be contemplated immediately. On the other hand, rising volumes represent an opportunity. They not only bring in more revenue but also decrease average cost per patient. Therefore, there is the opportunity for profit from more patients and for more profit from each patient. Profits ultimately allow the organization to replace buildings and equipment, add services, add staff, improve quality, and raise salaries.

In addition, in preparing budgets, nurse managers and executives should take into account the behavior of costs. The fact that certain costs vary in proportion while others are fixed may reorient the manager's thinking from the notion that a 10% increase in volume requires 10% more resources. This in turn can allow the manager to prepare budgets in a more sophisticated and exact manner.

Finally, managers and executives should remember that decisions to begin, continue, or stop a program are not made solely on the basis of profit-and-loss projections. Some programs are continued as a community service, and the institution makes a conscious decision to subsidize them from other sources of revenue. However, such decisions require as much information about anticipated profits or losses as possible.

✳ KEY CONCEPTS

Service unit   Basic measure of the product or service being produced by the organization, such as discharged patients, patient days, home care visits, ambulatory care visits, emergency department treatments, or hours of operations.

Direct costs   Costs that are incurred within the organizational unit for which the manager has responsibility, or costs that are directly related to patient care.

Indirect costs   Costs that are assigned to an organizational unit from elsewhere in the organization, or unit costs that do not directly relate to patient care.

Full cost   Total of all costs associated with an organizational unit or activity. This includes direct and indirect costs.

Average cost   Full cost divided by the volume of service units.

Fixed costs   Costs that do not change in total as the volume of service units changes within the relevant range.

Variable costs   Costs that vary directly with changes in the volume of service units.

Relevant range   Normal range of expected activity for the cost center or organization.

Marginal costs   Extra costs incurred as a result of providing care to one more service unit, such as for one extra patient day. If one considers the full or total costs incurred by an organization before it makes a change and the total costs after it makes the change, the difference in costs represents the marginal costs of that change.

Mixed costs   Costs that contain both fixed and variable cost elements.

Impact of volume on cost per patient   Average cost declines as the volume of patients increases, because more patients are sharing the fixed costs. Therefore, HCOs almost always find higher volume preferable to lower volume.

Marginal cost analysis   Decisions about changes should be based on the marginal costs of the change, not on full or average costs.

Cost estimation   Prediction of costs. This process is complicated by the necessity to divide historical mixed costs into their fixed and variable cost components and by the necessity to adjust historical costs for the impact of inflation to use them for predicting future costs.

Adjusting costs for inflation   Part of the change in costs over time is a result of volume changes, but part is attributable to inflation. To adjust for the impact of inflation, a historical cost must be multiplied by the current value of an appropriate price index divided by the value of that index when the cost was incurred.

Regression analysis   After historical costs have been adjusted for the impact of inflation, regression analysis can be used to estimate the fixed and variable costs. Costs are the dependent variable, and service units are the independent variable. The constant term of the regression represents fixed costs, and the coefficient of the independent variable represents the variable costs.

Multiple regression analysis and cost estimation   Technique that allows superior cost estimates by incorporating information from several independent variables rather than just one.

Break-even analysis (BEA)   Technique that allows the user to determine the volume of patients required for a program or service to be financially self-sufficient. At volumes above the break-even point, a profit is made; below that point, a loss occurs. BEA is based on the following formula:

$$\text{Break-Even Quantity (Q)} = \frac{\text{Fixed Costs (FC)}}{\text{Price (P)} - \text{Variable Cost per Patient (VC)}}$$

Contribution margin (CM)   Price minus the variable cost per service unit. This represents the additional financial benefit to the organization from each additional service unit. This benefit can be used to cover fixed costs or provide a profit. A weighted-average CM is used for break-even analysis when there is more than one type of service unit or more than one price for each type service unit.

✳ SUGGESTED READINGS

Cleverley W, Cleverley JO, Song PH: *Essentials of health care finance*, ed 7, Sudbury, Mass, 2010, Jones & Bartlett.

Finkler S, Ward D, Calabrese T: *Accounting fundamentals for health care management*, ed 2, Sudbury, Mass, 2012, Jones & Bartlett.

Folland S, Goodman AC, Stano M: *The economics of health and health care*, ed 6, Upper Saddle River, New Jersey, 2009, Prentice-Hall.

Gapenski L: *Healthcare finance: an introduction to accounting and financial management*, ed 4, Chicago, 2007, Health Administration Press.

Garber A, Phelps C: Economic foundations of cost-effectiveness analysis, *J Health Econ* 16(1):1-31, 1997.

Greene J, Metwalli A: The impact of activity based cost accounting on health care capital investment decisions, *J Health Care Fin* 28(2):50-64, 2001.

Hansen D, Mowen M: *Cost management*, ed 5, Cincinnati, 2005, South-Western Publishing.

Keown A, Martin J, Petty J: *Foundations of finance*, ed 7, Upper Saddle River, New Jersey, 2010, Prentice Hall.

Leister J, Strausberg J: Comparison of cost accounting methods from different DRG systems and their effect on health care quality, *Health Pol* 74(1):46-55, 2005.

McKeon T: *Home health financial management*, Gaithersburg, Maryland, 1996, Aspen Publishers.

McLean R: *Financial management in health care organizations*, ed 2, Albany, New York, 2002, Delmar.

Morrone A: Have another cup of coffee: another way to think about cost accounting for PPS, *Nurs Homes Long Term Care Manage* 48(4):22-26, 28-29, 81-82, 1999.

Pelfrey S: Cost-accounting techniques for health care providers, *Health Care Superv* 14(2):33-42, 1995.

Simione R, Simione K: Financial management of a hospice program, *Caring* 21(7):34-39, 2002.

Warner K, Luce B: *Cost-benefit and cost-effectiveness analysis in health care: principles, practice, and potential*, Ann Arbor, Mich, 1983, Health Administration Press.

Zelman W, McCue M, Milikan A, Gli N: *Financial management of health care organizations: an introduction to fundamental tools, concepts, and applications*, ed 3, Hoboken, New Jersey, 2009, Jossey-Bass.

Determining Health Care Costs and Prices

CHAPTER GOALS

The goals of this chapter are to:

- Clarify the difference between the types of cost information needed for external reporting and the information useful to managers
- Explain the traditional cost-finding methods as required in Medicare cost reports
- Describe approaches in assessing the cost of nursing care and provide examples of specific approaches in determining the cost of nursing care

- Describe the issues related to determining the costs of different patient product lines
- Introduce the concept of standard cost and discuss approaches designed to yield more accurate cost information
- Explain the various approaches to rate setting
- Discuss variable billing for nursing services

✳ INTRODUCTION

Chapter 8 discussed the foundations of cost analysis, including fixed, variable, average, and marginal costs, and explained which costs to use for different types of management decisions. In addition, methods were discussed for estimating future costs and for calculating whether a program or service would be financially self-sufficient. All of these elements are essential tools in routine management activities. One can think of that material as representing the trees. Now that the reader can identify each different type of tree, it is necessary to step back and look at the forest. This chapter looks at some broader, organization-wide costing issues as well as issues related to setting rates or prices for health care services.

The first section of this chapter considers the difference between cost information generated by the organization to help managers more effectively manage the health care organization (HCO) and cost information needed for reports provided to persons outside the organization. This is an important distinction because the needs of internal and external users of information differ significantly.

The requirements for external cost reporting are complex. Traditionally, health care institutions have calculated their costs in what is called a *cost-finding* process, which finds the costs of units of service such as laboratory tests, x-rays, or routine patient days based on an allocation of *non-revenue cost center* costs to *revenue centers*. That process generates the information needed to complete Medicare cost reports. Virtually all HCOs that receive some revenue from Medicare are

required to submit such reports. Historically, these reports formed the basis for cost accounting in HCOs. The information generated by such reports was used to determine department and patient costs.

However, such reports do not provide particularly useful information about the cost of nursing services. To understand the costs of caring for any specific type of patient, one must know the resources consumed by that type of patient and the cost of those resources. One of the most significant elements in that calculation is an understanding of the nursing resources consumed or assigned by each type of patient. In recent years, the nursing profession has placed an ever-greater stress on improving the ability to make such calculations. Understanding the costs of nursing services provides the manager with valuable information for decision making.

The chapter next turns to product-line costing. In the highly competitive health care marketplace, managers have found that to remain competitive, they must have information about the costs of running departments or units as well as the costs of treating different types of patients. This has led to a growing emphasis on what is called *product-line costing*. In product-line costing, an attempt is made to find the average costs for a given type of patient or group of similar patients. This is done for all costs, not just nursing service costs.

In recent years, HCOs have started to develop various *standard cost* approaches to provide improved cost information for managers, especially with respect to the cost of various types of patients. Product-line and standard costing are discussed in this chapter.

Setting prices and planning total revenues are also discussed. In the health care setting, pricing is often referred to as *rate setting*. Cost information is the most essential ingredient in the pricing decisions that HCOs make. When an organization sets prices for its services, it wants to be sure they are at least as high as the cost of providing those services. If they are not, losses will be incurred. The amount of revenue received in relation to the costs of providing care is critical to the continued existence of the organization.

Revenues are no longer the sole domain of the financial officer. In the past 20 years, there has been a shift in responsibility from finance to nursing for the planning and control of nursing costs. More recently, this shift in financial responsibility has included responsibility for revenues. Nurse managers need to become knowledgeable about the revenue process in HCOs. In some cases, revenues are set outside the organization. For example, the federal government sets Medicare Diagnosis Related Groups (DRG) rates. More often prices are negotiated by the purchaser (often the insurer) and the organization. Managers must be able to determine whether the revenue received in such cases will be sufficient to cover all of the costs of providing care.

In addition to general rate-setting issues, nurses also need to know about direct charging for nursing services. In home health care, for example, agencies primarily charge for nursing care. Accurate information on the cost of nursing services can be used as a basis for charging for nursing services. Nursing historically has not been a revenue center in hospitals because of a lack of accurate data about the nursing cost for different patient types. However, the increasingly prominent role nurses play in determining the financial well-being of HCOs suggests that this practice may change. With improved information, nursing can be a revenue department, similar to laboratory or radiology. These issues are also discussed in this chapter.

✳ COSTS FOR REPORTING VERSUS COSTS FOR MANAGEMENT CONTROL

Managers need to have cost information to manage their responsibility centers within large organizations or the entire operation of smaller organizations. Many decisions that managers must make require information about the costs their units incur. The correctness of the decisions depends to a great extent on the accuracy of the cost information available. Therefore, cost data collection for use by managers should have a high priority.

At the same time, HCOs are required to comply with a number of external reporting requirements. The financial statements for external reporting are discussed in Chapters 6 and 7. In addition to producing financial statements, most HCOs are also required to complete other reports that focus on the organization's costs. These external reports are most commonly prepared for Medicare, Medicaid, and other governmental agencies and for some insurance and managed care organizations. It is important to keep in mind that historically, many payments to HCOs have been based on costs incurred. As a result, payers often needed to know the organization's costs.

Most HCOs spend a great deal of energy generating reports that contain mandated cost information. Unfortunately, in some cases, the information contained in the external reports is used for internal management and decision-making without careful thought to how the needs of internal users differ from those of external users.

What types of information are inappropriately used for internal management purposes? Many types. Some of the problems that result from this practice are relatively easy to deal with; others are much more complex and are built into the underlying cost-accounting calculations used throughout the organization.

Consider an example of an easily solvable problem. Suppose you are a hospital or long-term care unit manager, and nurses are "floated," or sent from their home unit to work on another unit, based on staffing need (i.e., the home unit has too many nurses, the other has too few). In some organizations, the nurse's time is charged to the home unit even though the nurse spends his or her time working on another unit. This practice results in overcharges to the home unit for more resources than it consumed and undercharges to the unit where the nurse was floated.

For external reporting purposes, it may be adequate to simply show the total cost for the nursing staff. However, the organization needs its managers to control their costs. When it is time to contrast budgeted costs with actual costs, the actual costs should reflect the resources actually consumed on the unit. The scenario just described puts managers of both units at a disadvantage. The manager of the float nurse's home unit might be held accountable for the costs expended by all unit nurses who are floated, which, depending on the extent of floating, could put the home unit over budget. On the other hand, the manager of the unit to which the nurse floated is unable to document resources actually consumed and therefore may find it difficult or impossible to adequately justify and defend the additional staffing resources needed.

How can this problem be solved? A system needs to be put into place that tracks the "home" units where nurses are assigned to work each day and charges float costs to units where nurses actually work on any given day. Such systems are widely, although not universally, used.

A much more difficult problem concerns the use of cost reports for determining the costs of treating different types of patients. Cost reports are complex and difficult to complete. There are a number of problems with the information they contain. However, these problems become buried in the calculations, and many managers treat the cost report information as if it were more accurate than it really is. The next section explains the cost-finding process used to develop cost reports. The problems with the process that make its resulting information less than optimal for management use are discussed. Later sections of the chapter discuss alternatives that provide managers with more accurate information.

✳ TRADITIONAL COST-FINDING METHODS

Health care organizations consume a variety of resources in providing their services. Labor, supplies, and equipment are needed to provide care to each patient. The challenge faced by accountants in HCOs is both to accumulate cost information for all resources used and to find an efficient, economical way to accurately associate with each patient the costs incurred to treat that patient.

Practically speaking, assignment of perfectly accurate costs to each patient is an unreasonable expectation. To keep track perfectly would require constant observation of each patient to see how many towels are used, exactly how many minutes of nurse time and technician time are expended, and so on. Simply put, gathering cost information costs money. All HCOs therefore use accounting shortcuts to save money. However, there is a clear trade-off between how much is spent on gathering cost information and how accurate it is. It often costs more money to collect more accurate information. Each organization must decide when the level of information is "good enough." Expanded use of bar coding and computers makes it possible to collect more detailed and accurate information without substantially increasing the cost of data collection.

The simplest cost-finding approach is to divide the total dollars spent over a period of time by the number of patients treated over that period. The result is the average cost per patient. That average will be the same for all patients. Clearly, however, such an approach is not good enough. It would be impossible for managers to begin to determine which patients are profitable and which generate losses if such a method were used. If managers worked hard to treat a certain type of patient more efficiently, they would not have any sense of whether that goal was accomplished if the same cost was assigned to all patients regardless of resources consumed. The approach must be more sophisticated.

The Medicare Step-Down Approach

The approach most HCOs use for cost finding is the one mandated for Medicare cost reports. With that approach, all resource consumption is first associated with a cost center. Housekeeping, finance, medical records, pharmacy, an intensive care unit (ICU), the operating room (OR), and a coronary care unit (CCU) are examples of cost centers. Each cost center accumulates direct costs, such as labor and supplies used in the center.

The next step is to allocate all the costs of the non-revenue cost centers to the revenue centers. Recall from Chapter 3 that revenue centers are the organizational units that specifically charge for their services. For example, patients are generally charged a specific amount for a surgical procedure but not for security. Revenue center managers are responsible not only for the costs incurred in their unit or department but also for the revenues. Although this creates the burden of additional responsibility, it also adds benefits. If a unit or department is a revenue center, it can point to an explicit measure of the financial contribution that it earns for the organization. The revenue it generates can be used as an argument for giving additional resources to the center. If given the choice, most managers would want their departments to be classified as revenue centers.

How do HCOs distinguish between cost centers that are revenue centers and cost centers that are not? The key requirement for a revenue center is that it must be possible to measure different consumption of that center's services by different patients.

For example, each day each patient benefits equally from the presence of a security guard at the front door of the organization. Therefore, there can be one catchall charge per patient per day, called the *per diem,* which includes costs such as the security guard. However, if patients consume different amounts of a resource, specific charges are needed to reflect those differences. For example, if one patient has surgery and one does not, we need to be able to charge only the one who had surgery. And we need to be able to charge a greater amount to someone who had a more expensive operation than to someone who had a less expensive operation. Therefore, security is not a revenue center, but the OR is.

Examples of revenue centers in hospitals include pharmacy, radiology, OR, respiratory therapy, central supply, and the laboratory. Examples of non-revenue centers include dietary, administration, housekeeping, and medical records.

Why must the non-revenue center costs be allocated to the revenue centers? HCOs—or any type of service organization—get their revenues by charging for the services provided. When the prices or rates are set, the organization must consider all of its costs. Laundry is not a revenue center; it does not charge patients a fee for its services. ORs consume large amounts of scrubs and sheets, which must be laundered. If a hospital were to set its OR prices high enough to recover the cost of its OR nurses but did not consider the cost of the laundry, its prices might not be set high enough to recover all costs incurred by the organization. Therefore, to ensure that the organization sets prices high enough to recover all of its costs, the costs of the revenue centers must also include all of the costs of the non-revenue cost centers.

After all of the non-revenue center costs have been assigned to the revenue centers, each revenue center can in turn assign its total direct and indirect costs to the units of service that have been provided to the patients it has treated. The costs assigned to a specific patient by each of the revenue centers can be aggregated to determine the total cost of treating that patient.

Even though Medicare pays hospitals on the basis of DRGs (or the Medicare Severity DRG, or MS-DRG) rather than the hospital's cost, the Medicare cost report is still completed by hospitals. The cost information from the report is used by the federal government in its process of setting national payment rates for each DRG.

A Detailed Look at the Cost-Finding Approach

Accumulate Direct Costs for Each Cost Center

The first step in the cost-finding process is to accumulate the direct costs of the cost center. For example, consider an OR, which is a revenue center.

Direct costs in the OR include salaries and wages for regular staff. This includes all supervisory and staff personnel who work in the OR and are included in the OR budget. The OR manager, the scrub and circulating nurses, technicians, orderlies, clerks, and secretaries are all included. Employee benefits are also included in direct costs.

Other direct costs include the costs for supplies, seminars, agency per diem nurses, and all other items under the direct control of the OR that are normally considered its direct costs.

Determine Bases for Allocation

The laundry department is an example of a non-revenue cost center. After its direct costs have been accumulated, they must be assigned to revenue centers. Each center that uses laundry should be charged for a portion of the costs of the laundry. To do this, the manager must first decide on the basis for the allocation.

The cost of the laundry could be charged in equal shares to each department that uses it. However, that would be unfair to departments that use relatively little laundry. Such an allocation would not be good enough.

Other approaches to allocating the cost of laundry would be on the basis of pounds of laundry or pieces of laundry. In fact, most HCOs that have a laundry department assign laundry costs on the basis of the number of pounds of laundry. All dirty laundry is placed in a laundry cart, which is weighed. Then total laundry costs can be allocated based on the share of total pounds of laundry consumed by each department.

Is that an appropriate basis for the allocation? Clearly, it is not. A lab jacket may be more complicated to sort and fold than a sheet. Although four lab jackets together may weigh the same amount as one sheet, they no doubt require more labor than one sheet. Labor is one of the greatest expenses of the laundry department. Therefore, cost accuracy would improve if costing were done on the basis of the number of each type of laundry item. However, it costs much more to keep track of pieces than pounds.

Most HCOs have decided that pounds of laundry is a good enough measure. It effectively assigns all of the costs of the laundry to the revenue centers, and it uses an allocation basis that takes some, if not perfect, account of relative use by different cost centers. In any event, the only perfectly accurate measurement would require one staff member to constantly observe each patient to see exactly what laundry that patient used. The cost of that approach would obviously be prohibitive.

The problem of the specific basis to choose for allocating costs is not limited to the laundry. Other cost centers also make choices. For example, any HCO that has a building must allocate its annual depreciation to the various cost centers. That is usually done on the basis of square feet. A cost center that physically occupies many square feet would be charged more than one that has fewer square feet.

However, it actually costs more to build certain parts of a facility than other parts. For example, an OR costs much more per square foot than a patient room. By allocating an equal amount of depreciation per square foot, too little is assigned to the OR and too much to medical and surgical rooms. Ultimately, this means that medical patients are overcharged relative to their resource consumption, and surgical patients are undercharged. However, hospitals have generally decided that an equal depreciation charge per square foot is adequate.

Allocate from Cost Centers to Revenue Centers

All costs of the non-revenue cost centers are allocated to the revenue centers using the allocating bases previously discussed. Figure 9–1 provides a simplified example of what this type of allocation attempts. In the figure, housekeeping and laundry are non-revenue centers. The CCU and pharmacy are revenue centers. Each non-revenue center must ultimately allocate all its costs to the revenue centers.

Table 9–1 provides a highly simplified numerical example.[1] The numbers in this example are designed to show the impact of alternative allocation approaches and are not meant to be realistic dollar amounts or percentages. As in Figure 9–1, housekeeping and laundry are non-revenue centers, and the CCU and pharmacy are revenue centers. The first line in the table shows the direct cost incurred in each of the four centers; the next two lines show the allocation base and how much of the base is related to each department.

Housekeeping costs will be allocated on the basis of square feet and laundry on the basis of pounds. The table shows the percentage of all square feet that each cost center has and the percentage of all pounds of laundry used by each cost center. The square feet in the housekeeping department and the pounds of laundry done by the laundry for the laundry are excluded because no cost center allocates its own costs to itself. Thus, in this hypothetical example, housekeeping services are used 70% by the laundry, 25% by the CCU, and 5% by the pharmacy. Laundry services are used 20% by housekeeping, 10% by the CCU, and 70% by the pharmacy.

Table 9–2 shows an allocation of the direct costs to the revenue centers. The allocation in this table is called a *direct distribution*. In the direct distribution method, non-revenue center costs are allocated only to revenue centers. In making the allocation, a problem arises. Although 25% of the square feet are in the CCU and 5% are in the pharmacy (see Table 9–1), if those percentages are used for the allocation, the full $40,000 of housekeeping cost would not be allocated. This is because 70% of the square feet is in the laundry, and no cost is being allocated to the laundry. This problem is resolved by allocating to the revenue centers based on the remaining square feet after eliminating the non-revenue centers. Thirty percent of the square feet is in all the revenue centers combined, and 25% is

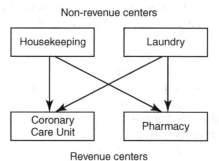

Non-revenue centers

Revenue centers

FIGURE 9–1. Allocating costs.

---

[1] These data are hypothetical and used for simplicity. They are not intended to reflect actual costs.

✳ **TABLE 9–1** *Cost-Base Information for Allocation*

| | Non-Revenue Cost Centers | | Revenue Cost Centers | | |
	Housekeeping	Laundry	Coronary Care Unit	Pharmacy	Total Cost
Direct cost	$40,000	$60,000	$500,000	$500,000	$1,100,000
Allocation statistics:					
Housekeeping (square feet)	—	70%	25%	5%	100%
Laundry (pounds)	20%	—	10%	70%	100%

✳ **TABLE 9–2** *Direct Distribution*

| | Non-Revenue Cost Centers | | Revenue Cost Centers | | |
	Housekeeping	Laundry	Coronary Care Unit	Pharmacy	Total Cost
Direct cost	$40,000	$60,000	$500,000	$500,000	$1,100,000
Allocation statistics:					
Housekeeping (square feet)	(40,000)	—	33,333	6,667	—
Laundry (pounds)	—	(60,000)	7,500	52,500	—
Totals	$ 0	$ 0	$540,833	$559,167	$1,100,000

in the CCU. Thus, 25% divided by 30% gives the proportion of the housekeeping cost allocated to the CCU. Similarly, 5% divided by 30% gives the housekeeping cost allocated to the pharmacy; 10% divided by 80% gives the laundry cost allocated to the CCU; and 70% divided by 80% gives the portion of the laundry cost allocated to the pharmacy. For example, 25% divided by 30% multiplied by the $40,000 housekeeping cost results in the $33,333 of cost allocated to the CCU.

There is an additional complexity because direct distribution fails to take into account the fact that some non-revenue cost centers provide service to other non-revenue centers. Housekeeping cleans the laundry. If all housekeeping costs went directly to revenue centers, none would be allocated to the laundry, and costs would be distorted. The possible distortion is so great that a direct allocation to revenue centers only is not considered good enough.

Instead, an allocation approach is used called the *step-down method,* shown in Figure 9–2 and Table 9–3. The step-down method requires the organization to allocate all of the cost of a non-revenue cost center to all other cost centers (both revenue and non-revenue). First one non-revenue center's costs are allocated to every cost center. Then another non-revenue center is allocated. As each center is allocated, its

cost balance becomes zero, and it no longer is part of the process. In other words, no costs can be allocated to a cost center after it has allocated its costs. Note in Figure 9–2 that housekeeping now would allocate costs to the CCU, pharmacy, and laundry. The laundry, however, would allocate costs only to the CCU and pharmacy. Therefore, some distortion still remains in the allocation process.

Other more elaborate allocation approaches eliminate most or all of the remaining distortion. These are called the *double distribution* and the *algebraic* or *matrix distribution* approaches. The algebraic or matrix distribution approaches are based on solving a set of simultaneous equations. Although the allocation that results from use of such methods is more accurate, it is also more complicated to understand and implement. The hospital industry generally considers step-down allocation good enough.

The use of step-down allocation creates another problem: Should housekeeping be allocated before or after laundry? The order of the allocation may affect the ultimate outcome. Table 9–4 changes the order of allocation. Laundry is now allocated using the step-down method before housekeeping is allocated. Look at what happened to the ultimate cost in each revenue center. The total CCU cost has risen by $28,333, from $521,000 in Table 9–3 to $549,333 in Table 9–4. The pharmacy cost has fallen by $28,333, from $579,000 to $550,667. This is an extreme example, but it demonstrates the distortion possible by changing the order of allocation. In a perfect allocation system, the ultimate cost in each revenue center would remain the same regardless of the order in which the non-revenue center costs are allocated.

Are the actual resources consumed by the organization any different because the order of allocation of non-revenue centers changed? No. The same total amount of money was spent. The same resources were used. However, the cost of the CCU and the pharmacy can vary because of the accounting method used. With the more sophisticated algebraic approach, such

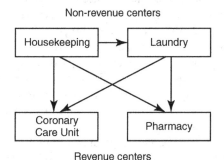

FIGURE 9–2. Allocating costs by the step-down method.

✳ TABLE 9–3 *Step-Down Distribution*

| | Non-Revenue Cost Centers | | Revenue Cost Centers | | |
	Housekeeping	Laundry	Coronary Care Unit	Pharmacy	Total Cost
Direct cost	$40,000	$60,000	$500,000	$500,000	$1,100,000
Allocation:					
Housekeeping (square feet)	(40,000)	28,000	10,000	2,000	0
Subtotal	$ 0	$88,000	$510,000	$502,000	$1,100,000
Laundry (pounds)		(88,000)	11,000	77,000	0
Totals	$ 0		$521,000	$579,000	$1,100,000

✳ TABLE 9–4 *Step-Down Distribution with Altered Order of Step-Down Allocation*

| | Non-Revenue Cost Centers | | Revenue Cost Centers | | |
	Housekeeping	Laundry	Coronary Care Unit	Pharmacy	Total Cost
Direct cost	$60,000	$40,000	$500,000	$500,000	$1,100,000
Allocation:					
Laundry (pounds)	(60,000)	12,000	6,000	42,000	0
Subtotal	$ 0	$52,000	$506,000	$542,000	$1,100,000
Housekeeping (square feet)		(52,000)	43,333	8,667	0
Totals		$ 0	$549,333	$550,667	$1,100,000

variation in costs does not occur. However, the step-down method, as noted, has been considered good enough.

It is possible that the step-down method has allowed HCOs to manipulate their cost reporting in an attempt to shift costs between revenue centers and in turn increase reimbursement. For example, many hospitals have both inpatients and outpatients. Medicare inpatients are paid on a fixed DRG payment scale. Outpatient payments for Medicare patients are not currently based on fixed DRG-type rates but on a prospective payment system called Ambulatory Payment Classifications (APCs), which pays hospitals for services provided that are similar clinically and in terms of resource use. If the order of the step-down allocation causes more costs to be allocated to the outpatient areas and fewer costs to departments that treat predominantly inpatients, total reimbursement will rise.[2]

Allocate Costs to Units of Service

Up to this point, the discussion has centered on allocating all costs of the organization into the cost centers that are revenue centers. The next part of the cost-finding process focuses on assigning each revenue center's costs to the units of service that it provides. For example, a laboratory assigns its costs to the various laboratory tests it performs, and an OR assigns its costs to the surgical procedures that take place. There are four approaches to allocating a revenue center's costs to units of service: the per diem or per visit, surcharge, hourly rate, and weighted procedure methods.

The *per diem method* is used if none of the other three methods reasonably applies. The per diem method divides the total costs of the center by the number of patient days, generating a uniform cost per patient day. Although some nursing cost centers do qualify for treatment using the other methods, this tends to be the exception rather than the rule. Most nursing costs are assigned ultimately to per diem categories. There are often different per diems for routine care as opposed to ICU or CCU. The major problem with such an approach is that it assumes that each patient consumes exactly the same amount of nursing (or other) resources per patient day. It takes no account of patient severity of illness or nursing requirements. However, the cost-finding process has treated this approach as being good enough.

The *surcharge method* is commonly used in the pharmacy and medical supplies cost centers. The revenue center compares its costs excluding inventory with the inventory cost and determines a surcharge. For example, if a pharmacy spends $10,000 on all costs except pharmaceuticals and $100,000 on pharmaceuticals, the surcharge would be 10% (i.e., $10,000 ÷$100,000). As each prescription is filled, the cost would be calculated as the cost of the drug itself plus 10%. The problem with this approach is that in reality, just because a drug costs 10 times as much to buy as another drug does not mean that it requires 10 times as much pharmacist time to process. Some organizations overcome this problem partly by using a minimum charge applied to all drugs dispensed. The proverbial $10 aspirin in the hospital is partly the result of charging a standard minimum amount for processing the aspirin order, storing the aspirin, and dispensing it.

The *hourly rate approach* measures the amount of service a revenue center provides by time. This method is used by respiratory therapy, physical therapy, ORs, and recovery rooms. For

---

[2]For more detailed information about cost reports or to download actual cost reports, see information available from the CMS at http://www.cms.hhs.gov/CostReports.

example, an OR would divide its total cost (after the step-down allocation) by the total number of hours of procedures to determine a cost per hour. Sometimes the calculations are done in minutes, yielding a cost per surgical minute. The logic of this method is that longer operations consume more resources.

This method is accurate for a service such as physical therapy in which generally only one therapist works with the patient. A problem with this approach in the OR is that an operation may require just one nurse, two nurses, or two nurses and a technician. Also, the supplies and equipment used may not bear a direct relationship to time. It is possible that a 2-hour operation might consume far more resources than a 3-hour operation. In the past, this method, although not very good, has traditionally been considered good enough. In recent years, however, ORs are trying alternative approaches. For example, many ORs keep track of person hours rather than just surgical hours to account for the number of staff members in the surgical suite.

The *weighted procedure method* (sometimes called the *relative value unit method*) is based on a special study of the center's costs, which establishes a relative costliness of each type of service the center performs. This method is commonly used in departments such as laboratory or radiology, where a specific and limited number of services are provided, and they are provided in a similar fashion each time. A base value is assigned to one type of procedure, and all other procedures are assigned a relative value. Thus, if blood gas analysis is twice as costly as a complete blood count (CBC), the CBC might be assigned a value of 1.0 unit of work and the blood gas a value of 2.0 units of work. In any given month, the values assigned to all of the services provided can be summed and divided into the total cost of the revenue center. This yields a cost per unit of work.

For example, suppose that the total costs of the laboratory revenue center after the step-down allocation of non-revenue centers costs is $5,000. If the laboratory performs 300 blood gas analyses and 400 CBCs, it performs a total of 1,000 units of work (300 blood gases × 2 units of work + 400 CBCs × 1 unit of work). The cost of $5,000 divided by 1,000 units of work is $5 per unit of work. Therefore, the $5,000 total laboratory costs would be assigned at a rate of $10 per blood gas analysis (2 units of work × $5 per unit) and $5 per CBC (1 unit of work × $5 per unit).

A problem with this approach is that it relies heavily on the assumption that a blood gas analysis is always twice as costly to perform as a CBC. This problem is exacerbated by the fact that many HCOs use standard relationships based on a survey of institutions rather than measuring the relative costs in their own facility. Because the personnel pay rates and the equipment used vary from one organization to another, the relative relationships are not likely to be exactly the same at all institutions. However, compared with having an accountant observe the resources used each time a lab test is performed, it is considered good enough.

Is Good-Enough Cost Finding Good Enough?

For the first 2 decades under Medicare and Medicaid, the good-enough approximations that resulted from the cost-finding system just described were considered acceptable. Most large third-party payers, such as Medicare, Medicaid, Blue Cross, and private for-profit insurers, had a large mix of patients so that if they were overcharged for one patient, they were likely to be undercharged for another. As long as the total costs were not overstated, overcharges and undercharges were likely to average out for large groups of patients. It was not sensible for third-party payers to require HCOs to spend substantially more money on improved cost accounting. They then would have had to bear the cost of the improved cost accounting in addition to the costs of patient care.

With the introduction of DRGs, however, incentives changed. DRGs place hospitals, in particular, at risk for the costs they incur. If patients cost more to care for than the DRG payment rate, the hospital suffers a loss. The growth of managed care has made it even more important for health care providers to measure patient costs more accurately.

This means that to the extent possible and still being mindful of the cost of collecting more accurate information, managers of HCOs would like to improve on the good-enough approximations. They would like to eliminate the inaccuracies of using pounds of laundry instead of pieces or using square feet instead of construction cost for depreciation. They would like to eliminate the distortions created by the order of allocation in the step-down process. They would like to remove the inaccuracies generated by weighted procedure and hourly, surcharge, and per diem assignments of cost.

Can this be done? There probably will never be a 100% accurate costing system. As automated systems have become more commonplace in HCOs, the potential exists to make great strides in more accurately assigning patient resource consumption. In the interim, many HCOs are taking at least intermediate steps to improve their costing. Some of the approaches used are discussed in the remaining sections of this chapter.

✳ COSTING OUT NURSING SERVICES

The essence of the costing problem is that nursing costs are often charged to patients as part of a general per diem charge rather than being charged separately on the patient's bill. As a result, all patients are assumed to receive the same level of care, consume the same "amount" of nursing care, and therefore receive the same charge for the nursing care they receive. Readers of this book are keenly aware that this is not the case. The reality is that patients receive very different levels of nursing care and they are cared for on very different types of patient care units—some receive care on an ICU, others receive care on a specialty unit, and yet others receive care on a general medical or surgical unit. Even patients on the same unit generally require different levels of care because their diagnoses differ, along with their prescribed treatments and nursing interventions.

In terms of providing management with an understanding of the cost implications for different patients, the per diem approach provides extremely poor information about the amount of nursing care and the resources different types of patients require or consume. This approach incorrectly assumes that all patients consume exactly the same amount of nursing care even though different patients have different nursing care requirements.

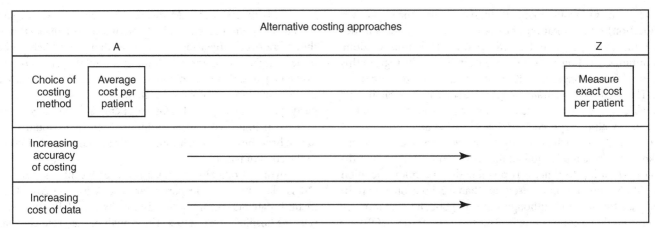

FIGURE 9–3.   The A versus Z extremes.

Hospitals interested in costing out nursing services have been faced with two extreme alternatives. One choice is to divide the total annual costs of nursing care by the number of patients treated for the year to determine the average cost per patient. At the other extreme, the hospital could hire a data collector to follow each nurse and determine exactly how much of the nurse's time was used by each patient. This detailed approach is generally referred to as *microcosting*. Figure 9–3 reflects this extreme choice: Whereas alternative A is simple and inexpensive, alternative Z is extremely detailed and expensive.

What hospital could afford to assign a data collector to each nurse to observe and gather detailed information on how much time was devoted to each patient and on all components of care delivered? The value of information should always justify its cost. Alternative Z in Figure 9–3 is labor intensive and generally too costly for most hospitals to undertake. Figure 9–4 adds a compromise. In most cases, a patient with a 3-day stay would consume less nursing care than a patient with a 15-day stay. If total nursing care costs are divided by total patient days, patients who are in the hospital for more days can be assigned more nursing cost than patients in the hospital for fewer days. This is alternative B. It is still not nearly so precise and accurate an approach as alternative Z; however, it is not much more expensive than alternative A and gives a much better approximation of the nursing care cost for different patients.

Under alternative B, the approach most hospitals use, the nursing cost is assumed to be the same for all patient days. More days imply more cost, but for the same number of patient days, all patients are assumed to use the same amount of nursing care. Thus, even though this is a much better option than alternative A, it is still a very poor measure of nursing cost.

Solutions to the Costing Problem

How can the cost of each individual patient be better measured without having an accountant follow every nurse? One solution that some hospitals are using is information systems. Health information technology is so important that CMS provides incentives for the use of electronic health records (EHRs) and the U.S. Department of Health and Human Services has an office devoted to the coordination of health information technology initiatives.[3] By taking advantage of available technologies such as computers in nursing stations and point of care technologies

[3] For more information, see information available from the CMS at https://www.cms.gov/ehrincentiveprograms/ and the U.S. Department of Health and Human Services, Office of the National Coordinator for Health Information Technology, at http://healthit.hhs.gov/portal/server.pt/community/healthit_hhs_gov__home/1204.

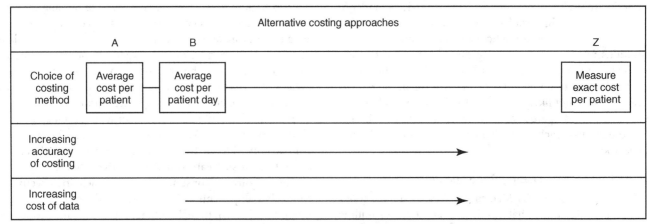

FIGURE 9–4.   Introduction of Alternative B.

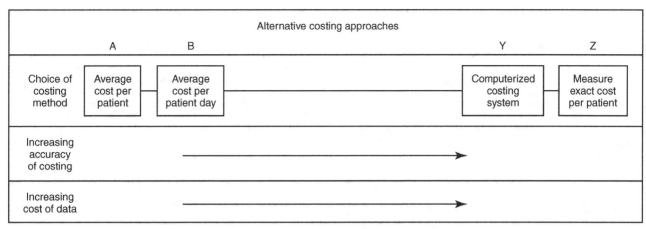

FIGURE 9–5. Introduction of Alternative Y.

(i.e., computers at each patient bedside or individual nurses with personal digital assistants [PDAs] or tablet personal computers [PCs]), nursing care can be delivered more efficiently[4] and its costs tracked more accurately.[5]

Figure 9–5 illustrates how computers have been added to the continuum from low-accuracy, low-cost information to high-accuracy, high-cost information. This is alternative Y. Using information systems, nurses electronically record when they are with each patient and what they are doing for that patient. The system then multiplies the nurse time spent by the salary of the particular nurse providing the care to determine the specific cost of nursing care for a particular patient. When nurses are doing some indirect activities, such as documenting in a patient's record, the computer can also assign that cost to the appropriate patient.

Substantial progress has been made in a variety of areas to ease the input of data into the computer. Uniform price codes (bar coding) are becoming more widely used on a variety of supplies consumed by hospitals. Bar coding is also being used in HCOs to track how nurses spend their time. For example, bar coding allows nurses to indicate when they enter and leave a patient's room, and thus, a determination can be made of how much time they spend with each patient. Although this technology does not document what nurses actually do when they are with patients, it complements the documentation feature in most information systems.

Note that alternative Y is close to alternative Z in several respects. The data to be gained are potentially quite accurate and clearly can be made patient-specific. These data would enable the hospital to assign costs (and ultimately charges) to patients based on their differing consumption of nursing resources.

Another approach to estimating the cost of nursing care is the use of a *patient classification system*. Patient classification systems require rating patients based on the likely nursing resource requirements resulting from the acuity of their illness. Sicker patients requiring more nursing care are assigned higher acuity or higher classification levels. Many hospitals have developed their own systems, and several commercial systems are widely used in hospitals throughout the United States. Patients are rated by nurses on scales such as 1 to 5; the higher the number, the greater the nursing resources consumed, and, in turn, the greater the cost of caring for patients with this rating. In other words, this system weights the costs of caring for patients based on a system of rating patients.

Patient classification generally is not a perfectly accurate measure of the resources needed for each patient. Some patients classified as level 2 will require more care than level 2 calls for, and some level 2 patients will require less care than would be expected based on that classification. If the system is functioning reasonably well, however, average patient resource consumption will match what is expected based on the classification system. And certainly it would generally be expected that a level 2 patient will consume resources closer to the level 2 average than to the level 1 or the level 3 average.

If a mechanism to determine patients' costs based on their classification can be established, it still will not provide the precise accuracy of alternative Z. It will not even provide the alternative Y accuracy that a computer system can generate. However, it can create a new alternative, X, as shown in Figure 9–6. Alternative X is inaccurate in that all patients are assigned the same nursing cost for a day at the same classification level. If two patients are both level 2 on a given day, their cost is assumed to be the same even though it is known that they will probably not consume exactly the same nursing resources. However, alternative X is much more accurate than alternatives A and B. Alternative B assumes that the cost is the same per patient day for all patients regardless of acuity.

[4]Turisco F, Rhoads J. 2008. *Equipped for Efficiency: Improving Nursing Care Through Technology*. California Healthcare Foundation. Retrieved at http://www.chcf.org/~/media/MEDIA%20LIBRARY%20Files/PDF/E/PDF%20EquippedForEfficiency.pdf.

[5]Birmingham SE. 2010. Evidence-based staffing: The next step. *Nurse Leader* 8(3):24-26, 35; Welton J, Zone-Smith L, Bandyopadhyay D. 2009. Estimating nursing intensity and direct cost using the nurse-patient assignment. *J Nurs Adm* 39:276-284; and Moss J, Saba V. 2011. Costing nursing care: Using the clinical care classification system to value nursing intervention in an acute care setting. *Comput Inform Nurs* 29(8):455-460.

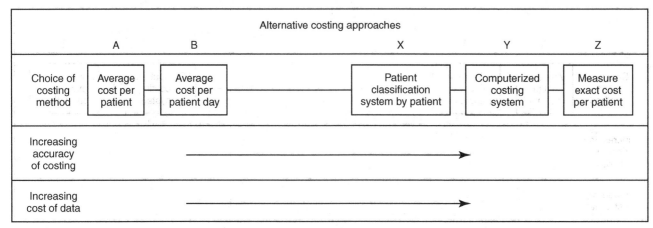

FIGURE 9–6.   Introduction of Alternative X.

Alternative X is an improvement because the cost is considered the same per patient day only for patients at the same acuity level. Different costs are assigned to patient days at different acuity levels. Users of alternative X must recognize that the information has some degree of inaccuracy. However, the system may be accurate enough, given the current high costs of using either alternative Y or Z. Therefore, patient classification systems can be the basis for a system that allows more accurate estimates of the cost a hospital incurs for nursing care for different types of patients.

Somewhere between X and Y on the scale from A to Z, one could place workload measurement tools. These are variants of patient classification. Workload measurement tools attempt to determine the nursing care time required for each patient each day. The approach is to identify the time required for each of the types of nursing interventions that take up most of the nurses' time. Each patient is evaluated each day to determine which interventions will be needed. Such tools can track required care hours specific to each patient. This is contrasted with patient classification systems that use an average hour figure for all patients within a broad category or level of care.

Such an approach is not as sophisticated as alternative Y, in which the actual care hours are entered into the computer as the patient receives the care. It is likely that some interventions will take longer than typical for some patients and less time for others. Therefore, the cost ultimately assigned to the patient will be based on average time, not actual time. However, the workload measurement approach is more sophisticated than alternative X, which uses average nursing care hours for all patients in a given patient classification category.

Although patient classification and workload measurement systems can be used to determine the cost of nursing, these systems were initially developed to predict staffing needs, not to determine costs. Nurse managers should be aware that although patients require a designated amount of care, this does not mean that they receive it. They should also be aware that secure electronic systems and wireless technologies are being used in HCOs to help nurses gain greater efficiency in their work. For example, many organizations give nurses pagers and secure cell phones so they can easily stay in touch with others on the health care team. This saves a great deal of nurses' time

spent navigating the system. Other hospitals are using PDAs and tablet PCs (e.g., iPads) so that nurses can record how they spend their time. This will help to make nurses' work more transparent and allow nurse managers to determine the amount of time nurses spend in direct and indirect care activities.[6] As systems evolve to better link nurses, the care they provide, the patients they care for, and the outcomes of their care, it will be possible to move closer to Alternative Z than we can imagine today.

Why Change the Costing Approach?

The mere fact that the ability to improve costing now exists does not in itself explain why a nurse manager would want to more accurately identify costs. What is to be gained from having a more accurate measure of the different costs for nursing care for different types of patients?

A critical benefit from improved costing of nursing services is that the organization can generate information for better management decisions. Is a particular service too costly? What price can be bid for a health maintenance organization or preferred provider organization contract? Hospital costing has long been based on averages and cross subsidizations. In the current environment, errors in calculations of costs become more serious as negotiations for discounted prices become more intense. Managers are being pushed along the increasing accuracy of the costing line in Figure 9–6, yet this also requires moving in the direction of increased cost of data.

In addition, as costing becomes more specific and more accurate, managers can not only deal better with pricing problems but also can be more efficient in the management of costs. Control of budgets improves as another measure of expected cost becomes available. Flexible budget systems can provide better analysis and control of costs, and productivity can be monitored better if more is known about costs. Not only is it possible to assess how costs should change based on changing numbers of patient days, but information about the cost per patient in a given DRG can also be used to assess costs as the number of patients in each DRG changes.

---

[6] *Ibid.*

Should Costing Be Linked to Diagnosis Related Groups?

If HCOs are going to move in the direction of more accurate costing of nursing services, one of the critical questions is how to categorize the cost. Should there be one nursing cost for medical patients and another for surgical patients? Should the cost for men as opposed to women be determined or for young people as opposed to old people? Should there be one nursing cost for each type of patient based on International Classification of Diseases (ICD) code? Should the cost be found by DRG?

The problem managers face is the definition of the product of nursing care. What do nurses "produce"? If a nurse changes a dressing or gives a patient a medication, are those the products of nursing care? Most people would probably consider those activities to represent only intermediate products or tasks. The ultimate product is the health and outcomes of the patient, not the tasks completed.

However, HCOs treat many different kinds of patients. They do not have only one final product. They have many final products represented by the different patients to whom nurses provide care. Yet currently, all patient costs are assessed for nursing care as if they were the same. That needs to change. Final products need to be defined so that nurse managers can assess the cost of each. Patients could be divided into categories called *nursing resource groupings* (NRGs), perhaps based on nursing diagnoses or some other categorization.[7] Ideally, patients should be divided into homogeneous NRGs based on nursing care consumed. Any patient in one NRG would consume a similar set of nursing resources as any other patient in that grouping.

What should be the basis for costing nursing services in the interim until a NRG type system is in use? One approach is to fall back on alternative X. A patient classification system can be used to determine how many days a given patient is rated at each classification level. If the cost of each day at each

classification level (discussed later in this chapter) can be determined, the manager can add up the costs to determine the patient's total nursing care cost.

However, this requires determination of the patient classification for every patient for every day. Some hospitals will find the advantages of being at alternative X on the costing accuracy scale sufficient to warrant this investment in data collection. Doing this will not only improve costing but will also collect information that can be used for calculating acuity variances.

However, many hospitals will not want to spend the resources needed to classify every patient every day. The alternative is to take a sample of patients from each DRG and determine the average nursing cost for patients in each DRG based on a sampling approach. All patients within a specific DRG will not consume the same nursing resources for each day at a specific patient classification level. Nor will all patients in one DRG have the same number of patient days at each classification level or even the same total number of patient days. This approach is based on average length of stay, the average number of days at each patient classification level, and the average nursing resource consumption within each patient classification level. However, the average amount of nursing resources for each type of DRG can be found.

For example, if a hospital uses a nursing patient classification system with a scale from 1 to 5, a group of patients from each DRG can be sampled to find out, on average, how many days of the patients' stay were at level 1, how many at level 2, and so on. Averaging all patients in a given DRG at a given hospital will not give a measurement alternative accurate enough to be labeled W on the scale from A to Z. Such an estimate of cost would probably be considered R on such a scale. It would not be nearly as accurate as X, but it would be substantially more accurate than A and B. This new alternative, R (Figure 9–7), would be substantially less expensive than alternatives X, Y, or Z.

Diagnosis Related Groups, although perhaps not ideal for the purpose of costing nursing care, are an adequate categorization for the assignment of average differential nursing costs. Many hospital decisions are based on particular DRGs or clusters of DRGs, so the DRG-based cost information generated will be of considerable management value.

---

[7]See, for example, the Center for Nursing Classification and Clinical Effectiveness developed by the faculty at the University of Iowa. Retrieved at http://www.nursing.uiowa.edu/excellence/nursing_knowledge/clinical_effectiveness/index.htm.

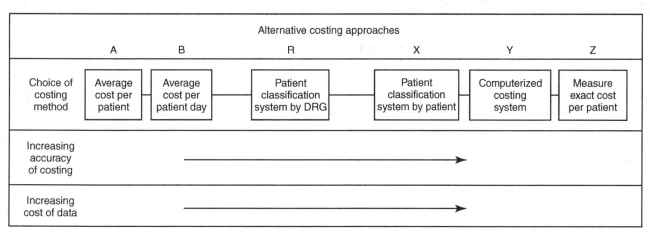

FIGURE 9–7. Introduction of Alternative R.

✳ SPECIFIC APPROACH TO COSTING NURSING SERVICES

Nursing care costs consist of the following:

- Direct costs of patient care (staff)
- Indirect costs of patient care (e.g., staff, supervisors, secretaries)
- Patient care-related costs (e.g., patient and unit supplies)
- Overhead costs (allocated from other departments)

Note that the cost of nursing care is more than just the hourly salary and benefits for the nurse giving care at the bedside. Nursing management, assessment, planning, evaluating, teaching, and discharge planning are also critical elements of nursing care. In addition, supplies, secretaries, and overhead are elements of overall nursing care cost. A manager could try to determine the costs of each of these elements separately for each category of patient or do the costing in some more aggregate fashion. Start with the assumption that all nursing department costs are aggregated.

The key element that allows for improved costing of nursing services is the fact that nursing patient classification systems are in place in almost every hospital. Without such systems, different patients may consume different amounts of resources, but the manager has no way to measure the differential consumption. With a classification system, after a patient has been classified, the manager has some idea of the nursing resources that patient will consume.

For example, suppose that a nursing unit has the following hypothetical patient classification resource guidelines:

Acuity Level	Hours of Care
1	3.0
2	4.0
3	4.8
4	6.6
5	9.0

In developing the patient classification system, various clinical indicators are used to determine if a patient should be classified as 1, 2, 3, 4, or 5. After the patient has been classified, the classification system tells how many hours of nursing care should be required to treat that patient. In this example, a patient classified as a 4 would typically require an average of 6.6 hours of care per day.

Note that the scale is not proportional. A patient classified as a 2 does not require exactly twice as many hours as a patient classified as a 1. Whereas a level 1 needs 3 hours of care, a level 2 needs 4 hours. Rather than double, this is only 33% more care. A level 3 patient needs 4.8 hours (i.e., 20% more than a level 2). A level 4 patient requires 38% more care than a level 3. As one moves from level to level, the amount of additional care does not change in proportion. It changes based on the specific classification system and the anticipated clinical needs of a patient at each level in that system.

This complicates the cost calculation. If the scale were strictly linear (i.e., a ratio scale with zero the lowest score and a score of 2 requiring twice as much care as a score of 1), one could add up all the patient days at each level and divide that sum into total nursing cost to get a cost per unit of patient classification. However, because the scale is not linear, it is necessary to create a relative value unit (RVU) scale. This scale helps determine how much care each level requires relative to the care needed for a typical level 1 patient. A patient classified as a 1 will be given a value of 1 on the *relative value scale*. Each other classification level would then be calculated in relative proportion. This can be accomplished by dividing the required hours of care for each level by the number of hours required for level 1. For example:

$$\frac{\text{Level 2}}{\text{Level 1}} = \frac{4.0 \text{ Hours}}{3.0 \text{ Hours}} = 1.33$$

Therefore, the relative value assigned to classification level 2 is 1.33. This value of 1.33 represents the fact that a level 2 patient consumes 0.33 more nursing care hours than a level 1 patient. Continuing for all classification (acuity) levels:

Acuity Level	Hours of Care	RVU
1	3.0	1.00
2	4.0	1.33
3	4.8	1.60
4	6.6	2.20
5	9.0	3.00

Assuming the following information, one can see how the RVU system can be used to develop cost information[8]:

Total nursing costs: $250,000

Acuity Level	Number of Patient Days
1	100 days
2	220 days
3	350 days
4	110 days
5	40 days

The first step is to determine the total amount of work performed by the nursing department. This is done by multiplying the RVUs for each acuity classification level by the number of days at that level. With the number of patient days and the RVUs calculated above, the total RVUs would be as follows:

Acuity Level	Patient Days	×	RVUs	=	Total RVUs
1	100	×	1.00	=	100.00
2	220	×	1.33	=	292.60
3	350	×	1.60	=	560.00
4	110	×	2.20	=	242.00
5	40	×	3.00	=	120.00
	820				1,314.60

---

[8]These data are hypothetical and used for simplicity. They do not reflect actual costs.

There were 1314.60 units of nursing work performed. We can divide this into the total nursing cost to find the cost for each RVU of nursing work.

$$\frac{\text{Total Nursing Costs}}{\text{Total RVUs}} = \text{Cost per RVU}$$

$$\frac{\$250,000}{1,314.60} = \$190.17 \text{ per RVU}$$

Here one can see that the nursing cost for a patient for 1 day with classification 1 would be $190.17. The cost for a patient with classification 4 would be $190.17 multiplied by 2.20 (the RVU for classification level 4).

How would a manager calculate the nursing cost for a patient from admission to discharge? Suppose that the average DRG 128 patient had a length of stay of 7 days, with 2 days classed as a 1, 4 days classed as a 2, and 1 day classed as a 4. The nursing cost for DRG 128 then would be as follows:

Acuity Level	Patient Days	×	RVUs	×	Cost per RVU	=	Total Cost
1	2	×	1.00	×	$190.17	=	$ 380.34
2	4	×	1.33	×	190.17	=	1,011.70
3	0	×	1.60	×	190.17	=	0.00
4	1	×	2.20	×	190.17	=	418.37
5	0	×	3.00	×	190.17	=	0.00
	7						$1,810.41

Would all patients in a given DRG be expected to consume the same resources? Not really, but the manager can still be confident that an approach such as this on average for any given DRG will give a much more accurate assignment of cost than simply assigning to every patient in a nursing unit the same daily cost for nursing care.

✳ LIMITATIONS OF THE RELATIVE VALUE UNIT APPROACH

Patient Classification versus Other Workload Measurement

The purpose of the RVU patient classification approach is to make a workable costing approach accessible to the majority of HCOs in the country. However, it does not generate perfectly accurate measures of cost and is subject to a variety of limitations.

The idea of an alternative to patient classification was discussed earlier. If a workload measurement tool is in place in a hospital and is being used on an ongoing basis to categorize resource needs of each patient each day, it can be used to provide potentially more accurate cost information. Rather than being limited to perhaps five patient classification levels for a given medical or surgical unit, such an approach collects indicators of hours of resource consumption for each patient. It is more patient-specific than the RVU approach. Putting such an approach in place and following through with it on a continuous basis may be a considerable undertaking. However, if it is used, the costing of nursing services is made much easier.

Under such an approach, the required interventions for each patient are translated into required hours of care. Total nursing care costs for direct and indirect expenses must be calculated as with the RVU system. Dividing total nursing costs by total hours of care generates a cost per hour of care. This cost per hour can be multiplied by the required hours of care for each patient for each day as determined by the system. This will give the cost per patient for each day in the hospital. If aggregate information is desired by DRG, it can be obtained by averaging the costs of each patient in that DRG. However, the majority of hospitals do not have patient-specific workload measurement systems in place.

Indirect Nursing Costs

A problem with both the RVU and more detailed workload measurement systems as described so far is the implicit assumption that all nursing costs vary in proportion to the hours of nursing care. Does that make sense for indirect costs? For example, will a sicker patient who requires more direct nursing care also require more indirect nursing care? More charting time? More supplies? More overhead? The answer to these questions depends on the specific situation of the institution.

Is it true that secretarial costs will be greater for more acutely ill patients? It may well be that a simple per diem allocation is a more appropriate way to allocate such costs. Costing could be improved, therefore, by dividing total nursing costs among those costs that vary with nursing care hours (e.g., RN staff, LPN staff, other patient care staff and perhaps clinical supplies) and those costs that do not vary with nursing care hours (e.g., office supplies, nurse manager time, and secretarial time). Costs that vary with nursing care hours would be allocated by the RVU or workload measurement approaches described previously. The other costs could be divided by total patient days and assigned to patients based on their number of patient days.

Staffing Mix

A significant problem is the fact that most hospital nursing classification systems provide required hours of care but do not specify the mix of care. If 30% of all nursing care hours are provided by LPNs, it is simply assumed that 30% of the care for each patient is provided by LPNs.

It is possible that one patient at level 2 might require 4 hours of RN care, but another might require 3 hours of LPN care and only 1 hour of RN care. Obviously, both of these patients do not consume the same amount of nursing care resources even if they consume the same number of hours of care. Therefore, there will be some distortion of costs unless the hospital uses a system that indicates not only how many hours of care are needed but also how many hours of care are needed by staff type.

This problem is not unique to costing, however. It represents a weakness of patient classification systems. If the hospital does not know the required mix of care providers, the classification system is not going to be useful for staffing decisions. Part of this problem stems from the fact that different hospitals have different views on which functions can be done by different types of staff. As patient classification systems improve, this mix problem should become less serious.

In the meantime, managers could attempt to separate the cost of RNs from LPNs and aides and assign those costs separately to patients. Special studies could be undertaken for each DRG to determine whether care was biased toward more than an average amount of RN care or toward more than an average amount of LPN care. Then the cost of nursing care for that DRG could be adjusted accordingly.

How complex are managers willing to make the costing system? Each HCO must decide how much it is willing to invest in refining its costing system, realizing that generally, the more accurate the costing system, the more expensive it is. Some managers believe that the historical average nursing cost per patient day is so inaccurate that an RVU-based system is a tremendous improvement even with the problems cited here.

We have used a hospital as an example. The same principles apply whether the cost determination is for nursing care delivered in a hospital, nursing home, outpatient setting, or patient's home. However, the costing is greatly simplified in home health care because patient records explicitly indicate the level of staff that provided the care.

✳ PRODUCT-LINE COSTING

One result of the work done on costing nursing services is that grouping all patients of one type and finding an average cost for that type of patient is possible. In other words, *product-line* costing is feasible with this method. A product line is a group of patients with some commonality that allows them to be grouped together, such as a common diagnosis. HCOs use product-line management as a way to achieve the best outcomes for a group of patients in the most cost-effective manner. Many organizations focus on providing care to patients with one disease, so-called disease management.[9] Often an organization cannot eliminate one product in a product line without eliminating the entire product line. For example, if a hospital sells its bypass pump because it is losing money on bypass surgery, it will no longer be able to do heart valve surgery. They are both part of the open heart surgery product line.

Many people believe that managers should be given hospital-wide responsibility for both the revenues and expenses related to specific patient product lines. For example, a manager might be responsible for the revenues related to the obstetrics product line. The manager is accountable for both the variance in the number of discharges and the revenue per discharge. Of course, the manager would be responsible for the budgeted and actual costs of the product line as well.

Before one takes the step of costing or budgeting by product line, it is necessary to question how the information will be used. In terms of running a nursing unit, will knowledge of the cost for all patients in a given DRG be useful? The answer depends a great deal on the types of decisions a manager or organization faces.

Cost information by DRG can be used as a way to promote efficiency. For example, the treatment patterns of two physicians who care for diabetic patients could be examined to determine if one approach is more effective or efficient than the other. If one approach achieves better outcomes at a lower cost, the approaches for managing patients with diabetes could be discussed and integrated to provide better care. Alternately, suppose that a hospital is trying to decide whether to accept a group of patients with diabetes from a certain insurer at a discounted price. Knowing the costs for that type of patient would certainly be advantageous in the negotiating process. Often product-line calculations include nursing costs simply as part of the overall per diem cost. The organization can have much better information about different types of patients if it relies on nurse costing approaches, discussed earlier in this chapter.

Direct Care Hours

Product-line information can be used not only for negotiations but also for budgeting. The direct care hours approach to product-line budgeting consists of dividing the patients for a given nursing unit into product lines, determining the number of hours of care required for each product line, and aggregating that information to find the total hours of care needed in the budget. This is a straightforward approach to using product-line information to improve budgeting capability. It represents an alternative to using acuity-adjusted patient days for determining nurse staff requirements (as will be discussed in Chapter 13).

In this approach, the first step is to separate all patients for a unit into specific groups. These groups, or product lines, could—but do not have to—conform to DRGs. The next step is to determine how many patients are expected in the coming period in each group. That information can be generated using the forecasting techniques discussed in Chapter 21. Using historical information, forecasting can also be used to predict the average length of stay of the patients in each group.

After the manager has predictions of the number of patient days in each group and the average length of stay, these two numbers can be multiplied to determine the total number of patient days expected in each product line. The number of patient days can be multiplied by the expected average direct care hours per patient day (HPPD) for patients in the product line to generate the total hours of direct care needed for each specific product line. The total direct care hours for each product line can then be aggregated to determine the total direct care hours needed for the unit for the coming year. Based on that information, the unit's budget for staff can be prepared. Table 9–5 presents a simplistic example of this process. In this example, sufficient staff must be budgeted to provide 24,300 direct care hours. The benefit of this process is that it has the potential to accurately provide information on the resources needed by the unit.

The major difficulty with this process is the determination of an accurate measure of average direct care HPPD by product line. If that information is inaccurate, the resulting total direct

---

[9]Disease management is defined as a system of coordinated health care interventions, communications, and services for populations with specific conditions in which patients' self-care efforts are significant. Retrieved August 14, 2011, at http://www.carecontinuum.org/dm_definition.asp.

✳ TABLE 9–5 *Product-Line Budgeting for Direct Care Hours*

	Forecast Volume of Patients	×	Forecast Average Length of Stay	=	Expected Patient Days	×	Expected Hours per Patient Day	=	Total Hours of Direct Care
Product line 1	200		3		600		5		3,000
Product line 2	50		5		250		6		1,500
Product line 3	100		4		400		3		1,200
Product line 4	300		7		2,100		6		12,600
Product line 5	500		3		1,500		4		6,000
									24,300

care hours needed will be inaccurate as well. Planning the budget based on a forecast of the number of patients in each product line may help the manager.

An alternative approach is to determine the total number of days at each patient classification level for all patients in each product line. Using information from the patient classification system, the nursing staff requirements for that product line can be determined. If this is done for all product lines, the total nursing requirements can be determined.

Standard Costs

Most industrial organizations establish standard costs against which performance can be measured. Standard costs represent expectations of what it should cost to produce a good or service, usually on a per-unit basis. They are targets, often established based on industrial engineering studies of the resources that should be consumed in the production of the good or service. Standard costing breaks the costs of each product down into its parts. These include direct and indirect costs, divided into their fixed and variable cost components.

It is important to isolate fixed and variable costs in standard costing so that the information can be used for decision making. By dividing costs in this manner, the manager can determine the likely change in costs resulting from changes in the number of patients treated. Historically, HCOs have not done much standard costing because providers have considered each patient to be unique, requiring a somewhat customized treatment.

A number of benefits could be realized from the use of standard costs, however. They present a basis for comparing actual results with a predetermined standard. They can be used when making decisions about contracts with insurers, expanding or contracting services, and revising the way services are offered in other areas. Even though patients are unique, there are standard approaches for most patients with specific problems. Those approaches can form the basis for development of standard costs.

A classic article on product-line standard costing overcomes much of the obstacle to standard costing by focusing on the idea that hospitals treat patients by providing them with a large number of intermediate products.[10] By carefully examining each department, one can make a list of the various intermediate products produced by that department. For example, a laboratory produces different types of tests.

Based on this approach, the set of intermediate products consumed by the average patient in a specific product line can be used to determine the standard costs of that product line. The set of intermediate products consumed by a patient in each product line is referred to as the standard treatment protocol (STP) for that product line.

In this system, each intermediate product line is called a service unit (SU). A chest x-ray would be one type of SU produced by the radiology department. A patient who has three chest x-rays receives three of that SU. A standard cost profile (SCP) must be established for each SU that indicates the cost of producing that SU. The profile would include direct and indirect costs and would identify fixed and variable costs.

Conceptually, this seems straightforward. The patient care provided by each department is broken down into intermediate products called SUs. The cost of each SU is determined. The average number of each SU from each department is found for each product line. Then the SUs consumed for a product line are multiplied by their cost to determine the total costs for patients in that product line.

A difficulty with this approach is determining SUs for nursing units. One could try to break down nursing care into the various specific activities and relate those to SUs. Administering a medication could be an SU. Taking a patient's vital signs could be an SU. Charting information about a patient could be an SU. With the use of hospital computer information systems, it is possible to disaggregate nursing care and assign it to patients in this manner.

An example of work in this area is the use of critical paths for a patient's hospital stay. With this approach, the standard care required for patients (usually by DRGs) is determined. During the course of the patient's stay, variances from this standard are noted. Some variances are acceptable; for example, a patient's health status changes, which is beyond the control of nursing. Other variances are not acceptable (e.g., if a patient is not ambulating because nurses did not provide care as outlined in the standard plan). With these data, it is possible to determine the ratio of outputs to inputs required (as determined by the standard) versus actual (as determined by the actual care provided). Because of the amount of data required to assess productivity in this way, successfully determining productivity for an episode of care usually requires the use of a computer.

For organizations with sufficiently sophisticated information systems in place, it is possible to determine the average

[10]Cleverley W. 1987. Product-costing for health care firms. *Health Care Manage Rev* 12(4):39–48.

number of vital signs taken for a patient in a specific product line. For most hospitals, such a detailed level of information is not currently cost-effective to collect. However, nursing SUs could be based on patient classification. Thus, a patient day at level 3 could be one SU, and a day at level 4 would be a different SU. When the STP is established, it would consider which nursing SUs are typically consumed and how many of each. The costs for those SUs could be determined by using the RVU method.

The RVU method is an ambitious approach to product costing, but it is used in more HCOs each year. It creates an ability to have very detailed information about each product line from all parts of the organization, including nursing. The management implications of such information are significant. By examining all the SUs consumed in each department, a team of clinicians might be able to find ways to more efficiently provide care. SUs with a lower SCP might be substituted for more expensive ones. Ways might be found to reduce the number of SUs in various departments. If one considers product-line costing broadly as a tool in the case management of the organization's product lines, the potential benefits of product-line standard costing are significant.

❊ NURSING INTENSITY WEIGHTS

Another approach to costing for nursing is Nursing Intensity Weights (NIWs). This approach, developed in New York State, was established as a way of accounting for patients' needs in the costing of nursing care. This approach allocates nursing costs to patients based on NIW scores. NIWs were developed by a panel of nurses using the Delphi technique (see Chapter 21) to score the amount of nursing care needed by patients in each DRG for each day of their hospital stay. The NIWs take into account five scoring dimensions: assessment, teaching, emotional support, medical, and physical assistance.

Nursing Intensity Weights are used in New York to determine the nursing care costs of different patients, separating those costs out from the per diem charges. A problem with NIWs, however, is that NIWs are not necessarily the same at all hospitals. To use NIWs to find costs at a given hospital, it would require the laborious process of having nursing staff establish weighted scores along the five dimensions for each day of a "typical" patient's hospital stay in each DRG. This is a very time-consuming process.

Another problem with NIWs is that, as originally developed, they do not take into account indirect nursing costs. That is, they account for the time nurses spend with patients. They do not, however, specifically take into account the time the nurse spends with family and physicians, the time preparing for patient discharge, record keeping time, and so on. That does not mean those costs are not included in the NIW costs. They are. However, they are included by being averaged in, in direct proportion to how direct time is spent. That might not be very accurate. It is possible that a patient might have less direct care needs but would still use as much indirect nursing time as a more acute patient who has greater direct care needs. NIWs could be established with separate computations of the direct and indirect nursing care needs. However, that would make the approach even more time-consuming. And when all is said and done, the results are based on the opinion (expert opinion, but still opinion) of a panel of nurses rather than on a more rigorous collection of actual cost data. As one study noted, "the future of NIWs is in doubt,"[11] and alternative approaches for determining patients' needs for nursing care, and, in turn, costing nursing services, are needed.

❊ ACTIVITY-BASED COSTING

Activity-based costing (ABC) is a relatively new approach to determining costs. The approach is based on the observation that costs are incurred because of specific activities. In most costing methods, costs are assigned to cost centers and patients based on some measure of volume, such as patient days or visits or hours. For example, OR costs are assigned to patients based on minutes in the OR. From an ABC perspective, it is not necessarily the amount of time but the specific activities that generate costs. Based on this notion, managers need to focus on the actions that drive costs higher. The activities of an organization that cause it to incur costs are referred to as *cost drivers*.

The use of cost drivers to assign costs has the effect of improving accuracy by focusing cost measurement more on a cause-and-effect basis. For example, suppose an HCO purchasing department orders many items on a routine basis and some items on a special order basis. The activity is placing orders. However, it is quite possible that a special order will be more costly than a routine order.

Purchasing departments are non-revenue cost centers. Their costs must be allocated to patients for the organization to recover its full costs. One common approach to such allocation is based on the number of purchase orders. Departments that generate a lot of purchase orders are assigned a greater share of the cost of the purchasing department. In turn, those costs are allocated to patients who use the department. This seems quite reasonable.

However, if a rush order is an activity that causes purchasing to spend extra money (e.g., time of the personnel in the department, express freight costs), then from an ABC perspective, one would argue that the departments that generate a large number of rush orders should be charged more than departments that do not, other things being equal. In other words, costs should not be assigned simply based on the number of purchase orders generated by each department. For the purchasing department, the activity of placing a rush order is more costly than the activity of placing a regular order. Rush orders drive costs higher.

The ABC approach requires the manager to analyze the activities of each cost center or department in an organization. The various activities that are cost drivers must be identified. Then costs can be assigned to departments and ultimately to patients based on the amount of the cost-driving activities they require.

---

[11] Mark BA, Harless DW. 2011. Adjusting for patient acuity in measurement of nurse staffing. *Nurs Res* 60(2):107-114.

For example, suppose that an OR has traditionally assigned its costs based on minutes of surgery. A patient with a 2-hour surgery is charged twice as much as a patient with a 1-hour surgery. However, one of the costs of surgery is cleaning and preparing the room after every surgery. Suppose that those costs are the same for each surgery regardless of the length of the surgery. The activity of cleaning and preparing the room should then be charged equally to each surgical patient.

This probably means that more allocation bases will be needed. The depreciation cost of the surgical suite may be charged to patients based on the length of the procedure. The cost of cleaning the room may be charged equally per patient. The cost of supplies consumed during the surgery should include the extra cost of any rush orders that were required for the procedure. This will complicate the costing process but will produce substantially more accurate information. ABC proponents argue that most industries really do not have a good sense of which of their products or services are profitable and which lose money. Furthermore, employees may be more cost conscious if they use ABC information.

Consider the purchasing department and OR examples just described. Surgical patients who require special order items are subsidized under the old costing system because costs of the rush orders are spread out over all departments that order supplies. This could cause a particular type of surgery to appear more profitable than it is because the true costs of the rush orders are not assigned to the departments and patients that caused the special orders.

However, after the ABC system is in place, that will change. The OR will be charged directly for each special order. It can then assign the cost of the rush order to specific patients who required the rush-ordered items. This in turn will provide more accurate information about the cost of care for each type of patient. Furthermore, seeing the higher costs resulting from rush orders, the manager of the OR may plan more carefully, avoiding the need for many of the rush orders. This will reduce the total costs for the patient, department, and organization.

In terms of routine medical or surgical nursing, using ABC requires an examination of what nurses do and why they do it. ABC works well with the concept of value-added costs. By examining everything we do to try to determine the cost drivers, we can also assess whether each activity adds value to the patient. If it does not, perhaps it can be eliminated. If it does add value, the cost of the activity should be assigned to the patient who directly benefits from it.

One problem with ABC is deciding how minutely to define activities. Is taking a pulse or blood pressure an activity? Certainly. However, should we determine the cost of that activity and track how many times it is done for each patient? This is not an easy question. From a clinical perspective, we already track such activities in the patient chart. However, until costing and clinical systems are fully linked, it would require additional data input to track the activity for costing purposes. And what about activities that are necessary but that are never entered in the clinical chart? With ABC, as with any approach to costing, we must always balance the value of more accurate information against the extra cost of collecting that information.

✳ SETTING PRICES

Nurse managers and executives today are becoming more directly involved in the revenue process of HCOs. It is no longer sufficient to simply control costs. For HCOs to prosper, their managers must have an understanding of the processes by which they receive their revenues. Rate setting is the element of financial management that focuses on setting the prices the organization charges for the services it provides.

Historically, rate setting has been outside the control of HCOs. The federal government sets hospital DRG rates for Medicare patients. In addition, many other rates of HCOs are mandated by governmental bodies, such as state-controlled Medicaid rates. With the proliferation of managed care, this process is changing. As Medicare and Medicaid recipients enroll in managed care organizations, hospital, home health care, and ambulatory care rates are being determined more and more on the basis of negotiation. Nevertheless, the process of developing a *charge master*—that is, a list of the organization's prices for each of its services—remains a critical element of the management process. Some patients still pay the prices set by the provider. And many negotiated rates are set as a percent of the organization's prices as listed in its charge master list.

Total Financial Requirements

Health care organizations strive to obtain the financial resources needed to meet their *total financial requirements* (TFRs). These requirements are the financial resources needed to meet the health care needs of the population served by the organization. Clearly, the financial requirements of any organization include sufficient money to cover the current costs of operations. On a broader perspective, however, the financial needs of the organization encompass the ability to replace facilities as they become obsolete and to adopt new technologies as they become available.

The total financial requirements of HCOs have been defined to include five categories[12]:
1. Costs of doing business
2. Costs of staying in business
3. Costs of changing business
4. Returns to capital sources
5. Costs of uncertainty

The *costs of doing business* are the routine operating costs of the organization, including salaries and expenses. If the organization provides education or research, it must recover enough to pay for those services in addition to patient care. If some payers pay less than the full costs generated on their behalf, other payers must be charged more if the organization is to recover the full costs of doing business.

The *costs of staying in business* are the financial resources all organizations need to operate, to replace assets, and to acquire new technologies. Most patients do not pay for their care until after they are discharged. However, the organization must

---

[12]Zelman W, McCue M, Glick N. 2009. *Financial Management of Health Care Organizations: An Introduction to Fundamental Tools, Concepts and Applications*, Hoboken NJ: Jossey-Bass.

acquire supplies before the patient arrives and must pay salaries concurrent with the patient stay. To stay in business, the organization must therefore have a reserve of cash available to tide itself over until revenues are received.

The *costs of changing business* are those expenditures that are required when organizations make modifications to existing services or add new services. Health care services do not remain stagnant over time. As the practice of nursing and medicine changes, HCOs must be flexible enough to delete outmoded services and to add new ones.

Returns to capital sources are the resources needed to repay those who provide the organization with the basic resources to be in business. This includes the money needed to establish the organization, as well as additional monies to allow the organization to acquire buildings and equipment over time. Some of this money is borrowed. In that case, return on capital refers to interest on the loan, as well as repaying the principal of the loan. For-profit entities have owners who have invested money. A return to those owners is generally in the form of dividends. In some cases, the organization is either community owned or voluntary, and its original resources came from tax dollars, philanthropic sources, or both. In such cases, the return on capital may come in the form of subsidized health care services for indigent patients.

The *costs of uncertainty* refer to the unexpected and unplanned expenses that organizations may incur simply as a result of being in business. These include the impact of adverse legal decisions, political decisions, regulatory changes, and similar occurrences.

A stable entity must set rates in such a manner that all these financial requirements are considered. Some payers (e.g., Medicare) can dictate their prices to the organization. The rates the organization charges the remaining payers must be adequate so that in total the organization has the financial resources it needs. This means that if the organization loses money on Medicare patients, it must attempt to charge a higher price to non-Medicare patients to offset the loss. This is sometimes referred to as a "plug-figure" approach. The organization decides the amount of revenue it needs, determines how much revenue it will receive from sources over which it has no ability to set prices, and then plugs in the charges for the remaining patients to achieve the desired revenue.

Unfortunately, this may require the organization to charge a high price for its services. Charging a high price is likely to result in increased bad debts as prices become higher than patients can afford. Increased bad debts mean that charges to the remaining payers must be even higher to offset that loss. This can create a vicious circle, with the organization unable to collect enough to remain financially viable.

Rate-Setting Approaches

There are three approaches typically used for rate-setting in health care: cost-based prices, negotiated prices, and market prices.[13]

_____
[13] *Ibid.*

Cost-Based Prices

Cost-based reimbursement generally relies on the traditional cost-finding analysis, discussed earlier in this chapter. Often cost-based payers, such as Medicaid, dictate that they will pay the lower of cost or charges. If for some reason the organization were to set its charges less than its costs, payers would reimburse the lower amount.

The cost-based approach requires knowledge of the cost of treating each patient. If one is to reimburse the organization for the cost of treating the patient, one must know that cost. However, rather than actually trying to capture the cost of treating any one patient, cost-based payers generally use what is known as the ratio of charges to charges applied to costs, often referred to as the *ratio of cost to charges* (RCC). In this approach, it is assumed that a given payer's costs and charges in any revenue center will be approximately the same. Thus, if 30% of all surgical charges are for Medicaid patients, Medicaid is responsible for 30% of all OR costs. That 30% can be applied to the total OR revenue center costs to determine the amount Medicaid must pay.

Looking at this calculation another way, suppose that the OR had total charges of $1 million and that 30% of those charges, or $300,000, were to Medicaid patients. Because Medicaid pays costs rather than charges, the costs of treating those patients must be determined. Suppose that the total costs of the OR were $800,000. Costs are 20% lower than charges (i.e., $800,000 is only 80% of $1 million). Therefore, Medicaid costs must be only 80% of the $300,000 of charges, or $240,000.

Negotiated Prices

Negotiated prices or rates are common in the health care industry. Managed care organizations, insurance companies, and even large employers actively negotiate directly with hospitals and other health care providers. Generally, guaranteed patient volume is offered in exchange for discounted prices. Based on the discussions of Chapter 8, to be acceptable to an HCO, negotiated prices should at least provide a positive contribution margin to the organization.

Market Prices

The market approach is based on the concepts of supply and demand introduced in Chapter 4. This is commonly how practitioners in private practice set prices. For example, suppose a nurse practitioner (NP) sets up a private practice. The NP might charge less than other practitioners in the area and initially not make a profit. However, if volume increases, the nurse practitioner will likely begin to make a profit. With this approach, the organization can set any price it wishes. However, if the price is high enough to earn a large profit, that would encourage competitors to enter the market and underbid the organization. If the price set is too low, the organization will lose money and eventually go out of business. HCOs therefore must walk a tightrope in setting prices.

There are also times when competition may cause the organization to lower some prices and raise others in order to not be perceived as an expensive provider. For example, suppose that two hospitals in the same area offer open heart surgery;

one hospital performs 500 per year but the other performs 50 per year. The charge at the hospital with the higher volume might be significantly less than at the one with low volume because of economies of scale. The low-volume hospital has fewer patients to share the fixed costs of doing open heart surgery (e.g., the expensive equipment required). It is not unreasonable to expect that the low-volume hospital will lower its charges to match the competition even if this means that it is charging less than cost.

How will the low-volume hospital survive in that case? It would probably raise charges on a low-cost high-volume item for all patients. For example, it might add a charge of $1 per test for all lab tests done for all patients to offset the reduced charge to open heart surgery patients for their surgery. In this way, it would avoid the possibility of being labeled as very expensive for a high-visibility program such as open heart surgery. If a policymaker questioned the wisdom of allowing a low-volume open heart surgery program to exist, the hospital could counter that it is so efficient that its charges are no higher than those of the high-volume program.

Major payers are aware of such influences on hospital rate setting. That is why cost-based payers often mandate that they pay only the lesser of cost or charges. This allows them to take advantage of competitive situations that result in prices below cost.

Rate setting is a critical area of health care management. Managers must take into account their total financial requirements, the patient mix by type of patient, and the patient mix by type of payer. Balancing these factors is often essential to organizational viability. It is particularly important for nurses in private practice.

✳ FINANCIAL REIMBURSEMENT FOR NURSING SERVICES

Despite the limitations of costing systems, great progress has been made in costing-out nursing services. It is now possible to recognize different nursing costs for different patients. That means that it is feasible for nursing to become a revenue center that charges directly for its services. The ability to recognize different consumption of resources by different patients and to charge accordingly is the essential ingredient for a revenue center. Establishment of nursing as a revenue center is feasible as long as different patient classification levels can be assigned different costs.

Clearly, nurses who work in home health are in a revenue center. Nurses in private practice, whether alone or in a group with physician providers, are revenue generators.

If an organization's patients are all fixed-fee patients, revenue centers make little sense. For example, a fixed DRG payment to a hospital will not vary if nursing, lab, or radiology varies its charges. If all patients were paid on a DRG basis, eventually there would be no revenue centers.

However, at present, most HCOs still have some patients who pay charges. Therefore, there are potential benefits if nursing is treated as a revenue center. First, it charges patients more fairly by charging on a closer approximation of their actual consumption of resources. Second, for hospitals, it clearly segregates nursing from room and board (the proverbial "black hole" of the per diem charge!). Third, it can help to alleviate the "nursing as a burden" misconception.

As HCOs find an ever-increasing need to manage themselves in a businesslike manner, a clearer understanding of both revenues and expenses will be required. The movement toward recasting the nursing function as a revenue center in hospitals can help in that evolution. Separate costing for different types of patients allows for *variable billing*—that is, the amount billed to each patient per patient day or per visit varies. Instead of simply charging all patients the same amount per day or per visit for nursing care, different patients are charged different amounts based on their differing resource consumption. After the different costs of caring for different patients are known, they can be charged accordingly. For example, in ambulatory care, it is common to charge more for a new patient visit than for a follow-up visit.

Variable billing may be a way to better justify hospital bills and in some cases increase overall revenues to the hospital. Variable billing may be beneficial to nursing because it dramatically shows the specific contribution that nursing makes to the overall revenue structure of the hospital.

Home health agencies generally charge on a per-visit basis, although nurse managers recognize that different patients require different amounts of care. For example, the diabetic patient who requires a glucose check and an insulin injection requires much less care (and time) than the HIV-infected patient who has opportunistic infections. Most managers assume that the variations will balance out. For each visit requiring a substantial amount of time, there will be an "in-and-out" visit to offset it. This approach was adequate in the past when most nurses were paid on a salaried basis. As more and more home health agencies are paying nurses on a per-visit basis, this approach may no longer prove workable. Billing may move to a variable basis depending on nursing resources consumed.

Pay for Performance (P4P)

Pay-for-performance (P4P) was introduced in Chapter 2 but has particular relevance to nursing cost and reimbursement issues. P4P is a method whereby payers reimburse providers for services delivered based on the provider's performance on certain quality of care outcome measures. P4P has the ability to transform the way in which care is delivered, the incentives inherent in our system of financing health care providers, and the way in which care is paid for. In the future, it very well may be that provider payments are differentiated based solely on performance.

Several quality initiatives are underway at the Centers for Medicare and Medicaid Services (CMS) to improve the care of Medicare patients, including the Nursing Home Quality Initiative (implemented in 2002), Home Health Quality Initiative (implemented in 2003), Hospital Quality Initiative (implemented in 2003), Physician Focused Quality Initiative (implemented in 2004), End Stage Renal Disease Quality Initiative (implemented in 2004), and Physician Voluntary Reporting Program (initiated in 2006). In all cases, data on evidence-based quality measures are gathered for reporting purposes and in some cases for payment purposes. These measures generally reflect the outcomes that result from the "process" aspects of quality (i.e., whether certain standard and recommended processes or treatments were carried out, whether they were done appropriately, and whether they were done in a timely fashion). Hospital Compare[14] provides information to consumers about hospital performance on 20 quality improvement measures, which allows them to compare the outcomes that are a function of processes carried out at different hospitals.

These quality initiatives have made HCOs rethink and in some cases redesign internal care processes. Because P4P measures are tied to payment, there is increasing pressure on hospitals to be efficient and effective in care delivery, to maximize revenues, and to reconsider how money is allocated internally. As hospitals and other HCOs simultaneously face declining reimbursements and increasing performance pressures, nursing may come under increasing pressure to improve performance, increase productivity, and even "do more with less." Under such financial pressures, it would not be unlike hospitals to consider cutting, or to actually cut, nursing staff to reduce costs; historically, this has happened because nurses are the largest professional group and represent the largest labor cost in most hospitals and are thus perceived as costly.

However, cutting nurse staffing today comes at a price. For example, evidence indicates that nurse staffing cuts that occurred in the 1990s adversely affected patient outcomes.[15] The question this raises is, given this evidence, how will hospitals choose to align their processes? Will they focus on costs exclusively, or will they strive to balance quality and costs?

Needleman and colleagues[16] declared an "unequivocal" business case for increasing nurse staffing. The business case indicates that under certain staffing scenarios, hospitals could reduce net costs by increasing RN staffing. Although not included in their analysis, increasing nurse staffing could also bring about cost savings that result from increased nurses' job satisfaction, decreased nursing turnover, and decreased turnover costs. The social case for increasing nurse staffing is the benefits that accrue to society resulting from improvements in quality—that is, decreased lengths of stay, adverse events, in-hospital deaths, and hospital readmissions.

The recognition of nurses' role in preventing health care–acquired conditions, the impact of nursing care on the financial bottom line of HCOs, and the P4P environment provides an opportunity for nursing to make great strides in this area. One report went so far as to say that nurses may become the new "rainmakers" in HCOs:

Employment changes and pay-for-performance reimbursement may combine to flip the workforce dynamic in hospitals. Traditionally, physicians were rainmakers who brought in revenue, and nurses were overhead. Through new, pay-for-performance programs that focus on clinical quality and patient satisfaction, nurses will have significant impact on the key metrics that will drive reimbursement updates.[17]

Although current P4P initiatives address important process aspects of health care quality, they still do not capture core processes related to nurses' work.[18] Some aspects of nurses' work that are critical to patient care quality, such as pain management and diabetes care management, are clearly overlooked.[19] Because these important aspects of nursing care are omitted from current performance measures, hospitals are not compelled to invest in routinely gathering data on and tracking these outcomes and in turn may not put efforts toward improving the quality of care in these areas.

It is ironic that the work of the largest group of health professionals has been overlooked in many of the CMS' P4P measures. However, identifying evidence-based measures that reflect nurses' work is difficult. Even the National Quality Forum's evidence-based nursing-sensitive performance measures (discussed in Chapter 5) do not reflect the complexity and reality of nurses' work. Until such evidence-based measures are available, hospitals will be challenged to adequately improve their processes that depend on nurses.[20]

Just as CMS links hospital payment to their performance, so too can hospitals and HCOs link nurses' payment to their performance. For organizational employees, incentives to improve performance may be directed toward groups (i.e., the organization or the work units) or to individual nurses and tied to performance evaluation. Similarly, incentives for nurse managers and executives may be linked to unit or departmental performance on measures such as patient satisfaction or staff nurse turnover. Concern has been expressed that these incentives may put financial gains above quality of care. Nurse managers and executives should be aware of the potential legal and ethical conflicts that may be associated with this practice and advocate for the use of financial performance incentives that do not compromise professional integrity and public trust.

✳ IMPLICATIONS FOR NURSE MANAGERS AND EXECUTIVES

Nurses who oversee nursing services have a responsibility to not only the units, departments and staff they manage but also

[14] Available at http://www.hospitalcompare.hhs.gov/hospital/home2.asp.

[15] Lankshear A, Sheldon T, Maynard A. 2005. Nurse staffing and health outcomes: A systematic review of the international research. *Adv Nurs Sci* 28(2):163-174.

[16] See, for example, Needleman J, Buerhaus P, Stewart M, et al. 2006. Nurse staffing in hospitals: Is there a business case for quality? *Health Aff* 25(1): 204-211.

[17] PricewaterhouseCoopers Health Research Institute. 2007. *What Works: Healing the Healthcare Staffing Shortage*. Retrieved at http://www.pwc.com/us/en/healthcare/publications/what-works-healing-the-healthcare-staffing-shortage.jhtml.

[18] Needleman J. May 12, 2006. Nursing and pay for performance. Presentation at the Alliance for Health Care Reform. Webcast retrieved July 12, 2006, at http://www.allhealth.org/briefing_detail.asp?bi=78.

[19] *Ibid.*

[20] *Ibid.*

a broader responsibility to the organization. It is imperative for nurse managers to understand the organization's perspective on cost finding and rate setting. This issue is particularly important for nurses in private practice.

Nurse managers and executives need to be aware that not all accounting methods and procedures will always be correct or appropriate. By understanding how the organization conducts its cost accounting, nurse managers and executives can identify situations in which the accounting data are inadequate for their needs. Perhaps all supplies are charged to the nursing department when paid for rather than when consumed. Although that would have little impact on the external reporting of costs, it makes monthly evaluation of performance difficult. Are the right amounts of supplies being used for the number of patients actually being cared for? That question cannot be answered without cost information related to monthly consumption of resources. Information about the amount paid in a given month for supplies is insufficient information for the nurse manager.

After such problems are identified, the organization's financial managers must be informed of the inadequacy of the existing information. Nurse managers and executives and financial managers can then work together to generate and use relevant information to improve the organization's overall management capabilities and results.

Nurse managers and executives cannot lose sight of the fact that a great deal of the organization's revenues depend on following the cost-finding requirements of external payers and providing them with external reports. The reasons for the cost-finding techniques should be understood lest they be condemned for their lack of perfection. At the same time, recognition of their limitations makes clear the need for the nursing profession to step forward and develop better approaches for costing out nursing services.

This need is made more critical by the introduction of fixed-payment systems such as DRGs, by capitation payments, and by insurer-negotiated rates for episodes of care or bundled payments. Prospective payment and P4P reimbursement makes knowledge about the cost of treating different types of patients essential. Improved costing of nursing services is a vital step toward getting a more accurate cost for each of the organization's product lines.

Whether this will in turn lead to variable billing for nursing services in hospitals on a universal basis is still unclear. Accurate costing information for nursing does, however, remove the roadblocks to variable billing.

Improving ways of costing of nursing services has become important to nurse managers and executives for several reasons. First, improved cost information can be used to better understand the contribution that nursing makes to the organization as a whole. Second, the information generated by improved costing can be used to help managers and executives make effective decisions and better control the costs of providing nursing services. Third, it can help to better understand and highlight the nursing resources needed by patients. Fourth, costing information is useful for examining changes in the way nursing care is provided. For example, the cost impact of various skill mixes on inpatient units or in ambulatory care centers can be examined, as well as the implications of making changes to skill mix. Finally, improved cost information can help nurse managers and executives understand the financial implications of errors and adverse events, including health care–acquired conditions.

The most accurate costing system requires continuous observation of all nurses by data collectors to derive detailed cost information. The cost of such highly accurate microcosting is prohibitive. However, one can think of a continuum of costing methods. In general, less expensive methods provide less accurate data; more expensive methods provide more accurate data.

Fully integrated information systems are used in many hospitals, and over time, software programs have been developed and perfected to make using these systems more efficient and effective. Many organizations are experimenting with various software programs to integrate clinical and financial systems. As the saying goes, however, "if it wasn't documented, it wasn't done." Nursing documentation systems are essential if we are to recognize and better understand nursing contributions to patient episodes of care and in turn capture and adequately measure nursing productivity. In the meantime, ABC and patient classification systems can be used to substantially improve the assignment of nursing costs to patients in an economical way.

Costing out nursing services is an extremely useful tool for product-line costing and budgeting. Information about product-line costs can show management where profits are being made and where losses are accruing. Product-line information can aid managers substantially in understanding which patients place the greatest burden on the unit and in helping the organization make appropriate decisions regarding changes in its patient mix.

The move to P4P system is changing the dynamics of care delivery, reimbursement, and resource allocation within HCOs. Unfortunately, the work of nurses is not adequately captured in current P4P measures. Leadership is needed from nurse managers to bring to light the importance of measuring and capturing the work of nurses and to work with researchers to develop such measures. Until evidence about the work of nurses is established, HCOs may miss important opportunities to improve certain internal processes that rely on the largest group of health professionals.

✳ KEY CONCEPTS

Cost information for reporting versus for management   Managers must be careful to use information appropriate to their needs. Cost information generated for external reports may provide managers with information that will lead to poor managerial decisions.

Traditional cost finding   Allocating the direct costs of non-revenue centers to other non-revenue centers and to revenue centers with the goal of ultimately allocating all of the organization's costs to its revenue centers. The total direct and indirect costs of the revenue centers are then allocated to units of service. Revenue centers are cost centers that charge for their services. To be a revenue center, the cost center must be able to distinguish the different amount of resources consumed by different patients. The steps in cost finding are:

1. Accumulation of direct costs for each cost center: Costs directly incurred within the cost center.
2. Determine basis for allocation: Costs must be allocated on some measurement basis such as pounds or square feet.
3. Allocate to revenue centers: The step-down method is widely used to assign non-revenue center costs to revenue centers.
4. Allocate revenue center costs to units of service: Using the weighted procedure, hourly rate, surcharge, and per diem methods.

Costing out nursing services   Process of determining the cost of providing nursing care for different patients. This cost has traditionally been included in the room-and-board charge.

Prospective payment   Patients are classified into a variety of categories. The health organization is paid a predetermined amount for patients in these various categories. The payment is not based on the amount of resources a patient uses.

Patient classification system   Scheme for grouping patients into categories. Each category contains patients who require similar amounts of nursing care. Some systems are commercially available; others are developed by individual HCOs.

Acuity   How acutely ill patients are. Usually used in conjunction with the nursing resources required to care for patients. The higher the acuity, generally the more resources needed for care.

Variable billing   Amount billed to each patient reflects the amount of resources consumed by that patient. Rather than billing a patient for a patient day of care, patients are billed an amount based on the nursing care hours and supplies actually used.

Inputs   Resources required to produce outputs. In nursing, inputs usually include personnel, supplies, and equipment necessary to care for clients.

Outputs   Products produced by nursing. Traditionally, these are identified as patient days of care, visits, and episodes of care. More recently, outputs are being defined as patient outcomes such as health or wellness.

Microcosting   The process of developing a detailed list of costs associated with each aspect of a patient's care that is attributed to nursing.

Product-line costing   Determination of the cost of providing care to specific types of patients. This approach is sometimes aided by the use of standard cost techniques such as Cleverley's model of STPs.

Activity-based costing (ABC)   An approach to costing based on cost drivers and measurement of the cost of activities rather than the cost of patients.

Rate setting   Process of assigning prices to the units of service of the revenue centers. Prices must be set high enough to recover the organization's total financial requirements.

✳ SUGGESTED READINGS

Aiken L, Clarke S, Sloane D, et al: Hospital nurse staffing and patient mortality, nurse burnout, and job dissatisfaction, *JAMA* 288:1987–1993, 2002.

Aiken L, Smith H, Lake E: Lower Medicare mortality among a set of hospitals known for good nursing care, *Med Care* 32:771–787, 1994.

Alvare C: Setting fees for service: are the dilemmas more acute for nurses? *Clin Nurse Spec* 10(6):309, 1996.

American Nurses Association: *Implementing nursing's report card: a study of RN staffing, length of stay, and patient outcomes*, Washington, DC, 1997, American Nurses Publishing.

American Nurses Association: *Nurse staffing and patient outcomes in the inpatient hospital setting*, Washington, DC, 2000, American Nurses Publishing.

Birmingham SE: Evidence-based staffing: the next step, *Nurse Leader* 8(3):24–26, 35, 2010.

Brannon R: Restructuring hospital nursing, *Int J Health Serv* 26(4):643–654, 1996.

Bruttomesso K: Variable hospital accounting practices: are they fair for the nursing department? *J Nurs Adm* 25(1):6, 1995.

Case J, Mowry M, Welebob E: The nursing shortage: can technology help? *California Healthcare Association* (website), 2002. www.chcf.org/documents/hospitals/NursingShortageTechnology.pdf.

Chiang B: Estimating nursing costs—a methodological review, *Int J Nurs Stud* 46:716–722, 2009.

Cho S, Ketefian S, Barkauskas V, Smith D: The effects of nurse staffing on adverse events, morbidity, mortality, and medical costs, *Nurs Res* 52:71–79, 2003.

Clements FM, Ghali WA, Donaldson C, Manns BJ: The impact of using different costing methods on the results of an economic evaluation of cardiac care: microcosting vs. gross-costing approaches, *Health Econ* 18:377–388, 2009.

Cleverley W: *Essentials of health care finance*, ed 5, Boston, 2002, Jones & Bartlett.

Crockett M, DiBlasi M, Flaherty P, Sampson K: Activity-based resource allocation: a system for predicting nursing costs, *Rehab Nurs* 22(6):293–298, 302, 1997.

Dietz D: The financial impact of resource-based relative value scale on US-based community health centers, *Res Healthc Financ Manage* 10(1):1–11, 2005.

Eastaugh S: *Health care finance and economics*, Boston, 2003, Jones & Bartlett.

Edwardson S, Nardone P: Resource use in home care agencies, *Appl Nurs Res* 4(1):25–30, 1991.

Finkler S: Costing out nursing services, *Hosp Cost Manage Account* 1(12):1–5, 1990.

Finkler S: The distinction between cost and charges, *Ann Intern Med* 96(1):102–109, 1982.

Finkler S, McHugh M: *Budgeting concepts for nurse managers*, ed 4, Philadelphia, 2007, WB Saunders.

Finkler S, Ward D, Baker J: *Essentials of cost accounting for health care organizations*, ed 3, Boston, 2006, Jones & Bartlett.

Forthman M: Episode treatment groups (ETGs): a patient classification system for measuring outcomes performance by episode of illness, *Top Health Inform Manage* 21(2):51–61, 2000.

Gardner K, Tobin J, Kamm J, Allhusen J: Determining the cost of care through clinical pathways, *Nurs Econ* 15(4):213–217, 1997.

Gold M, Siegel J, Russell L, Weinstein M: *Cost-effectiveness in health and medicine*, New York, 1996, Oxford University Press.

Green J. Metwalli A: The impact of activity based cost accounting on health care capital investment decisions, *J Health Care Financ* 28(2):50–64, 2001.

Hall L, Doran D, Baker G, et al: Nurse staffing models as predictors of patient outcomes, *Med Care* 41(9):1096–1109, 2003.

Hansen D, Mowen M: *Cost management: accounting and control*, ed 5, Cincinnati, 2005, South-Western Publishing.

Hendrickson G, Doddato T, Kovner C: How do nurses spend their time? *J Nurs Adm* 20(3):31–37, 1990.

Horngren C, Datar S, Foster G: *Cost accounting: a managerial emphasis*, ed 12, Upper Saddle River, NJ, 2005, Prentice Hall.

Iowa Intervention Project: Determining cost of nursing interventions: a beginning, *Nurs Econ* 19(4):146–160, 2001.

Jegers M: Cost accounting in ICUs: beneficial for management and research, *Clin Ther* 19(3):570–581, 1997.

Jones K: Standard cost accounting, *Semin Nurse Manage* 3(3):111–112, 1995.

Kovner C: Measuring indirect nursing costs, *Hosp Cost Account Advis* 1(3):6–7, 1989.

Kovner C: Public health nursing costs in home care, *Pub Health Nurs* 6(1):3–7, 1989.

Kovner C, Gergen P: Nurse staffing levels and adverse events following surgery in US hospitals, *Image J Nurs Sch* 30(31):5–21, 1998.

Kovner C, Jones C, Zahn C, et al: Nurse staffing and post surgical adverse events: an analysis of administrative data from a sample of U.S. hospitals, 1990–1996, *Health Serv Res* 37(3):611–629, 2002.

Lankshear A, Sheldon T, Maynard A: Nurse staffing and health outcomes: a systematic review of the international research, *Adv Nurs Sci* 28(2):163–174, 2005.

Lee R: Process-based costing, *J Nurs Care Qual* 18(4):259–66, 2003.

Leister J: Comparison of cost accounting methods from different DRG systems and their effect on health care quality, *Health Pol* 74(1):46–55, 2005.

Lichtig L, Knauf R, Milholland D: Some impacts of nursing on acute care hospital outcomes, *J Nurs Adm* 29:25–33, 1999.

Malloch K: Patient classification systems, part 1: the third generation, *J Nurs Adm* 29(7/8):49–56, 1999.

Mark B, Harless D, McCue M, Xu Y: A longitudinal examination of hospital registered nurse staffing and quality of care, *Health Serv Res* 39:279–301, 2004.

Mark BA, Harless DW: Adjusting for patient acuity in measurement of nurse staffing, *Nurs Res* 60(2):107–114, 2011.

Matthews C: Using linear programming to minimize the cost of nursing personnel, *J Health Care Fin* 32(1):37–49, 2005.

McLean R: *Financial management in health care organizations*, ed 2, Albany, NY, 2002, Delmar.

Moss J, Saba V: Costing nursing care: using the clinical care classification system to value nursing intervention in an acute care setting, *Comput Inform Nurs* 29(8):455–460, 2011.

National Quality Forum: *National voluntary consensus standards for nursing-sensitive care: an initial performance measure set. A consensus report*, Washington, DC, 2004, National Quality Forum.

Needleman J, Buerhaus P, Mattke S, et al: Nurse-staffing levels and the quality of care in hospitals, *N Engl J Med* 346:1715–1722, 2002.

Needleman J, Buerhaus P, Stewart M, et al: Nurse staffing in hospitals: is there a business case for quality? *Health Aff* 25(1):204–211, 2006.

Neumann B, Clement J, Cooper J: *Financial management: concepts and applications for health care organizations*, ed 4, Dubuque, Iowa, 1999, Kendall/Hunt Publishing.

Nyman J, Connor R: Do case-mix adjusted nursing home reimbursements actually reflect costs? Minnesota's experience, *J Health Econ* 13(2):145–162, 1994.

Pilette P: Presenteeism in nursing: a clear and present danger to productivity, *J Nurs Adm* 35 (6):300–303, 2005.

PricewaterhouseCoopers Health Research Institute: *What works: healing the healthcare staffing shortage* (website), 2007. www.pwc.com/us/en/healthcare/publications/what-works-healing-the-healthcare-staffing-shortage.jhtml.

Ross T: Analyzing health care operations using ABC, *J Health Care Fin* 30(3):1–20, 2004.

Rothberg M, Abraham I, Lindenauer P, Rose D: Improving nurse-to-patient staffing ratios as a cost-effective safety intervention, *Med Care* 43(8):785–791, 2005.

Saba V: Clinical care costing method for the clinical care classification system, *Int J Nurs Terminol Classif* 15(3):69–77, 2004.

Seago J: A comparison of two patient classification instruments in an acute care hospital, *J Nurs Adm* 32(5):243–249, 2002.

Spetz J: The cost and cost-effectiveness of nursing services in health care, *Nurs Outlook* 53(6):305–309, 2005.

Stone P: Economic evaluations and usefulness of standardized nursing terminologies, *Int J Nurs Terminol Classif* 15(4):101–113, 2004.

Turisco F, Rhoads J: Equipped for efficiency: improving nursing care through technology, *California Healthcare Foundation* (website), 2008. www.chcf.org/~/media/MEDIA%20LIBRARY%20Files/PDF/E/PDF%20 EquippedForEfficiency.pdf.

Unruh L: Licensed nurse staffing and adverse events in hospitals, *Med Care* 41:142–152, 2003.

Van Sylck A: Patient classification systems: not a proxy for nurses' "busyness," *Nurs Adm Q* 24(4):60–65, 2000.

Vincent D, Oakley D, Pohl J, Walker D: Survival of nurse-managed centers: the importance of cost analysis, *Outcomes Manage Nurs Pract* 4(3):124–128, 2000.

Welton J, Fischer M, Degrace S, Zone-Smith L: Nursing intensity billing, *J Nurs Adm* 36(4):181–188, 2006.

Welton J, Halloran E: Nursing diagnoses, diagnosis-related group, and hospital outcomes, *J Nurs Adm* 35(12):541–549, 2005.

Welton J, Meyer A, Mandelkehr L, et al: Outcomes of and resource consumption by high-cost patients in the intensive care unit, *Am J Crit Care* 11(5):467–473, 2002.

Welton J, Zone-Smith L, Bandyopadhyay D: Estimating nursing intensity and direct cost using the nurse-patient assignment, *J Nurs Adm* 39:276–284, 2009.

West D, Hicks L, Balas E, West T: Profitable capitation requires accurate costing, *Nurs Econ* 14(3):150, 162–170, 1996.

Zelman W, McCue M, Glick N: *Financial management of health care organizations: an introduction to fundamental tools, concepts and applications,* ed 3, Hoboken, NJ, 2009, Jossey-Bass.

Costs and Other Issues Related to Recruiting and Retaining Staff

CHAPTER GOALS

The goals of this chapter are to:

- Describe the relationship between the availability of nursing staff and budgeting
- Explain how to plan for variations in the availability of nursing staff
- Discuss retention as a strategy to maintain cost-effective nursing staff

- Analyze the costs of retention programs
- Discuss recruitment as a strategy to maintain cost-effective nursing staff
- Identify alternative solutions for care delivery to consider when nursing staff is in short supply

✳ INTRODUCTION

The largest part of most operating budgets for nursing departments and organizations consists of *personnel costs*. Justifying the need for a given level of staff requires careful calculations and a lucid argument. However, in the preparation of an operating budget, it is often assumed that hiring the amount of labor approved in the final budget is not a problem. That is not necessarily the case in nursing. Nursing shortages have occurred cyclically throughout the 20th century and into the 21st century. Sometimes the shortages are nationwide; other times only certain geographic areas are affected. Sometimes the shortages reach across all types of nurses and nursing positions; other times only certain segments of the nursing workforce are affected. To staff adequately in the face of a shortage increases the costs of recruiting and retaining nurses substantially. Even when there is no shortage, these costs are significant; during a shortage, staffing costs can be higher yet.

Recruitment of staff is a critical element in the overall management process. If positions are left unstaffed throughout the year, two potentially serious consequences could occur. First, remaining nurses working on a unit could begin to experience burnout from being overburdened. Shortages of staff lead to overwork, poor morale, increased sick leave, and other stress-related problems. This in turn tends to lead to staff turnover, which exacerbates the shortage on the unit. When this happens, additional turnover may occur as nurses who remain on the unit become overburdened and disillusioned because they lose their friends and social network. It becomes a self-fulfilling prophecy

of sorts, whereby a shortage brings about turnover, which intensifies the shortage.[1]

The second consequence is that the health care organization (HCO) may see less money being spent on nursing personnel than it has budgeted, and it may approve and budget for positions with the expectation that they will never be filled or that the funds will be used elsewhere in the organization. In that case, if nursing personnel becomes available to be hired, the organization may resist filling the positions because it has made its overall plans with the expectation that the money allocated for those positions would never be spent or it is unwilling to raise wages enough to attract available nurses. Although approved but vacant positions provide top management with a cushion to ease the impact of other unexpected financial demands throughout the year, these positions may be lost permanently. This could effectively lower the nursing care hours per patient day on a permanent basis.

The effects of these two consequences on the quality of patient care and on staff satisfaction are almost never examined and are rarely considered. However, their existence stresses the importance of attempting to understand and explicitly measure the costs of staff recruitment and retention.

Furthermore, an attempt must be made to make financial and budgeting decisions based on the expected *actual* staffing pattern. If 12 full-time equivalent (FTE) positions are authorized in a budget, the dollars in the budget should be based on the best expectation of how those 12 FTE positions will be staffed. Suppose that because of recruitment difficulties, the

---

[1]Jones C. 2004. The costs of nursing turnover, part 1: An economic perspective. *J Nurs Adm* 34(12):562-570.

unit will have 11 FTE positions filled with regular full-time employees and the 12th position filled with overtime or agency staff. In that case, the excess cost of overtime or an agency nurse, compared with a full-time employee, is a cost related to retention and recruitment.

Another approach to the problem of retention and recruitment of nursing staff has been to revise the manner in which nursing care was offered to use fewer professional staff. For example, in the past, nursing units have been reorganized to make greater use of alternative types of workers, such as unlicensed personnel. Information systems have been acquired with the expectation that the number of nursing hours needed for documentation would be reduced (this has not always proved to be the case). However, these changes and their costs are related to retention and recruitment, because they represent money spent to achieve and maintain an appropriate staffing level.

This chapter focuses on the actions that nurse managers and executives can take and issues they should be aware of in the management of nurse recruitment and retention efforts. When shortages occur, a given organization may be relatively helpless when it comes to overcoming the entire national or regional shortage in the supply of nurses. However, organizations have a great degree of control over recruitment and retention for their own organizations, and some organizations do exceptionally well attracting and retaining nurses. The recruitment and retention of nursing staff are important ongoing management concerns regardless of whether there is a shortage.

✳ RETAINING STAFF

Although some degree of *turnover* will keep an organization "healthy" by bringing "new blood" into the organization, the most effective personnel strategy an HCO can take is to minimize turnover by retaining its existing staff. An organization may not want to retain all staff. However, because some level of turnover will always exist in most HCOs, the overall goals should be to decrease undesired turnover and to keep turnover rates low. It is often the case that every nurse hired must be "hired away" from another organization or recruited from the pool of nonworking nurses. Therefore, recruiting nurses may be costly, especially under highly competitive market conditions. Major efforts should be made to reduce turnover. Both individual characteristics and organizational factors are postulated to be related to nurse *retention*. One key to staff retention is to have a high level of nurse satisfaction.

Nurse Satisfaction

Many factors are relevant to keeping nurses satisfied in their jobs. Studies have not shown any one consistent factor or any unique set of factors that are always present in satisfied staffs, and which, if absent, will necessarily lead to dissatisfied staff. Nevertheless, a number of elements are generally accepted as being related to nursing satisfaction. These elements are discussed next.

One primary element of nursing satisfaction is the development of professionalism in the delivery of health care services through a combination of increased autonomy and the availability of resource personnel for consultation. Nurses must feel like professionals and be treated like professionals to be satisfied in their employment. Time cards, for example, often thought to be demeaning for nurses, may contribute to nurses' dissatisfaction. Similarly, working as hourly workers does not generally result in the same level of satisfaction as working as salaried employees, having input to the work schedule, and having more scheduling flexibility.

A positive attitude toward nursing and professional treatment by the physician staff and the administration can be critical factors in having a satisfied staff. Nurses generally desire good communications and collaborative relationships with physicians and other colleagues, autonomy and control over their practice, input into decision making, and respect. Negative attitudes exhibited by physicians, administrators, or others toward nurses can cause staff dissatisfaction, and these negative attitudes toward nurses perpetuate problems with the overall perception of nursing's image. Although an organization may have little control over the national image of nursing, it can work toward creating a positive image internally and a work environment that fosters respect for nurses. The way nurses are treated and the way nursing is presented to patients can make a substantial difference in the attitudes of nurses as well as the rest of the organization's staff. Image building begins with actions taken by nurses and the nursing department to create and sustain a positive image.

The issue of financial payment is, of course, relevant. From an economic standpoint, nurses' salaries reflect their value to the organization. Although some would argue that pay is not as important as other factors related to satisfaction, and it may not be in all cases, some labor market studies indicate that nurses' behavior is sensitive to wage. Nurses also report that pay is important in determining their level of satisfaction. In 2005, the American Nurses Association reported that pay was one of three areas in which nurses were least satisfied (the other two areas were decision making and tasks).[2] Other researchers have also reported that pay is an important aspect of nurse satisfaction and the work environment.[3] We know from business and economics that higher salaries and good benefits will help keep staff from looking elsewhere, as will ample opportunity for career advancement, either into management or on a clinical track.

Flexible hours have also become a key to retaining staff. A wide variety of alternative working hour arrangements have been developed by organizations attempting to recruit new nurses. These flexible arrangements must be made available to existing staff as well, or they may become dissatisfied and move to an organization that offers such hours.

From a budgeting perspective, this can become quite complex. The use of four 10-hour shifts to create a 4-day work week is not a major budgeting problem. Although it may create a complicated staffing pattern for coverage, it still results in 40 hours of pay for 40 hours of work, the same as 5 days of

---

[2]American Nurses Association. April 1, 2005. Survey of 76,000 nurses probes elements of job satisfaction. Retrieved July 25, 2006, at http://www.nursingworld.org/pressrel/2005/pr0401.htm.

[3]See, for example, Kovner et al., 2007, and 2009, cited at the end of this chapter.

8 hours each. On the other hand, innovations such as three 12-hour shifts or two 12-hour weekend shifts for 40 hours of pay can create a variety of budgeting complications. Clear decisions must be made as to how many hours equals an FTE position. (See Chapter 13 for further discussion.)

What we do know about nurse satisfaction is that it is closely related to nurse turnover and retention. In fact, nurses' satisfaction pertaining both to their work and to their profession is predictive of intent to leave.[4-6]

Fringe Benefits

Clearly, one element of nursing satisfaction is related to the organization's employee benefits, commonly referred to as *fringe benefits*. How many weeks of vacation do staff get each year? How many paid holidays are there? Is free life insurance provided to employees? These are some of the most obvious employee benefits. Some benefits are required by law. For example, the employer must pay for FICA, a tax for Social Security, which eventually will provide the employee with a Social Security pension. Most benefits, however, are voluntary or the result of labor negotiations.

Other critical benefits concern the quality of the health insurance package offered to employees. Do nurses have to contribute to the cost of their health insurance? If so, how much? Are their family members covered? If so, is there additional cost to the nurse? Are staff members subject to *coinsurance* and *deductibles* on their health insurance? Coinsurance means that the insurer bears a portion of the cost (often 70% or 80%) and the employee bears the remainder (usually 30% or 20%). A deductible means that 100% of some amount (often $1,500 or more per beneficiary per year) must be paid first by the employee before any health benefits take effect.

Most employers also offer a variety of other benefits that are somewhat less obvious and are more responsible for the term "fringe benefits," as opposed to employee benefits. For example, if the chief executive officer (CEO) belongs to a golf club and the membership is paid for by the organization, that is a fringe benefit. If the CEO drives a hospital-owned car, that is another fringe benefit.

In terms of the budget, fringe benefits represent several different types of cost. The vacation and holiday time for each employee is already built into the annual salary cost for employees. There is no need to budget for that fringe benefit

except to make sure that there is adequate staff coverage for all days off. That is accounted for by budgeting additional personnel (see Chapter 13). On the other hand, the cost of life insurance, pension payments, Social Security taxes, health insurance, child care, and other fringe benefits that require cash outlays must be budgeted for explicitly.

In most organizations, the specific costs of fringe benefits are calculated by the finance office and are assigned to departments based on salaries, usually as a percentage. For example, a nursing unit might be charged 25% or 30% for fringe benefits for every dollar of salary paid to any staff member. Certainly, not all employees have the same cost to the organization per dollar of salary. That is simply an average. Is it fair? It might well be that certain fringe benefits are worth more to some employees than others. However, over the years, it has been decided that it is not worth the effort to get a more refined measure of costs. Therefore, budgeting for fringe benefits generally requires only the addition of a set percentage (provided by the finance office) to the budgeted salary amounts.

Many organizations are now offering a *cafeteria* approach to fringe benefits. The organization determines the amount of money it will contribute to fringe benefits for each employee. After the cost of each fringe benefit has been determined, employees choose their preferences from a list of benefit options, much as food is chosen in a cafeteria. Employees' desires for fringe benefits vary. A young new graduate might not care about life insurance but might prefer a low deductible on health insurance. A young mother might prefer child care and have no need for health insurance because her spouse has family coverage from his employer. The cafeteria approach is a more flexible option that allows employees to select the benefits that best meet their needs.

Retention Programs

The problems associated with nurse turnover are significant enough to warrant specific attention and programs aimed at staff retention. This should go beyond the basic notions of having competent managers, physicians who work on a collegial professional basis with nurses, autonomy in work, and the other elements of nurse satisfaction. Such programs should work toward making the institution one that shows caring for its staff, creates a loyalty bond that is hard to break, and in turn makes the institution a place where nurses and others want to work. Some such programs involve significant financial investment; others take relatively little. Before the development of a retention program, the manager should determine the desired retention goal and the actual retention level at the organization.

Proper design of retention programs first requires an understanding of the causes of turnover in the organization, both voluntary and involuntary. *Voluntary* turnover results when an individual leaves an organization as a personal choice—that is, in search of better pay or working conditions, career advancement, or relocation for personal reason. *Involuntary* turnover occurs when the organization decides the employee should leave or as a result of reasons other than personal choice, such as dismissal, layoff, disability, or even death. Although both voluntary and involuntary turnover can

[4]See, for example the publications by the research team of Kovner and Brewer cited at the end of this chapter, specifically Kovner C, Brewer C, Wu Y, et al. 2006. Factors associated with work satisfaction of registered nurses. *J Nurs Scholarsh* 38(1):71-79; Kovner CT, Brewer CS, Fairchild S, et al. 2007. Newly licensed RNs' characteristics, work attitudes, and intentions to work. *Am J Nurs* 107(9):58-70; Kovner C, Brewer C, Green W, Fairchild S. 2009. Understanding new registered nurses intent to stay at their jobs. *Nurs Econ* 27(2):81-98; and Brewer CS, Kovner CT, Greene W, et al. 2011. Predictors of turnover in a national sample of newly licensed registered nurses employed in hospitals. *J Adv Nurs* 67(8):1-18.

[5]Leveck M, Jones C. 1996. The nursing practice environment, staff retention, and quality of care. *Res Nurs Health* 19(3):331-343.

[6]Lynn M, Redman R. 2005. Faces of the nursing shortage: Influences on staff nurses' intentions to leave their positions or nursing. *J Nurs Adm* 35(5): 264-270.

be desirable or undesirable, voluntary turnover typically is the most concerning to managers.

Some basic information is needed for the development of a retention program. First, the retention goals for an organization or unit must be determined. Most organizations would be unhappy with 100% retention. Unless the organization expands its size or the programs and services it offers, this level of retention would leave no room for new staff to be hired or for internal advancement within the organization. New staff members are desired both because they bring new ideas to an organization and because new staff nurses are generally paid a lower wage than experienced nurses. Internal advancement opportunities allow talented and motivated staff to grow professionally and advance their careers. On the other hand, most managers would agree that 70% retention is too low. Orienting 30% of the staff each year is likely to be too costly and disruptive.

Second, the historical level of retention for the unit or organization must be determined. Most nurse managers determine turnover rates. This is defined as the number of employees who leave during a period of time divided by the average number of employees employed during the same period. An overall turnover rate can be calculated for the organization, along with specific turnover rates for job groups, such as registered nurses (RNs). The converse of turnover is often considered to be retention. If 10% of the staff terminate each year, retention is considered 90%. However, this approach is flawed and tells the manager little about the retention pattern of the nursing staff.[7] Who is leaving? When do they leave? Do most people leave within the first 3 months of employment? Is there an even distribution among staff with all levels of tenure? Actual retention rates can be determined with a "life tables" approach.[8]

This approach determines actual patterns of retention by first identifying all staff and then determining how long staff stays. For example, how many of the staff members stay more than 6 months? More than 3 years? More than 10 years? If 50% of the staff members leave within the first year and fewer than 5% of those who have been there more than 5 years leave, efforts can be directed at the former group rather than at the nurses who have been at the institution for more than 5 years. It could also be that nurses who have been at the organization for more than 5 years are now leaving because the organization raised salaries of entry level staff significantly but did not do so for incumbent staff, and a competing organization instituted a policy for increases in salary for every year of experience. After determining the organization's retention goal and the historical retention rate, a retention program can be developed to target specific groups of nurses who are leaving. It is important for nurse managers to stay current on the literature because many researchers are studying nurse retention, and new findings appear in the literature frequently.

A first step in the development of a retention program is acknowledging that employees should have a way of being recognized. There should be a formal mechanism that allows a pattern of exemplary work or even one good deed to gain recognition. There are a variety of ways that employee behavior can be recognized. A common method used in almost every organization is a one-on-one performance evaluation between the staff member and manager. Managers should maintain documentation about each employee's performance for the evaluation period, and they should solicit input from others with whom the employee interacts. Such evaluations need to make clear that poor performance will not be ignored or rewarded, but the overall tenor should be a strong focus on the positive aspects of performance. This may involve recognizing good performance or offering training in areas where performance could be improved. Rather than dwelling on poor past performance, a greater amount of time should be spent on discussing ways to improve future performance.

Performance evaluation meetings are often uncomfortable for both the evaluator and the one being evaluated. However, such meetings should not be taken lightly. Managers should use these meetings as an opportunity to reinforce information provided to the employee throughout the year, rather than providing "new information." Employees should have a sense of how they are performing on an ongoing basis as managers provide feedback throughout the year on employee performance. Employees should leave the meeting with a feeling that they understand what is expected of them, that their individual efforts make a difference in the overall performance of the unit, and that their positive contributions have been noted and specifically recognized by the organization.

Another key element of performance conferences should be to elicit input. What is going on that the employee likes, and what is going on that the employee objects to? Open lines of communication—with honest follow-up on suggestions and complaints—are likely to win over support and loyalty. A refusal to budge from "the way things are" is more likely to result in resentment and, in some cases, resignations.

In addition to meetings, specific actions may warrant letters of commendation. Such letters could be the result of favorable patient comments or could be based on recommendations from other staff. Commendations should be presented in staff meetings or in appropriate ceremonies or noted in organizational newsletters or on websites so that as many people as possible are made aware of them. This provides further psychological benefit to the recipient and perhaps serves notice to other workers that it is possible they, too, can gain such recognition. Achievement of such recognition should be within the reach of most staff members. Many nurse managers and executives are also adopting the strategy of writing personal, handwritten "thank you" notes that are mailed to nurses' homes. This allows staff to share the recognition with their families and goes a long way in building employee loyalty to the organization.[9]

[7]Waldman J, Arora S. 2004. Measuring retention rather than turnover: A different and complementary HR calculus. *Human Res Plan* 27(3):6-9.

[8]For a more detailed description of this process, see *ibid.* and Benedict M, Glasser J, Lee E. 1989. Assessing hospital nursing staff retention and turnover: A life table approach. *Eval Health Prof* 12(1):73-96.

[9]Studor, 2009. Retrieved September 4, 2011, at http://www.studergroup.com/tools/thank_younotes/ThePowerofThankYouNotes.pdf.

In providing motivation, the carrot or the stick can be used. Some schools of thought argue that the stick is more appropriate than the carrot. Poor performance is unacceptable, and that fact should be conveyed to workers. Other schools of thought argue that in the long run the carrot will have more positive results. Emphasizing the positive and deemphasizing the negative results in a happier and psychologically healthier work environment. In reality, a combination of the carrot and the stick is probably optimal. Employees who perform at a high level need reinforcement and encouragement so that their behaviors continue. Employees who perform at an average level of performance need to be encouraged and mentored so that their performance improves. Employees who perform at a low level need to be counseled so that they have clear parameters about how to improve their performance and they are held accountable for sub-par performance. By failing to address poor performers, a negative work environment can be created by an apparent tolerance for this kind of behavior; moderate performers may be encouraged to behave similarly, but high performers may get frustrated and leave.[10]

Another aspect of retention involves financial remuneration. Money is not a solution to all problems. Studies have shown that aspects of the work environment and working conditions (e.g., having adequate numbers of staff, nursing management support, respect, and input into decision making) are as, if not more, important to nurses than salary.[11] On the other hand, salaries, bonuses, and benefits are a reflection of the value placed on an employee by the organization and may be central to keeping good employees on staff if other aspects of the work environment (e.g., relationships with physicians and colleagues, advancement opportunities, career development) do not promote satisfaction. The reality is that financial compensation through competitive wages is necessary but not sufficient for nurse retention. Although money is not the solution to all problems, financial incentives have become a major competitive factor, requiring that nursing departments and HCOs offer competitive salaries as one aspect of their overall nurse retention program.

Higher wages are one type of financial incentive, but organizations are often reluctant to offer these because they can be a very costly long-term obligation. A recent report suggests that the average labor cost for RNs is about $45 per hour, which includes the cost of wages, insurance, recruiting, and nonproductive nursing costs. Of this amount, slightly more than three-quarters of this amount is nurses' wages.[12] Other types of financial incentives can be achieved without substantially higher cost to the institution. For example, it may be less expensive to pay nurses an annual salary than an hourly wage. This approach may also make nurses feel better about themselves and their institutions. Another financial approach is the use of bonuses. Bonuses generally are paid only out of cost savings. Thus, the institution can afford to pay for them because the payment is only part of a larger amount that would otherwise have been spent anyway. Bonuses had little use just a few decades ago but are becoming more and more widespread with the pay-for-performance movement (see Chapters 2 and 9).

Innovative employee benefits are another area that can be used to help retain nurses. For example, child-care centers at the HCO (perhaps with discounted or subsidized rates) can help in employee retention. In addition, such centers have the capacity to reduce sick leave substantially. Much sick leave is the result of a nurse's staying home to take care of a sick child. Therefore, sick leave can be reduced if the child-care center has facilities for mildly ill children.

These approaches to retention are already in the nursing and business literature. However, to be truly competitive, an organization must be innovative. For example, the implementation of self-scheduling on a unit and the use of a computerized nurse scheduling system are ways to better accommodate nurses' scheduling requests, give them more control and flexibility in their schedules, enhance communication and interaction among staff, and in turn retain nurses.[13] Also, strategies that empower nurses and foster a sense of family and community rather than strictly a workplace environment are likely to be viewed positively by nurses. For example, some nursing departments, patient care units, and service lines in HCOs are using social networking sites to stay connected. Nurses are likely to stay at an organization if they have a sense of family and if they have friends and network ties in the organization.

Having access to the supplies, equipment, and supports that nurses need to do their jobs is also important in retaining them. There is nothing that frustrates nurses more than not having access to the basic equipment they need to do their jobs—intravenous pumps, blood pressure monitors, and other equipment needed to deliver safe and timely care is essential. Other support services are also important in helping nurses do their jobs, such as lift teams to help move patients with limited mobility, intravenous infusion teams to start and help care for patient vascular access devices, and transportation services to take patients for prescribed therapies and treatments. These support services are critical to help nurses deliver the complex level of care required by patients today.

All of these issues can be boiled down to nine very basic nurse retention principles proposed by Runy.[14] These principles are grounded on nurses' desire for a safe, professional work environment that promotes quality of care:

1. Promote respectful collegial communication and behavior.
2. Create a communication-rich culture.
3. Create a culture of accountability.
4. Provide adequate numbers of qualified nurses.

[10]Studor, 2009. Retrieved September 4, 2011, at http://www.studergroup.com/dotCMS/knowledgeAssetDetail? inode5106533.

[11]See, for example, Groff Paris L, Terhaar M. December 7, 2010. Using Maslow's pyramid and the National Database of Nursing Quality Indicators™ to attain a healthier work environment. *Online J Issues Nurs* 16(1); Morgan J, Lynn M. 2009. Satisfaction in nursing in the context of shortage. *J Nurs Manag* 17(3):401-410; and Lynn M, Redman R. 2006. Staff nurses and their solutions to the shortage. *West J Nurs Res* 28(6):678-693.

[12]KPMG. 2011. *KPMG's 2011 U.S. Hospital Nursing Labor Costs Study.* Retrieved at http://kpmghealthcarepharmainstitute.com.

[13]Bailyn L, Collins R, Song Y. 2007. Self-scheduling for hospital nurses: an attempt and its difficulties. *J Nurs Manag* 15(1):72–77.

[14]Runy L. 2006. Nurse retention: An executive's guide to keeping one of your hospital's most valuable resources. *Hosp Health Netw* 80(1):53-57.

✳ **TABLE 10–1** *Managing the Multigenerational Nursing Workforce*

	Veterans	Baby Boomers	Generation Xers	Millennials
Recruitment	■ Like part-time work, shorter shifts, special projects ■ Bring experience ■ Hold "traditional" views about work ■ Seek good health benefits	■ Acknowledge experience and achievements ■ Like a challenge ■ Emphasize growth opportunities ■ Tend to like shorter shifts	■ Emphasize technology ■ Seek schedule flexibility ■ Like longer shifts, more time off	■ Emphasize flexibility, growth opportunities ■ Emphasize opportunity to take time off
Assimilating and integrating into the organization	■ Need time to learn the organization and the organization's story ■ Want to see how they fit in, contribute ■ Like to mentor others	■ Share strategy ■ Make linkages to budget ■ Emphasize relationships	■ Reinforce work–life balance ■ Train as future mentors	■ Promote equity ■ Provide support, mentors ■ Promote teamwork
Retention	■ Provide physical supports ■ Likely to remain unless the job does not fit	■ Reward with verbal recognition or salary increase, bonus ■ Involve in decision making ■ Prefer job stability but will change job for advancement	■ Provide work–life balance ■ Reward is time off ■ Provide skill development, promotion opportunities ■ View job change as necessity	■ Reward with competitive pay, benefits ■ Like to collaborate with others ■ View job change as expected

Adapted from Manion J: *Managing the multi-generational nursing workforce: managerial and policy implications*, Geneva, 2009, International Centre for Human Resources in Nursing, International Council of Nursing.

5. Make available expert, competent, credible, and visible leadership.
6. Share decision making at all levels.
7. Encourage professional practice and continued growth and development.
8. Recognize the value of nursing's contribution.
9. Recognize nurses for their meaningful contribution to the practice.

The provision of necessary supplies and equipment to care for patients is an important item to add to this list.

Nurse managers and executives are critical to nurse retention. As Hendren noted, "The old refrain says that employees don't leave organizations, they leave managers."[15] This is true especially in nursing, where nurse managers have been linked to nurse satisfaction and retention (Anthony et al., 2005; Leveck and Jones, 1996).

Managers are also in the best position to know what retains, satisfies, and motivates each employee and how they need to modify their approaches for different individuals. Although all nurses want a supportive work environment, an issue that managers need to be aware of is the generational differences that exist among nurses in practice today. Manion (2009) identifies four different generations of nurses in the nursing workforce: Veterans (born between 1922 and 1945), Baby Boomers (born between 1946 and 1964), Generation X (also called Gen-Xers, born between 1965 and 1979), and Millennials or Generation Y (born between 1980 and 2000). Nurses representing these four

different generations have different values, personal desires, and drives. For example, a Generation X nurse may not be motivated in the same way as a nurse from the Baby Boomer generation. Whereas Gen-Xers typically desire a schedule where they work longer shifts and spend fewer days at work, Baby Boomer nurses prefer to work shorter shifts and spread their time across a greater number of days.[16] Thus, the same retention efforts likely will not work for both groups. Table 10–1 outlines information managers need to know to manage a multigenerational workforce. Retention plans must be flexible and reflect the needs and wants of employees,[17] and managers must appreciate that a "one size fits all" approach will not always work.[18]

Clinical Ladders

A frequent complaint of staff nurses is that there is little room for advancement within the clinical ranks. Nurses can go into management. However, if they choose to pursue a clinical career by maintaining direct patient contact, there is little difference in reward for a nurse with 30 years of experience compared with one with 5 years. The concept of clinical ladders is one approach for overcoming this deterrent to nurse retention.

---

[15]Retrieved September 5, 2011, at http://www.healthleadersmedia.com/page-3/NRS-268201/5-Ways-to-Retain-New-Graduate-Nurses.

[16]Green J. 2005. What nurses want. Different generations. Different expectations. *Hosp Health Netw* 79(3):34-8, 40-2, 2. Retrieved September 5, 2011, at http://www.hhnmag.com/hhnmag_app/jsp/articledisplay.jsp?dcrpath=HHNMAG/PubsNewsArticle/data/0503HHN_FEA_CoverStory&domain=HHNMAG.

[17]*Ibid.*

[18]Swearingen S, Liberman A. 2004. Nursing generations: An expanded look at the emergence of conflict and its resolution. *Health Care Manag* 23(1):54-64.

There are a wide variety of clinical ladder models and different types of organizations that use them. Because career advancement is a feature in Magnet facilities, clinical ladders are often present in them. However, they are also common in non-Magnet facilities that seek to retain nurses through advancement at the bedside. Some clinical ladders are completely distinct from administrative career paths. Others integrate administrative duties into the clinical ladder. Also, some clinical ladders require on-the-job experience for moving up the ladder, but others require additional education, including advanced degrees. In some models, moving up the ladder requires community service, professional service, and/or publication. Another distinction among models is the amount of additional responsibility that must be assumed as one moves up the ladder.

There is a widespread belief that clinical ladders do improve nurse retention. Although there are obvious costs to the development and implementation of a clinical ladder program, such an approach improves the professional identity of the nurse, generates loyalty, and decreases turnover and its associated costs.[19] Advancement on the clinical ladder may also be associated with salary increases, with, for example, nurses earning 5% more per hour when they move to level 2, 7.5% when they move to level 3, and 10% more or higher when they advance to the highest rungs on the ladder. Thus, if nurses at higher levels on the clinical ladder in a given institution earn substantially more than those at lower levels in the organization, it makes it less likely that a nurse will leave, because it means giving up salary. It also becomes expensive if they have to give up seniority when they change employers. If that is the case, retention of the more experienced, expensive personnel becomes easier, but higher turnover rates may occur among nurses at the lower, less expensive rungs of the ladder. Over time, an organization could have a large proportion of its staff near the higher compensation end of the ladder. This makes it important for managers to pay attention to the distribution of nurses on the ladder and to develop a clinical ladder and retention plan that also recognizes the advancement needs of new or more inexperienced nurses.[20]

Why Nurses Leave

Nurses change jobs for a variety of reasons. Some of the reasons can be addressed by the organization; other reasons may not be as amenable to organizational intervention. It is critical, however, for nurse managers and executives to understand the various reasons that nurses might leave and to work toward creating an environment that addresses factors the organization can affect. As noted earlier, nurses' perceptions of job satisfaction, autonomy and control over practice decisions, the work environment, manager support, the technologies and support services available to them, career advancement opportunities, and salary and benefits offered by the organization are all factors that can influence nurses' decisions to leave. Many other organizational factors have also been reported to impact

nurse turnover such as short staffing, high workloads, the use of agency staff, long or inflexible work hours (e.g., mandatory versus voluntary overtime, lack of input into scheduling decisions), the type and structure of the unit, the cohesiveness of the patient care team, relationships with physicians and other health professionals, and the ability to deliver quality nursing care.[21]

Personal factors such as age, education, gender, nurses' attitudes about their work (including their intentions about leaving and their perceptions of burnout, job stress, or organizational commitment), their moral beliefs, their personal health, and their family situation can also influence nurses' decisions to change jobs. Although there may be little the nurse manager or executive can do about some personal factors (e.g., a nurse's family situation), others, such as age, can be addressed by targeting specific strategies to older or younger nurses. For example, an ergonomically friendly work environment might encourage older nurses to remain in the workforce, and working fewer hours might be of interest to younger nurses. The important point is that nurse managers and executives must be aware of the myriad of reasons nurses might leave, put strategies in place to address the factors that can be addressed, and plan for the financial costs of retaining nurses or the consequences of nurse turnover when it does occur.

Determining the Cost

What does it cost to retain staff? As with any decision in a health organization, the cost-benefit ratio of a retention program should be estimated in advance and evaluated after the program has been implemented. Having accurate data on current retention patterns and knowing the organization's goals provide the first step in determining the costs of the program. Although it is often difficult to associate a particular program with overall retention, some estimates can be made. If a new program such as free parking is instituted, its cost can easily be determined. Often, however, new programs have several goals and potential benefits. For example, a handheld computer system for home visits may be intended to attract and retain nurses who want to work in a "high-tech" environment where electronic charting may be easier. However, the computer system is also expected to improve the quality of patient care and to decrease the time nurses spend on documentation. Other programs aimed at improving retention may have additional benefits as well. Shared governance may be instituted to improve retention, and it may also improve patient care. Increasing salaries may retain staff in the short run, but as soon as the competitor across town increases its salaries, the benefits of such a program may disappear.

Determining the costs of turnover and therefore the benefits of decreasing turnover is somewhat more straightforward. The costs of turnover do not include just the costs of advertising for staff and the nurse recruiter's salary; they also include costs incurred by an organization before and after turnover. For example, turnover costs include productivity losses that

[19]Drenkard K, Swartwout E. 2005. Effectiveness of a clinical ladder program. *J Nurs Adm* 35(11):502-506.
    [20]*Ibid.*

    [21]See the work of Kovner and Brewer noted earlier; Lynn and Redman, 2005; and Strachota et al, 2003.

occur before and after turnover occurs, because the remaining unit staff may have to pick up the slack in staffing. A detailed study of nurse turnover costs identified costs associated with nurse turnover in the following areas.[22]

- Advertising and recruiting (e.g., interviewing prospective candidates, recruiter travel, and placing advertisements)
- Vacancy costs (e.g., agency nurses, overtime, and lost profits from closed beds while positions are vacant)
- Hiring costs (e.g., moving costs, signing bonuses, and administrative processing)
- Orientation and training (e.g., staff costs and materials used to familiarize new RNs with organizational policies and procedures)
- Newly hired RN productivity (productivity losses incurred during the learning period)
- Pre-turnover productivity (decreased productivity that may precede turnover)
- Termination costs

Using this method, the mean cost per RN turnover has been estimated to range from $62,000 for experienced and $67,000 for new graduates or even as high as $80,000 or more.[23] Brewer and colleagues[24] estimated that newly licensed RN turnover cost the U.S. health care system between $1.4 and $2 billion in 2006 alone.

Blaufuss and colleagues[25] present an alternative approach to evaluating turnover costs in response to a specific incentive. They do not include general advertising and recruiting costs in their calculations because, they argue, hospitals must advertise regardless of turnover rates, because there will naturally be some turnover in all organizations. They include interviewing, preparing for orientation, the orientation itself, and a learning period. Using a zero-base approach, they identify the individual cost of hiring each new staff member. In addition, they include estimated revenue enhancements as an offset to the recruiting cost. This is particularly important when increases in staff can lead to providing more home health care visits or in some other way to increasing the number of patients for whom nurses provide care. Essentially, if one looks at the cost of attracting new staff, the extra revenue the organization will earn if it has those new staff members must also be considered.

Others have estimated the mean cost per RN turnover to range from about $21,000 to $64,000.[26] Because it may not be

feasible to calculate the cost of RN turnover on an ongoing basis, managers can use "rules of thumb" to estimate the cost of nursing turnover. These rules of thumb range between 0.75 times salary (for hourly employees) to 2.0 times salary (for salaried employees).[27] It has been estimated that RN turnover costs are about 1.2 to 1.3 times the average RN annual salary.[28] Although these rules of thumb provide gross estimates of turnover costs, they can be useful to managers for estimating a "back of the envelope" cost of RN turnover.

The recruitment and replacement of nursing staff is inherently costly. Costs related to the retention or replacement of nursing personnel should be budgeted. The average duration of the vacancies should be anticipated, and the extra cost of overtime and agency nurses should be included in the coming year's operating budget. Newly hired employees are often less productive than experienced staff. This may require extra hours of nursing care per patient day, which may come in the form of overtime or hiring temporary staff. Sufficient nursing care hours should be budgeted to cover the time period while newly hired staff are being oriented and less productive than other staff. If relocation costs are charged directly to the unit, those costs should be included in the budget as well. Also, it is common for organizations to pay hiring bonuses of $10,000 or more to attract new nurses, especially for positions that are difficult to fill. Depending on the number of new nurses hired, the cost of paying bonuses could become quite high. Efforts should be made to anticipate turnover and its costs to adequately capture for those expenditures in the budgeting process.

✳ RECRUITING STAFF

No matter how effectively an organization works to retain its existing staff, some turnover must be expected. Some staff members will retire; others will move to another HCO or a different part of the country. Some replacement of staff will always be occurring. Concurrent with the nursing department's setting retention goals and working toward achieving them, there should be a *recruitment plan*. Recruitment is an ongoing process, not something that is done just at a time of staff shortage. Although recruitment strategies may change from shortage to shortage, successful organizations continually work to keep recruitment at the forefront of human resource planning.

Identifying the existing level of recruitment is the first step in developing a recruitment strategy. What are the current recruitment numbers? Are these acceptable to meet current organization needs? Are any changes in the organization (e.g., addition of a new unit) anticipated that will require changes in that level or an improvement in retention because of new initiatives in the organization?

[22]Jones C. 2005. The costs of nursing turnover, part 2: Application of the Nursing Turnover Cost Calculation Methodology. *J Nurs Adm* 35(1):41-49 and Jones C. 2008. Revisiting nurse turnover costs: Adjusting for inflation. *J Nurs Adm* 38(1):11-18.

[23]*Ibid.*

[24]Brewer et al., 2011.

[25]Blaufuss J, Maynard J, Schollars G. 1992. Methods of evaluating turnover costs. *Nurs Manage* 23(5):52-61.

[26]See, for example, Advisory Board Company. 1999. A misplaced focus: reexamining the recruiting/retention trade-off. *Nurs Watch* 11:1-14; O'Brien-Pallas L, Griffin P, Shamian J, et al. 2006. The impact of nurse turnover on patient, nurse and system outcomes: A pilot study and focus for a multicenter international study. *Policy Polit Nurs Pract* 7(3):169-179; Robert Wood Johnson Foundation. 2006. *Wisdom at Work: The Importance of the Older and Experienced Nurse in the Workplace.* Retrieved September 5, 2011, at http://www.rwjf.org/files/publications/other/wisdomatwork.pdf; and Waldman J, Kelly F, Sanjeev A, Smith HL. 2004. The shocking cost of turnover in health care. *Health Care Manage Rev* 29(1):2-7.

[27]See, for example, McConnell C. 1999. Staff turnover: occasional friend, frequent foe, and continuing frustration. *Health Care Manage* 18:1-13; and VHA, Inc. 2002. *The Business Case for Workforce Stability.* Retrieved November 26, 2006, at http://www.healthleadersmedia.com/pdf/white_papers/wp_vha_120103.pdf.

[28]Jones, *Op. cit.*, 2005.

The second step is to assess the external environment. What changes are occurring that will affect the level of recruiting? Is the market experiencing a shortage of nurses in general or of certain nurse specialties? Are nursing school enrollments increasing, making recruitment easier, or decreasing, making nurse recruitment highly competitive? Are current market conditions likely to continue? What specific factors in the environment may affect the organization's ability to recruit nurses? Have there been new hospitals or HCOs opened in the geographic area? Have there been salary increases at competing organizations? After assessing the external environment and determining a desired level of recruitment, managers can develop a specific nurse recruitment plan that targets organizational needs and ensures the organization's ability to deliver nursing care.

Marketing

An effective marketing strategy is a key element of recruiting nurses. As long as a limited supply of talented nurses exists, there will be a winner and a loser in the effort to recruit qualified personnel. Therefore, a plan must be developed to address the recruiting issue.

The essence of marketing is that the needs and desires of a group are determined on the basis of market research and then an effort is made to satisfy them. Notice that this definition does not revolve around advertising, which may or may not be part of a marketing effort. The first step is to find out what nurses want from their employment. Next, efforts must be made to ensure that the hospital meets those needs to the extent possible. Finally, it is necessary to be able to convey the fact that the needs have been met.

In performing market research, a decision should first be made concerning whom the organization wants to recruit. New nurses right out of school? Experienced nurses? Nurse managers? Specialists? Local nurses? Out-of-state nurses? Nurses from other countries? In trying to determine what the potential employee wants and needs, it is critically important to correctly evaluate the group that is to be the target of the marketing effort.

Because most HCOs already have some staff, the organization must have some attractive characteristics. In relative terms, all existing organizations have some strengths. Therefore, there should not be a hopeless attitude of "How can we compete with the rich research-oriented medical center in town?" Perhaps many nurses would prefer to provide care in a patient-oriented rather than research-oriented setting. It is important to identify the existing strengths of the organization so that the information can be conveyed to a target group.

At the same time, organizational weaknesses must be identified and a long-term plan designed to overcome as many of them as possible. Perhaps lack of convenient parking is the one overwhelming negative the organization has. In that case, replacing expensive advertising with a major fund-raising campaign to finance the building for an enclosed parking garage or a free and convenient park-and-ride shuttle service may be an appropriate marketing strategy. That is an example

of a one-time, expensive solution to a recruiting problem but one that helps recruitment over many years.

In other cases, solutions may be less expensive but require ongoing efforts. For example, a hospital could distinguish itself through a concerted effort to develop a system of shared governance. Such efforts are not necessarily expensive. They do, however, require tremendous internal cooperation and commitment. The potential result is that some media ads, search firm fees, and recruiter travel can be replaced with free news stories on the change at the hospital, with quotes from nurses on the benefits of shared governance. Nursing schools can be encouraged to have the organization's staff give lectures on the shared governance approach used by the organization. If the new system really provides something that nurses value, the word will eventually get out even without advertising. Advertising may be used to speed the communication process if desired.

Note, however, that marketing does not start with advertising but begins with identification of the need or desire and the filling of that need or desire. These elements must precede advertising. Only then can a specific plan be developed regarding the communication of what strengths the organization has to offer. Advertising in newspapers, on television or radio, or by direct mail is one approach to that communication. Another is college visits. Bonuses to existing employees who bring in new employees is another. Often it is this word-of-mouth approach—existing nurses telling other nurses about the organization—that is the best marketing tool for nurse recruitment.

Each of these approaches often results in inquiries by potential employees. The package of material that the organization develops to respond to those inquiries is a critical element of the overall marketing strategy. The marketing strategy should take into account all of the steps in the recruiting process. Generating inquiries without a strategy to follow up effectively is one critical mistake often made by those who view marketing only in terms of advertising. If a strategy is likely to generate inquiries, the organization should not appear unorganized or uncaring when it receives them. That is the point when the organization has the chance to reaffirm the feeling that caused the nurse to inquire about the position.

Suppose a hospital runs a newspaper ad that says, "Join the nursing staff at ABC Hospital, where nurses work in an environment of shared governance and shared commitment to the highest level of patient care." Some carefully planned literature must be available for the person who asks for more information about the shared governance program. The program's history, how it works, and the hospital's commitment should be included.

If the response to the inquiry leads to an interview, there should be some mechanism to make the interviewer aware that the candidate has inquired about the hospital's shared governance program. The interview should include at least some specific discussion that emphasizes or highlights the shared governance system, and if possible, a time should be arranged for the candidate to meet with nurses who participate on one or more shared governance councils.

Although advertising is not the first part of a marketing plan, in many instances, it is an effective mechanism for speeding the word-of-mouth process. Targeted advertising can reach a potential group of employees very effectively. This is particularly important in a competitive marketplace. If competing organizations are effectively communicating what they have to offer, your organization must be prepared to get its message to that group of potential employees as well.

One important element of advertising is that only a part of current advertising should be aimed at current recruitment. Another part, equally substantial, should be aimed at long-term image building. Often people associate with an organization because of its reputation. Such reputations are built over a period of years. They are built through an effort of getting the message out year in and year out. When there is a staffing shortage, the institution will want to advertise why it is a good place to work. It should also do so when there is no shortage of personnel. Image building is not a short-term response to shortages. By laying the groundwork over a long period, when the need for personnel occurs, the organization will have a head start over its competition.

Today, the Internet allows HCOs to market their organization and its services—including nursing—for relatively little expense. For example, a hospital that recently received Magnet recognition could acknowledge that achievement on its website. This recognition would signal nurses of the organization's commitment to attract and retain nurses and to deliver high quality of care. However, studies have reported that beyond advertising nursing employment opportunities, hospitals generally do not capitalize on using the Internet to communicate what they have to offer nurses.[29] This is an area in which nurse managers and executives should take advantage of the opportunity to collaborate with colleagues in their organization's marketing and information technology services departments to make sure that nursing information gets adequately communicated via the organization's website.

Murrow and Nowak[30] also present an interesting marketing approach to address nurse turnover. They view nurse employees as consumers of the job offerings of their employer. When viewed as such, organizations can consider the "switching costs" nurses face when they consider leaving or the value of certain aspects of their jobs (e.g., job satisfaction and personal relationships) that nurses will trade off by changing employers. Their findings support the notion that nurses are willing to change jobs even if doing so means that they incur short-term switching costs. Managers should thus devise strategies and internal programs that make switching costs high, which would serve as an impediment to nursing turnover.[31]

In keeping with a marketing perspective, organizations that adopt such an approach to nurse recruitment would identify tactics or specific actions that address the four Ps of marketing: *product, price, place,* and *promotion.* That is, the product being "sold" is vacant nursing positions and the opportunity to work in a progressive nursing department; the price is the salary offered in the market to nurses who might apply; the place is the organization and what it has to offer nurses who work there; and the promotion is how the organization goes about advertising and disseminating the product. How an organization addresses these four areas will impact its return on nurse recruitment efforts.

Recruiting and Retaining "Older" Nurses

There is no doubt: The nursing workforce is aging, along with our population. In fact, in 2008, the average age of the nursing workforce was about 47 years old, up a year from 2000 and up more than 4 years since 1996, when the average age of RNs was about 42 years.[32] Ironically, this "older" nursing workforce will be called on to care for our aging society at the same time that nurses are aging, retiring, and requiring health and nursing care themselves.

Buerhaus and colleagues[33] reported that one of the reasons for the growth in recent nursing employment was an increase in the number of nurses in the workforce who were older than the age of 50 years. In fact, their study indicated that nurses over the age of 50 years comprised about 77% of the total growth in RN employment between 2001 and 2008, the number of nurses 35 to 49 years of age declined, and the number of nurses 21 to 34 years of age increased considerably.

The growth in the number of nurses older than 50 years of age means that HCOs must be sensitive to the needs of nurses in that age group, create an environment that is known to be conducive to "older" nurses, and compete in the marketplace to recruit older nurses. Given that patients in hospitals today are generally sicker and stay in the hospital for shorter periods, the physical demands placed on nurses are great. Organizations that target the recruitment and retention of nurses older than the age of 50 years—or for nurses in any age group—need to create ergonomically safe environments with adequate staffing and technology to meet patient transport, lifting, and physical care needs. Some HCOs have also worked with older nurses to make sure they are assigned to work in more desirable environments that take advantage of their advanced skills, such as ambulatory surgery. Also, nurses of all ages are notorious for not taking breaks, and organizations are notorious for not requiring that they do so. However, managers have the ability to ensure that adequate breaks are provided so that nurses can get time off their feet and time away from the constant mental challenges of caring for patients. Buerhaus and colleagues[34] have noted that "older" nurses are

[29]Boyington A, Jones C, Wilson D. 2006. Buried alive: The presence of nursing on hospital Web sites. *Nurs Res* 55(2):103-109.

[30]Murrow J, Nowak P. 2005. What nurses want: Learn to reduce nurse turnover by using customer retention strategies. *Market Health Serv* 25(1):25-28.

[31]*Ibid.*

[32]U.S. Department of Health and Human Services. Health Resources and Services Administration. 2010. *The Registered Nurse Population: Findings from the 2008 National Sample Survey of Registered Nurses.* Retrieved September 5, 2011, at http://bhpr.hrsa.gov/healthworkforce/rnsurveys/rnsurveyfinal.pdf.

[33]Buerhaus P, Auerbach D, Staiger D. 2009. The recent surge in nurse employment: Causes and implications. *Health Aff (Millwood)* W4:657-668.

[34]Buerhaus P, Staiger D, Auerbach D. 2004. New signs of a strengthening U.S. nurse labor market? *Health Aff (Millwood)* W4:526-533.

responsive to wage increases, especially during times of economic downturns, when unemployment rates are high. Nurse managers and executives need to be aware of their market and take advantage of this opportunity to retain nurses from this age group. Nurse managers and executives should plan for the eventual retirement of this group of nurses from the nursing workforce.

Managers need to also be sensitive to the needs of recruiting and retaining nurses from different age groups and experience levels, and they need to target strategies to those groups. These two groups of nurses generally have different expectations about their work. Kovner and colleagues[35] report that older nurses have more positive perceptions of fairness in rewards, job satisfaction, organizational commitment, work group cohesion, and supervisory support than do younger RNs. Older nurses also perceived fewer organizational constraints, a lower workload, and a decreased desire to leave their jobs than younger RNs. These differences are important to consider in recruiting and retaining these two groups of nurses.

✳ USE OF ALTERNATIVE HEALTH CARE EMPLOYEES

Despite the efforts of organizations to retain nurses, nurse retention will be unable to solve all HCOs' nurse staffing needs. Recruitment more often results in nurses moving from one organization to another (particularly in local areas if recruitment is targeting experienced nurses) rather than increasing the overall supply. For example, although the rate of increase has varied, the number of nurses has increased over time and is currently at an all-time high.[36] However, nursing shortages have been predicted well into the year 2020[37] and beyond.[38] Thus, despite the best efforts to retain and recruit nurses, there will probably be some organizations with inadequate staffing. One suggested approach to solving this shortage is the use of alternative health care employees.

A variety of alternative health care employees are sometimes used. These include the following:

- **Agency nurses:** This approach is one in which organizations use nurses who are employed through a temporary or staffing agency. In this case, the RN is employed by the agency but hired under contract to the HCO. Agency nurses may also be referred to as traveling nurses or travelers if they are employed through an agency that provides staff under contract for an extended period of time (e.g., 3 or 6 months). Travelers are mobile and move around nationally and sometimes internationally to work in locations assigned by their employing agency. Agency

nurses may also be referred to as temporary or supplemental staff because they are hired on a temporary basis, or as a "supplement" to permanent staff.
- **International nurses:** This approach attempts to retain the concept of using RNs to the extent possible. In this case, nurses from another country come to the U.S. under contract to work in a HCO. This approach is one that has been used over decades to deal with national nursing shortages by looking for nurses to fill staffing needs from outside the United States.
- **Non-RNs:** This approach is one that has also been used to fill nurse staffing needs by using staff other than RNs to perform activities that in the past may have been performed by RNs.

Agency Nurses

One alternative that has been used frequently by HCOs is the hiring of agency nurses to fill vacant nursing positions. This is also a strategy that nurse managers can implement on short notice and with great flexibility. Agencies can often supply nurses with the specific training and experience that an organization needs.[39]

However, this flexibility comes with a cost—using large numbers of agency nurses or using agency nurses for long periods can be very expensive, in terms of both dollars and staff morale. One study reported that the use of agency nurses to fill vacant positions was the greatest cost of nursing turnover.[40] Also, because the organization may pay an amount for agency nurses that is two or more times the hourly rate earned by existing nursing staff, staff morale problems can occur if the situation persists. There are also concerns about differences in the quality of care provided by RNs who are employees of the organization versus those employed by agencies, yet research in this area is generally lacking. A recent study found that travel nurses experienced moderate levels of burnout and that their perceptions of job satisfaction and quality of care were higher when they worked in Magnet facilities.[41]

HCOs and managers should weigh the advantages and disadvantages of using agency nurses, especially if their use might extend for long periods. Table 10–2 outlines a just a few of these pros and cons. In some cases, it might be less expensive for an organization to use other methods to address vacancies, including paying existing staff overtime, closing beds, or diverting patients to other facilities. Agency nurses are often believed to impact morale on the unit, as well as physician

[35]Kovner CT, Brewer, CS, Cheng Y, Djukic M. 2007. Work attitudes of older RNs. *Policy Polit Nurs Pract* 8(2):107-119.

[36]U.S. Department of Health and Human Services. 2010.

[37]National Center for Workforce Analysis. April 2006. *What Is Behind HRSA's Projected Supply, Demand, and Shortage of Registered Nurses?* Health Resources and Services Administration, Department of Health and Human Services. Retrieved November 26, 2006, at http://bhpr.hrsa.gov/healthworkforce/reports/behindrnprojections/index.htm.

[38]Spetz J, Dyer J. June 2005. *Forecasts of the Registered Nurse Workforce in California*. Retrieved July 25, 2006, at http://www.futurehealth.ucsf.edu/pdf_files/forecasts2005.pdf.

[39]Aiken and colleagues (2007) examined the characteristics of agency nurses and reported that they were more likely to have a bachelor's degree, to be younger, and to be more ethnically diverse than the overall nurse population. They also reported that agency nurses were more likely to practice in intensive care units, where the nursing shortage is most severe. Thus, their use may be attractive to many organizations.

[40]Jones, 2005.

[41]Faller MS, Gates MG, Georges JM, Connelly CD. 2011. Work-related burnout, job satisfaction, intent to leave, and nurse-assessed quality of care among travel nurses. *J Nurs Adm* 41(2):71-77.

※ TABLE 10–2 *Pros and Cons of Hiring Agency Nurses*

Pros	Cons
■ Meet predictable, ongoing staffing levels (e.g., vacant positions, vacations) ■ Meet urgent or unexpected staffing needs (e.g., staff absences, sudden departure) ■ Provides flexibility in how staffing needs are met ■ Allows the organization to assess a potential future employee before committing to permanently hire ■ Save time and money ■ Obtain specialized skills for short-term projects	■ Meeting training needs ■ Decline in permanent staff morale and satisfaction ■ Concerns about safety ■ Legal concerns ■ Reliability of agency personnel ■ Increased supervision ■ Decreased productivity of permanent staff ■ Increased workload ■ Increased costs ■ Lack of commitment to organization ■ Decreased staff cohesion and teamwork

Data from Castle NG: Perceived advantages and disadvantages of using agency staff related to care in nursing homes: a conceptual model, *J Gerontol Nurs* 35(1):28–36, 2009; and Schaefer P: *The pros and cons of hiring a temp* (website), 2005. www.businessknowhow.com/manage/hire-temp.htm. Accessed September 12, 2011.

and patient satisfaction. However, when surveyed about agency nurse use, hospital executives indicated that the use of agency staff would likely increase in the future, to represent as much as 10% of a hospital's nursing workforce.[42] Given the potential impact on unit and organizational budgets, the use of agency nurses should be considered carefully, and if their use is anticipated, resources should be allocated for agency nurses in departmental budgets.

International Nurse Recruitment

Recruiting nurses from outside the United States is another approach for staffing a health care institution. During periods of nursing shortage, many HCOs rely on international nurse recruitment to fill a large gap in the numbers of nursing staff. However, this solution involves a number of difficulties ranging from regulatory to language barriers.

Another reason for the recent expansion in nursing employment has been the use of foreign-born nurses.[43] Buerhaus and colleagues[44] report that foreign-born nurses accounted for one-third of the total growth in the nursing labor market between 2001 and 2008 and represented more than 16% of the nursing workforce in 2008. Whereas foreign-born nurses have typically represented about 3,000 to 4,000 new RNs annually in

previous shortages, between 2001 and 2008, the total increase in the number of foreign-born nurses was more than 155,000. This is striking when one considers that the total increase in all RN FTE positions was 476,000!

According to preliminary findings from the National Sample Survey of Registered Nurses, about 5% of the 2008 nursing workforce was composed of foreign-trained nurses (referred to as "internationally educated nurses," or IENs), up from 3.5% of the workforce in 2004.[45] Of those foreign-trained nurses working in the United States, more than 70% were educated in either of two countries, the Philippines (50%) or Canada (12%), with the next highest numbers being trained in India (9.6%) and the United Kingdom (6%). Recruiting nurses from Canada, the United Kingdom, and other English-speaking countries is obviously advantageous to U.S. HCOs because they can minimize potential language problems. Northern states may be able to recruit in Canada relatively easily compared with other alternatives.

For recruiting outside the continent, expenses of travel and relocation can become substantial. An alternative to an organization's recruiting international nurses is to use an agency and pay a flat fee for each nurse hired. The more nurses hired, the more likely it will be cost-effective for the organization to undertake the entire recruiting project, rather than contracting with an agency.

If a strategy of international nurse recruitment is chosen, careful budgeting becomes essential. The choice for an organizations to conduct its own recruitment versus using a recruiting agency can have a dramatic financial impact. A budget allows considering the costs of each alternative. For example, suppose an agency charges 1 month's salary for recruiting an individual plus 1 month's salary for relocation expenses. It could easily cost well above $10,000 for each nurse recruited to process applications, prepare for the NCLEX exam, verify proficiency in English, and verify education.[46]

There are other recruiting costs as well. One cost of recruiting international nurses is that after they arrive in the United States, it may take additional time for them to complete requirements for practicing as an RN. This may take a few days, weeks, several months, or more. During this period, they may be paid but are not fully productive. Other costs may include providing convenient housing, helping the nurses get settled, and helping them to overcome language differences. Another cost is related to the loss of recruits between their recruitment and their arrival, because a fairly lengthy period is required to meet various visa and other requirements.

However, as Brush, Sochalski, and Berger (2004) note, the long-term costs of recruiting foreign-educated nurses may be less than nurses educated in the United States because they do not change jobs as often as U.S.-educated nurses, and the recruitment agencies tend to honor the contract if a foreign-educated nurse does not perform to expectations. It may also

---

[42]KPMG, 2011.

[43]Note that different sources report findings for "foreign-born" and "foreign-educated" (or "internationally educated") nurses. We recognize that there are actually three distinct groups of nurses: foreign-born and foreign-educated; foreign-born and U.S.-educated; and U.S.-born and foreign-educated. Specific data that allow the relative size of each group to be estimated are not available. However, most nurses recruited from foreign countries are likely to be foreign-born and foreign-educated. In this chapter, we use "international nurses" to refer to nurses who are foreign-born or foreign-educated unless specified otherwise.

[44]Buerhaus, Auerbach, and Staiger. 2009.

[45]U.S. Department of Health and Human Services. 2010.

[46]Reilly P. 2003. Importing controversy. *Mod Healthc* March:20-24.

be less costly to recruit and retain foreign-educated nurses than it might be to increase wages for nurses educated in the United States and the other economic incentives that might be needed to recruit and retain U.S.-educated nurses. They also highlight the benefits of hiring foreign-educated nurses in long-term care facilities. Because long-term care has experienced relatively severe shortages of both RNs and licensed practical nurses (LPNs), these facilities have received special legislative stipulations that have allowed them to hire foreign-educated nurses to fill vacancies.

The ability to recruit international nurses depends on certain "push" and "pull" factors. Push factors are generally a reflection of conditions in the country of origin that drive nurses to seek job opportunities elsewhere, including lack of nursing job availability, poor wages and working conditions, economic instability, and health and safety concerns.[47,48] Pull factors reflect conditions that attract nurses to the country to which they migrate, including higher wages, improved working conditions, greater opportunity for professional development, and a better lifestyle.[49,50] Together, these push and pull factors entice many international nurses to come to the United States on a temporary or permanent basis to improve their lifestyle and to earn more money than they could in their home country, often so that they can send money to support their families in their country of origin.[51]

The ability to recruit international nurses to the United States also depends on immigration laws. Immigrants who come to the United States are subject to the laws and regulations regarding the number of visas allotted for certain types of workers or to each country on an annual basis. When the quota of immigrants to the United States has been reached, no additional visas are granted. For example, between 2001 and 2004, immigration policies were tightened because of the terrorist attacks of September 11, 2001, which caused severe delays in the processing and receipt of visas for international nurses.[52] Exceptions were made in 2005 to allow additional nurses into the country, which cut the wait times (often 2 to 3 years) for getting foreign nurses into the United States.[53] However, this was an exception. International nurses attempting to come to the United States may face difficulties obtaining visas in the future, depending on the political climate.[54]

During recent years, several issues have been raised about the employment of international nurses. Recruiting international nurses, especially from countries that are unable to meet the health care needs of their people, raises ethical issues.

Although some nurses' countries of origin may have insufficient nursing jobs available, if nurses leave the country in large numbers, the country could be confronted with a nursing shortage of its own. Some international nurse recruiters have also been accused of "poaching" nurses to work in the United States and other industrialized countries from foreign countries that already have a shortage of nurses.[55] Others have recognized the "brain drain" associated with the depletion of experienced nurses from foreign countries when they relocate to the United States.[56,57] There are also reports of international nurses being placed in less desirable positions and being paid lower wages than their U.S. counterparts.

On the flipside, there are growing concerns about the technical and cultural competence of nurses who immigrate to the United States.[58] The Commission on Graduates of Foreign Nursing Schools was established to address these concerns, and this group verifies nursing educational credentials and skills as well as English language comprehension before nurse immigration. Concerns about potential differences in quality of care delivered and patient outcomes between U.S.- and foreign-educated nurses have also been raised, but lacking research in this area, there is no way of knowing if these concerns are warranted.[59]

The recruitment of international nurses into the United States is one of several short-term solutions to the address the cyclic shortages of nurses. Until such time as national and international health workforce policies are developed to guide the ethical recruitment and employment of international nurses, nurse managers and executives must be aware of the pros and cons of recruiting international nurses so they can make informed decisions when they are faced with staffing shortages. They must also create resources to support the transition of international nurses into U.S. nursing practice and help them learn our systems and cultures.

Alternative Care Givers

A drastically different approach to the use of foreign nurses is the alteration of the model of care within an HCO to assign more activities to non-RNs. Many organizations have made this shift. Although this was a movement away from all-RN staffing, it was based on recognition of the realities of nursing shortages.

Traditional alternative care givers include both licensed nursing staff, such as LPNs, and unlicensed assistive personnel (UAP) such as nurses' aides. A variety of other positions such as unit hosts or hostesses and clerks have also been developed to help organizations cope. Such a person introduces patients to the unit and responds to many of the nonclinical

[47]Aiken L, Buchan J, Sochalski J, et al. 2004. Trends in international nurse migration. *Health Aff* 23(3):69-77.

[48]Kline D. 2003. Push and pull factors in international nurse migration. *J Nurs Schol* 35(2):107-111.

[49]*Ibid.*

[50]Brush, Sochalski, Berger. 2004.

[51]Reilly. 2003.

[52]Fong T. 2005. Nurse visa crisis eases. *Mod Healthc* 35(24):28.

[53]Evans M. 2005. Easing the shortage. *Mod Healthc* 35(20):14.

[54]Evans M. 2006. Help from India Inc.: For-profit enterprises train nurses headed abroad. *Mod Healthc* 36(2):28.

[55]*Ibid.*

[56]Nullis-Kapp C. February 2005. Efforts under way to stem "brain drain" of doctors and nurses. *Bull World Health Org* 83(2). Retrieved at http://www.scielosp.org/scielo.php?pid=S0042-96862005000200004&script=sci_arttext&tlng=en.

[57]Brush et al. 2004.

[58]*Ibid.*

[59]*Ibid.*

needs and questions of patients and their families. There is little controversy about the use of alternative care givers to perform non-nursing functions such as transport and clerical activities.

There is, however, substantial controversy about using UAP to perform nursing activities. For example, the state of Ohio has approved the use of medication aides to deliver approved medications in long-term care facilities.[60] To be a medication aide, prospective applicants go through 6 weeks of training on medication administration that is approved by the Ohio Board of Nursing. In some cases, the RN is placed in a position of greater direct supervision of UAP, who provide more of the care. In other cases, "partnerships" are developed between the nurse and the UAP. In many cases, the ultimate impact of the use of UAP is less bedside time for the RN and more supervisory responsibility. The use of UAP means that RNs must have effective delegation skills to ensure safe, quality care and that RNs and UAP work together as a team.[61]

No single approach has emerged as the dominant path for providing nursing care in the future. There is little information about the costs of these alternative models. The main conflict seems to be a model that would have RNs serving as supervisors of UAP versus a model in which nursing activities are divided into an RN subset and a UAP subset. In the former, RNs have a decreasing bedside role but greater authority and responsibility for patient care. In the latter alternative, RNs may spend as much time as usual giving bedside care but perform only activities that require the clinical skills of an RN. The reality is that in many instances, RNs need staff support to provide care in today's fast-paced, complex care environments. When RNs and UAP work together as a team to deliver care, positive outcomes have been reported.[62]

❋ THE USE OF TECHNOLOGY

Changing how nursing care is provided because of a staff shortage is a less than ideal way for a profession to evolve. The changes are not the result primarily of an impetus to find better ways to give care; rather, they represent recognition of personnel availability constraints and the desire to provide care in a more cost-effective manner. If nursing shortages could be eliminated permanently, the approach to the delivery of nursing care might be substantially different. The use of computer technologies and the computerization of nursing units have been put forth as potential solutions.

Some claims have been made that as much as half of all nursing time is spent on documentation and that bedside computer terminals could save half that time. If true, as much as one-quarter of all required nursing time could be eliminated without taking any time away from nursing care provided to patients. Research suggests that nurses can spend as much as 30% more time with patients after the implementation of an electronic health record, although research findings are inconclusive.[63]

Highly touted for their timesaving potential, the financial returns to computer systems have not yet been fully realized. The *hardware* (equipment) capacity exists. Technological advances have reached a point at which terminals by each bedside are used in many hospitals. In fact, it would be surprising to see a new hospital without computer wiring to each room or wireless capabilities as part of the electrical plans. Gaining nurse acceptance for the use of unit or bedside computers has not turned out to be the problem that many predicted. On the other hand, developing the *software* (computer programs) and data integration has been a more complicated process.

Each health care institution tends to be unique in its procedures. This lack of industry standardization creates difficulties in the development of software that can be adopted by a wide range of HCOs. Furthermore, the process of recording the activities surrounding patient care and integrating patient care clinical and financial information with those activities is highly complicated.

It is likely that computer software advances will continue to evolve and that computer use by staff nurses will become common in most HCOs. In the long run, this will likely increase the quality of patient care because of more accurate and timely information while creating at least some efficiencies in the use of nursing time. Other technologies such as wireless communication devices, delivery robots, electronic workflow management systems, electronic medication administration via the use of bar coding, interactive patient systems, location systems, and electronic documentation systems with clinical decision supports hold great promise for improving the efficiency and effectiveness of nursing practice.[64] All of these technologies should release more RN time for patient care. To the extent that technologies reduce time spent on documentation relative to time spent in providing patient care, the integration of various technologies should work both to reduce nursing shortages and to increase nursing satisfaction. However, HCOs still struggle to allocate sufficient funds for information system implementation, maintenance, and upgrade—a challenge under normal conditions but a daunting task in an environment of declining reimbursements.

---

[60]See the information available at http://www.lorainccc.edu/Academic+Divisions/Allied+Health+and+Nursing/Allied+Health+and+Nursing+Programs/Medication+Aide.htm.

[61]Anthony M, Vidal K. May 31, 2010. Mindful communication: A novel approach to improving delegation and increasing patient safety. *Online J Issues Nurs* 15(2).

[62]Venturato L, Drew L. 2010. Beyond doing: Supporting clinical leadership and nursing practice in aged care through innovative models of care. *Contemp Nurse* 35(2):157-170.

[63]Banner L, Olney C. 2009. Automated clinical documentation: Does it allow nurses more time for patient care? *Comput Nurs* 27(2):75-81.

[64]Turisco F, Rhoads J. 2008. Equipped for efficiency: Improving nursing care through technology. California Healthcare Foundation. Retrieved at http://www.chcf.org/publications/2008/12/equipped-for-efficiency-improving-nursing-care-through-technology.

❋ NURSING SHORTAGES

This chapter began with a brief discussion of nursing shortages and their cyclic nature. A 2011 report indicates that the demand for RNs is up 53%.[65] However, the recent shortage of nurses is somewhat different than previous shortages, and this deserves elaboration. Aspects of the current shortage that distinguish it from previous shortages are the aging of the nursing workforce, general labor market shortages, and the global nature of the shortage.[66,67] Patient care has also changed, with patients being sicker, patients in the hospital for shorter times, and patients requiring more demanding care across a wider variety of patient care settings. The aging of the Baby Boomer generation is likely to exacerbate the shortage in the future. Technology also places demands on nurses to keep pace with rapidly changing technological advances, and although the use of technology is attractive to younger nurses, it may be a challenge for older nurses, who may find it difficult to learn new technologies. Moreover, although nursing school enrollments have increased annually since 2001, projections indicate that these increases will not meet demand for new nurses over the long run.[68]

This chapter has presented both short- and long-term strategies to address nursing shortages. Some of the short-term strategies include hiring temporary or agency staff, paying overtime to existing RN staff, closing beds, deferring patients to other providers, hiring international nurses, increasing wages and benefits, and paying bonuses.[69] Unfortunately, as Numerof and colleagues[70] note, money and benefits are important, but they may not satisfy nurses over the long run, and they may actually encourage undesirable behaviors, such as job hopping for wage increases or bonuses. That is not to say, however, that wages and benefits are not important. In fact, wages and benefits must keep pace with the market for an organization to be competitive.

Longer-term strategies to address nursing shortages are imperative. Although more difficult and probably more costly in the short run, these are needed if we are ever to get out of the cyclic shortage of nurses. Long-term strategies suggested to address nursing shortages include (1) improving the image of nurses through education and by valuing nursing contributions; (2) developing new models of nursing education and partnership to recruit and educate students in nursing; (3) focusing on retaining nurses through the use of creative scheduling, shared governance, clinical ladders, innovative models of care delivery, and other retention programs; and (4) knowing what satisfies nurses in the organization.[71] The federal government has also been actively engaged in supporting programs that encourage universities to start or expand nursing programs, to train nursing faculty, and to encourage retention in HCOs. The recent Institute of Medicine *Future of Nursing* report (discussed in earlier chapters) has recommended increasing the number of baccalaureate-prepared nurses from current levels (about 50% of the workforce) to 80% of the workforce by the year 2020, and doubling the number of nurses with doctorates to increase the number of nursing faculty. Achieving these goals means that not only must nursing be an attractive profession to enter, but there must also be enough slots in nursing programs and faculty to educate them.

Choosing between short- and long-term strategies to address the shortage is not an either–or situation. The reality is that organizations facing a shortage likely need to consider a combination of long- and short-term strategies to meet ongoing staffing needs. Some combination of these strategies will likely yield better returns over the long run than either short- or long-term solutions exclusively.

❋ IMPLICATIONS FOR NURSE MANAGERS AND EXECUTIVES

Retention and recruitment of staff are ongoing issues for organizations that employ nurses. A certain amount of turnover is expected and is in fact healthy for an organization. Historically, there have been national and local shortages of nurses. This cyclic pattern will likely continue. However, organizations should be concerned with recruitment and retention regardless of shortages.

The issue of recruiting and retaining staff members—whether RNs, LPNs, UAP, or other staff—is significant. There should be careful enumeration of all of the costs related to recruitment and retention. These include market research, consulting, advertising, travel, and relocation. They also include the costs necessary to make an organization attractive, such as training costs related to implementing a system of shared governance.

One fundamental point in this process is that for a specific organization to have an adequate staff, it must recognize a need to change over time. The environment of HCOs is in a constant state of change. Other career opportunities exist for potential staff. If a hospital job is not adequately attractive, a nurse can go into home health care or work in a physician's office. It is important to remain current in understanding what nurses desire from their employment in addition to a salary.

Successful HCOs will be aware of the desires of the nursing workforce, respond to those desires, and effectively communicate to potential employees the ways in which they meet those needs and desires. They must also become leaders in helping to change and improve the image of nursing, or face an ongoing shortage of nurses further into the future than ever imagined. Astute nurse managers and executives who understand these complex issues and how to address them will position their HCOs to become choice nursing workplaces in the future.

[65]Retrieved September 5, 2011, at http://www.wantedanalytics.com/insight/2011/06/10/nursing-shortage-continues-with-demand-for-rns-up-53-in-2011/.

[66]Nevidjon B, Erickson J. January 31, 2001. The nursing shortage: Solutions for the short and long term. *Online J Issues Nurs* 6(1):4. Retrieved at http://www.nursingworld.org/ojin/topic14/tpc14_4.htm.

[67]Lynn and Redman. 2005.

[68]American Association of Colleges of Nursing. July 2011. *Nurse Shortage*. Retrieved September 5, 2011, at http://www.aacn.nche.edu/media/factsheets/nursingshortage.htm.

[69]Jones C. 2004.

[70]Numerof R, Abrams M, Ott B. 2004. What works . . . and what doesn't? *Nurs Manage* 35(3):18.

[71]Nevidjon and Erickson. 2001.

✳ KEY CONCEPTS

Retention Continued employment of personnel. This is often measured as the converse of turnover or staff leaving an organization.

Fringe benefits Compensation in addition to wages; also called employee benefits. This usually includes such things as health insurance, life insurance, and disability insurance. Some organizations provide child care, free parking, and other benefits as a way to recruit and retain staff. Fringe benefits often cost as much as 20% to 25% of a worker's wages.

Cafeteria plan Method of providing fringe benefits in which the employee chooses from a variety of options those fringe benefits that the employee wants.

Retention programs Various approaches used by organizations to retain staff. These include clinical ladders, reorganization of the way care is provided, and a variety of compensation plans.

Clinical ladder Approach to promotion and compensation based on clinical excellence.

Recruitment Effort directed at getting potential employees to become employees. This process should be ongoing and not just developed in times of shortages of key workers.

Unlicensed assistive personnel (UAP) Employees who are less skilled than professional nurses but who may be able to assume some activities traditionally performed by RNs.

✳ SUGGESTED READINGS

Aiken L, Buchan J, Sochalski J, et al: Trends in international nurse migration, *Health Aff* 23(3):69–77, 2004.

Aiken LH, Xue Y, Clarke SP, Sloane DM: Supplemental nurse staffing in hospitals and quality of care, *J Nurs Adm* 37(7–8):335–342, 2007.

Anthony M, Vidal K: Mindful communication: a novel approach to improving delegation and increasing patient safety, *Online J Issues Nurs* 15(2), May 31, 2010.

Anthony MK, Standing TS, Glick J, et al: Leadership and nurse retention: the pivotal role of nurse managers, *J Nurs Adm* 35(3):146–155, 2005.

Bailyn L, Collins R, Song Y: Self-scheduling for hospital nurses: an attempt and its difficulties, *J Nurs Manag* 15(1):72–77, 2007.

Banner L, Olney C: Automated clinical documentation: does it allow nurses more time for patient care? *Comput Nurs* 27(2):75–81, 2009.

Blaufuss J, Maynard J, Schollars G: Methods of evaluating turnover costs, *Nurs Manage* 23(5):52–61, 1992.

Blegen M: Nurses' job satisfaction: a meta-analysis of related variables, *Nurs Res* 42(1):36–41, 1993.

Boyington A, Jones C, Wilson D: Buried alive: the presence of nursing on hospital Web sites, *Nurs Res* 55(2):103–109, 2006.

Brewer C, Kovner C, Wu Y, et al: Factors influencing female registered nurses' work behavior, *Health Serv Res* 41(3):860–886, 2006.

Brewer CS, Kovner CT: Work satisfaction among staff nurses in acute care hospitals. In Dickson GL, Flynn LR, editors: *Nursing policy research: turning evidence-based research into health policy*, New York, 2008, Springer, pp. 128–142.

Brewer CS, Kovner CT, Greene W, et al: Predictors of actual turnover in a national sample of newly licensed registered nurses employed in hospitals, *J Adv Nurs* 67(8):1–18, 2011.

Brewer CS, Kovner CT, Poornima S, et al: A comparison of second-degree baccalaureate and traditional-baccalaureate new graduate RNs: implications for the workforce, *J Prof Nurs* 25(1):5–14, 2009.

Brush B, Sochalski J, Berger A: Imported care: recruiting foreign nurses to U.S. health care facilities, *Health Aff* 23(3):78–87, 2004.

Buerhaus P, Auerbach D, Staiger D: The recent surge in nurse employment: causes and implications, *Health Aff (Millwood)* W4:657–668, 2009.

Buerhaus P, Staiger D, Auerbach D: Is the current shortage of hospital nurses ending? Emerging trends in employment and earnings of registered nurses, *Health Aff* 22(6):191–198, 2003.

Buerhaus P, Staiger D, Auerbach D: New signs of a strengthening U.S. nurse labor market? *Health Aff (Millwood)* W4:526–533, 2004.

Cangelosi J, Markham F, Bounds W: Factors related to nurse retention and turnover: an updated study, *Health Care Market Q* 15(3):25–43, 1998.

Castle NG: Perceived advantages and disadvantages of using agency staff related to care in nursing homes: a conceptual model, *J Gerontol Nurs* 35(1):28–36, 2009.

Cline D, Rosenberg M, Kovner C, Brewer C: Early career RNs' perceptions of quality care in the hospital setting, *Qual Health Res* 21(5):673–682, 2011.

Davidson H, Folcarelli P, Crawford S, et al: The effects of health care reforms on job satisfaction and voluntary turnover among hospital-based nurses, *Med Care* 35(6):634–645, 1997.

Drenkard K, Swartwout E: Effectiveness of a clinical ladder program, *J Nurs Adm* 35(11):502–506, 2005.

Ehrenberg R, Smith R: *Modern labor economics: theory and public policy*, ed 4, New York, 1991, Harper Collins.

Faller MS, Gates MG, Georges JM, Connelly CD: Work-related burnout, job satisfaction, intent to leave, and nurse-assessed quality of care among travel nurses, *J Nurs Adm* 41(2):71–77, 2011.

Greene J: What nurses want. Different generations. Different expectations, *Hosp Health Netw* 79(3):34–38, 40–42, 2, 2005.

Groff Paris L, Terhaar M: Using Maslow's pyramid and the National Database of Nursing Quality Indicators™ to attain a healthier work environment, *Online J Issues Nurs* 16(1), December 7, 2010.

Hendrikson G, Kovner C: Effects of computers on nursing resource use: do computers save nurses time? *Comput Nurs* 8(1):16–22, 1990.

Hospital staffing: How do agency nurses measure up? *Nursing* 36(1):35, January 2006.

Huey F, Hartley S: What keeps nurses in nursing: 3,500 nurses tell their stories, *Am J Nurs* 88:181–188, 1988.

Irvine D, Evans M: Job satisfaction and turnover among nurses: integrating research findings across studies, *Nurs Res* 44(4):246–253, 1995.

Joint Commission on the Accreditation of Hospitals: *Health care at the crossroads: strategies for addressing the evolving nursing crisis* (website), 2002. www.jointcommission.org/NR/rdonlyres/5C138711-ED76-4D6F-909F-B06E0309F36D/0/health_care_at_the_crossroads.pdf.

Jones C: The costs of nursing turnover, part 1: an economic perspective, *J Nurs Adm* 34(12):562–570, 2004.

Jones C: The costs of nursing turnover, part 2: application of the nursing turnover cost calculation methodology, *J Nurs Adm* 35(1):41–49, 2005.

Jones C: Revisiting nurse turnover costs: adjusting for inflation, *J Nurs Adm* 38(1):11–18, 2008.

Keepnews DM, Brewer CS, Kovner CT, Hyun Shin J: Generational differences among newly licensed registered nurses, *Nurs Outlook* 58(3):155–163, 2010.

Kimball B, O'Neil E: Health care's human crisis: the American nursing shortage, *Robert Wood Johnson Foundation* (website), 2002. www.rwjf.org/research/research-detail.jsp?id=1108&ia=137&gsa=1.

Kline D: Push and pull factors in international nurse migration, *J Nurs Schol* 35(2):107–111, 2003.

Kovner C, Brewer C, Yingrengreung S, Fairchild S: New nurses' views of quality improvement education, *Jt Comm J Qual Patient Saf* 36(1):29–35, 2010.

Kovner CT, Brewer CS, Fairchild S, et al: Newly licensed RNs' characteristics, work attitudes, and intentions to work, *Am J Nurs* 107(9):58–70, 2007.

Kovner CT, Brewer CS, Greene W, Fairchild S: Understanding new registered nurses' intent to stay at their jobs, *Nurs Econ* 27(2):81–98, 2009.

Kovner CT, Brewer CS, Kovner C, et al: Factors associated with work satisfaction of registered nurses, *J Nurs Scholarsh* 38(1):71–79, 2006.

KPMG: *KPMG's 2011 U.S. hospital nursing labor costs study* (website), 2011. kpmghealthcarepharmainstitute.com.

Leveck M, Jones C: The nursing practice environment, staff retention, and quality of care, *Res Nurs Health* 19(3):331–343, 1996.

Lucas M, Atwood J, Hagaman R: Replication and validation of anticipated turnover model for urban registered nurses, *Nurs Res* 42(1):29–35, 1993.

Lynn M, Redman R: Faces of the nursing shortage: influences on staff nurses' intentions to leave their positions or nursing, *J Nurs Adm* 35(5):264–270, 2005.

Lynn M, Redman, R: Staff nurses and their solutions to the shortage, *West J Nurs Res* 28(6):678–693, 2006.

Manion J: *Managing the multi-generational nursing workforce: managerial and policy implications*, Geneva, 2009, International Centre for Human Resources in Nursing, International Council of Nursing.

McClure M, Hinshaw A, editors: *Magnet hospitals revisited: attraction and retention of professional nurses*, Washington, DC, 2002, American Nurses Publishing, pp. 103–115.

McConnell CR: Staff turnover: occasional friend, frequent foe, and continuing frustration, *Health Care Manage* 18:1–13, 1999.

Morgan J, Lynn M: Satisfaction in nursing in the context of shortage, *J Nurs Manag* 17(3):401–410, 2009.

Mottaz C: Work satisfaction among hospital nurses. In Kovner A, Neuhauser D, editors: *Health services management: readings and commentary*, Ann Arbor, Mich, 1990, Health Administration Press, pp. 298–315.

Moulton P, Lacey L, Flynn L, et al: Addressing the complexities of survey research. In Dickson GL, Flynn LR, editors: *Nursing policy research: turning evidence-based research into health policy*, New York, 2008, Springer, pp. 43–69.

Murrow J, Nowak P: What nurses want: learn to reduce nurse turnover by using customer retention strategies, *Market Health Serv* 25(1):25–28, 2005.

Nevidjon B, Erickson J: The nursing shortage: solutions for the short and long term, *Online J Issues Nurs* 6(1):4, January 31, 2001. Available at http://www.nursingworld.org/ojin/topic14/tpc14_4.htm.

Nullis-Kapp C: Efforts under way to stem "brain drain" of doctors and nurses, *Bull World Health Org* 83(2), February 2005. Available at www.scielosp.org/scielo.php?pid=S0042-96862005000200004&script=sci_arttext&tlng=en.

Numerof R, Abrams M, Ott B: What works . . . and what doesn't? *Nurs Manage* 35(3):18, 2004.

O'Brien-Pallas L, Griffin P, Shamian J, et al: The impact of nurse turnover on patient, nurse and system outcomes: a pilot study and focus for a multi-center international study, *Policy Polit Nurs Pract* 7(3):169–179, 2006.

Page A, Institute of Medicine Committee on the Work Environment for Nurses and Patient Safety, Board on Health Care Services: *Keeping patients safe: transforming the work environment of nurses*, Washington, DC, 2004, National Academies Press, p. 4.

Pellico LH, Brewer CS, Kovner CT: What newly licensed registered nurses have to say about their first experiences, *Nurs Outlook* 57(4):194–203, 2009.

Pellico LH, Djukic M, Kovner CT, Brewer CS: Moving on, up, or out: changing work needs of new RNs at different stages of their beginning nursing practice, *Online J Issues Nurs* 15(1), 2010.

Powers P, Dickey C: Evaluation of an RN/co-worker model, *J Nurs Adm* 20(3):11–15, 1990.

Robert Wood Johnson Foundation: *Wisdom at work: the importance of the older and experienced nurse in the workplace* (website), 2006. www.rwjf.org/files/publications/other/wisdomatwork.pdf. Accessed September 5, 2011.

Robertson J, Herth K, Cummings C: Long-term care: retention of nurses, *J Gerontol Nurs* 20(11):4–10, 1994.

Runy L: Nurse retention: an executive's guide to keeping one of your hospital's most valuable resources, *Hosp Health Netw* 80(1):53–57, 2006.

Schaefer P: *The pros and cons of hiring a temp* (website), 2005. www.businessknowhow.com/manage/hire-temp.htm. Accessed September 12, 2011.

Spetz J, Dyer J: *Forecasts of the registered nurse workforce in California* (website), June 2005. www.futurehealth.ucsf.edu/pdf_files/forecasts2005.pdf. Accessed July 25, 2006.

Stamps P: *Nurses and work satisfaction: new perspective*, Chicago, 1997, Health Administration Press, p. 111.

Strachota E, Normandin P, O'Brien N, et al: Reasons registered nurses leave or change employment status, *J N Adm* 33(2):111–117, 2003.

Studor Q: High-middle-low performer conversations, *The Studor Group* (website), 2005. www.studergroup.com/dotCMS/knowledgeAssetDetail?inode=106533.

Studor Q: The power of thank-you notes, *The Studor Group* (website), 2009. www.studergroup.com/tools/tools_thank_you_notes.dot.

Swearingen S, Liberman A: Nursing generations: an expanded look at the emergence of conflict and its resolution, *Health Care Manage* 23(1):54–64, 2004.

Turisco F, Rhoads J: Equipped for efficiency: improving nursing care through technology, *California Healthcare Foundation* (website), 2008. www.chcf.org/publications/2008/12/equipped-for-efficiency-improving-nursing-care-through-technology.

U.S. Department of Health and Human Services, Health Resources and Services Administration: *The registered nurse population: findings from the 2008 national sample survey of registered nurses* (website), 2010. bhpr.hrsa.gov/healthworkforce/rnsurveys/rnsurveyfinal.pdf. Accessed September 5, 2011.

Venturato L, Drew L: Beyond doing: supporting clinical leadership and nursing practice in aged care through innovative models of care, *Contemp Nurse* 35(2):157–170, 2010.

Waldman J, Arora S: Measuring retention rather than turnover: a different and complementary HR calculus, *Human Res Plan* 27(3):6–9, 2004.

Waldman J, Kelly F, Sanjeev A, Smith HL: The shocking cost of turnover in health care, *Health Care Manage Rev* 29(1):2–7, 2004.

Yett D: The chronic shortage of nurses: a public policy dilemma. In Klaraman H, editor: *Empirical studies in health economics*, Baltimore, 1970, Johns Hopkins Press, pp. 357–389.

✳ PLANNING AND CONTROL

Planning and control are central to the success of any organization. Planning helps the organization set its future direction and develop a blueprint for getting there. Control helps to ensure that the adopted plan is carried out.

A long-standing definition of *planning* is "an analytical process which involves an assessment of the future, the determination of desired objectives in the context of that future, the development of alternative courses of action to achieve such objectives and the selection of a course (or courses) of action from among those alternatives."[1] *Control* has been defined as a "process that involves measurement and evaluation of the performance of organizational units, the identification of deviations from planned performance, the initiation of appropriate responses to these deviations, and the monitoring of remedial actions, all done with the intent of ensuring that managers' decisions and actions are consistent with planned organizational objectives."[2] These classic definitions link planning and control, and together, this linkage has developed into a strategic management process for the organization, operational budgeting, and control of the activities of an organization, department, or unit.

Strategic management is a field that is an outgrowth of the long-range planning movement of the 1950s. However, it goes beyond long-range planning, integrating strategic thought throughout the management process. Organizational success largely depends on the care with which the organization acts strategically. Knowing its strengths and weaknesses and being aware of its opportunities and threats are the critical elements upon which the field of strategic management has developed.

Strategic management is discussed in Chapter 11. We will address issues such as how strategic plans are defined, why they are prepared, and the benefits the organization can hope to gain from strategic management. The chapter also discusses some specific elements of strategic management, namely long-range plans, program budgets, and business plans.

The budgeting aspect of planning is explored in the next four chapters of this part of the book. Chapter 12 provides an overview of the various types of organizational budgets and the budget process. Chapter 13 provides greater depth on the preparation of the operating budget, and Chapter 14 focuses on revenue budgeting. Chapter 15 explores performance budgeting, an approach that allows the nurse manager and executive to plan for the amount of resources to be devoted to each of the major objectives of each unit or department in the organization.

Plans are of only limited usefulness unless actions are taken to ensure that the plans are followed to the extent possible. Chapter 16 discusses the issue of control. That discussion includes the provision of specific tools of variance analysis, which are used to help managers discover variations from the original plan and keep outcomes as close to the plan as possible. Chapter 17 provides more detailed information on variance analysis and provides examples of how and when the process is most useful for decision making. Chapter 18 discusses the use of benchmarking, productivity measurement, cost-benefit analysis, and cost-effectiveness analysis, all strategies used to varying degrees in health care organizations to find efficiencies in care delivery.

---

[1] Scott B. 1963. Some Aspects of Long-Range Planning in American Corporations with Special Attention to Strategic Planning, Ph.D. dissertation, Harvard University, Cambridge MA, p. 8.

[2] Camillus J. 1986. *Strategic Planning and Management Control.* Lexington, MA: Lexington Books, p. 11.

Strategic Management

CHAPTER GOALS

The goals of this chapter are to:

- Define *strategic management*, its importance to health care organizations, and the benefits of the strategic planning process
- Describe the evolution of strategic management from long-range planning to strategic planning to strategic management
- Distinguish between broad, long-term goals and time-oriented, specific, measurable objectives
- Introduce the concepts of total quality management and continuous quality improvement
- Discuss each element of a strategic plan, including a mission statement or nursing philosophy, a statement of long-term goals, a statement of competitive

strategy, a statement of organizational policies, a statement of needed resources, and a statement of key assumptions
- Stress the importance of strategic thought by all managers in carrying out all elements of their managerial responsibilities
- Explain the role of the long-range budget and the strategic plan in the planning process
- Define *program budgeting* and discuss the zero-base budgeting technique, stressing the importance of examining alternatives
- Outline the elements of a business plan
- Introduce the concept of pro forma financial statements

✳ INTRODUCTION

Strategic management is the process of setting *goals* and *objectives* for the organization, determining the resources to be allocated to achieving those goals and objectives, and establishing policies for getting and using those resources. This process includes an environmental assessment and depends heavily on data concerning the organization's external environment. The strategic management process is critical to the organization's success. Managers and their staff must not only do the things they do well but also carefully decide what must be done.

One planning text quotes Henry Thoreau: "It is not enough to be busy—the question is, what are we busy about?"[1] This simple question should cause nurse managers to pause and consider their role in the management process. Day-to-day routine activities often cause nurse managers to become overloaded. In fact, managers can become so busy that they have little time to plan for the future, to introduce innovations, or to feel like a "player" at the table. In some cases, their view may not be sought. In other cases, their work limits the

degree to which they can or perceive that they can take part in strategic planning. However, it is important for nurse managers and executives to structure their jobs so that planning is not pushed aside by the pressing day-in and day-out issues. Nurse managers and executives bring a vital perspective to developing the strategic plan and are key in communicating that plan to those at the point of care who will actually fulfill the plan.

Planning theory indicates that the higher a manager is in the organization's chain of command, the greater the portion of time that should be spent on planning. Planning should not be simply a rote process repeated each year; rather, it should focus on change and on improvement. A considerable amount of the chief executive officer's (CEO) time should be spent on planning and much less on day-to-day operations. The chief nurse executive (CNE), as the chief strategist for nursing, should also devote considerable time to planning and innovation. The proportion of time spent on planning decreases as one moves down through the ranks of nursing management because of their closer proximity to the point of care, but it should never become an insignificant amount. The key role that nurses play in health care organizations (HCOs) today,

---

[1]Ellis D, Pekar P. 1980. *Planning for Nonplanners.* New York: Amacom, p. 24.

particularly their role in shaping organizational reimbursements, requires that nurse managers and executives at all levels actively engage in the strategic planning process.

From a historical perspective, businesses began to place growing reliance on *long-range planning* in the middle of the 20th century. Long-range plans focus on general objectives to be achieved by the organization, typically over 3 to 5 years. By the 1960s, the term *strategy* became common, and long-range planning began to be referred to as *strategic planning*. It was contrasted with operational planning, the development of a detailed plan for the coming year.

When strategic planning was introduced, the concept of strategy was that operational planning is tactical, whereas long-range planning is strategic. Under strategic or long-range planning, an organization prepares a set of goals, and a strategy is developed for accomplishing them. That strategy is formalized into a plan of action generally covering a horizon of 3 to 5 years. This recognized the fact that major change and improvements to an organization often cannot be achieved within a time horizon of 1 year. Without having a plan that looks beyond 1 year, organizations severely limit their ability to innovate and thrive.

In the late 1980s and early 1990s, experts in the field began to use the more generic term *strategic management* to better define the role of strategic thought in organizations.[2] Such experts argued for a broad view of strategic planning. The primary focus remains the identification of broad, long-term goals and the creation of plans to achieve them. However, the current view of strategic management or strategic planning relies on the use of strategic thought in guiding all plans and actions in an organization. This relates to short-term operational plans as well as long-range plans.

Strategic planning is no longer simply long-range planning with a new name, as it has been in the past. Strategic management "stresses three points: that the strategic planner is clearly the advisor and facilitator to line management decision-makers; that the program executive, not the strategic planner, is the key strategist; and that strategic planning is always integrated with other functions of the program management process-program design, organizing, budgeting, staffing, controlling, and evaluating."[3] Long-range planning is still a part of strategic planning, but it is one of several integrated features.

In health care, changes in reimbursement and continued pressure to reduce costs have, over time, shaped the strategic focus in HCOs. For example, consuming acute care services was "encouraged" with the introduction of Medicare and Medicaid in the mid-1960s. At that time, fee-for-service was the predominant reimbursement mechanism, and organizations focused on providing inpatient services because they would be paid for doing so. With the introduction of Diagnosis Related Groups (DRGs) in the 1980s, the shift to prospective payment was initiated, and decreasing the consumption of costly acute and inpatient care was emphasized. Organizational planning

efforts followed suit, focusing on the provision of ambulatory and outpatient services to replace inpatient care and reduce costs. With today's emphasis on pay-for-performance and nonpayment of the care provided to deal with hospital- or health care–acquired conditions (HACs), the strategic focus in HCOs has shifted to identifying ways in which organizations can provide value through the provision of quality care. Over time, HCOs have been faced with a landscape of political, social and regulatory changes and have had to deal with the implications of those changes on incentives and competition.

Thinking strategically should not be the sole domain of the strategic planners in HCOs. Planning by planners is important but insufficient. Strategic thought should be an element of the job description of all managers throughout the organization. Nurse managers have a central role in strategic planning.[4] Today, the way a nursing unit is organized to provide care and the way staffing patterns are established to provide care should be conveyed by the unit-level nurse manager as part of the strategic planning process. The nurse manager's role in communicating information needed in the development of financial budgets is basic to managing at the unit level. It is a critical element in the unit's gaining authorization for adequate resources to provide care. The principal change from earlier views of strategic planning is the emphasis on bringing all managers into the direct process of working to achieve the organization's primary goals, rather than focusing narrowly on specific short-term objectives.

This chapter first discusses quality management as a part of strategic planning and then moves on to the definition, aims, and benefits of strategic planning and strategic thought. It then focuses on several specific aspects of strategic management, namely, long-range plans, program budgets, and business plans.

✳ QUALITY MANAGEMENT

A theme for the provision of health services in the 21st century is improving quality of care and controlling cost. In fact, a major focus in the provision of care in the 21st century is providing *value*, defined as quality relative to costs (see Chapter 5). The focus on quality, costs, and value reflects the quality management movement that evolved during the 20th century and that is a prominent aspect of our health care system today. One would be hard pressed to find an HCO that did not have a current focus on quality management, and that focus has, over time, become prevalent at the level of the health care system.

The changes to the health care system resulting from the Affordable Care Act (ACA) (discussed in Chapter 2) make quality management essential. Although at the time this book was written there was uncertainty about exactly how this law will fare during its legal challenges, some, if not many, aspects of the law may remain. Even in a modified form, the ACA will present quality management challenges. Quality management strategies must take into account the incentives and responsibilities faced by consumers who receive care, the payers that reimburse for

[2]Koteen J. 1989. *Strategic Management in Public and Nonprofit Organizations*. New York: Praeger, pp. 19-21.
[3]*Ibid*, p. 21.

[4]Kerfoot K. 2006. On leadership. Megatrends, the annual report, possibilities. *Nurs Econ* 24(1):47-49.

that care, and the organizations that deliver the care. These changes resulting from the ACA may be potentially transformational because HCOs will be held accountable for costs and outcomes of care, and reimbursements will be determined by the organization's actions and quality performance.

There are many quality models used in HCOs today: FOCUS-PDCA (Find, Organize, Clarify, Understand, Select-Plan, Do, Check, Act), the Institute for Healthcare Improvement's (IHI) Breakthrough Series, ISO (International Organization for Standardization) 9000, lean principles, Six Sigma, and others.[5] However, these models are generally associated in some way with two prominent quality approaches: total quality management (TQM) and continuous quality improvement (CQI). These represent philosophies concerning the production of an organization's goods and services. Although distinct, TQM and CQI are often used interchangeably because they both address the strategic management of quality in organizations with a consumer orientation. McLaughlin and Kaluzny[6] even warn: "Don't be fooled—whether it is called [TQM], [CQI], or some other term, TQM/CQI is a structured organizational process for involving personnel in planning and executing a continuous flow of improvements to provide quality health care that meets or exceeds expectations." The terms *quality improvement* and *performance improvement* are often used to refer to both TQM and CQI approaches and the tools and techniques that are associated with them.

Arikian[7] notes that "TQM emphasizes a preventive approach to management, one that addresses problems before they arise, and handles concerns with a studied, long-term commitment to continuous improvement in product and service." From a strategic management perspective, production in the United States has been dominated by an attitude of getting it done and then fixing it if it is wrong. Observations of the Japanese production process, where TQM was "imported" from the United States by scientist and statistician W. Edward Deming, have taught us that if more time is spent on planning, less will be wrong, and less will have to be fixed. This philosophy is apparent in HCOs through the use of failure modes and effects analysis (FMEA), which recognizes that a weakness in one part of the process can cause serious quality and safety problems throughout the system.

Over time, many U.S. corporations have learned this lesson as they have lost some of their competitive edge. To regain that edge, corporations have adopted procedures that focus on avoiding the costs associated with poor quality. Examples of the change in attitude are apparent in the slogans adopted by corporations. A quick search of the Web shows that many companies have taken a "get it right the first time, every time" approach to quality and adopted the slogan "Quality is job one."

As discussed in Chapter 5, ensuring quality care requires that HCOs devote time and money to address related concerns.

However, failing to address quality may cost as much as – or more – than dealing with related concerns in the first place. TQM focuses on the issue of being responsive to the needs of customers while reducing waste. Kirk[8] notes in an examination of Japanese firms, "The most significant discovery related to their determination to *build quality into the product (or service)* rather than to inspect for errors and assume that error removal would lead to quality. Many Japanese managers bought into the concept of planning and followed through on it—unlike many American managers who avoid this concept like the plague, in preference to the ready-fire-aim approach. 'We don't have time to plan,' some American managers say. Contrarily, many Japanese businessmen say, 'We don't have time *not* to plan.'"

Continuous quality improvement is a health care quality improvement approach that integrates structure, process, and outcomes into a system of quality analysis.[9] Readers may associate this structure–process–outcome approach with the seminal work of Avedis Donabedian, who is recognized as bringing a critical focus on quality into health care. CQI focuses on processes, not people, and seeks to understand processes that contribute to process failures and poor quality.[10] CQI recognizes that quality management is an ongoing process, not an activity in which an organization engages only when there are problems.

There are philosophical and structural elements of CQI, as well as health care–specific methods used for managing quality.[11] One common CQI method used in health care is rapid cycle improvement (RCI). This method brings a sharp focus to quality improvement that circumvents some of the failed traditions in health care quality processes. For example, quality processes have typically moved at glacial speed in health care. This was not because health care professionals have not cared about quality; rather, quality was assumed to be a part of health care delivery often without question, and quality efforts generally resulted in long and arduous processes, very little (if any) change, and frustrated and apathetic clinicians.

RCI does not mean doing things hastily and without thought. Rather, it means doing things in an intensely focused, systematic, and disciplined way to improve and streamline processes that bring about change more quickly.[12] RCI is a hallmark of IHI's Breakthrough Series, which has been well received by health care clinicians and demonstrated as successful in improving quality of care.[13] At the heart of RCI is the rapid improvement team. These teams are different than

[5]Ransom S, Joshi M, Nash D. 2005. *The Health Care Quality Book: Vision, Strategy and Tools*. Chicago: Health Administration Press.

[6]McLaughlin C, Kaluzny A. 2005. *Continuous Quality Improvement in Health Care*. Gaithersburg, MD: Aspen Publishers.

[7]Arikian V. 1991. Total quality management: Applications to nursing service. *J Nurs Adm* 21(6):46.

[8]Kirk R. 1992. The big picture: Total quality management and continuous quality improvement. *J Nurs Adm* 22(4):24.

[9]Nash D, Evans A. 2005. Physician and provider profiling. In Ransom S, Joshi M, Nash D, editors. *The Health Care Quality Book: Vision, Strategy and Tools*. Chicago: Health Administration Press.

[10]*Ibid.*

[11]McLaughlin and Kaluzny. 2005.

[12]Plesek P. 1999. Section 1: Evidence-based quality improvement, principles, and perspectives. Quality improvement methods in clinical medicine. *Pediatrics* 103(1) (Suppl), 203-213. Retrieved February 19, 2012 at http://www.directedcreativity.com/pages/PlsekPeds.pdf.

[13]Wagner E, Glasgow R, Davis C, et al. 2001. Quality improvement in chronic illness care: A collaborative approach. *J Comm J Qual Improv* 27(2): 63-80. See also http://www.ihi.org.

patient care teams, although not mutually exclusive. Rapid improvement teams bring together organizational participants—clinicians, managers, and others—who are focused on a specific quality topic of concern. Alemi and colleagues[14] offer several suggestions to guide the development and work of these teams:

- **Identify the right problem:** Delay benchmarking if the problem is obvious; define the problem from the customer's perspective; communicate throughout the organization from the outset; restate the problem from different perspectives; break large problems into smaller units.
- **Hold rapid meetings:** Identify uninvolved facilitator to conduct meetings; connect with team members before the meeting to identify relevant issues and concerns; delay evaluation of individual ideas until all ideas are on the table; think it through again.
- **Plan rapidly:** Start with the end and work backward; focus on the future.
- **Collect data rapidly:** Plan carefully; collect only data needed; sample representative patients; if quantitative data are lacking, rely on estimates provided by those familiar with processes.
- **Make rapid, whole-system change:** Change membership on cross-functional teams to diffuse information; get outside perspectives; use storyboards and other media to disseminate message; go beyond self-interests.[15]

Alemi and colleagues[14] argue that by using these guidelines, rapid improvement teams can bring about change more quickly with a minimum of problems along the way. Whereas the IHI's Breakthrough Series typically convenes larger groups of professionals from multiple HCOs to form collaboratives targeting rapid system changes on a variety of topics, rapid improvement teams generally operate to carry out local changes within organizations.

Various authors have identified different elements of TQM and CQI. Deming,[16] the pathfinder in the field, established 14 points related to TQM. These include such factors as a focus on education and training of employees, viewing employees not only as providers but also as customers, quality assurance, and a constant focus on finding ways to continuously improve quality.

TQM and CQI are not financial management tools per se, so we do not go into a detailed analysis of the methods here.[17] However, TQM and CQI have tremendous financial implications. Historically, HCOs have minimized planning and maximized control over day-to-day operations. The lesson of TQM and CQI is that managers will more likely achieve their objectives if they can redesign their work to allow much more time for planning and innovating. Such activities are not occasional but should be viewed as a major element of the management function. The quality management field tells us that a focus on improving the service we provide rather than on simply making sure we provide it is key to organizational success. From the writings on lean management, we know that planning to eliminate "waste" in organizational processes promotes quality and improves efficiencies. Thus, organizational spending should focus on activities that add value because all non–value-added functions represent wasted resources. In the long run, increased focus on improvement of quality may well lead to more satisfied staff and patients, higher quality of care, and lower costs.

✳ STRATEGIC PLANNING

Strategic planning calls for setting objectives, allocating resources, and establishing policies concerning those resources. With this strategic planning approach, all managers become involved in this process.

To establish and achieve goals, strategic planners have found it useful for the managers of an organization to focus on a series of key questions. The following questions are the most essential an organization must consider:

- Why does the organization exist?
- What is the organization currently?
- What would it like to be?
- How can we make the transformation to what it wants to be?
- How will it know when it is done?

These questions in turn lead to many other questions. What are the organization's strengths? Its weaknesses? Its opportunities? Its threats? Who are the organization's primary customers? Are they being well served? Who are its stakeholders? Does the organization learn from its mistakes and promote a culture of trust or does it seek to place blame when errors occur? Does the organization have a vision for the future? These questions are related to the organization as a whole, but they also relate to each department and unit within the organization.

Managers need to step aside from the current day-to-day activities and assess the nature of the existing organization. Has the organization over the years lost track of its reason for existence? Is the current status of the organization the desired one? If not, the organization needs to formally address the issue of how it can change things to become the type of organization it believes it should be. Again, this is true for departments and units as well as for entire organizations.

Strategic planning asserts that the way to become the type of organization desired is to establish a set of clear goals and objectives and then a plan for achieving them. Goals are defined as the broad aims of the organization; objectives are specific targets to be achieved to attain those goals.[18]

[14]Alemi F, Moore S, Hedrick L, et al. 1998. Rapid improvement teams. *J Comm J Qual Improv* 24(3):119-129.

[15]Modified from Alemi et al. 1998.

[16]See McLaughlin C, Kaluzny A. 2005. *Continuous Quality Improvement in Health Care.* Gaithersburg, MD: Aspen Publishers; Ransom S, Joshi M, Nash D, editors. *The Health Care Quality Book: Vision, Strategy and Tools.* Chicago: Health Administration Press; Cartin T. 1993. *Principles and Practices of TQM.* Milwaukee: Quality Press; and Jones S. 1995. Quality improvement in hospitals: how much does it reduce healthcare costs? *J Healthc Qual* 17(5):11-23.

[17]Interested readers are referred to the readings on the topic listed at the end of this chapter.

[18]The planning literature is inconsistent in the definition of goals and objectives. In some instances, the definition used here for goals is assigned to objectives and vice versa.

After goals and objectives have been identified, specific tactics can be designed to move the organization toward those goals. Tactical plans require resources. Often in the segregation of strategic planning into long-range planning versus operational planning, short-term operating resource allocations fail to match the allocation needed to reach long-term strategic goals. That is one reason that strategic management now takes a more global perspective.

In developing a short-term operating budget for the coming year, the unit manager must decide whether to place more emphasis on short-run profits or long-term growth. Spending extra money on quality improvements now will generate expenses not offset by revenues. But the reputation for quality will generate more revenues in the future. The dichotomizing of strategic plans and operating budgets forces managers with responsibility for operating expenses to focus on reducing short-run expenses. That tends to be exactly counter to the long-run strategic goals of the organization as designed by preparers of the strategic plan. Therefore, managers must balance the short-term objectives of their units or departments with a long-range vision for the organization.

It is not clear whether any organization will ever get to where it wants to be. The target goals tend to be modified over time in reaction to changes both inside and outside the organization. However, to make progress toward goals, the organization should constantly attempt to answer the questions asked earlier and to take necessary actions based on the answers to the questions.

Nurse managers and executives should not only be involved in the strategic planning process. They should also use elements of the strategic plan to guide the overall development, implementation, and evaluation of nursing initiatives that are consistent with the organization's values.[19]

The Elements of a Strategic Plan

Strategic plans must be adapted to specific situations. The elements of a plan for one organization may not be perfectly suited to another. Different organizations face different environmental issues, such as legal, political, regulatory, and demographic concerns. Over time, the environmental issues faced by an HCO may also change, and these environmental issues must be considered in the strategic planning process. In fact, flexibility in addressing a changing environment is a positive attribute in the strategic planning process. For most organizations, however, the basic elements of a strategic plan include the following:

- Mission statement or philosophy
- Statement of long-term goals
- Statement of competitive strategy
- Statement of organizational policies
- Statement of needed resources
- Statement of key assumptions

Mission Statement or Philosophy

The first step in strategic management is the development of a *mission statement* for the organization, department, or unit. What is the purpose of the organization or unit? An organization cannot begin to plan goals effectively and allocate resources sensibly until it first clearly determines its reason for existence. Strategic planners refer to an organization-wide statement of purpose or focus as the mission statement. In the department of nursing, this may be referred to as the *philosophy statement.*

A great deal of care should be taken in developing a mission statement. The mission statement should focus the organization by defining what it does. Some HCOs set their mission statement either too broadly or too narrowly. At one extreme, they wind up running restaurants or other non-health facilities that sap time and energy and often fail because the organization lacks expertise in that area. At the other extreme, growth and change are not encouraged by the statement, and the organization stagnates.

Some degree of limitation in the mission statement is beneficial because it forces the organization to concentrate on what it knows how to do. At the same time, the mission statement should allow growth and diversification. The mission statement should be defined in such a way as to prevent the organization from exceeding its manageable boundaries but to encourage exploration within those boundaries. Camillus[20] notes:

> An HCO engaged in providing eye-care services can describe itself as fulfilling the mission of examining eyes and writing prescriptions for corrective lenses or the mission of protecting and improving human vision. The first statement is essentially a description of activities in which the organization is engaged. The second statement, in contrast, identifies consequences rather than activities and thus leads to the identification of such possibilities as opening clinics where eye surgery is carried out, engaging in the development and possibly the manufacture of devices for rectifying faulty vision, and running programs for educating the public about the proper care of eyes.

The key to designing the mission statement is to focus not on what the organization does at a given point in time as much as to think about the range of possible types of activities one would see as a logical extension for the organization over time. Several examples of mission statements are shown in Exhibits 11–1 to 11–4.

Statement of Long-Term Goals

Goal setting is the organization's attempt to set the direction for itself as it tries to meet its mission. Often an organization will have both quantitative and qualitative goals. Quantitative goals may relate to financial outcomes, such as rates of growth in the number of patients served and in revenues, or quality of care

[19]Ingersol G, Witzel P, Smith T. 2005. Using organizational mission, vision, and values to guide professional practice model development and measurement of nurse performance. *J Nurs Adm* 35(2):86-93.

[20]Camillus J. 1986. *Strategic Planning and Management Control.* Lexington, MA: Lexington Books, p. 47.

✳ **EXHIBIT 11–1** *Examples of Simplified Mission Statements*

Hospital
Narrowly defined mission: To provide short-term acute hospital care to the community in the geographic area immediately surrounding the hospital.
Broadly defined mission: To improve the overall health of community members.
Overly broadly defined mission: To provide health care and other services and products to all potential patients and customers.

Hospital Nursing Department
Narrowly defined mission: To deliver high-quality care to the hospital's patients.
Broadly defined mission: To deliver high-quality nursing care at a reasonable cost to the citizens of the community.
Overly broadly defined mission: To promote the well-being of the organization and its clients by undertaking such activities as might be in the organization's interests.

✳ **EXHIBIT 11–2** *Mission Statements of the North Shore–LIJ Health System and Its Institute for Nursing*

The North Shore–LIJ Health System strives:
    To improve the health and quality of life for the people and communities we serve by providing world-class service and patient-centered care.
North Shore–LIJ Health System Institute for Nursing Mission:
    To promote health and quality patient care through the advancement of nursing science at every level of practice by integrating nursing research, education, professional growth and outcome studies.
    To empower nurses to share and enhance their knowledge, expertise and potential within a supportive and focused environment.
    To facilitate a system-wide standard of care and a national model for nursing practice.

Available at http://www.northshorelij.com/NSLIJ/About+Us+Mission+Statement; and http://www.northshorelij.com/NSLIJ/Institute+for+Nursing+ Welcome+-+Professionals. Retrieved September 17, 2011.

✳ **EXHIBIT 11–3** *Mission Statement of Lutheran Medical Center**

LUTHERAN MEDICAL CENTER

Mission Statement:
    Lutheran HealthCare has no reason for being of its own; it exists only to serve the needs of its neighbors. Lutheran HealthCare defines health as the total well-being of the community and its residents. Beyond the absence of individual physical illness, this includes, at least, decent housing, the ability to speak English, employment, and educational opportunities and civic participation. Lutheran HealthCare understands a hospital not as a collection of buildings, machines and beds, but a staff of talented, creative and committed people who serve the community as they are needed. Lutheran HealthCare works in partnership with its neighbors, each relying on the other as friends who care about and assist each other. Motivated to serve by its own history within the biblical tradition of faith and teaching, and organized as a not-for-profit organization according to the uniquely American heritage of democratic voluntary association, Lutheran HealthCare's purpose is to serve as the corporate vehicle for its trustees, medical and dental staff, nurses, employees, volunteers and others to care for the needs of our neighbors.

*This mission statement was formally adopted by Lutheran Medical Center's Board of Trustees at their regular meeting held on October 24, 1990, and has been reaffirmed annually since. Lutheran HealthCare adopts this mission and vision.
Available at http://www.lmcmc.com/AboutUs/MissionStatement. Retrieved September 17, 2011.

✳ **EXHIBIT 11–4** *Mission Statement for Family Home Care Services*

Mission Statement:
    The mission of Family Home Care Services (FHCS) is to be an excellent provider of home care services to clients with a commitment to improving their quality of life. FHCS will enable clients to be cared for safely and with dignity. FHCS will respond to changing health care needs; provide an atmosphere of mutual respect and growth for every employee; and ensure long-term financial viability for the Agency in order to continue to provide quality services in the future.

Available at http://www.fhcsny.com/about.html. Retrieved September 17, 2011.

outcomes, such as decline in the rate of catheter-associated bloodstream infections. Qualitative goals may relate to patient satisfaction and general reputation.

In developing the long-term goals of the organization, their timeless nature should be kept in mind. Objectives are intended to be attained within a specific time frame. Goals tend to stay in force over long periods. Providing the needs of an increasing percentage of the community's citizens is a long-term goal. Increasing the number of patients by 8% in the coming year is a specific measurable objective.

Although statements of objectives are necessary, the statement of goals is of greater concern in strategic management. As managers attempt to respond in their operations to specific, time-oriented objectives, they should bear in mind the overriding goals that the organization wants to achieve. Innovations that allow the organization to make major steps toward achieving its long-range goals should constantly be sought by all managers.

Statement of Competitive Strategy

The organization's competitive strategy is its plan for achieving its goals—specifically, what services will be provided and to whom. The development of this strategy relies to a great extent on a thorough internal and external review. What are the organization's strengths and weaknesses, its opportunities and threats?

Competitive strategy is the planning of what care will be provided and to whom. To develop such a plan, the organization must consider what competitors are or are not doing and what expertise the organization does or does not possess. On the basis of that information, the organization can decide where it should expand and perhaps where it should pull back. This in turn helps to guide the allocation of resources.

Essentially, the organization must evaluate its mission and goals in light of its particular strengths and weaknesses and in light of the demand for services and competition in the external environment. Based on that evaluation, it can make a plan that will take advantage of opportunities that present themselves and plan a reaction to threats that exist.

Statement of Organizational Policies

The role of policies is to specify what practices are and are not acceptable for the organization. The establishment of a mission and objectives incorporates a set of values. It integrates the values of the organization's founders, the values of its management and staff, and the values of the community. These values should be incorporated in the decisions made by the organization.

In most organizations, no single person can review each and every decision and determine if it is appropriate. A set of policies that clearly indicates what actions are appropriate and what actions are not removes an unreasonable burden from managers throughout the organization. It also removes the necessity for guesswork by individual managers in many specific situations. Policies are often driven by regulations and requirements handed down by regulatory groups (e.g., The Joint Commission), but organizational values shape the actual policies developed.

Policy statements are substantially different from mission statements, statements of goals, and statements of competitive strategy. In each of those earlier statements, there is a need to encourage creativity. Each one leaves room for the organization to innovate or grow. In contrast, policy statements are generally limited to specifically guiding actions and acceptable behaviors. They provide the constraints that the organization *wants* to place on managerial discretion.

Surprisingly, such constraints can ultimately enhance organizational growth. Without specific policies, managers may find that they are chastised for specific actions without any rhyme or reason. They become uncertain as to when it is acceptable to take initiative and make changes and when higher levels of management want things done just the way they always have been done. This high degree of uncertainty will lead managers over time to become reluctant to innovate in any respect. The availability of specific procedures clearly delineates where innovation is not allowed. However, that also provides the manager a sense of where innovation is allowed and welcomed.

Statement of Needed Resources

Strategic planning cannot be conducted apart from the reality of the resources needed to carry out the plan. These include resources in terms of personnel, the facilities for the personnel to work in and with, and the other requirements for accomplishing the goals of the organization. Without linkage between the plan and the resources to carry it out, there can be little hope of achieving the organization's goals.

Statement of Key Assumptions

Part of the planning process is development of a statement of key assumptions. Because strategic management calls for decentralization of the planning process, there must be a set of common guidelines that all managers use. For example, if management expects to have additional contracts with managed care organizations that will affect the entire organization, the same assumption about such contracts should be used consistently by all managers. This will make plans consistent and will improve coordination of plans throughout the organization. It will also help in determining whether variations from the plan are due to carrying out the plan or the accuracy of the underlying assumptions.

Benefits of the Strategic Planning Process

One can think of a number of benefits that result from having a strategic planning system. One of the predominant benefits is that it forces the organization to determine its long-run goals and come up with an approach to accomplish them. Establishing long-run goals forces managers to decide what the organization's purpose is and to formalize that purpose. Many HCOs were established long before any of the current employees worked for the organization. The original goals of the organization can easily become lost among the personal needs and desires of the current management and staff. The process of establishing a formalized mission and goals gives a sense of direction to the organization.

A strategic planning system also promotes efficiency. Managers working toward clear goals are less likely to be inefficient. When everyone clearly knows what the organization is trying to achieve, there is a greater likelihood that less effort will be spent on unnecessary activities.

The strategic planning process provides a means of communication among the various hierarchical levels of the organization. In large organizations (and sometimes even in relatively small ones), communication among organizational levels becomes difficult. The managers on the lower rungs may know that things are not being done efficiently. The managers on the upper rungs may believe that the systems they have in place do generate efficiency. Inadequate channels exist for moving information up or down through the ranks. Innovation in such cases is expected to be dictated from the higher levels of the organization. In fact, often the need and opportunities for improvements are most visible at the lower levels. A strategic management process should allow new ideas to flow down or up much more smoothly.

Managers at lower levels in the organization will learn more about why changes are taking place if they share the strategic plan and can see how changes relate to achieving the plan's goals. This will facilitate their buy-in to strategic initiatives and enable them to more easily communicate these initiatives to staff. Higher level managers will receive better information if lower level managers focus some of their attention on factors that affect the organization's long-term goals. In general, this process should help both lower- and higher-level managers gain a better understanding of the importance of their respective roles in the strategic planning process.

The strategic planning process develops management skills at all levels throughout the organization. Management skills are developed primarily by giving managers the opportunity to make decisions and to handle things that are not part of the routine. Out-of-the-ordinary activity requires skilled management even more than repetitive tasks.[21] By working at the planning process, managers develop skills needed to deal with change and with unusual events.

The strategic planning process provides managers an improved sense of the needs of the organization and of its environmental constraints. It has often been found that a partnership approach to management works better than a dictatorial approach. Managers who are told they must operate within constraints may resist them, but managers who are asked to become part of the team to address the constraints learn to understand the challenges presented by the constraints and are more willing to work cooperatively instead of as adversaries.

The strategic planning process increases the level of organizational creativity in addressing problems. Successful and highly reliable organizations encourage rather than resist change.[22] Things are done differently now than they were 20 years ago. Change, however, does not occur at some arbitrary point every

20 years. It occurs gradually in an evolutionary process. The fact that most organizations do things now in a way that is different from the way they did them 20 years ago indicates that someone tried a new approach and found it superior. Who is that someone? Is it the lucky one who accidentally fell upon an improved approach?

Generally, this is one area in which organizations create their own destiny. Creativity cannot be forced on people. One cannot tell employees to be creative and to develop innovative improvements. However, creativity can be either fostered or stifled. A strong commitment to strategic management throughout the organization will convey the organization's view of creativity as positive rather than negative.

One can summarize strategic management as the process that adds creative vision to all other processes of the organization. In a now classic book to guide nurses in the development of business skills, Strasen[23] defines vision as "the ability to set goals that are not limited to what is presently inevitable. In order to be meaningful, goals must stretch the imagination and efforts of the individual or organization setting them. If goals are inevitable occurrences in the future, they are set too low and are no real measure of progress or accomplishment." This definition is still relevant today. After the vision of the future is in place and is clearly communicated, the organization's managers can work creatively on changes to bring that vision to fruition.

Implementing a Strategic Management Process

This chapter has alternatively referred to the strategic plan and to the strategic planning or strategic management process.

The specific development of a strategic plan is discussed in the next section. However, strategic management relies not just on a plan but on a broad planning process. That process is one of making managers aware of the need to think strategically as they carry out all of their management activities. In developing a long-range plan, managers must relate the plan to the mission. In designing specific program budgets or business plans, the manager must consider how the program will help the organization achieve its goals. In developing the specific details of the operating budget, the manager again should be trying to link the details with how they help the organization reach its long-term aims.

The remainder of this chapter focuses on some long-range elements of strategic planning, specifically long-range planning, program budgets, and business plans. As readers proceed to the remaining chapters in Part IV, the notion of trying to link operational activities with strategic thought should be kept in mind.

❋ LONG-RANGE PLANNING

In developing the long-range budget, the organization begins the process of translating its general goals and objectives into a specific action plan. Long-range budgets or plans are often

---

[21]Bazerman M, Watkins M. 2003. Predictable surprises: The disasters you should have seen coming and how to prevent them. *Harv Bus Rev* 81(3):72-80.

[22]Weick K, Sutcliffe K. 2001. *Managing the Unexpected*. San Francisco: Jossey-Bass.

[23]Strasen L. 1987. *Key Business Skills for Nurses*. Philadelphia: JB Lippincott, p. 208.

referred to as the organization's *strategic plan*. Such plans generally cover a period of 3 to 5 years.

Given a strategic management process that calls on managers to focus on the organization's goals, is a strategic plan essential? Yes, clearly. Long-range planning is critical to the vitality of an organization. For organizations to thrive, they must move forward. The staff of an organization should be able to look back and see the progress that has been made over an extended period. Budgeting for 1 year at a time does not allow for the major types of changes that would take years to plan and implement. Yet that lengthy process is needed for the efforts that will substantially move the organization forward.

For example, suppose that one goal of the organization is to move from being a primary care community hospital to a regional tertiary care center. This cannot be accomplished by having each department attempt to modify its operating budget. An overall organizational plan is needed. Which of the new tertiary services can or should be added in the next 5 years? Which programs already exist but need to be expanded in the next 5 years to accommodate the changing role of the organization? These questions are specifically addressed in the strategic plan or long-range budget.

Because nursing is such a large part of the services provided by HCOs, nurses and nurse leaders should be involved in this planning process. The success of the plan will depend on how well it is carried out. If the plan does not have adequate nursing input when it is prepared, it is unlikely that the nursing staff will fully support it. Nurses must push their organizations to incorporate nursing leadership into the planning process, not only for the good of nurses and nursing but also for the good of patients and ultimately the success of the organization. Figure 11–1 illustrates a collaborative care model that was adopted by a nursing organization in an integrated health system (the missions of both were presented earlier). This model serves the dual purposes of guiding organizational leaders in planning for nursing services and guiding nurse managers, executives, and clinicians as they put that plan into action.

The strategic plan may lay the groundwork for a fundraising campaign to precede and parallel expansion of services. Or the plan may indicate that each year for 5 years, growth in specified existing profitable areas must be undertaken to offset start-up losses incurred in the introduction of major new programs. Specific dollar amounts of additional revenue and new program cost may be projected only as extremely rough estimates. Although general, such a plan does give the organization enough specific information about the implications and requirements for expansion into a tertiary care center to allow for development of specific programs to move the organization toward that ultimate goal.

The strategic plan may be somewhat more detailed, showing projections of the dollar amounts expected to be available (and their sources) as well as which specific programs will be adopted and what their approximate costs will be. Because a strategic or long-range plan projects at least 3, and up to 10, years into the future, it is unlikely that revenue and cost estimates will be highly accurate. Therefore, although rough estimates are often included in such plans, they are generally not overly detailed or refined.

The plan should not focus only on major program additions. The services and programs that already exist are equally important to an organization. Expanding, downsizing, or even eliminating a program or service requires the same consideration and planning as adding a program or service. A part of the planning process should be to explicitly address whether those services and programs that make up a majority of operations of the organization are being retained at a steady-state level or whether they are to be contracted or expanded in scope.

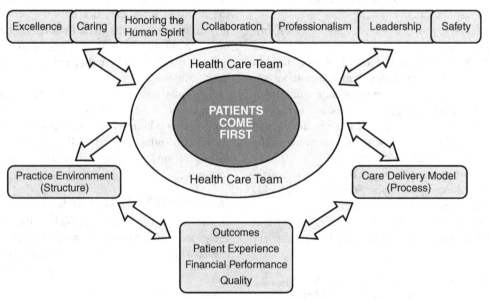

FIGURE 11–1. Collaborative Care Model©, North Shore–Long Island Jewish Health System. (Used with permission from North Shore–LIJ Health System.)

One serious potential problem arises if this issue is ignored in preparing strategic plans. If existing programs are implicitly assumed to continue unchanged, a plan that includes a number of new programs may appear feasible. However, it may not be feasible when technological and other changing factors are explicitly considered for the ongoing operations of the organization. Therefore, expectations regarding existing programs should be explicitly reviewed and included as part of the plan.

After the plan has been finalized and formalized, it serves as a guide for a number of years. Long-range plans are typically prepared only once every 3 or 5 years. Creating a new plan each year would only lead to constant changes in the organization's direction. This would lead to wasted efforts and frustrated managers. However, such plans should be reviewed each year. Assumptions may turn out to be wrong. A new cancer treatment that shifts care from the inpatient to the outpatient setting could drastically change patient volume. The external environment can change dramatically. An influx of refugees could change the demand for services in certain areas. Annual reviews allow the organization to adjust the strategic plan to react to current events.

Each year, elements of the plan are brought into the current activities of the organization. To make the transition from the plan into operations, many proposed additions or changes require thorough evaluation. This may be accomplished through the development of a program budget.

✳ PROGRAM BUDGETING AND ZERO-BASE BUDGETING

Program budgeting is the part of the overall strategic planning process that focuses on all of the costs and benefits associated with a specific program. The program may be an existing one that the organization is considering whether to expand, contract, or eliminate, or it may be a new program that the organization is thinking of adding. Program budgeting examines alternative programs to meet the organization's objectives and examines feasible alternative ways to accomplish each program.

Some program budgeting is done within a nursing unit or department. Often, however, the program changes generated by a strategic plan have interdepartmental impact. Such program changes are much more complicated because of the need for coordination among departments. It is vital that nursing participate fully in such interdepartmental planning. Working on key committees is essential not only to protect the interests of nursing but also to ensure that any plans developed make sense from a nursing perspective and can be supported by the nursing staff.

In most cases, program budgets relate directly to the strategic planning of the organization. The projects being evaluated are under consideration because they relate directly to moving the organization toward achievement of its long-term goals.

Program budgets are substantially different from other types of budgets. Long-range budgets or strategic plans look in general terms at the entire organization over a period of years. Their information is based on rough approximations rather than on details. Operating and cash budgets look in great detail but only at the coming year. A program budget combines a great amount of detailed information for one specific program for a long projected period. Furthermore, whereas most budgets focus on a given department's revenues and costs, program budgets compare revenues and expenses for an entire program, cutting across departments or cost centers.

A program budget compares all associated costs and benefits to evaluate the entire program's effect on the organization over its lifetime. In doing this, the program budgeting methods identify costs and benefits of different programs aimed at the same purpose or of different approaches to one program. Because resources are limited, program budgeting often focuses on trade-offs; that is, program budgeting considers the extra benefit to be gained by spending additional money on a program. Alternatively, program budgeting considers how much of the benefit of a program would be lost if less money were spent on the program.

Zero-Base Budgeting

Zero-base budgeting (ZBB) is a popular program budgeting technique that gained fame for its strong push toward analysis of all costs. ZBB accounts for all costs, starting at a base of zero; from this base, each and every cost must be justified. Until the introduction of ZBB, it was common for budget negotiations to revolve around the appropriate amount of increase in a budget. How much more should be spent next year than was spent in the current year? Implicitly, such an approach assumes that all current-year spending continues to be reasonable and justified for the next year. Only the amount of the increment is subject to examination and discussion.

In reality, as technology and diseases change, some departments have growing financial needs, but other departments can get by with decreasing resources. The concept of requiring zero-base evaluation is attractive because it means that budgets are not allowed to become "fat" over time. Some organizations use ZBB analysis to see exactly how money is being spent within a unit or department. Such an approach requires existing programs to justify their continued existence. Rather than basing the future budget on the past budget, the program must demonstrate why all expenditures in the proposed budget are needed.

In addition, the ZBB approach pays great attention to the alternative ways in which any one given program can be offered. ZBB collects information regarding a program into a *decision package*. A decision package contains documentation in support of the program and summaries of the analyses performed. In that sense, the decision package is just a mechanism to ensure a formal, systematic review of each budget.

Each package (Figure 11–2) contains a statement of the purpose of the program, the consequences of not performing the program, and the ways that the costs and benefits of the program can be measured. More interestingly, the package also includes statements of alternatives. These statements are the heart of ZBB.

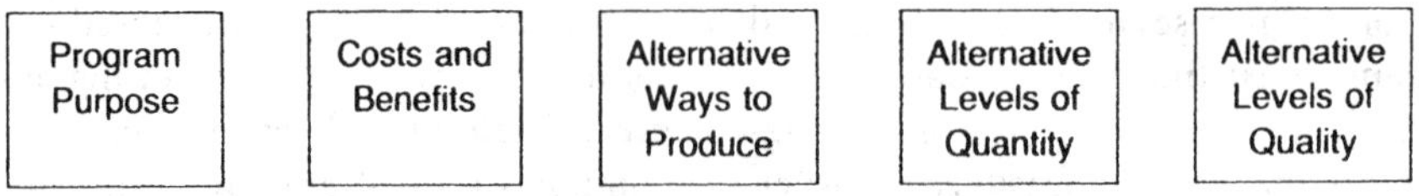

Program Purpose	Costs and Benefits	Alternative Ways to Produce	Alternative Levels of Quantity	Alternative Levels of Quality

FIGURE 11–2. Elements of a zero-base budgeting decision package.

ZBB provides a great degree of sophistication in the analysis of alternatives. ZBB not only compares different programs with separate decision packages but also compares three major types of alternatives within the decision package for each individual program. The first alternative involves ways to produce the treatment, service, or other output. The second set of alternatives relates to the quantity of treatments, service, or output to be provided. The third set of alternatives considers varying levels of quality.

For many nurses, considering trade-offs such as these is counterintuitive to their traditional education. Nurses, as health care professionals, are trained to provide the best possible care to each patient. At the larger level of organizational planning, however, it must be acknowledged that no health care provider can provide everything to everyone. There simply are limited resources. ZBB forces recognition of the need to determine the greatest overall good that can be provided to the entire population served by an organization, in contrast with the view of providing care to a specific individual. Considered this way, ZBB is consistent with the idea that organizational policy, planning, and budgeting should be connected with the needs of those who receive care. Table 11–1 illustrates some of the distinctions between traditional and ZBB approaches.

Perhaps the best way to understand how these alternatives are examined is to work through a potential program budget problem.

Zero-Base Budgeting Case Study: Hemodialysis

Suppose that the hypothetical Wagner Hospital has decided on the basis of its environmental review that there is a pressing need for additional hemodialysis services in the community. In Wagner's long-range plan, the introduction of a hemodialysis program has been included, although the plan does not include much in the way of specifics other than to note that some form of hemodialysis program should be fully instituted within the next 5 years. This program was highly placed when priorities were established, although it would have to vie for funds with several other important new programs that were also included in the long-range plan, such as a new primary care center.

Wagner has compiled a decision package for the hemodialysis program. The formal documentation in the package first notes the name of the program (hemodialysis) and the sponsoring department within the hospital (internal medicine). The stated purpose of the program is to reduce levels of mortality and morbidity currently experienced in the community because of insufficient hemodialysis facilities. The resources needed for the program are stated in general terms. They include dialysis machines, physicians, nurses, technicians, supplies, and overhead items such as electrical power and physical space.

If Wagner were not a user of ZBB, it is likely that the renal specialists in the hospital would have designed a first-class hemodialysis center, perhaps as a new hospital wing, with five machines to satisfy all community needs. The proposal would have been a take-it-or-leave-it package, with strong political emphasis on its acceptance.

There is nothing wrong with wanting everything to be first-class. It is not wasteful to provide top-quality care. However, that does not mean that an organization can afford to provide that care. Having a first-class hemodialysis center may mean that there will not be enough resources left for adequate cancer treatment.

Because Wagner Hospital uses ZBB, the hemodialysis plan cannot be approved until an analysis is performed that examines a number of alternatives. The first issue concerns the level of output. How much treatment will be provided? Suppose that five machines would take care of the entire community demand now and for the foreseeable future. Suppose that the estimated annual cost of this alternative were $2 million, including depreciation, supplies, personnel, overhead, maintenance, and so on. A second alternative may be to purchase only four machines. Suppose that at this level, it would still be possible to eliminate mortality and morbidity, but some of the machines might have to operate two or three shifts per day, causing some inconvenience for nurses and physicians.

✳ **TABLE 11–1** *A Comparison of Traditional Budgeting and Zero-Base Budgeting Approaches*

Traditional Budgeting Approach	Zero-Base Budgeting Approach
Focuses on increases to what was spent in prior year rather than the resources needed	Justifies all spending starting at a base of zero
May not account for waste, workloads, or cost drivers; only amount of increment is subject to examination	Focuses on the elimination of waste and obsolete operations; programs must demonstrate why expenditures are needed
Typically does not engage users or encourage buy-in	Typically engages users, motivates, and communicates strategic plan
May not be connected to overall organizational strategy	Connected to strategy by considering alternatives for delivering a program or service
Assumes current year spending is justified for the next year	Assumes resources allocated based on needs and benefits

Deborah Lessard, RN, BSN, MA, JD, CPHRM, information modified from personal communication from her review of the third edition of this book, to assist us in preparation for this new edition.

Four machines might cost a total of $1,700,000. Note that although the number of machines would decrease 20%, from five to four, the costs would fall only 15%. That is possible because some costs associated with the program are likely to be fixed. As discussed in Chapter 8, fixed costs do not change as the output level increases. Does this mean that five machines would be better than four because the hospital would get 20% more machines for only 15% more cost? Not necessarily. That is the wrong comparison. The goal is to provide cost-effective, high-quality health care to the community, not to buy unnecessary equipment to minimize the cost per machine.

The alternative of four machines instead of five would save $300,000. Although there would be some inconvenience, the reduced cost would not result in higher mortality or morbidity. The extra convenience gained by having five machines must be compared with the benefits from spending $300,000 for some other program. Would the extra machine generate additional revenue? Or would it affect only scheduling?

Other alternative levels of output might be the use of three machines, which would eliminate 100% of mortality and 50% of morbidity for a cost of $1,400,000; two machines, which would eliminate only 80% of mortality at a cost of $1,100,000; and one machine, which would eliminate only 40% of mortality at a cost of $800,000.

Itemizing the costs and benefits of the alternative output levels is informative. Unlike the usual all-or-nothing presentation for a new program, either five machines or no program at all ("We don't practice second-class medicine here!"), the choice is not that dramatic. In fact, in a constrained environment, it may well be that after a review of all the alternatives, the choice will be between three or four machines. Fewer than three may be considered inadequate to accomplish the long-run objectives; more than four may raise questions of priorities.

It is not only the amount of output that is a question here. The ZBB system requires that alternative ways to produce the output also be considered. Is there a choice? Is it hemodialysis machines or nothing? Perhaps the answer is yes, but one of the major roles of ZBB is to ask questions such as that. The next question might be whether hemodialysis has to be performed in a hospital setting. The answer is no. Although one alternative would be to perform all dialysis in the hospital, another alternative would be to perform all dialysis in one clinic location. Another alternative would be to have a series of external locations spread throughout the community, one location for each machine. It is also possible to use one mobile van for each machine, allowing dialysis to be performed at many locations. Each of these alternatives would be matched with one, two, three, four, and five machines.

Other options must also be considered. Can a patient be on the machine for a shorter period, thus increasing the number of patients who have access to it? Can money be saved by buying machines with fewer accessories? Such questions almost certainly hit upon issues of quality. However, the trade-offs between quality and cost must be examined.

Trade-offs are always made, and they sometimes affect the quality of care. If one cardiac patient dies, it may be because insufficient resources were devoted to having the very latest open heart surgery equipment. That person suffered from a lack of high-quality care. More resources devoted to updating heart surgery equipment might have saved that individual. Perhaps the hospital should cut back in another area and pursue the very best in heart surgery. In the vast majority of cases, that would simply result in other people dying in another area. The program budgeting system must attempt to select a set of projects that are carried out in a way that minimizes the overall negative impact on quality. That may mean undertaking two new services, each at less than the optimal level of care, rather than totally sacrificing either service so the remaining one can be run on an optimal basis. Table 11–2 provides a summary of the hemodialysis decision package and its focus on trade-offs in this hypothetical example.

❋ TABLE 11–2 *Zero-Base Budgeting Decision Package: Hemodialysis*

1. Name of program: Hemodialysis
2. Department: Internal Medicine
3. Purpose: Reduce mortality and morbidity because of a lack of hemodialysis facilities
4. Resources required: Dialysis machines, physicians, nurses, technicians, supplies, overhead
5. Quantity or level of output alternatives

Level	Health Implications	Cost
Five machines	Eliminates all mortality and morbidity; no inconvenience to staff	$2,000,000
Four machines	Eliminates all mortality and morbidity; some inconvenience to staff	1,700,000
Three machines	Eliminates all mortality and 50% of all morbidity	1,400,000
Two machines	Reduces mortality by 80%	1,100,000
One machine	Reduces mortality by 40%	800,000

6. Alternative ways to produce output: This section should consider the various approaches to providing the product and the cost of each. For instance, it should consider providing the care in the hospital, in clinics, or in mobile vans. For each way of providing the output, each output level (i.e., one machine, two machines, etc.) should be considered.
7. Alternative levels of quality of care: This should consider the cost of using different types of machines or changing the amount of time each patient is on the machine for each way of producing the output and for each level of output in terms of the number of machines.

The difficult part of the analysis is to explicitly and creatively seek and examine trade-offs from alternatives. Specifically, it is necessary to ask whether more lives could be saved by the organization if it spent $300,000 less on hemodialysis and got four machines instead of five. Could even more lives be saved in some other program if dialysis was cut to three machines and the $600,000 was spent on other programs? Three machines might mean less care and lower-quality care or less time on the machine for each noncritical patient. What could $600,000 do elsewhere in the organization? Would $600,000 spent elsewhere provide enough benefit to justify less care and lower quality of care in this area?

Suppose that in addition to hemodialysis, a primary care center has been proposed. A first-class primary care center might cost $1 million per year (the numbers here are hypothetical). This primary care center is envisioned to provide access to care for 50,000 visits per year (or about 12,000 patients). However, a ZBB review of primary care indicates that for $600,000, a total of only 35,000 visits could be handled. All children in the community could get immunizations, but some older patients would have to travel extra minutes to go to an existing clinic.

Because of the large capital investment, Wagner Hospital does not have sufficient cash to establish both a primary care center and a hemodialysis service at the ideal first-class levels. It is highly likely that without a ZBB review, the hospital might well select either hemodialysis or primary care. The choice often comes down to politics. The well-being of the community can get lost in the struggle between vested interest groups within an organization.

There might, however, be enough resources to provide both hemodialysis and primary care at slightly reduced levels of care. The hospital could add three dialysis machines and a primary care unit.

The key to the ZBB review is that it forces the examination of alternatives. It forces recognition of the fact that more lives would be saved by scaling back the levels of hemodialysis and primary care and providing both services. Given the explicit information contained in the ZBB reviews, both vested interest groups are likely to be more willing to accept the resulting compromise.

Ranking Decision Packages

Because the resources of the organization are always limited, it is rare that all proposed packages can be accepted. Therefore, ZBB requires each manager to rank the alternative decision packages. The best alternative is ranked number 1.

During the process of budget review and negotiation, managers at higher levels of the organization will receive ranked decision packages from a number of subordinate managers. For example, a clinical nursing director with responsibility for multiple units in a service line might receive packages from each unit nurse manager. The packages from all of the different units must be ranked in order of importance by the clinical nursing director. Then the packages will continue up through the organization. The CNE may first consider all nursing departmental packages and make recommendations for an overall ranking based on a planning session of all clinical nursing directors; then the organizational administrative staff will make a final ranking of all the packages received from all the different clinical areas.

In large organizations, the ranking process can become quite tedious. However, it is a necessary evil if the goal of the program budgeting process is to compare all of the alternatives available to the organization and to ultimately allocate the organization's resources to projects that best help the organization attain its goals.

✳ BUSINESS PLANS

One approach to program budgeting that became widely used in the 1980s is the business plan. This technique, commonly used in industry, became popular in health care as it became clear that HCOs would have to take a more business-like approach to providing their services in an ever more difficult financial environment. It is a method that is supported in almost all types of HCOs.

What Is a Business Plan?

A *business plan* is a detailed plan for a proposed program, project, or service, including information to be used to assess the venture's financial feasibility. Often the plan is used as a sales document that makes the case for undertaking a new project. However, despite its advocacy role, the plan should provide an honest appraisal of the project. If in fact the proposed project is not good for the organization, that should be determined at the planning stage rather than after a large financial investment has been made to implement it.

The first step in planning a new program should be to understand which organizational goals the program promotes. Does the proposed project fit with the organization's mission statement? In developing the plan, sufficient information must be gathered to indicate whether and how the proposed program will move the organization closer to its goals. In evaluating the plan, it is important not to lose sight of the original organizational goal to which the project relates.

For example, one business plan might relate to the development of a community education program for patients with diabetes; another plan might focus on providing home health care. Both of these new programs might fit nicely within a mission of providing health care services to the community. It is possible, however, that the program on community education would not be expected to be financially self-sufficient. It fits into the element of mission that concerns providing important services on a charitable basis. On the other hand, the home care plan may be based on the notion of earning profits to be used to subsidize the charitable elements of the organization's mission. The organization cannot provide some services at a loss unless it provides some at a profit.

Even the program aimed at the charitable mission would require a business plan. The fact that it is not expected to earn a profit does not remove the need to understand just how large a subsidy it might require. At the same time, if home care is being proposed to earn profits to subsidize the other operations of the organization, we should not lose sight of that fact during the planning process. Business plans are discussed in greater detail in Chapter 22.

✳ IMPLICATIONS FOR NURSE MANAGERS AND EXECUTIVES

Often nurse managers at all levels of the organization have insights that can result in significant operational changes that will move the organization closer to its strategic goals. That is why strategic management takes the view that strategic planning is not limited to the development of the long-range plan and program budgets. Strategic management must exhibit itself through strategic thought by managers throughout the entire organization. All nurse managers and executives should make themselves aware of their organization's mission and goals as well as its specific objectives and policies. Knowing the philosophical statement of the nursing department alone is not sufficient. Familiarity with the organization's mission and vision will equip nurse managers and executives to negotiate from a stronger position for their programs areas within the overall context of the organization.

Because strategic management does not occur within a vacuum, it helps to think of the process within the overall context of quality management. As discussed in Chapter 5, quality has tremendous financial implications. TQM and CQI are both common approaches used to manage quality in HCOs that encourage managers to focus on planning and innovation to improve organizational processes. These approaches recognize that quality management is an ongoing function that adds value to services provided. These approaches also help position organizations to survive in a pay-for-performance or value-based purchasing environment. In the long run, this process will certainly lead to more satisfied patients and staff and improved quality of care. However, in the pay-for-performance environment, quality management can also help HCOs determine ways to lower costs and maximize reimbursements.

The organization-wide goals developed in the strategic management process are used as a point of reference in assessing where the organization has been, where it is going, and what it hopes to accomplish in the coming years. These goals help organizations put their mission and vision for the future into action.

Strategic management requires a significant effort from managers at all levels. However, that effort is rewarded by reducing the extent to which managers must operate in "crisis mode." It promotes the efficient use of resources and the financial health of the organization. It results in goal setting and the establishment of a vision for the organization. Strategic planning helps ensure that managers will identify opportunities and take reasonable risks to take advantage of those opportunities. Strategic management promotes organizational change within a stable framework of constant mission and goals.

Some of the benefits of strategic planning follow:

- Forces the organization to determine its long-run goals and devise an approach to accomplish them
- Promotes efficiency
- Provides a means of communication among the various hierarchical levels of the organization
- Develops management skills at all levels throughout the organization
- Provides managers with an improved sense of the needs of the organization and of its environmental constraints
- Increases the level of organizational creativity in addressing its problems
- Reduces the extent to which managers move from crisis to crisis
- Promotes the efficient use of resources and the financial health of the organization
- Results in goal setting and establishment of a vision for the organization
- Helps ensure that managers identify opportunities and take reasonable risks to take advantage of those opportunities
- Promotes organizational change within a stable framework of constant mission and goals

The strategic plan or long-range budget indicates which programs are to remain at a steady state, which are to be downsized or eliminated entirely, which are to be expanded, and which are to be added. This process gives impetus to specific program budgets in which a unit, department, or program undergoes a complete assessment.

Using a method such as ZBB, an organization's managers can systematically examine all of the implications of a program over its lifetime. The program can be compared with others that would achieve the same end. The program can also be assessed in terms of alternative ways to produce the output, alternative levels of quality, and alternative levels of quantity of output.

Program budget analyses can uncover unneeded costs in existing programs. There is waste in HCOs, as in virtually all organizations. Furthermore, program budgeting can help the organization to make effective choices as to how best to use limited resources. Trade-offs among various alternatives can be assessed more clearly with the increased information program budgets provide about the impact of different available options.

The organization can settle for a less-than-first-class bedside computer system but can also have new unit-based patient educational materials and Web-based educational materials. Alternatively, it can have a new first-rate bedside computer system and forgo development of Web-based materials. This textbook cannot say which of the choices would be best. However, there should be an awareness that alternatives do exist. The organization should not blindly get a first-rate bedside computer system because of internal political pressure and then simply concede that there is no money for more advanced patient educational capabilities. The alternatives should be considered and an explicit choice made.

Program budgeting techniques are equally effective for reviewing the operations of an ongoing unit and for evaluating a new program. The way a nursing unit performs its tasks may go unchanged from year to year. A ZBB review, however, can force the nurse manager to consider whether there are alternative ways or levels of effort that could be used to accomplish the unit's goals.

Performing a ZBB review for a nursing unit is expensive. It takes a substantial amount of time to evaluate all of the cost elements of a budget. It is much simpler to indicate that the next year's operating budget will be 5% more than that of the current year. Despite the flaws inherent in this approach, it is the path of least resistance and the one more often taken. However, the chances of making a significant positive gain for the organization are much higher when a thorough justification of each and every expenditure is undertaken. Managers tend to accept the status quo. Instead, organizations should position managers to spend less time on day-to-day routine activities and more time on innovation. Examining all aspects of a unit's operations can result in significant and lasting benefits for the unit and the entire organization.

Business plans are documents that are becoming essential for the introduction of new programs. Such plans help managers complete a comprehensive examination of a proposed program. By making such a thorough review, the manager and the organization gain an in-depth understanding of the program as well as its financial implications for the organization.

In today's health care environment, change is a given. HCOs are constantly faced with changing political, social, and regulatory demands. These pressures often place organizations in the position of responding quickly to an ever-changing environment. The uncertainty from these changes can cause managers and executives within them to feel like they are on a rollercoaster. However, having a longer-term view attained through strategic management enables the organization and its managers and leaders to respond in a manner that is consistent with its mission, vision, and goals.

Strategic management has broader implications than just for use in specific areas such as ZBB reviews or business plans. Managers should be creative in their applications. For example, there are many models for the delivery of nursing services. Each has financial, quality, and other implications. Nurse managers and executives who understand strategic management can apply its principles when their organization makes choices among alternative delivery care models. In this way, the choice made will reflect consideration of the wide range of factors that relate to that decision.

✳ KEY CONCEPTS

Strategic management   Process of setting the goals and objectives of the organization, determining the resources to be allocated to achieving those goals and objectives, and establishing policies concerning getting and using those resources. The current view of strategic management or strategic planning relies on the use of strategic thought by all managers in guiding all plans and actions of an organization. Strategic thought requires managers to balance the short-term objectives of their units or departments with a long-range vision for the organization. Nurse managers have a central role in strategic management under this new planning philosophy.

Goals and objectives   Goals are the broad, timeless ends of the organization meant to aid the organization in accomplishing its mission. Objectives are specific targets to be achieved to attain goals. Planning calls on each organization to establish a set of clear goals and objectives and a plan for achieving them.

Elements of a strategic plan   Basic elements of a strategic plan include:

- Mission statement
- Statement of long-term goals
- Statement of competitive strategy
- Statement of organizational policies
- Statement of needed resources
- Statement of key assumptions

Mission statement   Statement of the unit's, department's, or organization's purpose or reason for existence. The mission statement should be defined in such a way as to prevent the organization from exceeding its manageable boundaries but to encourage exploration within those boundaries.

Competitive strategy   Organization's plan for achieving its goals—specifically, what services will be provided and to whom. The development of this strategy relies to a great extent on a thorough internal and external review. What are the organization's strengths and weaknesses, its opportunities and threats?

Policy statements   Limiting statements indicating what managers can or cannot do as they work to carry out the organization's mission by attainment of goals and objectives.

Long-range budget (long-range plan)   Often referred to as the organization's strategic plan. Such plans generally cover a period of 3 to 5 years.

Program budgeting   Part of the overall strategic planning process that focuses on all costs and benefits associated with a specific program. A program budget combines a great amount of detailed information, cutting across departments, for a long-term period.

Zero-base budgeting (ZBB)   Popular program budgeting technique that gained fame for its analysis and justification of all costs. From a program budgeting perspective, ZBB is especially useful because of its strong focus on an examination of alternatives.

Business plan   Detailed plan for a proposed program, project, or service, including information to be used to assess the venture's financial feasibility. The plan should clearly state the objectives of the proposed project and provide a linkage that shows how the plan's objectives will lead to accomplishment of the organization's goal.

❊ SUGGESTED READINGS

Abrams R, Kleiner E: *The successful business plan: secrets and strategies*, ed 4, Palo Alto, Calif, 2003, Planning Shop.

Alemi F, Moore S, Hedrick L, et al: Rapid improvement teams, *Joint Comm J Qual Improve* 24(3):119–129, 1998.

Alexander J, Weiner B, Shortell S, et al: The role of organizational infrastructure in implementation of hospitals' quality improvement, *Hosp Topics* 84(1):11–20, 2006.

Anderson R, Ammarell N, Bailey D, et al: Quality improvement in long-term care. The power of relationship for high-quality long-term care, *J Nurs Care Qual* 20(2):103–106, 2005.

Arikian V: Total quality management: applications to nursing service, *J Nurs Adm* 21(6):46, 1991.

Arkebauer J: *Guide to writing a high-impact business plan*, New York, 1995, McGraw-Hill.

Asantewa D: Holistic budgeting: a process, *Info Outlook* 7(8):14–18, 2003.

Baier R, Gifford D, Patry G, et al: Ameliorating pain in nursing homes: a collaborative quality improvement project, *J Am Geriatr Soc* 52(12):1988–1995, 2004.

Bazerman M, Watkins M: Predictable surprises: the disasters you should have seen coming and how to prevent them, *Harv Bus Rev* 81(3):72–80, 2003.

Beauvais B, Wells R: Does money really matter? A review of the literature on the relationships between healthcare organization finances and quality, *Hosp Topics* 84(2):20–28, 2006.

Camillus J: *Strategic planning and management control: systems for survival and control*, Lexington, Mass, 1998, Lexington Books.

Castaneda-Mendez K: Value-based cost management: the foundation of a balanced performance measurement system, *J Healthc Qual* 19(4):6–9, 1997.

Clark J: Improving hospital budgeting and accountability: a best practice approach, *Healthc Financ Manag* 59(7):78–83, 2005.

Cortes T: Zero-based budgeting for a radiology service: a case study in outsourcing, *Hosp Cost Manag Account* 8(2):1–6, 1996.

Dillon R: *Zero-base budgeting for health care institutions*, Gaithersburg, Md, 1979, Aspen Publishers.

Drenkard K: Creating a future worth experiencing: nursing strategic planning in an integrated healthcare delivery system, *J Nurs Adm* 31(7/8):364–376, 2001.

Drenkard K: Invest the time to develop a "business" plan, *Pat Care Staff Rep* 2(1):6–7, 2002.

Finkler S, Ward D, Baker J: *Essentials of cost accounting for health care organizations*, ed 3, Boston, 2007, Bartlett & Jones.

Fredrickson J: *Perspectives on strategic management*, New York, 1990, Harper Business.

Fuchs V, Emanuel E: Health care reform: why? what? when? What it might take to effect comprehensive change, *Health Aff* 24(6):1399–1414, 2005.

Gitlow H, Gitlow S: *The Deming guide to quality and competitive position*, Englewood Cliffs, NJ, 1987, Prentice Hall.

Gladwell M: *The tipping point: how little things can make a big difference*, Boston, 2000, Little, Brown.

Hough D, Bolinger J: *Developing a managed care business plan*, Chicago, 1998, American Medical Association, p. 111.

Ingersol G, Witzel P, Smith T: Using organizational mission, vision, and values to guide professional practice model development and measurement of nurse performance, *J Nurs Adm* 35(2):86–93, 2005.

Kerfoot K: On leadership. Megatrends, the annual report, possibilities, *Nurs Econ* 24(1):47–49, 2006.

Kirk R: The big picture: total quality management and continuous quality improvement, *J Nurs Adm* 22(4):24–31, 1992.

Kleckner M: Blending hospital economics with quality of care: a case study (includes abstract), *Healthc Financ Manag* 58(12):64–68, 70, 2004.

Kovner, CT, Lusk EJ: The sustainability budgeting model: multiple mode flexible budgeting using sustainability as the synthesizing criterion, *Nurs Econ* 28(6):377–385, 2010.

Lynn M, Osborn D: Deming's quality principles: a health care application, *Hosp Health Serv Adm* 36(2):111–119, 1991.

Mackey T, Cole F, Lindenberg J: Quality improvement and changes in diabetic patient outcomes in an academic nurse practitioner primary care practice, *Am Acad Nurse Pract* 17(12):547–553, 2005.

Magiera F, McLean R: Strategic options in capital budgeting and program selection under fee-for-service and managed care, *Health Care Manag Rev* 21(4):7–17, 1996.

McKeon T: Performance measurement: integrating quality management and activity-based cost management, *J Nurs Adm* 26(4):45–51, 1996.

McLaughlin C, Kaluzny A: *Continuous quality improvement in health care*, Gaithersburg, Md, 1999, Aspen Publishers.

Nash D, Evans A: Physician and provider profiling. In Ransom S, Joshi M, Nash D, editors: *The health care quality book: vision, strategy and tools*, Chicago, 2005, Health Administration Press.

Nedd N, Nash M, Galindo-Ciocon D, Belgrave G: Quality improvement in long-term care. Guided growth intervention: from novice to expert through a mentoring program, *J Nurs Care Qual* 21(1):20–23, 2006.

Omachonu V: *Total quality and productivity management in health care organizations*, Norcross, Ga, 1991, Industrial Engineering and Management Press, Institute of Industrial Engineers.

Pace K, Marren J, Harrington C, Kluger M: Nursing counts. Focus on: quality improvement in home health care, *Am J Nurs* 106(1):38, 2006.

Papp E: Starting a business as a nurse consultant: practical considerations, *AAOHN J* 48(3):136–144, 2000.

Pelfrey S: Managing financial data, *Semin Nurse Manag* 5(1):25–30, 1997.

Plesek P: Section 1: Evidence-based quality improvement, principles, and perspectives. Quality improvement methods in clinical medicine, *Pediatrics* 103(1)(Suppl):203–213, 1999. Available at www.directedcreativity.com/pages/PlsekPeds.pdf. Accessed February 19, 2012.

Pyhrr P: *Zero-base budgeting: a practical management tool for evaluating expenses*, New York, 1973, Wiley-Interscience.

Ransom S, Joshi M, Nash D, editors: *The health care quality book: vision, strategy and tools*, Chicago, 2005, Health Administration Press.

Reinertsen J: Outcomes management and continuous quality improvement: the compass and the rudder, *Qual Rev Bull* 19(1):5–7, 1993.

Rosen J, Mittal V, Degenholtz H, et al: Organizational change and quality improvement in nursing homes: approaching success, *J Healthc Qual Prom Excel Healthc* 27(6):6–14, 21, 44, 2005.

Sales A, Moscovice I, Lurie N: Implementing CQI projects in hospitals, *Joint Comm J Qual Improve* 26(8):476–487, 2000.

Schmidt K, Beatty S: Quality improvement: the pursuit of excellence, *Qual Manag Health Care* 14(3):196–198, 2005.

Scott-Cawiezell J: Quality improvement in long-term care. Are nursing homes ready to create sustainable improvement? *J Nurs Care Qual* 20(3):203–207, 2005.

Seymour D, Guillett W: Connecting the dots: grounding quality improvement and cost cutting initiatives in strategic planning, *J Healthc Res Manag* 15(7):14–19, 1997.

Sorensen D, Sullivan D: Business. Managing trade-offs makes budgeting processes pay off, *Healthc Fin Manag* 59(11):54–58, 60, 2005.

Stiles R, Mick S: Components of the costs of controlling quality: a transaction cost economics approach, *Hosp Health Serv Adm* 42(2): 205–219, 1997.

Strasen L: *Key business skills for nurses*, Philadelphia, 1987, JB Lippincott.

Suver J, Neumann B, Boles K: *Management accounting for healthcare organizations*, ed 3, Westchester, Ill, 1992, Pluribus Press.

Turner S: Transitioning yourself into the new health care business, *Orthop Nurs* 17(2):30–32, 1998.

Wagner E, Glasgow R, Davis C, et al: Quality improvement in chronic illness care: a collaborative approach, *Joint Comm J Qual Improve* 27(2):63–80, 2001.

Walsh J: Quality improvement strategies for hypertension management: a systematic review, *Med Care* 44(7):646–657, 2006.

Weick K, Sutcliffe K: *Managing the unexpected*, San Francisco, 2001, Jossey-Bass.

West T: Comparing change readiness, quality improvement, and cost management among Veterans Administration, for-profit, and nonprofit hospitals, *J Health Care Fin* 25(1):46–58, 1998.

Budgeting Concepts

CHAPTER GOALS

The goals of this chapter are to:

- Define *budgeting* and *control*
- Describe some benefits of budgeting
- Introduce and describe the various types of budgets, including master, operating, capital, long-range, program, and cash
- Discuss the generation, justification, and evaluation of capital budget proposals
- Introduce the concepts of the time value of money, discounting, net present value, and internal rate of return

- Distinguish between revenue and expense and between cash inflows and outflows
- Outline the steps in cash budget preparation and provide a cash budget example
- Describe the budgeting process
- Provide an example of a budget timetable
- Discuss specific steps in the budgeting process
- In a technical appendix, the chapter discusses time-value-of-money computations

✳ INTRODUCTION

A *budget* is a plan. The plan is formalized (written down) and quantified (e.g., stated in dollars, another currency, or the number of patient days or other measure of the amount of service provided). It represents management's intentions or expectations. In financial terms, an organization-wide budget generally compares expected revenues with expected expenses to ascertain the organization's expected profit or loss for the coming year.

Preparation of a budget forces the organization's managers to plan ahead. Management experience has shown that, in general, actively managed organizations will do better than those that just let things happen. A budget forces managers to establish goals. Without goals, organizations tend to wander aimlessly, rarely improving the results of their operations or the services they offer.

By requiring managers to prepare a budget at least annually, organizations compel their management to forecast the future. Changes in nursing and medical practice, technology, and demographics can be anticipated and their impact predicted. For example, the manager should consider the changes in patient mix if a new manufacturer moves into the area and large numbers of factory workers are employed in the community. They should also consider the resource effects if a new program or service is added or if a competing health care facility opens across town. These considerations allow managers to anticipate changes that will affect the organization and to plan actions

accordingly. When one responds to changes after the fact, alternatives may be limited. By looking at the impact of changes during the planning phase, the broadest possible range of alternative actions can be considered. Often the result of careful planning is that more cost-effective approaches can be found and put into place.

In the budget process, after plans are established, an effort is made to meet or exceed the goals of the plans. This latter effort is referred to as the *control* process. Control of costs requires a concerted effort by both managers and staff. Control techniques such as variance analysis (and others discussed in Chapters 16 and 17) uncover problems that may have a negative financial impact on the organization and allow actions to be taken to correct those problems at an early stage.

Budgets can be used to provide both managers and staff with the motivation to work positively for the organization. They can also show how well both management and units or departments are performing. However, budgeting requires effort and commitment from all levels of management. Often a budget committee (which should include the chief nurse executive [CNE]) is formed to ensure maximum cooperation and coordination throughout the budget process.

Many organizations produce a "budget calendar" that indicates the various specific activities to be carried out in the budget process, identifies the responsible individuals (e.g., financial managers, unit or department managers, board of trustees), and provides deadlines for completion of each budget activity. Larger organizations have budget manuals. These manuals include uniform instructions and forms to be used throughout the organization, a copy of the budget calendar, and a statement of organizational mission. They also generally include a variety of other pieces of information relevant to the process of budget preparation. For instance, inflation rates, specific measurable goals, and an environmental statement are often included to help guide the process. Budget manuals or packages are institution-specific, differing substantially from one organization to another.

The budgeting process in any organization depends as much on the specific individuals working in that organization as it does on the formalized steps involved in budget preparation and use. The role of individuals in the budget process cannot be overemphasized. Organizations not only have their own forms and procedures but also tend to have specific philosophies of fiscal affairs. The amount of participation that any individual manager has in the budget process depends on the approach or philosophy of the organization's top management. Some organizations are very traditional and centralized and use a top-down approach, allowing unit managers very limited control over their budget. Other organizations are more decentralized and delegate substantially all budget preparation and control duties to the unit-level manager.

Teachers of budgeting often stress the importance of participation in the budget process by individuals at all levels in the organization. If the budget is expected to be a useful tool for managing, it must be realistic. It is often not possible for top-level managers to be aware of all of the specific circumstances and conditions that exist in the day-to-day operations throughout the organization. Unit managers have experience, judgment, and specific information about their units that let them provide valuable input to the budget.

❋ TYPES OF BUDGETS

Many managers tend to think of the budget as simply a cap on expenses that instructs them regarding how much they may spend. This is a very limited view of just the *operating budget*. The operating budget, in turn, is only a small part of the overall budget of the organization. A well-managed organization has a *master budget*. The master budget is a set of all of the major budgets in the organization. It generally includes the *operating budget*, a *long-range budget*, *program budgets*, a *capital budget*, and a *cash budget*. Some organizations use *product-line budgets*. From time to time, the organization will also need to budget for some additional special project that is not part of the organization's normal activities. In those cases, it will prepare a *special purpose budget*.

An operating budget typically plans for the revenues and expenses of the organization for the coming year. A long-range budget covers a period of 3 to 5 years. Program budgets look at specific programs that cut across a number of departments. Such budgets take a multi-year perspective. Capital budgets look at proposed equipment and building acquisitions that will be used by the organization for more than 1 year. Cash budgets look specifically at the organization's cash inflows and cash outflows. Product-line budgets focus on groupings of specific types of patients rather than on budgets for cost centers. Special purpose budgets are used to develop a plan for any specific special purpose not covered by one of the other types of budgets. Each of these will be discussed to lay the groundwork for discussions in future chapters.

Operating Budget

The operating budget is the plan for day-to-day operating revenues and expenses for the organization. It generally covers a period of 1 year. If the budget shows an excess of revenues over expenses, it means that the organization expects to make a *profit* from its activities for the year. If the organization is a for-profit company, some of the profits can be paid to the owners of the company in the form of a *dividend*. However, even not-for-profit organizations need to earn profits. In their case, profits can be used to replace worn-out equipment and old buildings or to expand the services available to the community. If any health care organization (HCO), for-profit or not-for-profit, consistently fails to earn profits, it will not be able to add new technologies, programs, or services and continue to provide high-quality care. Chapter 13 provides a detailed discussion of the operating budget and its preparation.

Long-Range Budgets

Budgets help managers plan for the future. Operating budgets give a detailed plan but just for the coming year. Many changes in an organization require a long lead time and take a number of years to be fully implemented. To avoid suffering from shortsightedness, many organizations use a long-range plan or budget. Such a budget is often referred to as a strategic plan (strategic plans are defined and discussed in Chapter 11). Such 3-, 5-, or even 10-year plans allow management to temporarily ignore the trees and focus on the forest. This is a very important endeavor for organizations because it helps them think through questions such as: Where is the organization relative to its peers? What improvements can or must be made over the next 3, 5, or 10 years? What must be done each year to move toward those goals?

In many organizations, managers tend to look at the current year and then add an increase for inflation and produce a budget for the next year. The problem with this approach is that it contains no vision. There is no way to make a major leap forward because what has been done in the past is simply being projected into the future. If one would like to be able to look back 5 years from now and say, "Look at how far we have come," it is necessary to have a way to make major strides forward. Otherwise, 5 years into the future, organizational leaders will look back and wonder why the organization has made little, if any, advancement.

That is where long-range or strategic plans are helpful. Their focus is not on how to get through next year but on the overriding organization goals and on the major changes that ought to be made over the coming years to achieve those goals. Long-range plans help to give the organization a sense of commitment to the future. Such plans serve a vital function in allowing the organization to prepare each year's detailed operating budget on the basis of an overall sense of purpose and direction.

The operating budget becomes more than just next year's survival plan; it becomes a link between where the organization has been and where it is going. Long-range budgets are discussed as part of strategic management in Chapter 11.

Program Budgets

Program budgets are special budgeting efforts analyzing specific programs. Generally, the orientation is toward evaluating a planned new program or closely examining an existing program rather than merely planning the revenues and expenses for a program in the coming year. Often the program involved is in some way optional. The purpose of the program budget is to make a decision. Should the new program be undertaken or not? Should an existing program be continued, modified, or discontinued altogether?

Program budgets are often developed for specific programs as a result of the long-range budgeting process. The long-range budget or strategic plan may determine that three tertiary care services should be added over the next 5 years. Because new services often require 1 year to plan and sometimes more than 1 year to implement once the planning phase is complete, one result of the long-range plan may be to immediately select one new service to be added. Frequently, new services involve labor and equipment from numerous departments. By setting up a program budget process for the new service, all of the information related to the addition of that service can be considered and evaluated.

Because program budgets often cut across departments, they generally must be developed with committee input from at least the major departments that will be affected by the service. Program budgets also cut across years. The financial impact of the service needs to be assessed not just in the coming year but over a reasonably long period. Because the operating budget is a 1-year budget, this is another reason for special budget treatment for new programs or services.

In recent years, business plans have become a vital tool for program budgeting. The elements of such plans are discussed along with long-range budgets and other aspects of program budgeting in Chapter 11.

Capital Budgets

A capital budget is a plan for acquisition of long-term investments. These investments can range from those as small as acquiring a new intravenous infusion pump to projects as large as completely rebuilding a hospital at a new location. The key element in capital budgeting is that the building or piece of equipment being acquired has a lifetime that extends beyond the year of purchase. Capital budget items are often referred to as *capital assets, long-term investments, capital investments,* or *capital acquisitions.* The money used to purchase long-term investments is often referred to as *capital.*

These assets are treated separately from operating budget expenses because of their multi-year nature. They are only partly used up in any one year, and in any one year, the organization earns only part of the revenues that the capital assets generate over their useful lifetimes. If these assets were included in the operating budget, their entire acquisition cost would be compared with revenues only in the year the asset was purchased. Many capital assets that are good financial investments over their entire useful lifetime would appear to lose money when only one year's worth of revenues is considered. By having a separate capital budget, multi-year assets can be evaluated on the basis of their implications for the organization over their entire useful life.

Capital assets are generally purchased to replace older items of a similar nature, to improve productivity (substituting equipment for more expensive labor), to improve quality of care (often the addition of newer technology), or to provide needed equipment for a new service or expansion of an existing service. A variety of other reasons to acquire capital assets will also arise from time to time, such as the need for equipment that will improve employee or patient safety.

Capital assets are often quite expensive. However, high cost is not a required element for an asset to be classified and treated as a capital asset. The only requirement is that the capital asset must be able to provide useful service beyond the year it is first put into use. For pragmatic purposes, most organizations set a minimum dollar limit for inclusion in the capital budget. It is not worth the extra effort to analyze and track relatively inexpensive items over a period of years. Items that have a low cost are treated as part of the operating budget even if they have a multi-year life. Most HCOs have a minimum cost requirement of anywhere from $2,500 to $5,000 for an item to be included in the capital budget.

Generation of Capital Budget Proposals

The starting point in the capital budgeting process is the identification of proposed investments. The nurse manager in a home health agency may propose the acquisition of several company cars to reduce travel time between patients, because available public transportation is inadequate for efficient use of staff time. The nurse manager in a hospital's coronary intensive care unit (CICU) may request a particular piece of equipment to improve the efficiency of care delivery, or the nurse manager in the operating room may request a particular piece of equipment because a leading surgeon has requested it.

Exhibit 12–1 presents an example of the type of worksheet a nurse manager or executive would use to list capital proposals. The first column represents the manager's priority ranking for the request. The most important acquisition is ranked number 1. The second column indicates the type of capital item being requested. These include *c*onstruction or *r*emodeling (CR), *r*eplacement of an *e*xisting item (RE), *r*eplacement and *u*pgrading of an existing item (RU), an item that is an *a*ddition to *s*imilar existing items and adds to their capacity (AS), or an *a*dditional item that is *n*ot currently available in the unit (AN). The third column is the quantity being requested. For example, you might want to purchase one CICU bedside monitor to replace one that has not been working well, or you might want to purchase 20 monitors to replace all of the monitors in the CICU. The unit cost in the fifth column is the cost for each unit to be acquired, such as the cost per monitor, and the extended cost in the sixth column is the unit cost multiplied by the quantity.

✳ EXHIBIT 12–1

CAPITAL BUDGET WORKSHEET

Fiscal Year_____

COST CENTER _____

PRIOR. #	TYPE: CR/RE/RU AS/AN	EQUIP.	DESCRIPTION	UNIT COST	EXTENDED COST	COMMENTS

In proposing a capital acquisition, the manager must provide financial information with respect to the asset. A required piece of information is the likely cost of the asset. In addition, to the extent possible, information must be collected about how much cash will be spent or received each year over the life of the investment or project. The difference between the cash received and the cash spent in any given year is referred to as the *net cash flow* for that year.

The nurse manager or executive can generally seek the aid of financial managers of the organization for the specific estimates of annual cash inflows and outflows. Cash inflows can be particularly difficult because the entire billing process is often handled outside the control of the nurse manager or executive. On the other hand, with respect to estimating costs, the nurse manager or executive is more likely than any financial manager to be able to estimate what resources will be needed and when. The payroll and purchasing departments can be a great aid in converting the raw resource information into dollars based on projected salaries and prices. This estimating process should be done separately for each year during which the capital asset is expected to provide useful service. Having information on the annual cash flows as well as the acquisition cost will make it easier for the organization's managers to make a decision about whether or not to acquire the asset.

Justification of Capital Requests

Sufficient resources are not usually available to allow an organization to acquire all of the items it desires. The capital budget facilitates choices that have to be made in deciding how to spend the organization's limited resources. In describing proposed capital expenditures, the nurse manager or executive provides a priority ranking. It is also appropriate to justify each requested purchase by giving a description of the item, its cost, its impact on operating expenses and revenues, and the justification for acquiring it. Exhibit 12–2 is an example of the documentation needed for a justification of a capital asset acquisition.

The justification should be thorough and should specifically indicate the consequences if funding for the item is not made available. Equipment costs include not only the purchase price but also shipping and installation. Construction costs should be reviewed by the planning and engineering departments. In all cases, vendor estimates or proposals should be included if possible. The impact on operating costs should include salaries, fringe benefit costs, maintenance costs or maintenance contracts, utilities, supplies, and any interdepartmental impact. Incremental revenue to be generated by the capital asset, if any, should be described and estimated to the extent possible.

Evaluation of Capital Budget Proposals

The capital budgets for all departments are evaluated in light of available cash. An investment that seems to make a lot of sense to a clinical department manager may have to be deferred for a year, or indefinitely, simply because the organization does not have enough cash to make the purchase.

✳ EXHIBIT 12–2

CAPITAL JUSTIFICATION FORM

Fiscal Year _____

COST CENTER _____   **PRIORITY ITEM** _____

Description of item or project:

_____

Justification:

_____

Construction Costs: **Equipment Costs:**

Fees   _____   Purchase Price _____

Construction   _____   Installation   _____

Contingency   _____

Total   _____

Date of Estimate _____   By _____

_____

Impact on Operational Expenses:

_____

Impact on Revenues:

_____

Even if sufficient cash is available to make a capital acquisition, the organization may choose not to acquire the item because of its financial evaluation of the asset. In recent years, the financial analysis of capital assets has grown more sophisticated. Organizations have started to adopt investment analysis techniques used in other industries.

One widely used approach is the *payback* method. The payback approach calculates how many years it will take for the profits from a capital expenditure to repay the initial cash outlay. The less time it takes to recover the initial investment, the better the project.

The payback method does have some severe weaknesses. First, it ignores what happens after the payback period is over. Thus, one might fail to select a very profitable project that does not earn substantial profits until after the payback period in favor of a less profitable project with a shorter payback period. Second, it ignores the timing of cash flows within the payback period. Two projects would be considered equal if they both have a 3-year payback period. However, if one pays back the bulk of the investment in the second year and the other pays back the bulk of the invested cash in the third year, they are not equally good.

Another approach that is often used in evaluating proposed capital projects is *return on investment* (ROI). The ROI uses a ratio to help determine whether an investment should be made. The ratio is calculated as follows:

$$ROI = \frac{Profits\ from\ Investment}{Amount\ Invested}$$

The manager would consider a project for which the ROI is positive, and the higher the ROI, the better. If a manager is comparing the ROI of several alternative projects, the projects with a higher ROI should be considered unless there are other compelling reasons to choose a lower ranked project (e.g., improved health care for a disadvantaged group, goodwill in the community, reputation). The advantage of using the ROI method is that it is very easy to calculate; the disadvantage is that similar to the payback method, the ROI does not take into account the timing of cash flows.

Both the payback method and ROI are often used for the first appraisal of a project. If a proposed investment cannot pay back its cost within a reasonable period or if it has a negative or low ROI, it should be rejected to the extent the decision is based on financial merit. If an investment passes the payback test or has a positive ROI, a more sophisticated evaluation is still needed to determine if a specific proposal is acceptable.

The more sophisticated methods used to overcome the problems of the payback and the simple ROI methods are called *discounted cash flow methods.* These methods consider the cash flow over the full life of the capital asset rather than just the payback period. They also consider the timing of cash flows or the *time value of money.* The time value of money is a concept based on the notion that "a dollar today is worth more than a dollar tomorrow." In other words, money paid or received at different points in time is not equally valuable. One would always prefer to receive money sooner and to pay it out later. By receiving money sooner, one can use the money for current needs or invest it and earn interest.

When a nurse manager or executive looks at alternative investment opportunities, there must be consideration of not only how much the organization will put in and how much it will get out but also *when* money will be spent and received. Financial managers can calculate the economic viability of a project by using discounted cash flow techniques. *Discounting* is the reverse of compounding interest. A $100 amount today would be worth $121 in 2 years with 10% compound interest. In the first year, $10 of interest is earned on the $100 investment (i.e., 10% of $100 = $10). In the second year, the $10 of interest earned in the first year itself earns interest. Therefore, the original $100 plus the $10 of interest earned in the first year equals a total of $110. Ten percent interest in the second year would be $11 (i.e., $110 × 10%). The $110 plus the $11 would total $121. When interest earns interest, it is referred to as *compound interest.* In just the reverse process, $121 received 2 years from now would be worth just $100 today if one were to *discount* the interest earned in the two intervening years.

Discounted cash flow techniques are designed to take future receipts and discount the interest to find out what those receipts would be worth today. The receipts can then be compared with current cash outlays to determine if a project is financially worthwhile. The two most common discounted cash flow models are *net present value* (NPV) and *internal rate of return* (IRR).

The NPV approach requires the manager to indicate a specific interest rate, called the *discount rate.* It is sometimes called the *required rate of return.* Under this method, the cash outlay to acquire an asset must be recovered, plus a return at least equal to the discount rate. The discount rate is usually set at the rate that the bank would charge the organization if it borrowed money. Thus, the capital asset must recover not only its cost but also the interest the organization would have to pay the bank if it borrowed the money necessary to buy the asset. If the project earns a positive NPV, it is earning at more than its cost plus interest. Therefore, it is profitable. If the NPV is negative, the project does not recover the investment plus the interest cost, so it is unprofitable.

The IRR method does not require the manager to indicate a specific discount rate. Instead, the method looks at how much cash is required to acquire the capital asset and how much cash will be received and determines the rate of return (called the *internal rate of return*) the asset earns. If that rate is higher than the organization's discount rate, acquisition of the asset is financially acceptable. Obtaining an IRR greater than the discount rate is one of several hurdles that must be passed before a decision is made to acquire the asset. An organization might decide not to acquire a capital asset even if it has a favorable IRR. There may be other proposed capital acquisitions that are either more profitable or more critical for improving the quality of care provided, and the organization will likely have only a limited amount of money available to spend on capital for the coming year. The decision about whether to acquire a capital asset or not must be based on a number of considerations The technical details of calculating NPV and IRR are discussed in the Appendix to this chapter.

Many times HCOs acquire capital assets that cannot be connected clearly to specific inflows of cash. Replacing old monitors in the intensive care unit with a newer type may improve quality of care rather than increasing revenues. The use of formalized, quantitative approaches to capital investment evaluation should not and does not rule out the acquisition of assets that cannot be evaluated on a profit basis or even those that seem to result in losses. The evaluation of capital budget requests should consider both the quantitative and qualitative benefits that any asset provides the organization and its community.

Product-Line Budgets

A product (or service) line is a group of patients with some commonality that allows them to be grouped together, such as a common diagnosis. Budgeting in HCOs is largely focused on departments and units. In hospitals, for example, radiology has a budget, dietary has a budget, and nursing has a budget. However, there may also be a budget for cardiac patients or women's services or other product-line groupings of patients.

Prospective payment, pay-for-performance, bundled payments, and newer organizational structures have brought about a focus on budgeting for groups of patients based on a cost per case or service. Because the Diagnosis Related Group (DRG) system has a fixed payment rate for each group of patients, it becomes of great managerial interest to be able to budget for the planned revenues and expenses of specific patient groups. Such an approach has the potential to reveal the profitability of different types of patients.

The move toward product-line budgeting has also gained impetus from the active pressure by managed care organizations to negotiate discounted rates for providing care to specific groups of patients, especially in hospitals. It is difficult to negotiate sensible revenue rates unless the related costs of the patients are known. HCOs have been moving in a product-line budgeting direction while not abandoning departmental budgets. Product-line costing was discussed in Chapter 9.

Cash Budgets

Cash is the lifeblood of any organization. Survival depends on the ability to maintain an adequate supply of cash to meet monetary obligations of the organization as they come due.

Operating budgets focus on the revenues and expenses of the organization. If the organization is expected to lose money, that will be reflected in the operating budget. It is possible, however, for the organization to have a cash crisis even if it is not losing money. Many expenses an organization incurs are paid in the present. Wages are typically paid at least monthly and frequently biweekly or weekly. However, revenues may take several months to collect because of the internal lags in processing patient bills and the external lags before insurers such as Blue Cross or Medicare make payment. Thus, an organization can literally run out of cash even though it is making a profit!

Another cash problem relates to major capital expenses. Suppose the organization budgets to add a wing for $30 million, and it is expected to have a 20-year life. The full $30 million will not be an operating budget expense in the coming year's budget. However, the entire $30 million will have to be paid in cash in the coming year.

For these reasons, a cash budget is prepared. Cash budgets plan for the monthly receipt of cash and disbursement of cash from the organization. If a shortage is predicted for any given month, appropriate plans can be made for short-term bank financing or longer term bond financing (see Chapters 19 and 20).

Cash budgeting is as vital as program, capital, and operating budgets to the survival and well-being of the organization. For this reason, the nurse manager should have a reasonable understanding of cash budgets and the cash budgeting process. In addition, cash budget constraints often force a need for modifications in the budgets nurse managers prepare. Although the organization's managers should pursue various ways to get the cash for worthwhile investments—whether they are worthwhile because they are profitable or simply because they are good for the patients—there is a responsibility to the well-being of the organization not to spend the money until it is first determined that there will be sufficient cash available.

Cash Budget Preparation

In HCOs, the cash budget is generally prepared for the entire coming year on a monthly basis. Each month begins with a starting cash balance. The expected cash receipts for the month are added to this. These receipts may be broken down into categories such as inpatient, outpatient, other operating, and non-operating or by payer (e.g., Medicare, Medicaid, Blue Cross, other insurers, self-pay patients, donors, cafeteria sales). The starting cash balance is added to the total receipts to get a subtotal of available cash.

Expected cash payments are subtracted from the available cash. The principal categories of payments include salaries, payments to suppliers, payments for capital acquisitions, and payments on loans. The result of subtracting total payments from the available cash is a tentative cash balance. This balance is considered tentative because the organization will generally have a minimum desired cash balance at the end of each month. That minimum balance is used for cash payments at the beginning of the next month and serves as a safety net for any required but unexpected cash outlays.

If the tentative balance exceeds the minimum desired balance, the excess can be invested. If the tentative cash balance is less than the minimum desired balance, the organization will borrow funds to meet the minimum level if its credit is good enough. The final cash balance is the tentative cash balance less any amount invested or plus any amount borrowed. The ending cash balance for one month becomes the starting balance for the next month.

Cash Budget Example

A hypothetical example of a cash budget for the first quarter of a year is presented in Table 12–1. In the example, the beginning cash balance for January is $20,000. With the $385,000 expected in receipts during January, there is $405,000 available in cash. With expected disbursements of $375,000, the tentative cash balance is $30,000. Assuming that $20,000 is desired as a safety cushion, there is $10,000 available to invest. In February, cash payments have risen by $25,000 to a total of $400,000, but cash receipts have risen even more. The result is that an additional $18,000 is available for short-term investment.

In March, cash receipts are down and cash payments are up. What could logically cause this result? Does it indicate a serious problem? Quite possibly not. It is reasonable to assume that during December, substantially fewer elective procedures were done because of the Christmas holiday. The March cash receipts from Medicaid, Medicare, and Blue Cross are likely to be influenced by what happened in December. On the other hand, because January, February, and March may have colder weather, they are quite possibly very busy months, with high salary payments for overtime and per diem or agency nurses. Thus, it is not surprising to see lower cash receipts in a given month and at the same time see cash payments rising during that month. Frequently, HCOs find that in any given month, their payments reflect that month's activity, but their receipts are more influenced by what happened in earlier months.

The March tentative balance indicates a cash deficit of $27,000. In addition, there is a desired $20,000 ending balance. The organization needs $47,000 of additional cash for March. This need can be met in several ways. The organization could simply borrow $47,000. More likely, the $10,000 invested in January and the $18,000 invested in February will be used to reduce the amount needed to $19,000; then the $19,000 will be borrowed. In Table 12–1, the $28,000 from March noted in the *Less amount invested* row indicates a use of money that was previously invested.

Planning for necessary borrowing should take place well in advance. The plan developed should also include a projection of when it will be possible to repay the loan. Lenders are much more receptive to an organization's needs if it has specific plans and projections than if it simply tries to borrow money when an immediate cash shortage becomes apparent. From the lender's perspective, an organization that can plan reasonably well is more likely to be able to repay a loan than one that does not even know several months in advance that a cash shortage is likely.

✳ **TABLE 12–1** *Cash Budget for One Quarter*

	January	February	March
Starting cash balance	$ 20,000	$ 20,000	$ 20,000
Expected receipts			
Medicare	$120,000	$140,000	$115,000
Medicaid	80,000	90,000	75,000
Blue Cross	90,000	90,000	85,000
Other insurers	42,000	40,000	45,000
Self-pay	40,000	38,000	41,000
Philanthropy	5,000	10,000	8,000
Other	8,000	10,000	9,000
Total receipts	$385,000	$418,000	$378,000
Available cash	$405,000	$438,000	$398,000
Less expected payments			
Labor costs	$170,000	$180,000	$190,000
Suppliers	25,000	30,000	40,000
Capital acquisitions	0	10,000	15,000
Payments on loans	180,000	80,000	180,000
Total payments	$375,000	$400,000	$425,000
Tentative cash balance	$ 30,000	$ 38,000	$ (27,000)
Less amount invested	(10,000)	(18,000)	28,000
Plus amount borrowed			19,000
Final cash balance	$ 20,000	$ 20,000	$ 20,000

Special Purpose Budgets

A budget is a plan. There is not a great deal of rigidity in the definition of a budget. Therefore, there is also not a great limitation placed on the types of possible budgets. Any HCO can prepare a budget for any activity for which it desires a plan.

In recent years, a number of HCOs have offered screening for high cholesterol, colon cancer, diabetes, and human immunodeficiency virus (HIV) infection. In some cases, these screenings have been free; in others, there has been a charge. What will it cost to provide the service for free (i.e., to help the community and at the same time get some favorable press)? How much would an HCO have to charge to just cover the costs of such a program?

These programs are often not part of the yearly operating budget. They are special programs put together in response to a current need or as a public relations effort. A special purpose budget can be prepared any time a plan is needed for some activity that is not already budgeted as part of one of the ongoing budget processes. The budget does not have to have any formal system or set of forms, but it often makes use of some of the techniques used in the budgeting process (e.g., determining payback). It is desirable to anticipate the impact on staffing and on the morale of the staff. One would want to specify the resources needed for the special program and determine if a profit, loss, or neither is anticipated. The key to development of a special purpose budget is to rationally consider all of the human and financial consequences of the proposed activity.

✳ THE BUDGET PROCESS

Although a budget is simply a plan, the budgeting process in HCOs has become quite complex. To compile all of the information necessary for the organization to complete a master budget, most HCOs require completion of a number of complicated documents. Often a budget timetable is developed that outlines the deadlines for completion of various parts of the budget process.

Throughout the budget process, it is important to remember that the budget is carried out by all employees of the organization. Therefore, it is essential to involve all employees—especially nursing staff—in all aspects of budgeting. Their input should be solicited as the budget is prepared, as it is implemented and carried out, and after the fact as well.

One of the first steps that must be taken in the annual budgeting process is the establishment of the foundations for budget preparation. The foundations of the budgeting process consist of an environmental scan; a statement of general goals, objectives, and policies; a list of organization-wide assumptions; specification of program priorities; and a set of specific, measurable operating objectives. The information developed in these foundations provides the direction needed by unit and department managers in preparing their own budgets. In addition, strategic plans and program budgets must be developed early in the process to provide further input needed by managers in completing budgets for specific parts of the organization.

After that information is available, unit and department managers prepare budgets for their individual areas. That information in turn is used to compile a cash budget. After the initial round of budget preparation, it is often found that budget requests exceed resources available to the organization. Negotiation and revisions follow in an attempt to arrive at an acceptable budget. After a budget has been approved, the organization must work to control results and keep to the plan as closely as possible.

Budget Timetable

It is important to have a plan for the planning process itself. Managers should have a road map that tells them what steps must be taken in the planning process and when they should be undertaken. Table 12–2 presents a sample budget calendar or timetable. Each organization will have its own timetable. In small organizations, the entire process described by the timetable may take only several weeks. In large hospitals, the budgeting process often takes more than 6 months from start to finish.

Just as the length of time to complete the budget process varies from organization to organization, so do the specific elements of the budget timetable. Table 12–2 assumes a budget process for an organization with a July 1 through June 30 fiscal year. Different organizations may have fiscal year timetables, such as an October 1 through September 30 fiscal year. This sample timetable lays out a general plan for completing certain budget-related activities, and it reflects the complex nature of the process. It also highlights the importance of deadlines along the way to ensure that tasks are completed to obtain the necessary approvals.

The first step is the appointment of the supervisory budget committee. This committee is usually selected by the chief executive officer but may be appointed by the board. It is especially important for the CNE to be a member of this committee. This selection process should take place as early as feasible, and the committee should meet promptly. In this example, it is assumed that the committee first meets no later than January, a full 6 months before the next fiscal year. The committee must ensure that department heads will have the information needed to prepare their budgets. In this example, 2 months is allowed for that process.

During the month of March, the strategic plan must be reviewed and specific programs considered. The decisions regarding these programs must be known early in the budget process so that each department head can take the impact of new programs or of program changes into account in preparing their operating and capital budgets. In actuality, the strategic plan and new programs are generally considered at some length even before the budget process begins. The month of March in this example is used to finalize decisions based on months of deliberations, data collection, and analysis.

Unit managers will have started preparing their budgets in early March. However, the revisions to the strategic plan and the new program budgets may result in some changes. This leaves just 2 weeks for unit nurse managers to finish preparing a first draft of their unit's budget. This is followed by a brief but intense period of negotiation between the nursing department and its units. In this example, only 1 week is available for this negotiation process, but in reality, this process is usually allowed considerably more time. If this period of time can be expanded, there would be less likelihood of an atmosphere of crisis and more time for reasoned discussions.

The nursing department has 1 week in this timetable to compile all of the unit budgets into a final nursing department budget. Finance has 2 weeks to take the information from all of the hospital budgets and develop a cash budget. One month is then allowed for organization-wide negotiation and budget revision. If all goes well, the budget can be approved by the board at its June meeting so it can be put into effect July 1. Even with this 7-month process, delays would not be unusual (especially in negotiation and revision), which may prevent the final approval of a budget by July 1. To avoid such a situation, the process could be started earlier. However, to start the process any earlier would mean that the information collected at the very start of the budget process would be outdated by the start of the year.

Because many aspects of the budgeting process cannot be undertaken without information generated by one of the previous activities, the budget timetable becomes a crucial guide in the budget process. Failure to meet one deadline may have an impact on all of the remaining deadlines.

Statement of Environmental Position

No organization exists in a vacuum. The community, its economy, shifting demographics, inflation, the role of a key employer, the socioeconomic setting, and other external factors play vital roles in the organization's success or failure. Each organization must understand its position within the community and its relative strengths and weaknesses. Based on knowledge of the needs of the community, the characteristics of the population, the existing competition, and other similar factors, the organization can determine its relative strengths and weaknesses and set its overall goals and objectives.

The lessons of strategic management (see Chapter 11) tell us that it is inadequate to review the environment only when the strategic plan is being formulated once every 3 to 5 years.

✳ **TABLE 12–2** *Sample Budget Timetable*

Activity	Responsibility	Deadline
1. Appointment of budget committee	Chief executive officer	December
2. First meeting of budget committee	Budget committee chair	January
3. Complete budget foundations activities and communicate to department heads	Budget committee	February 28
4. Complete long-range and program budgets	Budget committee and subcommittees	March 31
5. Unit capital and operating budgets	Unit managers	April 15
6. Negotiation between nursing units and nursing administration	Chief nurse executive	April 22
7. Compilation of all nursing unit budgets	Chief nurse executive	April 30
8. Development of cash budget	Chief financial officer	May 15
9. Negotiation and revision process	All managers	June 15
10. Approval and implementation	Board of trustees; all managers	June 16

Each year, the external environment must be evaluated, and changes in the environment must be factored into the planning process.

What data can a nurse manager collect to contribute to the organization's environmental review? Although much of the demographic data will be collected by marketing and other nonclinical staff, nurse managers can contribute critical information. For example, they can get a sense of changing physician attitudes toward the use of the organization's facilities as opposed to a competitor's. Based on their industry contacts, they may be aware of changes taking place at other organizations that will affect the competitiveness of their facilities. Information of this type provides part of the overall picture that the organization requires to correctly assess its position in the community.

The annual environmental analysis serves as a good review of where the organization is and where it is possible to go. On the basis of this review, the budgets prepared by its managers are more likely to merge the organization's desired long-term direction with its range of reasonable possible actions. The result should be a plan that is within the organization's capabilities and strives to achieve its strategic goals.

General Goals, Objectives, and Policies

After the organization's position in the environment is understood, the overall goals of the organization can be established. These goals are broad, long-term objectives, reassessed in light of the organization's strengths and weaknesses. It is not likely that goals will change annually. Over time, however, factors may arise that will cause goals to change.

For example, based on the environmental review, a home health agency may decide that the adjacent communities are underserved and that it is consistent with its mission to initiate a 5-year period of geographic expansion. A nursing home may set a goal of establishing a life-care community. A hospital may decide to phase out its maternity service.

The key to long-run goal setting is that it is basically more of a *qualitative* direction-setting process than a quantitative exercise with specific numerical objectives. The detailed numbers can be worked out later. First, the overall direction must be set. The overall goals, objectives, and policies of the organization may not change each year. They should be reviewed annually, however, if only to remind budget preparers about these broader considerations in making decisions about specific items.

Organization-Wide Assumptions

Throughout the budget process, it will be necessary for all managers to work on the basis of some explicit assumptions. How large will salary increases be during the next year? What will be the impact of inflation on the purchase price of supplies? Will the government change its policies with respect to reimbursement of Medicare and Medicaid patients? Probably the most crucial assumptions concern workload. What will be the occupancy or patient volume in the coming year? These assumptions are critical in the budgeting process and must be prepared annually.

Specification of Program Priorities

The next step is to establish a set of priorities for the entire organization. It is not unusual for the strategic plan, program budget, and capital budget to contain proposed spending for more things than the organization will be able to afford. There is a tendency to want to achieve all elements of a long-range plan immediately. When it becomes clear that the organization cannot do everything, a choice must be made between what is done and what is postponed.

It is advisable to try to set a generalized hierarchy of priorities at an early stage before detailed program budgets are developed. When it is necessary to make choices, top management can use the formalized guidelines that have been developed from the perspective of long-term growth and development, as opposed to letting "power politics" rule the budgeting process. Prioritization should be designed so that resources are allocated to areas that best promote the organization's long-term goals.

Specific, Measurable Operating Objectives

One of the most frustrating elements of budgeting for unit and department managers occurs when they are expected to develop a budget, totally unaided by any communicated guidelines, and then find the budget rejected because it does not provide for adequate achievement of objectives such as improved efficiency or reduced cost per patient day.

Organizations should provide a set of specific, measurable objectives that the budget should accomplish. This set of objectives should be communicated before the units and departments prepare their budgets. Managers can then attempt to prepare a budget that achieves those objectives. If the objectives are unattainable, managers can be prepared to explain why they believe that is the case.

The established objectives should be consistent with the overall general policies and goals of the organization, but they should be much more specific. For example, staffing reductions of 5% or ceilings on spending increases of 3% provide firm, specific objectives.

Budget Preparation

After the foundations have been laid, the organization can establish its various budgets. Strategic plans and program budgets must be completed first. Decisions made about new programs or changes in existing programs will have a specific impact on the capital and operating costs of the various departments throughout the institution. After that information is available, the next step in the budget process is preparation of unit and departmental budgets. The operating and capital budgets are generally prepared at the same time. Decisions concerning one budget are also likely to affect the other. For example, if the capital budget includes computer upgrades for the nurses' station, there may be some impact on staffing.

Having completed an operating and a capital budget, the next step in the budget process is preparation of a cash budget by the finance office. This is followed by budget negotiation and revision.

Budget Negotiation and Revision

As a result of limitations on the resources available to HCOs, budgets often cannot be accepted as submitted. Some needs will be so critical that certain departments will have to receive larger-than-average increases. However, such increases may necessitate cuts in other departments. This results in a series of negotiations, with managers having to defend why their proposed budgets should not be cut. This creates substantial complexity, because most of the budgets that constitute the organization's master budget are interrelated. Changes in one type of budget can have direct ramifications on the other budgets of the organization.

For example, the capital budget for the various units and departments of the organization cannot be finalized until all program budgets have been prepared. This is because a new program may require departments to purchase additional capital items. The operating budget, in turn, must contain revenues and expenses related to capital items to be purchased during the coming year. And the cash budget cannot be prepared until after the operating budget is established.

The cash budget may show an unacceptable cash shortfall. This will necessitate a reevaluation of which programs and capital budget items provide the most benefit and which can be postponed or disapproved. These changes may result in an acceptable set of budgets that constitute the master budget. On the other hand, there may be so many vital capital expenditures that it is preferable to go back and increase revenues or cut the operating budget expenses. Or perhaps more borrowing will be planned.

Eventually, negotiation with all departments, followed by budget revisions, will result in a budget that top management feels is acceptable. Such a budget may be far from optimal. However, it represents the overall management attempt to accomplish organizational goals to the extent possible, given the limited resources available to the organization. The completed budget is sent to the board for review and approval.

Control and Feedback

The last steps in the budget process are control and feedback. Control relates to actions taken to help the organization follow its plan. Feedback relates to using actual results to improve the accuracy and usefulness of future budgets.

The control process is one in which managers attempt to keep the organization operating in an efficient manner. Much of the control process centers on variance analysis, which is discussed in Chapters 16 and 17. Variances compare actual results with the budget. The underlying causes of differences between actual results and the budget are determined. If the cause is something managers can control, actions are taken to eliminate the variance in the coming months. If the causes are beyond the control of managers, that information goes into the feedback process.

Feedback should provide any information about actual results, which is then used to improve future plans. During the year, many things will not happen according to budgeted plans. Some variations from the budget will be attributable to random uncontrollable events that establish no pattern. Other actual results will indicate that certain factors were not adequately considered in making the current budget. Those factors must be given more weight in the preparation of the next budget. Other elements will simply change from past patterns. Those changes will also have to be accounted for in future budgets.

✳ IMPLICATIONS FOR NURSE MANAGERS AND EXECUTIVES

Budgeting consists of planning and controlling. The planning phase of the budget process requires that all managers and executives think ahead, anticipate changes, establish goals, forecast the future, examine alternatives, communicate goals, and coordinate plans. The controlling phase of budgeting requires that managers work to keep actual results close to the plan, motivate employees, evaluate performance of staff and units, alert the organization to major variances, take corrective actions, and provide feedback for future planning.

Each organization has its own approach to budgeting and its own philosophies regarding the budget process. Some HCOs treat budgeting as a highly centralized process. That approach tends to generate frustration by the managers asked to carry out the budget. Other organizations call for more participation by managers throughout the organization. Such budgets tend to gain more support by both managers and staff alike and are more likely to result in targets that are achieved.

The actual budgeting process requires that the organization consider its environment; define goals and policies; make assumptions for use throughout the organization; specify priorities; and define specific, measurable objectives. Each of the various types of budgets in the master budget must be prepared, and they are generally not approved without a process of review, justification, and revision. Finally, after budgets have been approved and are in place, a system must be created to control the results of operations.

The approved budget is often more constrained than one would like. However, it is necessary to balance the long-term financial needs of the organization with the short-term quality-of-care needs for patients and the needs of the organization's employees. The final budget is a result of a compromise of these and other factors that affect the organization.

❋ KEY CONCEPTS

Budget plan The plan is formalized (written down) and quantified (e.g., stated in dollars, another currency, the number of patient days). It represents management's intentions or expectations.

Control Effort to meet or exceed the goals of the plans.

Operating budget Plan for day-to-day operating revenues and expenses for the organization. It generally covers 1 year.

Long-range budget or strategic plan Covers a period of 3, 5, or 10 years. Serves a vital function as a link between where the organization has been and where it is going.

Program budgets Special budgeting efforts analyzing specific programs. They cut across departments and look at programs over their expected lifetime rather than 1 year.

Capital budget Plan for the acquisition of investments that will be used by the organization beyond the year they are acquired. Such assets are excluded from the operating budget because of their multi-year nature.

Payback method Calculation of the number of years it will take for the profits from a capital expenditure to repay the initial cash outlay. The less time it takes to recover the initial investment, the better the project.

Return on investment (ROI) Ratio used to determine whether an investment should be made. ROI is calculated as follows:

$$ROI = \frac{\text{Profits from Investment}}{\text{Amount Invested}}$$

A project should be considered if the ROI is positive; the higher the ROI, the better.

Time value of money Any specific amount of money is worth more today than the same amount in the future. Capital assets often require large cash outlays in the budget year. To assess the financial impact of those outlays, one must consider the time value of money.

Discounted cash-flow techniques Capital investment analysis techniques that incorporate the time value of money. The two most common are net present value and internal rate of return.

Net present value (NPV) Method that determines whether a proposed investment earns at least a predetermined rate of return.

Internal rate of return (IRR) Method that determines the specific rate of return earned by a proposed investment.

Qualitative analysis Evaluation of capital budget requests should consider the qualitative benefits that the asset provides the organization and its community.

Product-line budget Budget for a group of patients with some commonality that allows them to be grouped together, such as a common diagnosis.

Cash budgets Budget for the cash receipts and cash payments of the organization. Because capital expenditures require large cash outlays and revenues are often received in cash after expenses are paid, it is vital for the organization to have a plan for its cash flows.

Budget process Organization develops a statement of environmental position, a statement of general goals, objectives, and policies, a list of organization-wide assumptions, specification of program priorities, and a set of specific, measurable operating objectives. Then long-range and program budgets are prepared. Next, unit and departmental budgets are compiled. Based on those budgets, a cash budget is prepared. Based on information from all of these elements, a process of negotiation and revision generally precedes budget approval. A final essential element of the budget process is control of actual results and feedback.

✳ SUGGESTED READINGS

Cavouras C, McKinley J: Variable budgeting for staffing analysis and evaluation, *Nurs Manag* 28(5):34–36, 39, 1997.

Finkler S, McHugh M: *Budgeting concepts for nurse managers,* ed 4, Philadelphia, 2007, WB Saunders.

Finkler S, Ward D, Baker J: *Essentials of cost accounting for health care organizations,* ed 3, Sudbury, Mass, 2007, Jones & Bartlett.

Finkler S, Ward D, Calabrese T: *Fundamentals of accounting for health care organizations,* ed 2, Burlington, Mass, 2013, Jones & Bartlett.

McLean R: *Financial management in health care organizations,* ed 2, Albany, NY, 2002, Delmar.

Moss M, Shelver S: Practical budgeting for the operating room administrator, *Nurs Econ* 1(1):7–13, 1993.

Pelfrey S: Financial techniques for evaluating equipment acquisitions, *J Nurs Adm* 21(3)15–20, 1991.

Pelfrey S: Managing financial data, *Semin Nurse Manag* 5(1):25–30, 1997.

Ratcliffe J, Donaldson C, Macphee S: Programme budgeting and marginal analysis: a case study of maternity services, *J Public Health Med* 18(2):175–182, 1996.

Sengin K, Dreisbach A: Managing with precision: a budgetary decision support model, *J Nurs Adm* 25(2):33–44, 1995.

Shelver S, Moss M: Operating room budget factors: a pocket guide to OR finance, *Nurs Econ* 12(3):146–152, 1994.

Swansburg R: *Budgeting and financial management for nurse managers,* Sudbury, Mass, 1997, Jones & Bartlett.

Time Value of Money

✳ INTRODUCTION

The concept of the *time value of money* requires sophisticated analysis to calculate the profitability of a proposed investment. The critical issue is that money received at different points in time has a different value. One would much rather have $100 today than 1 year from now. If you have the money today, then at the very least, the $100 could be put in a bank and earn interest. A year from now, the money you invested would be worth more than $100.

Suppose that two investments are being considered. One investment requires an outlay of $10,000 today, and another requires an outlay of only $7,500. Over the life of the investment, the operating costs will be $3,000 each year for 5 years for the first alternative but $3,600 per year for the second alternative over the same period.

	Alternative 1	Alternative 2
Initial outlay	$10,000	$ 7,500
Year 1	3,000	3,600
Year 2	3,000	3,600
Year 3	3,000	3,600
Year 4	3,000	3,600
Year 5	3,000	3,600
Total cost	$25,000	$25,500

Which alternative is less expensive?

Note that there is no revenue in this example. Often in health care, the focus is on cost-efficient ways to accomplish an objective. Suppose different types of air conditioners are being compared. Over the 5-year life of the air conditioners, the organization will spend $25,000 for the first alternative. The second type of air conditioner is less expensive but not as energy-efficient. It will cost $25,500 in total. Which alternative is cheaper? The first project requires the organization to spend $500 less over its lifetime. But it does require spending $2,500 more at the beginning. That $2,500 could have been earning interest, thus offsetting some of the extra operating costs.

A way is needed to compare dollars spent at different points in time. Then one would be able to consider not just how much cash is involved but also when it is received or spent. Rather than solving the problem of the air conditioners now, put it aside for the time being. Let us focus on the methods for dealing with cash flows at different points in time. Then it will be possible to solve the problem of the air conditioner investment later in this Appendix.

✳ TIME-VALUE-OF-MONEY CALCULATION MECHANICS

In time-value-of-money (TVM) calculations, the amount of money spent or received today is referred to as the *present value* (PV). The *interest rate*, or the rate charged or paid to use money, is referred to as i%. The *number of interest compounding periods*, or the points at which interest is compounded (e.g., monthly, annually), is referred to as N. There are several TVM calculation formulas. The most fundamental is:

$$FV = PV \, (1 + i\%)^N$$

This formula allows a one-step determination of the future value (FV) of some amount of money invested today, the PV, at an interest rate (i%) for a period of time equal to N. Many handheld business calculators, personal digital devices such as tablets, and computer spreadsheet programs have this and other TVM formulas built in. Calculators are relatively simple to use for this process. One should be sure to coordinate N and i%. If N is years, then i% is the annual interest rate. If N is months, then the annual interest rate must be divided by 12 to get a monthly i%.

So far, this discussion has focused on finding out how much an amount of money held today would grow to in the future. Discounting requires that one be able to take an amount of money to be received in the future and determine what it would be worth today. That requires reversal of the compounding process. The interest rate used in the calculation is called the *discount rate*.

What if it is expected that some money will be received or spent every year rather than all at once at one point of time in the future? For instance, what is the value today of receiving $100 every year for the next 3 years? One way to solve this problem is to take the PV of $100 to be received 1 year from now plus the PV of $100 to be received 2 years from now plus the PV of $100 to be received 3 years from now.

Obviously, this has the potential to be a rather tedious process. Any time payments are to be made or received and the payments are exactly the same in amount and evenly spaced in time, those payments are referred to as an annuity *payment* (PMT). To calculate the PV of $100 received every year for 3 years, the PMT = $100, N = 3, and i% = 10. A calculator or spreadsheet could be used to determine the PV, which is $248.69. Note that FV does not enter into this calculation because there is not one single FV but rather a series of payments, all considered by the term PMT.

✳ THE PRESENT COST APPROACH

To return to the problem raised earlier, recall that there are two potential air conditioners. One will cost $10,000 and will have operating costs of $3,000 per year for 5 years. The other will cost $7,500 and will have operating costs of $3,600 per year for 5 years. The problem of choosing one or the other concerns the fact that the total cost of the first alternative is $25,000, whereas the second alternative costs $25,500, but the alternative with the lower total cost has the higher initial cash outlay.

In today's dollars, the first alternative is $10,000 plus the PV of an annuity of $3,000 per year for 5 years. The second alternative is $7,500 plus the PV of $3,600 per year for 5 years.

Assume that the discount rate is 10%. At N = 5, i% = 10, and PMT = $3,000, the PV is $11,372. When the PMT = $3,600, the PV is $13,647. Combined with the initial outlays, the PV of the first alternative is $21,372, and for the second alternative, it is $21,147. Therefore, other things being equal, the second alternative would be chosen, because it is less expensive when one considers the time value of money.

This method is the present cost approach. It considers the PV of the costs of alternative projects that accomplish the same end. Assuming that both projects are just as effective in terms of accomplishing the desired outcome, the alternative with the lower cost in PV is superior.

❋ THE NET PRESENT VALUE APPROACH

The *net present value* (NPV) method of analysis determines whether a project earns more or less than a desired rate of return, which is used as the discount rate in the calculations.

It is reasonable to assume that any investment that can earn more than the rate for borrowing money should be accepted, assuming the organization has a good enough credit rating to be able to borrow the necessary funds. Therefore, the interest rate that the organization would pay on a loan is often used as the discount rate.[1]

The NPV method can be used to assess whether a project is acceptable. The NPV method compares the PV of a project's cash inflows with the PV of its cash outflows, as calculated at a particular hurdle rate, or the minimum acceptable rate of return on a project. In equation form, NPV can be defined as follows:

$$NPV = PV \text{ inflows} - PV \text{ outflows}$$

If the NPV is greater than zero, the inflows are greater than the outflows when evaluated at the hurdle rate. If the NPV is less than zero, the organization is spending more than it is receiving. If the NPV is exactly zero, the inflows are equal to the outflows, and the project is earning exactly the hurdle rate. In most cases, financial managers rather than nurse managers or executives perform the actual calculations. Nevertheless, nurse managers and executives should understand that the evaluation process of capital projects requires obtaining prior approval.

To find the NPV, first sum the PVs of the cash received in each year. Then find the sum of the PVs of the cash spent each year. Then compare the sum of the PVs of the inflows to the sum of the PVs of the outflows.

For example, suppose that a hospital is considering adding a new wing. There is an initial cash outflow of $10 million. Assume that the money for the wing could be borrowed at 10%. Suppose that the operating cash expenses (including information about the costs relating to nursing, which you have contributed to the analysis) and the cash revenues for each of the 20 years of the useful life of the wing are as shown in Table 12A–1. Without considering the timing of the cash flows, a total of $16,570,000 is being spent, and $35,435,192 is being received. The project appears to be very profitable. Note, however, that a large amount

❋ **TABLE 12A–1** *An Example of Project Cash Flows and Present Values*

	Cash Flow		Present Value	
	Cash Expenses	**Cash Revenues**	**Cash Expenses**	**Cash Revenues**
Start	$10,000,000		$10,000,000	
Year 1	200,000	$ 1,000,000	181,818	$ 909,091
2	230,000	1,020,000	190,083	842,975
3	250,000	1,081,200	187,829	812,322
4	270,000	1,146,072	184,414	782,783
5	270,000	1,214,836	167,649	754,318
6	280,000	1,287,726	158,053	726,888
7	290,000	1,364,990	148,816	700,456
8	310,000	1,446,889	144,617	674,985
9	310,000	1,533,703	131,470	650,440
10	320,000	1,625,725	123,374	626,787
11	330,000	1,723,269	115,663	603,995
12	345,000	1,826,665	109,928	582,032
13	355,000	1,936,265	102,831	560,866
14	370,000	2,052,440	97,433	540,472
15	380,000	2,175,587	90,969	520,818
16	390,000	2,306,122	84,875	501,879
17	400,000	2,444,489	79,137	483,628
18	410,000	2,591,159	73,742	466,043
19	420,000	2,746,628	68,673	449,096
20	440,000	2,911,426	65,403	432,765
Totals	$16,570,000	$35,435,192	$12,506,777	$12,622,639

---

[1] In addition, assets that earn less than the rate for borrowing money might be acquired if they have strong social merit and there are sufficient funds available to the organization to acquire the asset.

of money is spent at the beginning of the project, but revenues are earned gradually over the 20 years.

By using PV methods, the PV of each cash flow can be calculated; then the PVs of the inflows and the outflows can be summed. The result is that the total PV of the inflows is $12,622,639, and the PV of the outflows is $12,506,777. The NPV, equal to the PV of the inflows less the PV of the outflows, is $115,862. Because this is greater than zero, the project is earning more than 10% and is acceptable. However, it is not nearly as profitable as it appeared to be at first glance.

✳ THE INTERNAL RATE OF RETURN APPROACH

The principal objection to the net PV approach is that it does not indicate the specific rate of return that a project is earning. This creates problems if several capital assets exceed the hurdle rate and the projects conflict, or if there are insufficient funds to undertake all the projects with a positive NPV. The *internal rate of return* (IRR) method is a mathematical formulation that sets the PV of the inflows equal to the PV of the outflows. That equation is true only at the exact interest rate that a project is earning. If the equation is solved for the interest rate that makes it hold true, that is the rate of return that the project is earning.

The mathematics for calculating the IRR are complex. This is particularly true when the cash flows are not the same from year to year. However, business calculators, computers, and other digital devices can be used to solve for the IRR with variable cash flows.

The IRRs calculated can be used to rank projects by profitability. The IRR method tells the specific interest rate that each project is expected to return. Even if the organization is a not-for-profit one, it must consider that the projects with the highest return on investment, or rate of return, will provide the largest amount of cash coming into the organization in the future. That cash in turn can be used to allow for additional projects. By listing projects in order from the highest rate of return to the lowest, this ranking makes the project selection process far easier.

Handheld electronic devices and calculators that compute TVM calculations are readily available to most managers. The computations can also be performed easily using a computer spreadsheet program.

✳ USING COMPUTER SPREADSHEETS FOR TIME-VALUE-OF-MONEY COMPUTATIONS

A number of different computer spreadsheet software programs are available that can be used to solve TVM problems. These programs are particularly useful for some of the more complicated calculations. This Appendix provides examples of how to solve TVM problems with Excel.[2] The approach of other spreadsheets is similar. We would also like to note that there are often multiple ways to do the same computation, even within the same software program. The various approaches may also be a

bit different in each different version of a software program, particularly the PC versus MAC versions. We will be discussing one approach to TVM computations in Excel. Readers should feel free to use the Excel help icon to explore other approaches, such as the use of the "Formulas" menu option.

Consider finding the FV of $100 invested for 2 years at 6%. Using Excel, you begin by entering the data that will be used to solve the problem. Note that Excel uses *Nper* rather than N for the number of compounding periods and *Rate* rather than i for the discount rate. In this example, the problem could be set up as shown in Figure 12A–1. This screen shows the data you have, the variable, FV, that you are looking for and indicates where the answer will be shown. After data have been entered, you move the cursor to the cell where you want the solution to appear. In this case, that is cell D9.

Note that Excel follows the logic that if you pay out something today, you will get back something in the future. So if the FV is to be a positive amount, representing a receipt of cash, the PV must be entered as a negative amount, representing a payment of cash.

In Excel, you would put your cursor in the cell where you want your FV to appear and type "=FV(". As soon as you type the open parenthesis, an Excel formula will appear as follows:

FV(rate, nper, pmt, [pv], [type])

Figure 12A–2 shows how this appears in Excel.

The FV can be solved by simply entering the cell numbers for each of the variables into the formula. When this approach is used to solve the problem above, an extra comma should be inserted for the *pmt* variable. The value for the *type* can be omitted completely. For example, given the cell location of the raw data in the worksheet shown in Figures 12A–1 and 12A–2, the formula to solve the above problem would be:

=FV(D5,D6, ,-D4)

Finally type the close parenthesis, as shown in Figure 12A–3.

If you prefer, rather than inserting two consecutive commas, you may insert a value of 0 for the pmt variable because

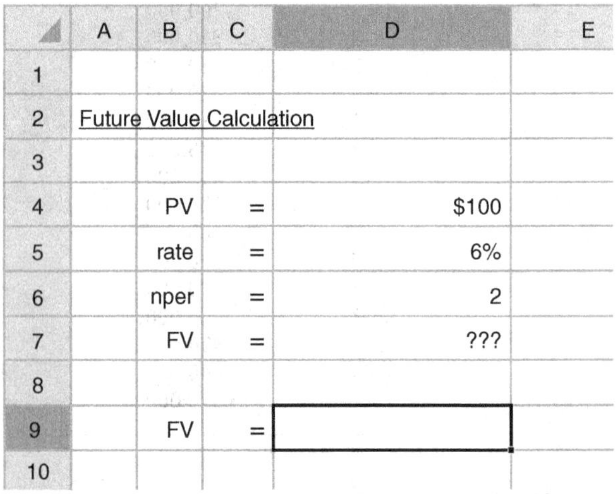

◢	A	B	C	D	E
1					
2	Future Value Calculation				
3					
4		PV	=	$100	
5		rate	=	6%	
6		nper	=	2	
7		FV	=	???	
8					
9		FV	=		
10					

FIGURE 12A–1. Initial data entry. Excel® Spreadsheet Software. (Microsoft product screen shot reprinted with permission from Microsoft Corporation.)

[2]The Excel approach used in this chapter is based on Microsoft Excel 2010. Other versions of Excel may differ somewhat in the exact approach, steps, or formulas used or in the exact appearance of the screen.

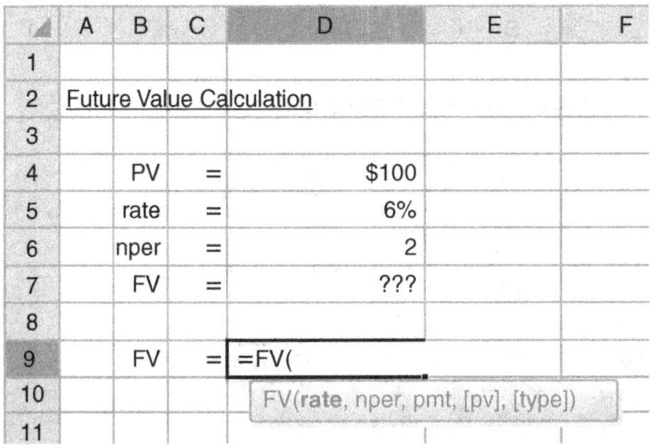

FIGURE 12A–2. The Formula window, future value (FV). Excel® Spreadsheet Software. (Microsoft product screen shot reprinted with permission from Microsoft Corporation.)

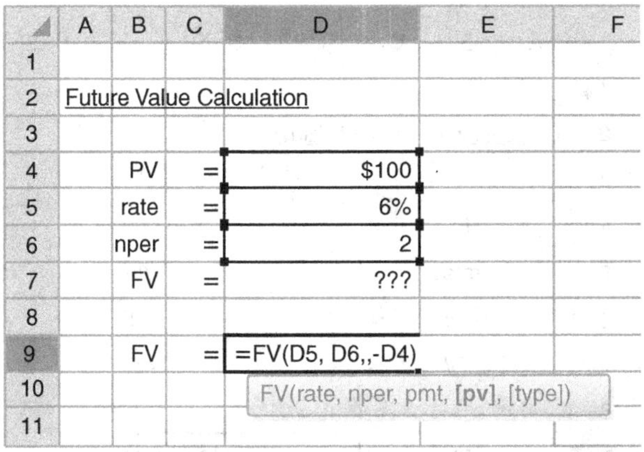

FIGURE 12A–3. Cell references entered into formula window, future value (FV). Excel® Spreadsheet Software. (Microsoft product screen shot reprinted with permission of Microsoft Corporation.)

there is no repeating payment, and the formula would appear as:

$$=FV(D5,D6,0,-D4)$$

After the formula is typed, click the "Enter" key to get the solution for FV, shown in Figure 12A–4.

An advantage of a formula that uses the cell references is that it will automatically recalculate the FV if the numeric value in any of the indicated cells is changed. If we were to change the rate in cell D5 from 6% to 8%, a new FV would immediately appear on the worksheet.

However, another approach is to show the numeric values for the raw data in the Excel formula, such as:

$$=FV(6\%,2,0,-100)$$

The advantage of this approach is that it not only will calculate the answer in your Excel spreadsheet but can be communicated to a colleague, who can tell exactly what information you have used and what you are trying to calculate. Anyone can insert this formula into their spreadsheet to compute the PV without needing your full spreadsheet. They will get the correct

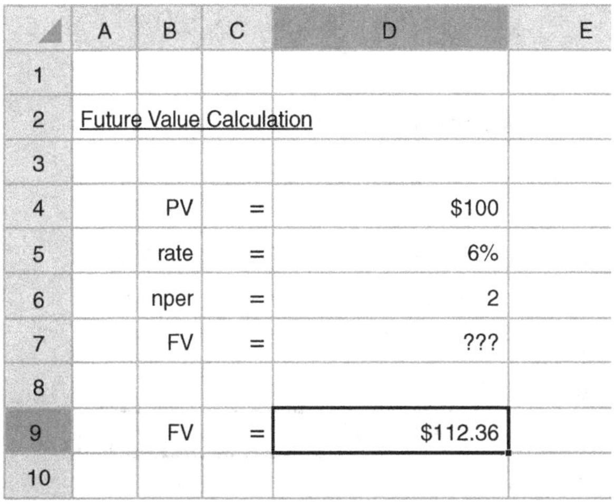

FIGURE 12A–4. Solving for future value (FV). Excel® Spreadsheet Software. (Microsoft product screen shot reprinted with permission from Microsoft Corporation.)

PV and will also know the values for all of the variables used to compute it.

For the remainder of this appendix, TVM Excel problems are discussed in both the form of the basic Excel formula for a variable and also the *numeric value formula*, such as:

$$=FV(rate, nper, pmt, pv, type)$$

$$=FV(6\%,2,0,-100)$$

Note that if you enter =FV(6%,2,0,-100) into an Excel spreadsheet cell, the solution of 112.36 will automatically be calculated.

Examples

The previous example started with information about the PV, rate, and number of compounding periods and solved for the FV. Using Excel, one can solve for any of these variables if the other information is available. As you type an equal sign followed by the variable you are looking for and an open parenthesis in any cell, Excel will display the respective formula for each variable. The formulae are:

$$=PV(rate, nper, pmt, fv, type)$$

$$=Rate(nper, pmt, pv, fv, type, guess)$$

$$=Nper(rate, pmt, pv, fv, type)$$

$$=PMT(rate, nper, pv, fv, type)$$

$$=NPV(rate, value1, value2, . . .)$$

$$=IRR(values, guess)$$

Present Value

Suppose that we can buy a capital asset that will result in our receiving $15,000 5 years from now and that we believe an appropriate discount rate for this specific piece of equipment is

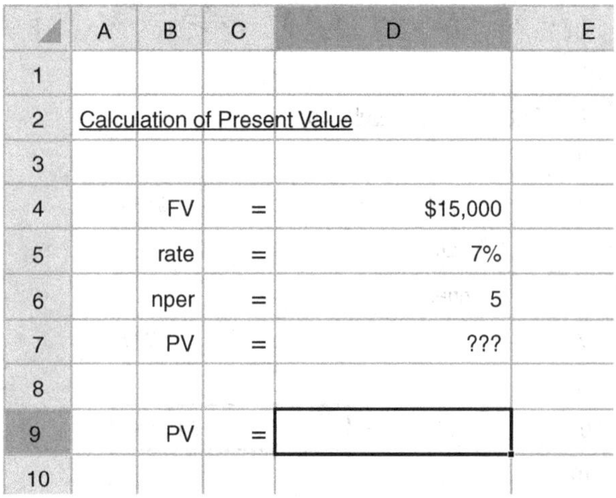

FIGURE 12A–5. Present value (PV)—data. Excel® Spreadsheet Software. (Microsoft product screen shot reprinted with permission from Microsoft Corporation.)

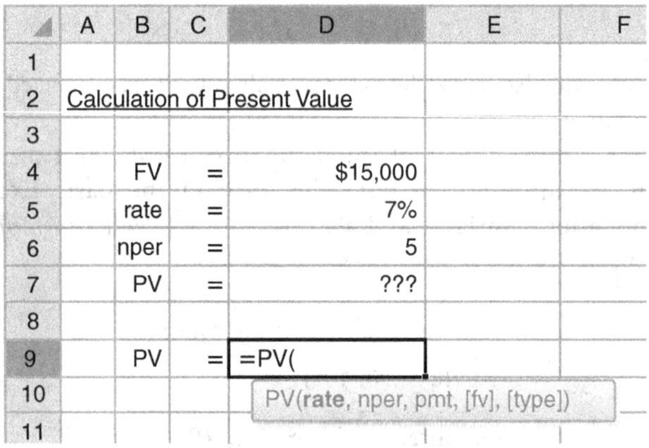

FIGURE 12A–6. Formula window, present value (PV). Excel® Spreadsheet Software. (Microsoft product screen shot reprinted with permission from Microsoft Corporation.)

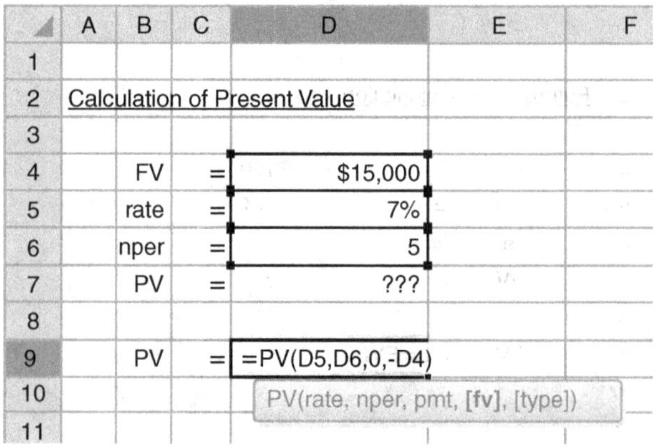

FIGURE 12A–7. Cell references entered into formula window, present value (PV). Excel® Spreadsheet Software. (Microsoft product screen shot reprinted with permission from Microsoft Corporation.)

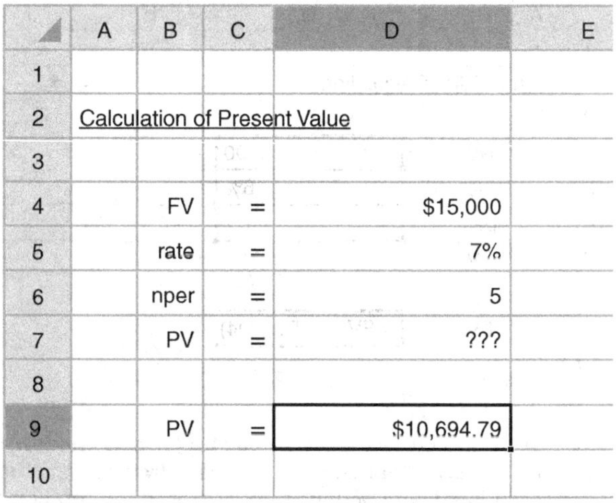

FIGURE 12A–8. Present value (PV) solution. Excel® Spreadsheet Software. (Microsoft product screen shot reprinted with permission from Microsoft Corporation.)

7%. We need to decide the most that we would pay for that asset. What is the PV of that future receipt?

We can start the solution by recording the raw data in an Excel spreadsheet (Figure 12A–5). The formula is shown in Figure 12A–6. Note that we can see in that screen that the formula for the PV is PV(rate, nper, pmt, fv, type). Enter the cell references for the Rate, Nper, and FV.[3] If you want the solution to appear as a positive number, enter a minus sign before the cell reference for the FV. This will generate Figure 12A–7. Be sure to hit the Enter key to solve the problem. The resulting screen would appear as in Figure 12A–8, and the PV is $10,694.79. If we wished to show the formula with numeric values, it would be:

$$=PV(7\%,5,0,-15000)$$

---

[3]The cell references can be inserted directly into the formula shown on screen by holding down the "Ctrl" button and clicking on the cells that are used in the calculation; in this case, these are D5, D6, and D4. A negative sign would then be inserted in front of D4.

Rate

Suppose that we have $10,000 today, could invest it for 6 years, and need to have $20,000 at the end of that time period. What rate would have to be earned? The data setup would be similar to the problem just solved except that we are looking for the rate rather than the PV. After "=Rate(" is typed, the remaining portion of the equation appears as "nper, pmt, pv, [fv], [type], [guess])." We would then enter the cell references as shown in Figure 12A–9. Note that either the PV or the FV must be a negative number. The rate that must be earned for $10,000 to grow to $20,000 in 6 years, 12%, is shown in Figure 12A–10. The formula for this with numeric values would be =Rate(6,0, -10000,20000). There is a zero for PMT because there is no periodic repeating payment in this problem. We do not need to enter any values for type or guess.

Number of Periods

Suppose that we can earn only 9% per year. How many years would it take before our $10,000 will grow to become $20,000?

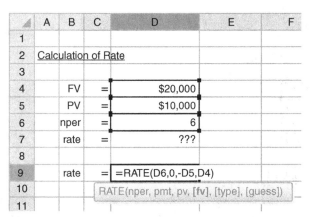

FIGURE 12A–9. Cell references entered into formula window, rate example. Excel® Spreadsheet Software. (Microsoft product screen shot reprinted with permission from Microsoft Corporation.)

FIGURE 12A–11. Cell references entered into formula window, number of periods example. Excel® Spreadsheet Software. (Microsoft product screen shot reprinted with permission from Microsoft Corporation.)

FIGURE 12A–10. Rate solution. Excel® Spreadsheet Software. (Microsoft product screen shot reprinted with permission from Microsoft Corporation.)

FIGURE 12A–12. Cell references entered into formula window, periodic payments in arrears. Excel® Spreadsheet Software. (Microsoft product screen shot reprinted with permission from Microsoft Corporation.)

After typing "=Nper(" and entering the cell references (as shown in Figure 12A–11), then hit the Enter key. The result is 8.04, or a little bit longer than 8 years. The formula with numeric values would be =Nper(9%,0,-10000,20000).

Periodic Payments (in Arrears)

Assume that you can invest money every year for 7 years at 8%. If you need $20,000 at the end of the 7 years, how much would you have to put aside each year? Assume you make the payments at the end of each year. After setting up the data, the formula is PMT(rate, nper, pv, fv, type) as shown in the Excel screen in Figure 12A–12. We find that we would have to invest $2,241.45 each year. The formula with numeric values would be =PMT(8%,7,0,-20000).

Periodic Payments (in Advance)

However, what if we could put aside money at the beginning of each year rather than the end? That is called an *annuity in advance*. When payments come at the end of each period, as

they do in an ordinary annuity or annuity in arrears, the value for "type" is 0. If we leave it blank, as we have so far, Excel assumes that it has a value of 0. For an annuity in advance, we must indicate the "type" as being 1 in the formula. Figure 12A–13 shows how this would appear. If the periodic payments are made at the start of the year, we would need to put aside only $2,075.41 each year. The formula with numeric values would be =PMT(8%,7,0,-20000,1).

Net Present Value

Suppose that we can invest $1,000 today in a capital asset and will receive $500, $700, and $800, respectively, at the end of each of the 3 years of the asset's life. Our discount rate for the project is 6%. What is the NPV? After typing "=NPV(" the formula appears as NPV(rate,value1,value2, . . .). The appropriate cell references can then be entered. Note that the initial outlay should *not* be entered as one of the values. The initial outlay must be subtracted from the Excel NPV calculation. Figure 12A–14 shows the problem set up and cell references. Press the Enter key to see the result, 1,766.39. After subtracting the outlay of $1,000, the NPV is $766.39.

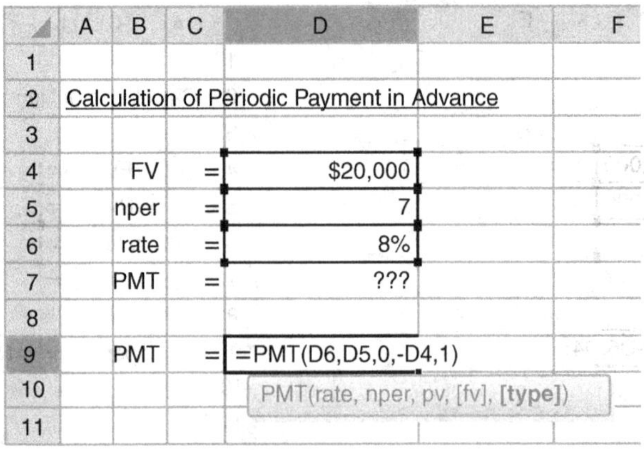

	A	B	C	D	E	F
1						
2		Calculation of Periodic Payment in Advance				
3						
4		FV	=	$20,000		
5		nper	=	7		
6		rate	=	8%		
7		PMT	=	???		
8						
9		PMT	=	=PMT(D6,D5,0,-D4,1)		
10				PMT(rate, nper, pv, [fv], [type])		
11						

FIGURE 12A–13.   Cell references entered into formula window, periodic payments in advance. Excel® Spreadsheet Software. (Microsoft product screen shot reprinted with permission from Microsoft Corporation.)

	A	B	C	D	E	F	G	H
1								
2		Calculation of Net Present Value						
3								
4		PV	=	($1,000)				
5		Year 1	=	500				
6		Year 2	=	700				
7		Year 3	=	800				
8		rate	=	6%				
9		NPV	=	???				
10								
11		NPV	=	=NPV(D8,D5,D6,D7)				
12				NPV(rate, value1, [value2], [value3], [value4], [value5],...)				
13								

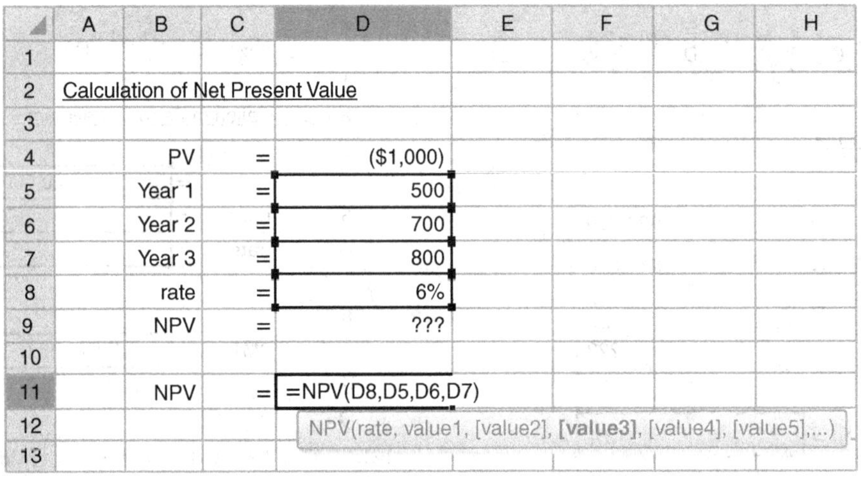

FIGURE 12A–14.   Cell references entered into formula window, net present value (NPV). Excel® Spreadsheet Software. (Microsoft product screen shot reprinted with permission from Microsoft Corporation.)

Internal Rate of Return

What is the IRR of the cash flows described in the previous NPV example? After typing in, "=IRR(" the formula appears as IRR(values, guess). This time, all values should be entered, *including* the initial outlay. In this respect, the IRR formula works differently than the NPV function. Also provide Excel with an initial guess for the rate; here we used 15%. After hitting Enter, the solution can be determined. Figure 12A–15 shows the problem setup and cell references. The formula result is .404. This means that the IRR for the capital asset would be 40.4%. If you are entering numeric values for the variables directly into the formula, you must insert them in curly brackets: =IRR({-1000,500,700,800},15%).

Each of the major spreadsheet programs handles the TVM process slightly differently. In fact, within any program from one version to the next, very minor changes in the process tend to occur. And to some extent, the spreadsheet approaches are quirky. For example, not allowing the initial, time zero, outflow to be directly included in the NPV calculation seems odd. Nevertheless, spreadsheets can handle the more complicated

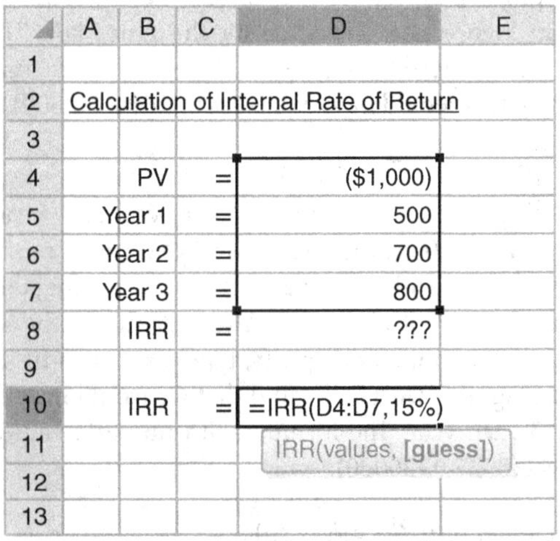

	A	B	C	D	E
1					
2		Calculation of Internal Rate of Return			
3					
4		PV	=	($1,000)	
5		Year 1	=	500	
6		Year 2	=	700	
7		Year 3	=	800	
8		IRR	=	???	
9					
10		IRR	=	=IRR(D4:D7,15%)	
11				IRR(values, [guess])	
12					
13					

FIGURE 12A–15.   Cell references entered into formula window, internal rate of return (IRR). Excel® Spreadsheet Software. (Microsoft product screen shot reprinted with permission from Microsoft Corporation.)

numbers found in real-world situations with ease, and most organizations now rely almost exclusively on computer spreadsheets for their TVM calculations.

✳ SUMMARY

Discounted cash flow techniques—including present cost, NPV, and IRR—account for the time value of money. The present cost approach is useful for comparing alternative ways to accomplish the same goal. The method does not evaluate revenues. Both the NPV and IRR methods determine whether the cash inflows are adequate to justify the cash outflow from a strictly economic point of view. The IRR method additionally allows for a ranking of projects by rate of return on investment.

✳ KEY CONCEPTS

Time-value-of-money (TVM) calculation mechanics   Amount of money spent or received today is the present value (PV), interest rate is i%, number of interest compounding periods is N, and

$$FV = PV\,(1 + i\%)^N$$

where FV is the future value.

Net present value (NPV) approach   Comparing the present value of a project's cash inflows with the present value of its cash outflows, as calculated at a particular hurdle rate, this method determines whether a project earns more or less than a stated desired rate of return.

Internal rate of return (IRR) approach   Method sets the present value of the inflows equal to the present value of the outflows and solves for the interest rate at which that is true.

Operating Budgets

CHAPTER GOALS

The goals of this chapter are to:

- Explain the various factors related to preparation of an operating budget
- Define the elements of workload
- Provide a technique for calculating personnel service requirements and costs
- Provide a technique for calculating other-than-personnel service requirements and costs

- Describe the process of budget submission, negotiation, and approval
- Consider issues related to the implementation of the operating budget

❊ INTRODUCTION

The operating budget is a plan for the organization's revenues and expenses. It generally covers a period of 1 year. Preparation and control of the operating budget is probably the single most time-consuming aspect of most nurse managers' involvement with financial management.

In most organizations, the manager of each cost center is directly involved in preparation of the operating budget. The finance office of the organization provides support as needed throughout the budget process. The budgets for the costs centers are consolidated, and the organization's executive management team, including the chief nurse executive, makes final decisions on a budget to be submitted to the board for approval.

For nurse managers to begin the process of preparing operating budgets for their cost centers, they need a variety of information. Much of this information is generated by the budgeting foundations process, discussed in Chapter 12. Specifically, the information generated by the organization's environmental review and by its development of general goals, objectives, policies, organization-wide assumptions, program priorities, and specific measurable objectives is essential to the manager in preparing a budget.

That information will accomplish two primary objectives: It will enable the manager to understand the forest before becoming immersed in the trees, and it will provide specific budget preparation guidance. The environmental review and the general goals, objectives, and policies allow the manager to understand what the organization wants to accomplish and what it believes it will be able to accomplish. Program priorities

provide the manager with information about the level of importance that will likely be assigned to various types of budget requests. These pieces of background information will help the manager focus on what the specific cost center should be trying to accomplish.

The organization-wide assumptions and specific measurable objectives then provide the manager with information needed to start preparing the specific details of the budget. Inflation rates and likely changes in patient volume and mix are examples of assumptions that are critical for the manager in determining likely resource requirements and costs. Measurable objectives such as an overall 3% maximum increase in unit costs provide a target to aim for in the budget development process. They also serve notice to the manager that it will be necessary to justify any proposed budget expenses that exceed those specified in the objectives or revenue categories that fall short of stated objectives.

Within nursing administration, additional background data are needed before nurse managers and executives can commence cost center and division budget preparations. Specifically, the organization's approach to delivering nursing care must be clearly understood by all nurse managers and executives. To what extent does the organization rely on licensed practical nurses (LPNs) as opposed to registered nurses (RNs)? What are the roles of nursing assistants (NAs) and other unlicensed personnel? What proportion of staff works on each shift, and what variations are there between weekday and weekend shifts? Is the mix of staff different on different shifts, and if so, how? The answer to these questions may vary from unit to unit. After being resolved, these guidelines may remain unchanged for a number of years (although they should be reviewed annually for needed changes).

Information from long-range and program budgets (discussed in Chapter 12) should also be available to unit managers as they begin their budgeting process. The addition of new services or programs will have a direct bearing on the planning of the budget for each cost center affected, even if only indirectly. For example, the addition of certain types of surgeries may result in increased demands on the recovery room, postsurgical intensive care units (ICUs), or even the general medical/surgical units.

Similarly, if other units or departments of the organization are planning changes in procedures, that information must be communicated to all relevant cost centers. For example, if the pharmacy asks nurses on patient care units to reconstitute more drugs on the unit, this will save money in the pharmacy but may increase nurse staffing needs on the units and the number of medication errors. On the other hand, if pharmacists are dispatched to patient care units to consult with nurses and physicians and to teach patients about their discharge medication regimens in an effort to reduce medication errors, it may reduce nurse staffing needs but increase staffing requirements in the pharmacy. Coordination, cooperation, and communication are vital to arrive at an operational plan that is best for the organization as a whole and allows managers to develop cost center budgets according to the work requirements.

After the background information required to commence the budget process is available, nurse managers can move forward to prepare the three primary elements of the operating budget: the expense budget for personnel, the expense budget for costs other than personnel services, and the revenue budget. All nursing cost centers have expense responsibility. Many hospital nursing units are not required to prepare revenue budgets. However, some cost centers managed by nurses, such as the operating room (OR), do have revenue responsibility. The role of nursing with respect to revenue management is growing and is discussed in the next chapter. After the budget is prepared, it must be submitted and possibly negotiated before approval. After it is approved, it must be implemented and controlled.

The development of the operating budget discussed in this chapter is one possible approach to calculating the elements of the budget. Health care organizations (HCOs) often have their own customized forms and specific step-by-step procedures. Therefore, the forms used in this chapter and the order of the steps taken in developing the budget should not be viewed as the focal points; rather, one should try to understand the elements of the budget—what items must be included and why. A conceptual understanding of the operating budget will allow readers to adapt to a wide variety of types of organizations and to the specific procedures of any organization.

❋ WORKLOAD BUDGET

To prepare the revenue or expense portions of the operating budget, the first step is to ascertain the volume of work for the coming year. The amount of work performed by a unit is referred to as its *workload*. Nurses often think of workload as the number of patients they care for on a given shift, or the patient-to-nurse ratio. In budgeting terms, workload is typically measured as *units of service*. A unit of service is the measurement of the work performed by the cost center. Workload may be measured in a variety of ways, such as the number of patients, patient days, deliveries, visits, treatments, or procedures. Each cost center must determine the measure that is most appropriate for its unit of service.

Units of service can provide a meaningful basis for both revenue and expense calculations. For example, a patient who undergoes surgery will be charged based on the number of hours an operation takes. In this case, the duration of the surgical procedure in hours (or portions of hours) represents the unit of service. That measure may also be used as a starting point in developing the staffing needs for the OR.

After a cost center defines its key unit or units of service, it must predict the number of units of service that will be provided in the coming year. This will allow development of the operating budget. In some organizations, nurse managers may be told a specific number of units of service to use in their budget. In many cases, however, the nurse manager will have to forecast that number. In fact, given the specific knowledge a unit manager has about a specific cost center, probably the nurse manager is in the best position to forecast units of service for the cost center. (See Chapter 21 for specific forecasting techniques.)

In addition to units of service, it may be necessary to forecast things such as the average length of stay or the mix of patients by Diagnosis Related Group (DRG) or severity of illness. After these forecasts are made, the nurse manager will translate the work that must be done into a set of personnel and other-than-personnel resource requirements.

Activity Report

One aid in forecasting the coming year budgeted workload is the *activity report*. This report measures key statistics concerning current activity. It centers on both the number of units of service and the relative proportion of the organization's capacity that is being used. For example, in a hospital or nursing home, the most common measure of capacity is the number of beds available for patients in total. The *census* represents the number of these beds occupied each day at a certain point in time (usually midnight). The *occupancy rate* is the percentage of total beds filled, or the number of beds filled divided by the total number of beds available on the unit. For example, if a nursing home has 120 beds and on average 108 of them are occupied, it has a 90% occupancy rate (i.e., 108 filled beds ÷ 120 total beds × 100%).

Two other statistics commonly found in an activity report are the *average daily census* (ADC) and the *average length of stay* (ALOS). The ADC is the average number of patients cared for per day over a period of time. A *patient day* is an accounting term that represents the notion of one patient cared for during a 1-day or a 24-hour period. The ADC is calculated by dividing the number of patient days over a certain time period by the number of days in the period. The ALOS is the average number of days for which each patient is in the hospital or nursing home. It is calculated by dividing the total number of patient days by the total number of admissions. Outpatient providers of health care collect similar data, such as the average number of visits or treatments.

The activity report is valuable, but it must be used with care. Patients tend not to be homogeneous. Thus, knowing the number of patient days is inadequate for planning purposes. A more useful budget for a medical-surgical unit would be developed if the manager knows the type of patients cared for on the unit and can project their severity of illness rather than just the number of patient days. An OR needs to know the different types of procedures to be performed rather than simply the number of hours of operations. The same total number of patients in two different years can have widely differing nursing care costs if they represent a different mix of patients. The unit of service often needs adjustment for patient mix in the budget process, whether we are considering inpatient surgery or home health visits.

Adjusting Units of Service

As a consequence of the heterogeneity of patients, whenever possible, budgeting should be based on adjusted units of service. For example, in the case of a hospital, the number of patient days for a general medical-surgical unit can be adjusted using a system for classifying patients into categories based on the resources they are expected to use; this is often referred to as patient acuity, or *patient classification* (see also Chapter 9).

The most general approach to using patient classification is to determine workload based on required hours of nursing care. Suppose that a medical-surgical unit expects to have 9,000 patient days for the coming year. Rather than trying to determine a budget based solely on the number of patient days, an estimate can be made based on the acuity level of the 9,000 patient days. For example, assume that a unit classifies patients into one of five categories from 1 to 5, with a rating of 1 representing patients that require the fewest hours of nursing care. Based on historical data and expected changes in patients and the services provided, the 9,000 patient days might be projected across the five categories as follows:

Patient Classification	Number of Patient Days
1	1,500
2	3,700
3	2,400
4	900
5	500
Total	9,000

Segregating the 9,000 patients into the five classifications allows the operating budget to be developed based on the resource requirements of the specific mix of patients expected for the unit.

Calculating Workload

For the separation of patient days or visits or treatments by classification level to be valuable for budgeting, there must be a way to differentiate resource consumption by patients in each category. Patient classification systems generally provide information on the average required care *hours per patient day* (HPPD) per 24 hours for each level or per visit or treatment. The number of hours of care is based on a specific staff mix (i.e., proportion of RNs, LPNs, and NAs needed to deliver care). If the staff mix changes, the required hours of care at any patient classification level also change.

Using expected patient classification information, it is possible to determine the number of care hours for these 9,000 patient days. For example, assume the average care hours are as shown in Table 13–1.

In this case, the total care hours required for the year, based on the organization's patient classification system, are 60,820 for this unit. Based on 9,000 patient days, the average HPPD are:

$$60,820 \text{ care hours} \div 9,000 \text{ patient days} = 6.76.[1]$$

Note, however, that one cannot assume that for this particular nursing unit, 6.76 HPPD is a permanent standard. The 6.76 care hours result is sensitive to the expected mix of patients each year. Suppose, for instance, that the mix of patients had been as follows:

Patient Classification	Number of Patient Days
1	1,100
2	3,000
3	2,600
4	1,400
5	900
Total	9,000

---

[1]An alternative approach to measuring workload is to use a relative value unit (RVU) system. In such an approach, a specific level of patient classification is chosen to be assigned an acuity index value of 1. All other levels are assigned RVUs based on the amount of hours of care they require relative to the index level. For example, if classification level 2 was set to a relative value index of 1 and if classification level 5 required four times as many care hours as level 2, then level 5 would be assigned a relative value of 4. The advantage of the RVU scale over the average required hours scale is that whereas the RVU scale describes the patient population, the average required hours scale focuses on the resources required to treat the population. For a further discussion of using RVUs for acuity and staffing, see Graf C. 2007. The operating budget. In Finkler S, McHugh M. *Budgeting Concepts for Nurse Managers*, 4th edition. Philadelphia: WB Saunders.

✳ **TABLE 13–1** *Required Patient Care Hours*

Patient Classification	Number of Patient Days	×	Average Care Hours per 24-Hour Period	=	Total Unit Workload
1	1,500		2.5		3,750
2	3,700		4.7		17,390
3	2,400		8.0		19,200
4	900		12.2		10,980
5	500		19.0		9,500
Total	9,000				60,820

※ **TABLE 13–2** *Required Patient Care Hours for Revised Patient Mix*

Patient Classification	Number of Patient Days	×	Average Care Hours per 24-Hour Period	=	Total Unit Workload
1	1,100		2.5		2,750
2	3,000		4.7		14,100
3	2,600		8.0		20,800
4	1,400		12.2		17,080
5	900		19.0		17,100
Total	9,000				71,830

In that case the total workload is 71,830 care hours, as calculated in Table 13–2.

The total care hours of 71,830 is then divided by 9,000 patient days to determine that 7.98 HPPD are needed. Without the total number of patient days having changed at all, the change in the mix of patients calls for an 18% increase in nursing care HPPD, from 6.76 to 7.98! On average, patient resource requirements have risen from 6.76 hours of care per patient day to 7.98 hours. To accurately budget for expenses, it is essential that the anticipated workload be specified as accurately as possible. That is the purpose of adjusting units of service for the specific anticipated mix of patients. Similar calculations can be made in ambulatory settings. All that is required is a method to classify patients into different categories and to estimate the average resource consumption for patients in each category.

※ EXPENSE BUDGET: PERSONNEL SERVICES

After the manager has a workload forecast, the next step is to start the process of determining the staffing requirements for the unit. These requirements include projecting the numbers and type of personnel needed to care for patients on the unit, usually RNs, LPNs, NAs or other unlicensed personnel, and clerical staff. In addition, other types of licensed and unlicensed employees, such as nurse navigators, nurse educators, technicians, orderlies, and patient escorts, may be part of the unit staffing.

At the time of this writing, one state, California, has legislated minimum nurse staffing levels, 15 states plus the District of Columbia have enacted legislation or adopted regulations to address nurse staffing, and five states require disclosure or public reporting of nurse staffing levels.[2] The American Nurses Association has also developed Principles for Nurse Staffing,[3] and attempts have been made to pass federal legislation based on these principles. However, there are generally no universally accepted standards for determining specific nurse staffing levels. Each institution has unique physical plant characteristics, a unique mix of services offered, varied types of patients cared for, and its own philosophy concerning the appropriate provision of care. Therefore, the mix of staff and standard care hours deemed appropriate vary from one HCO to another.

The growing body of evidence on the relationship between nurse staffing levels and patient outcomes (see references at the end of the chapter) and the attention focused on the issue with regard to patient care quality and safety have made the processes by which units and organizations determine the numbers and types of personnel needed and then deploy them increasingly important. All organizations must document and provide rationale regarding how they set staffing levels to meet requirements set by The Joint Commission and other state and federal regulatory standards.[4] The patient classification system in place provides managers and executives with an assessment of the care hours required per patient by classification level, but it often does not address the mix of staff needed.

Calculation of staffing requires more than simply knowing the total number of hours of care to be provided per patient day on average. To explain how staffing needs can be determined, we will use an example. Assume that the number of hours of care needed by a 30-bed medical-surgical unit is 71,830. This number was calculated earlier for an expected workload of 9,000 patient days spread across five different patient-classification levels. With these numbers in mind, the following sections illustrate a step-by-step process for calculating unit staffing. This information, in turn, can be used in the budgeting process. The reader should keep in mind that there are staffing software programs available to perform some or all of these calculations. However, an understanding of these fundamentals will enable nurse managers and executives to appropriately converse with financial staff and other organizational leaders.

Average Daily Census and Occupancy Rate

Assuming that the unit is open 365 days of the year, we can start by calculating the ADC and the occupancy rate.

$$\text{ADC} = 9,000 \text{ patient days} \div 365 \text{ days per year}$$
$$= 24.7 \text{ patients per day}$$

$$\text{Occupancy} = 24.7 \text{ patients per day} \div 30 \text{ beds} \times 100\%$$
$$= 82\%$$

[2]See Nurse Staffing Plans and Ratios, retrieved October 9, 2011, at http://www.nursingworld.org/MainMenuCategories/ANAPoliticalPower/State/StateLegislativeAgenda/StaffingPlansandRatios_1.aspx.

[3]Retrieved October 9, 2011, at http://www.nursingworld.org/MainMenuCategories/ThePracticeofProfessionalNursing/NursingStandards/ANAPrinciples/UtilizationGuide.aspx.

[4]See, for example, Jones C, Pink G. 2008. Nurse workload, staffing and measurement. In Fried B, Fottler M, Johnson J, editors. *Managing for Success: Human Resources in Health Care*, 3rd edition. Chicago: Health Administration Press, pp. 393-431.

This information is important to managers because it indicates the capacity of the unit to expand its service. Recall from Chapter 8 that because some costs are fixed and some are variable, volume is critical. As volume rises, revenues tend to rise in direct proportion. Costs also rise but less than proportionately, which means that increases in patient volume are especially profitable. The 82% occupancy rate seen here indicates that there is still substantial physical capacity for expansion of the services provided by this unit.

Outpatient providers can also calculate an "occupancy" or utilization type of statistic if they believe their capacity is limited. The volume of patients would be divided by the number of days per year the organization provides service. It might be closed Sundays and holidays. If so, those days are excluded in calculating average patients per day. The average number of patients per day is divided by the capacity to find the occupancy equivalent for the organization.

Staffing Requirements and Full-Time Equivalents

Next we need to consider staffing requirements for the number of expected hours. In this case, 71,830 hours of care are required. How many staff members will be needed to provide that care? Some staff work full time; others work part time. A way is needed to distinguish between those who are full-time workers and those who are not. The approach that has been developed is to distinguish between *positions* and *full-time equivalent* (FTE) employees. A position is defined as one person working for the organization for any number of hours per week to perform specific job duties. One person who works the number of hours that is considered to be full-time is considered a full-time employee. Any number of positions (or individuals) that combine to provide the hours of work of one full-time employee is an FTE.

Thus, one employee working full-time is one FTE. So are two employees each working halftime. They occupy two positions but generate only one FTE of work. Staffing calculations must first determine how many FTEs are required. Then those FTEs can be filled with any number of positions that add up to the number of FTEs needed.

One FTE gets paid for full-time work. The commonly accepted definition of an FTE is one individual working 8 hours per day, 5 days per week, 52 weeks per year, or a total of 2,080 hours per year.[5] However, the staff needed to provide the 71,830 required care hours cannot be determined by simply dividing 71,830 by 2,080. That would assume that all 2,080 paid hours per FTE were productive hours. The 2,080 paid hours actually include productive and "nonproductive" time. For a nurse, productive time reflects the actual time spent providing care to patients and on nursing care–related activities. Vacations, sick leave, holidays, and any other non-worked time are considered nonproductive hours. The organization may also count time worked, but spent away from direct patient care or the nurse's unit, as nonproductive (e.g., time spent on professional development, such as attending educational seminars). Because the 71,830 hours represent needed care hours, we must relate them to productive hours rather than paid hours. Organizational policy determines the amount of nonproductive time that is paid to individuals. The amount of nonproductive time is often based on years of service.[6]

Productive versus Nonproductive Hours

How can one distinguish between productive hours and nonproductive hours? This information is generally available from reports that payroll provides to each unit. The report shows the total paid hours as well as the number of non-worked hours or worked but nonproductive hours in each category. Based on paid and worked hours over the past 12 months, the nurse manager can determine an average number of productive hours per FTE. This requires dividing total worked hours by total paid hours and multiplying by 100% to arrive at a percentage of paid hours that are productive. For example, assume the following for our hypothetical unit for the previous 12 months:

$$\text{Productive Hours:} \quad 75,480$$
$$\text{Paid Hours:} \quad 94,350$$
$$(75,480 \div 94,350) \times 100\% = 80\%$$

This means that 80% of paid hours are productive. There are 0.8 productive hours for every paid hour.

Using a standard 2,080 paid hours per FTE, we could then determine how many productive hours one would expect for each FTE:

$$2,080 \text{ Paid Hours} \times 80\% = 1,664 \text{ Worked or}$$
$$\text{Productive Hours per FTE}$$

The total care hours, 71,830, can be divided by the 1,664 productive hours per FTE to find the number of FTEs needed.[7] In this example, the result of that division is 43.17 FTEs. Based on decisions made by the organization, that FTE total will be separated into different types of nursing staff members (e.g., RNs, LPNs, NAs) and assigned to different shifts. Those 43.17 FTEs will be responsible for providing direct and indirect care to patients 24 hours per day, 7 days per week, all year long.

Assignment of Staff by Type and Shift

One should not assume that there will be 43.17 staff members working each day. The 43.17 FTEs represent an adequate

---

[5]In some geographic areas, it is common for employees to work a 7.5-hour day. This totals to 37.5 hours per week or 1,950 paid hours per year per FTE. Some organizations use three 12-hour shifts per week for an FTE, which totals 1,872 paid hours per year; other organizations may use seven 10-hour shifts per 2-week period for an FTE, which adds up to 1,820 paid hours per year. The point is that each organization can set its own standard number of paid hours per FTE, and an organization can use different FTE standards for certain positions. However, the organization's standards should be used as the basis for budgeting and scheduling.

[6]Strasen L. 1987. *Key Business Skills for Nurse Managers*. Philadelphia: JB Lippincott.

[7]As noted in footnote 5, not all organizations use 2,080 paid hours for one standard FTE. Regardless of the number of paid hours per FTE for a specific organization, the percentage of productive paid hours can be multiplied by the total paid hours per FTE to find how many productive hours are provided per FTE. This result can be divided into the total hours of care needed to determine the number of FTEs needed.

❋ TABLE 13–3 *Allocation of Staff by Type and Shift*

Staff Type	Staff Allocation	7 AM–3 PM Shift	3 PM–11 PM Shift	11 PM–7 AM Shift	Total
	100%	45%	35%	20%	
RN	65%	7.2	5.6	3.2	16.0
LPN	25%	2.7	2.2	1.2	6.1
NA	10%	1.1	0.9	0.5	2.5
Total		11.0	8.7	4.9	24.6

❋ TABLE 13–4 *Final Allocation of Staff by Type and Shift*

Staff Type	Staff Allocation	7 AM–3 PM Shift	3 PM–11 PM Shift	11 PM–7 AM Shift	Total
	100%	44.9%	36.7%	18.4%	
RN	65.3%	7.0	6.0	3.0	16.0
LPN	24.5%	3.0	2.0	1.0	6.0
NA	10.2%	1.0	1.0	0.5	2.5
Total		11.0	9.0	4.5	24.5

number to provide care 7 days per week every week. On any given day, some staff members are sick or on vacation, take a holiday, or are on a scheduled day off. How many staff members will actually be working each day? The total hours of care required was 71,830 over a period of 1 year. Dividing the 71,830 by 365 days in a year produces the required care hours per day on average.

71,830 Care Hours ÷ 365 Days per Year = 197 Hours of Care per Day

Assuming that employees work 8-hour shifts results in 24.6 person-shifts per day (197 hours per day divided by 8 hours per shift = 24.6 shifts).[8] These 24.6 person-shifts per 24 hours must be allocated by shift and by type of employee. Suppose that this medical-surgical unit has a predetermined pattern that requires approximately 65% RN staff, 25% LPN, and 10% NAs. Assume further that the scheduling standard is 45% days, 35% evenings, and 20% nights. These numbers, similar to the others in this chapter, are hypothetical. In practice, these standards must be established by the nursing unit or department based on its decisions about the most appropriate division of staff for a specific unit.

Table 13–3 spreads the available 24.6 person-shifts across the various staff categories and shifts. First, the total number is calculated for each type of staff. Because 65% of shifts are to be covered by RNs, 65% of the 24.6 is allocated to the RN staff nurse category, generating the 16.0 in the total column for the RN staff nurse row (65% × 24.6 = 16.0). Then 25% and 10% are used to allocate 6.1 total LPNs and 2.5 total NAs (25% × 24.6 = 6.1; 10% × 24.6 = 2.5) . (Some of these numbers, and those below, contain slight rounding errors. In practice, you

should carry all computations out at least several decimal places to reduce the impact of rounding).

The next step is to take 45% of the total for each type of staff and allocate that to the 7 AM to 3 PM (or day) shift. Of 16 RNs, 45% is 7.2 (45% × 16.0 = 7.2), so there will be 7.2 RNs on the 7 AM to 3 PM shift each day. Continuing, 45% of 6.1 is 2.7 (45% × 6.1 = 2.7), and 45% of 2.5 is 1.1 (45% × 2.5 = 1.1). This step is repeated for the 3 PM to 11 PM (evening) shift and 11 PM to 7 AM (night) shift using 35% and 20%, respectively. The results of these calculations fill in the numbers of staff on each shift by type of staff as shown in Table 13–3.

This provides a basic guideline for the manager. However, the manager will next need to make some minor modifications to determine the actual number of people to be on duty on each shift (Table 13–4). In this case, the manager might decide to decrease the number of RNs on the 7 AM to 3 PM day shift to an even 7 instead of using the exact 7.2 that had been calculated. The number of RN staff nurses on the 3 PM to 11 PM shift was increased to 6, and the number on the 11 PM to 7 AM shift was decreased to 3. This leaves the total number of RNs at 16 per day. The LPN category, on the other hand, is increased somewhat on the day shift and reduced on the other two shifts. The total coverage has also been reduced by 0.1. Similar changes are made in the NA category. The total number of shifts per day has been reduced from 24.6 to 24.5.

After the manager modifies the categories, the percentages are recalculated. This allows the manager to see how far from the guidelines the actual proposed staffing pattern has varied as a result of the adjustments. The new total for each shift is divided by the new total shifts, and the new total for each type of staff is divided by the new total for all shifts to get the updated percentages. For example, in Table 13–4, there are now 4.5 total employees on the night shift. Dividing 4.5 by 24.5 total shifts gives 18.4% compared with the guideline of 20%. Most of the percentage changes for both shift and staff type were reasonably small in this example; large variations from the guidelines would require specific justifications.

---

[8]Alternatively, 197 divided by 10 equals 19.7 10-hour shifts per day. Use of 10- or 12-hour shifts instead of 8-hour shifts does not create a problem for finding the number of persons needed on duty each day. However, if the length of shift creates overlapping shifts (the second shift comes on duty before the first shift goes off duty), then the manager must plan work activities with care to ensure that patients receive all required care and productivity levels are maintained.

It is important to bear in mind that the required total staffing hours are based on the hours needed per patient at differing patient classification levels. However, the hours per patient are established based on a specific staff mix. If the staff mix changes substantially, the required hours might change as well. In this example, the changes in actual staff mix from that pre-established total are minor and would not require any adjustment.

The patterns developed here also assume that staffing is the same throughout the week. If some days are particularly busy or slow, it would be possible to have a daily staffing guide. In that case, the total number of shifts per week would be kept at approximately the target level (i.e., 24.6 shifts per day × 7 days per week = 170.2 shifts per week). However, these 170.2 shifts per week could be allocated so there would be more than 24.6 shifts on some days of the week and fewer on others.

Fixed Staff

In addition to the staff calculated above, there are employees whose numbers do not vary with patient volume, such as the unit manager, perhaps nurse educators, and clerical staff. Such staff members are budgeted in addition to the staff retained to directly fill the 71,830 required hours of care. Often such staff members are not replaced when they are sick or on vacation. In those cases, there is no need to calculate sufficient hours to provide coverage when they are out, as was done with the staff FTEs.

Table 13–5 adds fixed staff to the patient care staff in the example. In the table a nurse manager, a nurse educator, three unit clerks (one per shift), and one administrative assistant have been added. Note that it is assumed that there is only one manager, with no coverage when that manager is not present on the unit. This clearly represents fixed staffing. On the other hand, a clerk is required during all three shifts every day. Therefore, enough FTEs will have to be hired to ensure that the clerk position is filled every single day. Nevertheless, the clerks are still fixed staff because they do not vary with the number of patients. Were the expected 9,000 patient days to increase or decrease by 5%, 10%, or 15%, the unit would not employ more or fewer clerks.

Converting Staff and Full-Time Equivalents to Positions

At this point, the number of shifts per day and the number of FTEs needed have been calculated. The next step is to convert this information into the specific positions that will be needed to provide that care. Specifically, it is necessary to determine how many full- and part-time employees will be needed, as well as how much overtime and agency staff time are needed.

Calculating FTEs by Type and Shift

To establish staff positions, it is necessary to calculate the relationship between shifts per day and FTEs. If the manager divides the 43.17 required FTEs by the 24.5 daily staff shifts, it turns out that each person-shift calls for employing 1.76 FTEs. Recall that one FTE will provide coverage one shift per day, 5 days per week, 52 weeks per year (less vacation, holiday, and other nonproductive time). An adequate number of FTEs are needed to provide for the other 2 days out of 7 per week plus the vacations, holidays, and so on. It is important to note that the staff who were hired to fill in 2 days per week—plus vacation, holidays, and other nonproductive time—will *themselves* be taking vacations, holidays, and so on. Therefore, it is not unreasonable to find that coverage of one shift for 365 days per year would require the organization to employ 1.76 FTEs.

Table 13–6 converts the number of staff who are needed to the number of FTEs to be employed. For the employees for whom coverage is not provided when they are on vacation or are otherwise being paid for nonproductive time, the number of person-shifts from Table 13–5 is identical to the number of FTEs in Table 13–6. For example, the one nurse manager shown in Table 13–5 remains as one FTE in Table 13–6.

For each position that must be covered 365 days per year, the number of person-shifts from Table 13–5 is multiplied by 1.76.[9] For example, the 7 person-shifts for RNs from 7 AM to 3 PM

---

[9]Note that 1.76 is not an industry standard. It depends on the portion of paid time that is productive at a specific institution. In this example we want to cover each position 8 hours a day for 365 days per year. That means we need 2,920 productive hours (365 × 8). On the basis of our productive/total paid time ratio of 0.8, we determined that we get 1,664 productive hours/FTE (2,080 paid hours/FTE × 0.8). If we divide 2,920 required hours by 1,664 productive hours/FTE, we find that we need 1.76 FTEs for each position covered one shift for 365 days per year.

✳ **TABLE 13–5** *Staff by Type and Shift (Including Fixed Staff)*

Staff Type	7 AM–3 PM Shift	3 PM–11 PM Shift	11 PM–7 AM Shift	Total
Fixed Staff				
Nurse manager	1.0			1.0
Nurse educator	1.0			1.0
Administrative assistant	1.0			1.0
Clerk	1.0	1.0	1.0	3.0
Subtotal	4.0	1.0	1.0	6.0
Variable Staff				
RN	7.0	6.0	3.0	16.0
LPN	3.0	2.0	1.0	6.0
NA	1.0	1.0	0.5	2.5
Subtotal	11.0	9.0	4.5	24.5
Total	15.0	10.0	5.5	30.5

✳ **TABLE 13–6** *Full-Time Equivalents by Type and Shift (Including Fixed Staff)*

Staff Type	7 AM–3 PM Shift	3 PM–11 PM Shift	11 PM–7 AM Shift	Total
Fixed Staff				
Nurse manager	1.0			1.0
Nurse educator	1.0			1.0
Administrative assistant	1.0			1.0
Clerk	1.8	1.8	1.8	5.4
Subtotal	4.8	1.8	1.8	8.4
Variable Staff				
RN	12.3	10.6	5.3	28.2
LPN	5.3	3.5	1.8	10.6
NA	1.8	1.8	0.9	4.5
Subtotal	19.4	15.9	8.0	43.3
Total	24.2	17.7	9.8	51.7

(see Table 13–5) when multiplied by 1.76 becomes 12.3. This procedure is carried out for each type of staff member for each shift.

Establishing Positions

The 12.3 FTE RNs could be provided by hiring 12 RNs to work full-time and having those 12 nurses additionally share a total of 0.3 FTEs of overtime. Or it could be staffed with 24 half-time RNs and 0.3 FTEs of RNs working per diem (i.e., on an as-needed basis). Or it could be staffed by any of a wide variety of other combinations. Managers should consider that some nurses want to work full time, others want to work part time, and yet others want to work per diem. These personal desires provide the manager flexibility in how a unit is actually staffed.

After the manager knows how many FTEs are needed for each shift and for each type of employee, the next step is to divide the FTEs into straight time and overtime, as shown in Table 13–7. This division will depend on organizational policy and on practical realities. In this example, the policy of the organization is to never use overtime for more than 0.5 FTE for any type of employee on any shift. It is assumed that if more

than 0.5 FTE is needed, it can be supplied by hiring a half-time employee, which would be less costly than paying an overtime premium to a full-time employee. For example, a total of 1.8 FTEs are needed for LPNs on the 11 PM to 7 AM shift. It is assumed that 1.5 FTEs will be filled at straight time, probably by using one full-time employee and one half-time employee. The remaining 0.3 FTEs will be filled by overtime.

In some cases, it is assumed that there is even more flexibility that allows overtime to be avoided. For example, 1.8 FTEs are needed for clerks on each shift. However, the straight-time versus overtime breakdown differs from that used for the LPN on the 11 PM to 7 AM shift. It is assumed by the organization in this example that clerks are easier to hire on a part-time basis than clinical staff. Therefore, no overtime is planned. It must be expected that the organization can hire clerks who will work part of an FTE as needed by the organization. A similar assumption is made about NAs.

After the separation of straight time and overtime is made, the FTEs shown in Table 13–7 can be converted into specific numbers of positions, as shown in Table 13–8. This budget is a link between resources required to care for patients and the cost of the resources. By converting FTEs into the specific

✳ **TABLE 13–7** *Full-Time Equivalents Divided by Straight Time and Overtime*

Staff Type	7 AM–3 PM Shift			3 PM–11 PM Shift			11 PM–7 AM Shift			Total		
	ST	OT	Total	ST	OT	Total	ST	OT	Total	ST	OT	Total
Fixed Staff												
Nurse manager	1.0		1.0							1.0		1.0
Nurse educator	1.0		1.0							1.0		1.0
Administrative assistant	1.0		1.0							1.0		1.0
Clerk	1.8	—	1.8	1.8	—	1.8	1.8	—	1.8	5.4	—	5.4
Subtotal	4.8	—	4.8	1.8		1.8	1.8		1.8	8.4	—	8.4
Variable Staff												
RN	12.0	0.3	12.3	10.5	0.1	10.6	5.0	0.3	5.3	27.5	0.7	28.2
LPN	5.0	0.3	5.3	3.5		3.5	1.5	0.3	1.8	10.0	0.6	10.6
NA	1.8	—	1.8	1.8	—	1.8	0.9	—	0.9	4.5	—	4.5
Subtotal	18.8	0.6	19.4	15.8	0.1	15.9	7.4	0.6	8.0	42.0	1.3	43.3
Total	23.6	0.6	24.2	17.6	0.1	17.7	9.2	0.6	9.8	50.4	1.3	51.7

OT, overtime; ST, straight time.

✳ **TABLE 13–8** *Positions and Hours Budget*

Position Title	Shift	Number of Positions	ST FTEs	ST Hours	OT FTEs	OT Hours	Total FTEs	Total Hours
Fixed Staff								
Nurse manager	7 AM–3 PM	1	1.0	2,080	0.0	0	1.0	2,080
Nurse educator	7 AM–3 PM	1	1.0	2,080	0.0	0	1.0	2,080
Administrative assistant	7 AM–3 PM	1	1.0	2,080	0.0	0	1.0	2,080
Clerk: FT	7 AM–3 PM	1	1.0	2,080	0.0	0	1.0	2,080
Clerk: PT	7 AM–3 PM	1	0.8	1,664	0.0	0	0.8	1,664
Clerk: FT	3 PM–11 PM	1	1.0	2,080	0.0	0	1.0	2,080
Clerk: PT	3 PM–11 PM	2	0.8	1,664	0.0	0	0.8	1,664
Clerk: FT	11 PM–7 AM	1	1.0	2,080	0.0	0	1.0	2,080
Clerk: PT	11 PM–7 AM	4	0.8	1,664	0.0	0	0.8	1,664
Subtotal		13	8.4	17,472	0.0	0	8.4	17,472
Variable Staff								
RN: FT	7 AM–3 PM	11	11.0	22,880	0.3	624	11.3	23,504
RN: PT	7 AM–3 PM	2	1.0	2,080	0.0	0	1.0	2,080
RN: FT	3 PM–11 PM	10	10.0	20,800	0.1	208	10.1	21,008
RN: PT	3 PM–11 PM	1	0.5	1,040	0.0	0	0.5	1,040
RN: FT	11 PM–7 AM	5	5.0	10,400	0.3	624	5.3	11,024
RN: PT	11 PM–7 AM	0	0.0	0	0.0	0	0.0	0
LPN: FT	7 AM–3 PM	5	5.0	10,400	0.3	624	5.3	11,024
LPN: PT	7 AM–3 PM	0	0.0	0	0.0	0	0.0	0
LPN: FT	3 PM–11 PM	3	3.0	6,240	0.0	0	3.0	6,240
LPN: PT	3 PM–11 PM	1	0.5	1,040	0.0	0	0.5	1,040
LPN: FT	11 PM–7 AM	1	1.0	2,080	0.3	624	1.3	2,704
LPN: PT	11 PM–7 AM	1	0.5	1,040	0.0	0	0.5	1,040
NA: FT	7 AM–3 PM	1	1.0	2,080	0.0	0	1.0	2,080
NA: PT	7 AM–3 PM	1	0.8	1,664	0.0	0	0.8	1,664
NA: FT	3 PM–11 PM	1	1.0	2,080	0.0	0	1.0	2,080
NA: PT	3 PM–11 PM	1	0.8	1,664	0.0	0	0.8	1,664
NA: FT	11 PM–7 AM	0	0.0	0	0.0	0	0.0	0
NA: PT	11 PM–7 AM	2	0.9	1,872	0.0	0	0.9	1,872
Subtotal		46	42.0	87,360	1.3	2,704	43.3	90,064
Total		59	50.4	104,832	1.3	2,704	51.7	107,536

FT, full time; FTE, full-time equivalent; OT, overtime; PT, part time; ST, straight time.

number of full- and part-time positions, the manager can start to assign specific individuals to positions to provide patient care. By determining the number of hours that each position will be paid for at straight time and overtime, the manager is beginning to develop the specific information that will be needed to determine the cost of the personnel resources. Often the current-year positions budget is used as a guide in preparing the positions budget for the coming year.

Table 13–8 is derived by taking the information from Table 13–7 that indicates the number of FTEs needed on each shift by type of employee. The FTEs are split between full- and part-time employees according to the manager's perception of staffing needs. In some cases, full-time employees are desired for continuity of care; in others, part-time employees are desired because they allow the manager greater flexibility in filling in for vacations, holidays, and other nonproductive time.

According to the number of positions column of Table 13–8, 59 individuals will be hired by the unit, either full or half time. However, that is not always the case. A variety of staffing patterns are observed. For example, under fixed staff in Table 13–8, note that it is assumed that one clerk can be hired to work 0.8 FTEs on the 7 AM to 3 PM shift. On the 3 PM to 11 PM shift, it is expected that two part-time employees will split 0.8 FTEs, and on the 11 PM to 7 AM shift, four employees will make up 0.8 FTEs. Under variable staff, it is noted that even though 12 full-time RNs could have been hired for the 7 AM to 3 PM shift, 11 full-time and two half-time positions are used. This may provide a greater degree of staffing flexibility for the manager.

Calculating Labor Cost

After the positions have been identified, the next step is to determine the labor cost. This will include straight-time hours, overtime hours, differentials, premiums, and benefits.

Straight-Time and Overtime Salaries

Table 13–8 indicates the paid hours related to the positions. These hours are calculated based on the number of FTEs for each position at a rate of 2,080 paid hours per FTE. For example, two part-time NA positions have been established on the 11 PM to 7 AM shift. Those two positions total 0.9 FTEs. Multiplying 0.9 by 2,080 hours results in a total of 1,872 paid straight-time hours for that employee type. It is important to know the paid hours for overtime separately from total paid hours, because overtime is generally paid at a higher rate.

✳ Table 13–9 *Personnel Cost Budget*

Position Title	Shift	Column: A ST Hours	B Average Rate	C Shift Premium	D Total ST Rate (B + C)	E Total ST $ (A × D)	F OT Hours	G OT Rate (D × 1.5)	H Total OT $ (F × G)	I Total $ (E + H)
Fixed Staff										
Nurse manager	7 AM–3 PM	2,080	$38.00	$0.00	$38.00	$ 79,040	0	$ N/A	$ 0	$ 79,040
Nurse educator	7 AM–3 PM	2,080	27.00	0.00	27.00	56,160	0	N/A	0	56,160
Administrative assistant	7 AM–3 PM	2,080	15.00	0.00	15.00	31,200	0	22.50	0	31,200
Clerk: FT	7 AM–3 PM	2,080	12.00	0.00	12.00	24,960	0	18.00	0	24,960
Clerk: PT	7 AM–3 PM	1,664	11.00	0.00	11.00	18,304	0	16.50	0	18,304
Clerk: FT	3 PM–11 PM	2,080	12.00	1.00	13.00	27,040	0	19.50	0	27,040
Clerk: PT	3 PM–11 PM	1,664	11.00	1.00	12.00	19,968	0	18.00	0	19,968
Clerk: FT	11 PM–7 AM	2,080	12.00	2.00	14.00	29,120	0	21.00	0	29,120
Clerk: PT	11 PM–7 AM	1,664	11.00	2.00	13.00	21,632	0	19.50	0	21,632
Subtotal		17,472				$ 307,424	0		0	$ 307,424
Variable Staff										
RN: FT	7 AM–3 PM	22,880	$24.00	$0.00	$24.00	$ 549,120	624	$36.00	$22,464	$ 571,584
RN: PT	7 AM–3 PM	2,080	25.00	0.00	25.00	52,000	0	37.50	0	52,000
RN: FT	3 PM–11 PM	20,800	23.00	3.45	26.45	550,160	208	39.68	8,252	558,412
RN: PT	3 PM–11 PM	1,040	25.00	3.75	28.75	29,900	0	43.13	0	29,900
RN: FT	11 PM–7 AM	10,400	23.50	4.70	28.20	293,280	624	42.30	26,395	319,675
RN: PT	11 PM–7 AM	0	25.00	5.00	30.00	0	0	45.00	0	0
LPN: FT	7 AM–3 PM	10,400	15.00	0.00	15.00	156,000	624	22.50	14,040	170,040
LPN: PT	7 AM–3 PM	0	17.00	0.00	17.00	0	0	25.50	0	0
LPN: FT	3 PM–11 PM	6,240	15.50	2.33	17.83	111,228	0	26.74	0	111,228
LPN: PT	3 PM–11 PM	1,040	16.00	2.40	18.40	19,136	0	27.60	0	19,136
LPN: FT	11 PM–7 AM	2,080	15.00	3.00	18.00	37,440	624	27.00	16,848	54,288
LPN: PT	11 PM–7 AM	1,040	15.50	3.10	18.60	19,344	0	27.90	0	19,344
NA: FT	7 AM–3 PM	2,080	10.00	0.00	10.00	20,800	0	15.00	0	20,800
NA: PT	7 AM–3 PM	1,664	10.00	0.00	10.00	16,640	0	15.00	0	16,640
NA: FT	3 PM–11 PM	2,080	10.00	1.50	11.50	23,920	0	17.25	0	23,920
NA: PT	3 PM–11 PM	1,664	10.00	1.50	11.50	19,136	0	17.25	0	19,136
NA: FT	11 PM–7 AM	0	10.00	2.00	12.00	0	0	18.00	0	0
NA: PT	11 PM–7 AM	1,872	10.00	2.00	12.00	22,464	0	18.00	0	22,464
Subtotal		87,360				$1,920,568	2,704		$88,000	$2,008,568
Total		104,832				$2,227,992	2,704		$88,000	$2,315,992

FT, full time; OT, overtime; PT, part time; ST, straight time.

As a check in the process, it would be appropriate to determine if the number of care hours budgeted is approximately the number that had been calculated earlier as being required. Recall that for these 9,000 patients, it was determined that 71,830 care hours were needed. From Table 13–8, it is noted that the variable staff subtotal for total hours is 90,064. These represent paid hours. Because 80% of paid hours are productive, according to the earlier calculations, 80% of 90,064 is the budgeted number of care hours. Multiplying 80% by 90,064, the result is 72,051. This is almost exactly the required care hours.[10]

On the basis of hours by type of employee, a cost budget can be prepared. This can be done either by using an average wage rate by category or by listing each of the individuals who will fill the positions and specifying their exact pay rate. The latter approach is more time-consuming but also more accurate.[11] In Table 13–9, the straight-time and overtime hours are taken from Table 13–8, and an average wage is used for each class of employee for each shift. That average would generally be based on the manager's knowledge of the specific individuals making up each category.

The rates used in the budget should be based on the anticipated rates for the coming year. That rate includes any raises over current rates. In some cases, raises are an across-the-board percentage; in other cases, raises may differ by type of employee or even employee by employee.

---

[10]The difference of 221 care hours over the course of the year is a rounding error. We had originally expected to need 43.2 FTEs. The actual plan resulted in 43.3 FTEs, a minor difference.

[11]See Graf C. 2007. The operating budget. In Finkler S, McHugh M. *Budgeting Concepts for Nurse Managers,* 4th edition. Philadelphia: WB Saunders.

Top management may also change the amount of raises built into the operating budget. They may either raise or lower the amount of raises calculated in the initial preparation of the budget. This action may require recalculation of the entire budget. It is advisable to prepare all budgets on a computer, using a spreadsheet program. If such a program is used, hourly rates used in the budget preparation can be changed and a new budget generated without the manager having to manually re-compute the entire budget. Such a computerized approach is also advisable because it will ease the process of budget revision necessitated by any other changes in the budget.

Note that the wage rates for the same type of employee tend to vary by shift and by whether the employee is full-time or part-time. Because part-time employees may not receive the same benefits as full-time employees (perhaps no pension, life insurance, and so on), it may be necessary to pay a higher hourly wage to attract sufficient numbers of part-time employees. In some cases, the less desirable shifts may be staffed by less senior staff, and therefore their base rate is lower than for those working on the day shift.

Such rate differences tend to be highly idiosyncratic. For instance, in this example, the base pay rate for NAs is the same on all shifts for both full- and part-time employees. Part-time clerks receive a lower hourly base wage than full-time clerks. Part-time RNs and LPNs receive a higher hourly wage.

If positions are vacant, care must be exercised in selecting an appropriate pay rate. Will those positions most likely be filled by entry-level employees at the lowest wage rates or by experienced employees at higher pay levels? Managers should try to assess who will be hired, to keep the budget as accurate as possible.

That assumes that vacancies are filled. In some cases, positions may remain open for some time. According to Graf, "If float, per diem or agency staff are used only rarely to cover temporarily vacant positions, then the dollars allocated to the vacant positions can be assumed to cover the alternate staff and the nurse manager can be authorized to hire into all positions."[12]

If it is known that agency staff time will be used even if positions are not vacant, those hours should be converted to FTEs and budgeted for in addition to the staffing shown in Table 13–8.

Differentials and Premiums

Table 13–9 provides a calculation of personnel cost based on average wage rates. Average rates can be obtained from the personnel or payroll offices or by simply averaging the specific rates paid to current staff members. It is common for HCOs to provide a higher wage for evening and night shifts and sometimes for weekend shifts. There are two common approaches for including these costs in the budget. One is to calculate the total lump-sum cost of the differentials to the unit. The other approach is to adjust the hourly wage of employees to include the differential.

To calculate differentials on a lump-sum basis, it is necessary to calculate the number of evening and night hours by class of employee for all the days per year and multiply that by the differential for the class of employee. For example, in the shift premium column in Table 13–9, we note that clerks on the night shift receive a $2 per hour differential. There are 2,080 and 1,664 total night hours scheduled for full-time and part-time clerks, respectively. That adds up to 3,744 hours for the year. At $2 per hour differential, the night clerk differential will be $7,488 ($2 per hour × 3,744 hours). That amount and the differential for each other class of employee must be added into the total personnel cost. The lump-sum approach is especially useful if differentials are stated by the organization on an annual basis per FTE rather than on an hourly basis.

The alternative approach is to calculate the differentials as shown in Table 13–9. This figure specifically adjusts the straight-time hourly wage of each class of employee (column B) based on the appropriate shift differential (column C). This adjustment results in a total straight-time rate (column D) including the differential (Column B + Column C = Column D).

In this example, some differentials are a flat dollar amount and some are based on a percentage of base salary. In the case of clerks, there is a $1 per hour premium for working the 3 PM to 11 PM shift and a $2 per hour premium for working the 11 PM to 7 AM shift. Some clinical staff members in this example receive a 15% differential for the 3 PM to 11 PM shift and a 20% differential for the 11 PM to 7 AM shift. For example, note in column C of Table 13–9 that whereas a full-time 3 PM to 11 PM shift LPN, paid a base wage of $15.50, earns a shift differential of 15%, or $2.33 per hour, a full-time 11 PM to 7 AM shift LPN, paid a base wage of $15.00, earns a shift differential of 20%, or $3.00 per hour. The straight-time rate from column D, which includes the differential, is multiplied by the straight-time hours from column A (taken from Table 13–8) to find the cost of straight-time wages (column E).

An overtime rate is calculated in column G by multiplying the column D straight-time rate by 1.5, or time and a half. The resulting overtime rate is multiplied by the column F overtime hours, which came from Table 13–8, to find total overtime dollars (column H). The column I combination of straight-time and overtime wages gives the total of these two cost elements.

Overtime in some organizations may be calculated differently. For example, the straight-time salary may be increased by 50% for overtime, and then the shift differential is added to that number. If the differential is added to the straight-time salary and then the rate is increased by 50%, the resulting wage is higher than if the differential is added after the salary has been multiplied by 150%.

Weekend differentials, holiday premiums, and on-call premiums create additional complexities in the calculations of personnel cost. A complete budget considers all factors that affect the total salary received by each employee in each position. The specific approach to calculating these premiums differs from organization to organization. Effectively, however, the manager must determine the hourly differential or premium; the number of weekend, holiday, and on-call shifts per year; the number of employees on each of those shifts; and the

[12]Ibid, pp. 202-203.

total cost of those differentials. That total cost must be added into the budget for the unit.

Fringe Benefits

An additional element of personnel cost is fringe benefits. Fringe benefits are employee costs that are in addition to salary. Fringes typically include health and life insurance, pension costs, Social Security (Federal Insurance Contributions Act [FICA]) payments, and other employee benefits. Generally, an average fringe benefit rate is calculated and applied on a uniform basis to payroll costs. The calculation of the fringe benefit rate itself is generally performed by the finance or payroll departments. In some organizations, those departments adjust the budgets of each department or unit to include fringe benefits. In other cases, they communicate the rate, and the unit or department managers increase their budgets by the amount of the fringe benefits.

For example, Table 13–10 shows the addition of fringe benefits to personnel costs in our example. In this organization, two different fringe benefits rates are used: one for full-time and one for part-time personnel. Frequently, part-time employees receive substantially fewer benefits than full-time employees. By calculating two rates to be used, the manager realizes the financial impact on the organization of the decision to use full- versus part-time personnel to provide the needed FTEs. Keep in mind, however, that there is a trade-off, as noted earlier. Although part-time employees have a lower fringe benefit cost to the organization, they may have a higher hourly base salary, to make up for the lower fringe benefits.

In Table 13–10, the total personnel costs before fringe benefits (column A) are taken from the last column in Table 13–9 (column I). These costs (column A, Table 13–10) are multiplied by the appropriate fringe benefit rate to find fringe benefit costs (column C). The cost before fringe benefits (column A) plus the fringe benefit cost (column C) is the total personnel cost (column D).

Special Situations

A variety of specific situations may require that the manager make additional calculations. An important element of the budget process is for the manager to think about various

✳ **TABLE 13–10** *Personnel Cost Budget (Including Fringe Benefits)*

Position Title	Shift	Column: A Total Cost before Fringes	B Fringe Rate	C Fringe $ (A × B)	D Total Personnel Cost (A + C)
Fixed Staff					
Nurse manager	7 AM–3 PM	$ 79,040	23.5%	$ 18,574	$ 97,614
Nurse educator	7 AM–3 PM	56,160	23.5	13,198	69,358
Administrative assistant	7 AM–3 PM	31,200	23.5	7,332	38,532
Clerk: FT	7 AM–3 PM	24,960	23.5	5,866	30,826
Clerk: PT	7 AM–3 PM	18,304	14.5	2,654	20,958
Clerk: FT	3 PM–11 PM	27,040	23.5	6,354	33,394
Clerk: PT	3 PM–11 PM	19,968	15.5	3,095	23,063
Clerk: FT	11 PM–7 AM	29,120	23.5	6,843	35,963
Clerk: PT	11 PM–7 AM	21,632	14.5	3,137	24,769
Subtotal		$ 307,424		$ 67,053	$ 374,477
Variable Staff					
RN: FT	7 AM–3 PM	$ 571,584	23.5%	$134,322	$ 705,906
RN: PT	7 AM–3 PM	52,000	17.5	9,100	61,100
RN: FT	3 PM–11 PM	558,412	23.5	131,227	689,639
RN: PT	3 PM–11 PM	29,900	17.0	5,083	34,983
RN: FT	11 PM–7 AM	319,675	23.5	75,124	394,799
RN: PT	11 PM–7 AM	0	18.0	0	0
LPN: FT	7 AM–3 PM	170,040	23.5	39,959	209,999
LPN: PT	7 AM–3 PM	0	14.3	0	0
LPN: FT	3 PM–11 PM	111,228	23.5	26,139	137,367
LPN: PT	3 PM–11 PM	19,136	14.3	2,736	21,872
LPN: FT	11 PM–7 AM	54,288	23.5	12,758	67,046
LPN: PT	11 PM–7 AM	19,344	14.3	2,766	22,110
NA: FT	7 AM–3 PM	20,800	23.5	4,888	25,688
NA: PT	7 AM–3 PM	16,640	14.3	2,380	19,020
NA: FT	3 PM–11 PM	23,920	23.5	5,621	29,541
NA: PT	3 PM–11 PM	19,136	14.3	2,736	21,872
NA: FT	11 PM–7 AM	0	23.5	0	0
NA: PT	11 PM–7 AM	22,464	14.3	3,212	25,676
Subtotal		$2,008,568		$458,052	$2,466,619
Total		$2,315,992		$525,105	$2,841,096

FT, full time; PT, part time.

additional costs that are incurred every year but not included or accounted for in the budget. Such hidden costs can result in a failure to meet the budget. However, the failure is not the result of poor control of operations but rather poor planning. To avoid such problems, it is essential that managers understand how their staff uses its time and whether any factors are not adequately accounted for in the existing budget formulation.

✳ EXPENSE BUDGET: OTHER-THAN-PERSONNEL SERVICES

The personnel budget is often by far the largest part of the operating budget for a nursing unit, nursing department, or home health agency. However, a complete budget also requires inclusion of a budget for expenses for other-than-personnel services (OTPS). The nurse manager should exercise care in this portion of the budget even if it is substantially smaller than the personnel budget. Miscalculations made in this element of the budget may lead to a need to cut back costs during the year. Often such cutbacks can only be made in the area of personnel. Thus, an underestimated budget for clinical supplies may negatively affect a nursing unit's ability to provide high-quality care.

The nonpersonnel portion of the operating budget, the OTPS budget, includes a wide variety of items, such as clinical supplies, office supplies, minor equipment (noncapital budget items), seminars, books, and a variety of *overhead* items. Overhead represents indirect costs charged to the unit or department from other departments. Some overhead, such as the cost of laundry, is at least partly controllable by the unit. The more laundry used by a department, the higher the overhead charge

for laundry. Other elements of overhead are completely outside the unit manager's control, such as administrative salary and building depreciation charges.

OTPS expenses may be for either fixed or variable items. Clinical supplies, for example, are variable. Their cost should be determined based on the expected number and mix of patients. Publications for the nursing department are a fixed cost. Assuming that publications (e.g., management, specialty practice journals, newsletters) are ordered by the organization for the use of managers and clinicians, the number of patients would have no effect on that cost. Managers must determine a budgeted amount for subscriptions on a somewhat more subjective basis.

Table 13–11 provides a budget worksheet for OTPS costs. This worksheet is generally a summary of information from detailed supporting schedules providing calculations for each of the lines in the worksheet. The worksheet provides information on actual costs incurred to date, the budget for the current year, a projection of total costs for the current year, and the proposed budget for the coming year.

The projection for the current year can be done in one of two ways. The simpler approach is to divide the current year-to-date actual result by the number of months it covers to get an average monthly amount. That amount could then be multiplied by 12 to get an annual projection. A more accurate approach would be to assess whether the remaining months of the year are likely to be busier or slower than the year has averaged up to the current time. The projected annual totals could be estimated after adjusting for expected activity levels. These two approaches are primarily useful for variable costs.

✳ Table 13–11 *Costs for Other-Than-Personnel Services (OTPS)*

	Year-to-Date Actual	Current Year Budget	Current Year Projection	Proposed Budget
Direct Unit Expenses				
Medical-surgical supplies	$126,533	$187,546	$ 191,249	$216,237
Office supplies	8,348	12,493	13,021	15,027
Noncapital equipment	14,325	17,094	17,000	18,255
Seminars	23,450	28,000	27,655	30,000
Publications	1,788	2,000	2,000	2,100
Other	7,351	10,000	10,000	10,500
Total direct unit OTPS	$181,795	$257,133	$ 260,925	$292,119
Overhead Expenses				
Administration	$ 28,345	$ 42,517	$ 43,394	$ 45,234
Depreciation—buildings	34,592	51,888	51,888	51,888
Depreciation—equipment	18,492	27,738	27,738	29,956
Laundry	13,295	21,340	22,431	24,390
Pharmacy	8,391	12,309	13,125	14,150
Laboratory	11,090	14,398	15,232	16,342
Duplication	3,113	4,310	4,100	4,100
Communications	14,321	19,430	19,834	21,079
Other	8,310	12,321	12,500	12,857
Total overhead OTPS	$139,949	$206,251	$210,242	$207,139
Total OTPS	$321,744	$463,384	$471,167	$499,258

For fixed costs, the manager must determine the typical expenditure patterns. If these costs are incurred reasonably evenly throughout the year, the average monthly approach is adequate. If all seminars and meetings take place during certain months of the year, a specific calculation of remaining seminars will need to be made to project the current year total. Similarly, if publications and equipment are all purchased near the beginning of the year (to have their benefit throughout the year) or near the end of the year (after the manager has a feeling for whether spending cuts will be needed near year-end), the manager will have to take those factors into account in making the current year projection.

Developing an accurate current year projection is worth a reasonable amount of effort because it is an important starting point in planning the OTPS costs for the coming year, which is often based on an increase or decrease compared with current-year spending. For example, if the level of photocopying stays the same from year to year, this year's actual duplication costs serve as a primary guide to developing next year's budget.

Costs for the coming year can be developed based on sophisticated forecasting techniques (see Chapter 21), which rely on historical and current information as well as the manager's knowledge and intuition. A simpler, although possibly less accurate, approach is to project next year's budgeted cost as being the current-year cost increased by a percentage for inflation.

In some instances, the manager will be able to prepare a budget based on specific circumstances. If turnover is expected to be unusually high because of planned retirements or maternity leave, a higher budget for filling vacancies and training new staff may be necessary. The specific number of individuals who will be needed and the training that will be needed can be estimated and a budget developed. That number may not bear much relation to costs incurred currently or in the recent past. Rather, the costs will relate primarily to the number of new staff. As Graf points out:

> *The key to budgeting nonsalary expenses . . . is to identify the most reasonable predictor . . . and to make expense projections based on that predictor. In some cases, more than one predictor may be needed. For example, assume that the delivery room's disposable linen account includes linen packs for . . . deliveries and . . . scrub clothes packs for fathers attending deliveries. The predictor for the linen packs is logically the number of deliveries . . . The predictor for the scrub clothes packs, however, may be the attendance at prepared childbirth classes.*[13]

The predictor approach will be quite useful for some OTPS accounts, but noncapital equipment typically requires a more direct approach. During the current year, managers should accumulate lists of noncapital equipment needed for the unit. Any such items that cannot be accommodated during the current year within the existing budget would be explicitly included in the operating budget for the coming year. In addition, at budget preparation time the manager should consider and specify equipment needs. Therefore, this category is less likely to be just a repeat of the prior year adjusted for patient volume or inflation, in contrast to a category such as medical-surgical supplies.

✳ BUDGET SUBMISSION, NEGOTIATION, AND APPROVAL

The three elements of the operating budget—personnel services expenses, OTPS, and revenues—must be compiled into a coherent total document for submission. The budget may not be accepted as submitted, in which case a period of negotiation and budget revision will take place. Finally the budget is approved.

The submitted budget should include an overview page that summarizes the revenues and expenses of the unit or department. In some cases, only expenses are calculated at the unit or department level, and revenues are not part of the operating budget process. In addition to the budget's overview or summary page, detailed schedules should support the requested amounts. Each number from the summary page should be easily traceable to its supporting documentation through titles on the supporting schedules or by a series of references.

The supporting schedules should contain not only numerical calculations, such as those in Tables 13–3 through 13–11, but also narrative support. The narrative defines the unit of service used to develop the budget, the sources of projections for the coming year, and explanations of why the requested amounts are needed. It should also discuss the ramifications of denying the full requested amounts.

Negotiation of the budget usually follows its submission. Because HCOs' resources are limited, requests for funds are often in excess of the amount available. The subsequent reductions in the budget requests should be done in a way that best allows the organization to accomplish its goals and objectives. The budget negotiation process was discussed in Chapter 12.

After the negotiation and revision processes are completed, the budget can be approved by top management and the board. If they do not approve the submitted budget, it must be further revised until it is approved. The manager must then implement the approved budget.

✳ IMPLEMENTING THE APPROVED BUDGET

The development of the operating budget and its ultimate approval are in many ways just the beginning of the budget management process. The manager must convert the approved resources into a working document to guide specific staffing decisions throughout the year.

The manager must address a number of specific problems. First, a staffing schedule must be developed to allow the number of positions approved to be used to fill the daily staffing need. Recall from the example that there was a need for 30.5 shifts per day on average (including fixed staff [see Table 13–5]) and a total of 59 staff positions to fill those shifts. It is necessary to determine when those 59 individuals will be working.

Although there are scheduling programs available to assist the manager, an appreciation of the fundamentals is essential

---

[13]Ibid, p. 212.

to understand that this is a complicated task. Not only must there be coverage 7 days per week, but holiday and vacation coverage must also be planned. Furthermore, there must be flexibility to deal with sick leave, which does not occur on a planned basis. If turnover is expected, the manager must also be able to deal with potential disruptions in unit operations while positions are vacant, followed by low productivity of new workers during their orientation period.

An additional complicating factor is the seasonal nature of many HCOs. There are busy periods and slow periods. Adequate staff must be available to work the busier periods; that requires maintaining a lower staffing level during slower periods. Sometimes a staffing problem can be somewhat offset by using supplemental staff from a per diem or centralized staffing office, which gives a unit flexibility to cover staffing needs during busy periods without hiring staff on a permanent basis or through a contract agency.

Finally, a key element of the implementation process is control. An attempt must be made to keep as close as possible to the approved plan. Control aspects of budgeting are discussed in the next chapter.

✳ SUMMARY OF STEPS IN THE OPERATING BUDGET PROCESS

The following steps are involved in the development of an operating budget:

1. Identify the unit of service that will be the key workload measure for the budget.
2. Calculate workload using the acuity system.
   a. Determine the total nursing care requirements for the year and the number of hours of care needed per patient day.
3. Determine staff requirements.
   a. Calculate the average number of productive hours per FTE.
   b. Determine the number of FTEs needed.
   c. Assign staff by type and shift.
4. Convert staff and FTEs to positions.
   a. Determine positions and how many days per year must be covered.
   b. Determine straight-time and overtime needs.
   c. Determine number of positions and the full- and part-time employees needed to fill them.
5. Calculate labor costs, including shift differentials and overtime.

Completing this process requires knowledge of the organizational assumptions that may be needed at each step.

✳ IMPLICATIONS FOR NURSE MANAGERS AND EXECUTIVES

The operating budget often consumes more of a nurse manager's time than any other aspect of financial management; for that reason, it is worthy of special attention. The three aspects of operating budgets are revenues, personnel expenses, and OTPS. Revenue budgeting is addressed in the next chapter.

The largest element of a nursing unit's operating budget is usually labor. Personnel costs dominate, largely because the clinical care provided by nurses is essential to the process of providing health care services. To account for labor costs as carefully as is warranted requires a lengthy and complicated budgeting process. A workload budget must be developed specifying care hours needed. The workload estimate must be as accurate as possible, adjusting for patient mix whenever possible. Care hours are converted to FTEs and positions. FTEs and positions are converted to dollar costs.

The process as described in this chapter is laborious for the manager and consumes a great deal of time. However, it is essential. Two critical things are at stake in the proper preparation of the personnel budget for nursing. One is the ability of the organization to survive; the other is the ability of the organization to provide patients with high-quality care.

Budgets not prepared with the greatest measure of care may lead to wasted resources. Overstaffing on one shift or one unit is a mistake that may lead to understaffing elsewhere because of inadequate total resources. The budgeting process attempts to allocate the organization's scarce resources to the areas where they are most needed to achieve the organization's objectives. Any resources allocated to a unit where they are not essential represent a failure to allocate those resources to parts of the organization where patients may have had a greater need for them.

The goal of budgeting is neither to maximize nor to minimize a budget. Thus, it is important for managers to overcome the adversarial impulse that naturally arises in the budgeting process. The budgeting process should not be a fiercely competitive exercise. Instead, the process requires a whole systems view of the organization that attempts to take the needs of all areas into account. The goal of budgeting is to develop a plan that places the organization's available resources in the appropriate places where the sum total accomplishment of the organization goals will be the greatest.

✳ KEY CONCEPTS

Operating budget   Plan for the day-to-day operating revenues and expenses of the organization, generally prepared for a 1-year period.

Workload   The amount or quantity of work performed by a unit.

Workload budget   Budget that indicates the amount of work performed by a unit or department, measured in terms of units of service. This information is used to prepare expense budgets.

Unit of service   Measure of the work performed by the cost center, such as number of patients, patient days, deliveries, visits, treatments, or procedures.

Activity report   Measures key statistics concerning current activity. It centers on the number of units of service and the relative proportion of the organization's capacity being used.

> **Census**   Number of beds on a patient care unit that are occupied each day at a certain point in time (usually midnight).

> **Occupancy rate**   Percentage of total beds filled on a patient care unit or an entire organization (i.e., the number of beds filled divided by the total number of beds available).

> **Average daily census (ADC)**   Number of patients cared for per day on average over a period of time.

> **Average length of stay (ALOS)**   Average number of days that each patient is in a hospital or nursing home.

> **Patient day**   Accounting term that represents the notion of one patient cared for during a 1-day or a 24-hour period.

Adjusted units of service   Whenever possible, budgeting should be based on expected workload units of service adjusted for the specific mix of patients expected.

Patient acuity (or patient classification system)   System for categorizing categories based on the resources they are expected to use.

Care hours calculation   Determination of the average required care hours per patient per 24 hours for each classification level and the total required care hours for all patients.

Expense budget: personnel services   Budget for all personnel under the manager's direction, generally within a cost center.

Variable staff   Staff needed to provide the required number of care hours, whose time and work vary with volume or service. Variable staff is calculated as follows:

1. Determine the number of paid hours per FTE.

2. Determine the percentage of productive hours to total paid hours.

3. Multiply the number of paid hours per FTE by the percentage of productive hours to find the number of productive hours per FTE.

4. Divide required care hours by productive hours per FTE to find the required number of FTEs.

5. Divide the required care hours by the number of days per year that the unit has patients to find care hours, per day. Divide that result by hours per shift to find the number of person shifts needed per working day.

6. Assign person shifts per working day by staff type and among required shifts.

Fixed staff   Employees on the unit whose time does not vary with patient volume.

FTE   Full-time equivalent, typically defined as 8 hours per day, 5 days per week, 52 weeks per year, for a total of 2,080 hours per year. The determination of the hours that constitute an FTE may vary by organization, but FTE always represents full-time work. FTEs can be filled with any combination of people working in positions for varying amounts of time that add up to the required number of FTEs.

Position   One person working for the organization for any number of hours per week to perform specific job duties. Daily staff requirements can be met by a variety of full-time and part-time positions that add up to the required number of FTEs. The breakdown between full-time and part-time is at the manager's discretion.

Productive time   Time spent by staff delivering care to patients, communicating with other staff about patients, obtaining supplies needed by patients, and engaging in other patient care–related activities.

Nonproductive time   Time paid to staff as a benefit that is not spent delivering care to patients. Nonproductive time includes sick, vacation, holiday, and often professional development days.

Calculating labor cost   Each position's hours must be converted to a dollar basis considering straight-time salary, overtime rate, differentials, raises, and fringe benefit costs for each employee type.

Expense budget: other-than-personnel services (OTPS)   Budget for all non-personnel expenses (e.g., supplies, minor equipment), including both direct unit or department expenses and indirect overhead expenses.

Budget submission   Revenue and expense portions of the budget must be summarized and submitted for review together with detailed supporting calculations and narrative justification. Budget revisions may be required as the result of a series of negotiations over the submitted budget.

Budget implementation   Managers must address a number of issues in implementing an approved budget, including development of a staffing plan that provides coverage for staff weekends, holidays, vacations, and sick leave as well as busy and slow periods.

✳ SUGGESTED READINGS

Aiken LH, Clark SP, Sloan DM, et al: Hospital nurse staffing and patient mortality, nurse burnout, and job dissatisfaction, *JAMA* 288(16):1987–1993, 2002.

Aiken LH, Sloan DM, Cimiotti JP, et al: Implications of the California nurse staffing mandate for other states, *Health Serv Res* 45(4):904–921, 2010.

Bolton LB, Aydin CE, Donaldson N, et al: Mandated nurse staffing ratios in California: a comparison of staffing and nurse-sensitive outcomes pre- and post-regulation, *Policy Polit Nurs Pract* 8(4):238–250, 2007.

Bolton LE, Aydin CE, Donaldson N, et al: Nurse staffing and patient perceptions of nursing care, *J Nurs Adm* 33(11):607–614, 2003.

Budreau G, Balakrishnan R, Titler M, Hafner M: Caregiver-patient ratio: capturing census and staffing variability, *Nurs Econ* 17(6):317–324, 1999.

Carruth A, Carruth P, Noto E: Financial management. Nurse managers flex their budgetary might, *Nurs Manage* 31(2):16–17, 2000.

Cavouras C, McKinley J: Variable budgeting for staffing analysis and evaluation, *Nurs Manage* 28(5):34–36, 39, 1997.

Cho SH, Ketefian S, Barkauskas VH, Smith DG: The effects of nurse staffing on adverse events, morbidity, mortality, and medical costs, *Nurs Res* 52(2):71–79, 2003.

Corley M, Satterwhite B: Forecasting ambulatory clinic workload to facilitate budgeting, *Nurs Econ* 11(2):77–81, 114, 1993.

Douglas D, Mayewske J: Census variation staffing, *Nurs Manage* 27(2):32–33, 36, 1996.

Dreisbach A: A structured approach to expert financial management: a financial development plan for nurse managers, *Nurs Econ* 12(3):131–139, 1994.

Edwardson S, Giovannetti P: Nursing workload measurement systems, *Annu Rev Nurs Res* 12:95–123, 1994.

Finkler S, McHugh M: *Budgeting concepts for nurse managers*, ed 4, Philadelphia, 2007, WB Saunders.

Finkler S, Ward D, Baker J: *Essentials of cost accounting for health care organizations*, ed 3, Boston, 2006, Jones & Bartlett.

Goodard N: The five most common flaws in healthcare staffing and personnel budgeting, *Nurse Leader* 1(5):44–48, 2003.

Henderson E: Continuing professional development: budgeting. Budgeting: part one, *Nurs Manage (Harrow)* 10(1):33–37, 2003.

Henderson E: Continuing professional development: budgeting. Budgeting: part two, *Nurs Manage (Harrow)* 10(2):32–36, 2003.

Hernandez C, O'Brien-Pallas L: Validity and reliability of nursing workload measurement systems: review of validity and reliability theory, *Can J Nurs Adm* 9(3):32–50, 1996.

Horn SD, Buerhaus P, Bergstrom N, Smout RJ: RN staffing time and outcomes of long-stay nursing home residents: pressure ulcers and other adverse outcomes are less likely as RNs spend more time on direct patient care, *Am J Nurs* 105(11):58–70, 2005.

Institute of Medicine: *Keeping patients safe: transforming the work environment of nurses*, Washington, DC, 2004, National Academies Press, p. 237.

Kane RL, Shamliyan T, Mueller C, et al: *Nurse staffing and quality of patient care*, Rockville, Maryland, 2007, Agency for Healthcare Research and Quality. AHRQ Publication 07-E005.

Kirkby M: Number crunching with variable budgets, *Nurs Manage* 34(3):28–34, 2003.

Kovner C, Gergen PJ: Nurse staffing levels and adverse events following surgery in U.S. hospitals, *Image J Nurs Sch* 30:315–321, 1998.

Kovner C, Jones C, Zahn C, et al: Nurse staffing and post-surgical adverse events: an analysis of administrative data from a sample of U.S. hospitals, 1990-1996, *Health Serv Res* 37(3):611–629, 2002.

Kutney-Lee A, McHugh MD, Sloane DM, et al: Nursing: a key to patient satisfaction, *Health Aff* 28(4):669–677, 2009.

Lake E, Shang J, Klaus S, Dunton N: Patient falls: association with hospital Magnet status and nursing unit staffing, *Res Nurs Health* 33(5):413–425, 2010.

Mark BA, Harless DW: Nurse staffing and post-surgical complications using the present on admission indicator, *Res Nurs Health* 33(1):35–47, 2009.

McGillis Hall L, Doran D, Pink GH: Nurse staffing models, nursing hours, and patient safety outcomes, *J Nurs Adm* 34(1):41–45, 2004.

McLean R: *Financial management in health care organizations*, ed 2, Albany, New York, 2002, Delmar.

Needleman J, Buerhaus P, Mattke S, et al: Nurse staffing levels and the quality of care in hospitals, *N Engl J Med* 346(22):1715–1722, 2002.

Needleman J, Buerhaus P, Pankratz V, et al: Nurse staffing and inpatient hospital mortality, *N Engl J Med* 364(11):1037–1045, 2011.

O'Brien-Pallas L, Irvine D, Peereboom E, Murray M: Measuring nursing workload: understanding the variability, *Nurs Econ* 15(4):171–182, 1997.

Ray C, Cavouras C: Managers forum. Budgeting education costs, *J Emerg Nurs* 30(3):267–268, 292–297, 2004.

Rogers AE, Hwang W, Scott LD, et al: The working hours of hospital staff nurses and patient safety, *Health Aff* 23(4):202–12, 2004.

Rothberg MB, Abraham I, Lindenauer PK, Rose DN: Improving nurse-to-patient staffing ratios as a cost-effective safety intervention, *Med Care* 43(8):785–791, 2005.

Samuels D: *The healthcare financial management and budgeting toolkit*, Burr Ridge, Ill, 1997, Richard D. Irwin.

Sengin K, Dreisbach A: Managing with precision: a budgetary decision support model, *J Nurs Adm* 25(2):33–44, 1995.

Shelver S, Moss M: Operating room budget factors: a pocket guide to OR finance, *Nurs Econ* 12(3):146–152, 1994.

Sochalski J: Is more better? The relationship between hospital staffing and the quality of nursing care in hospitals, *Med Care* 42(Suppl 2):1167–1173, 2004.

Sochalski J, Konetzaka T, Zhu J, Volp K: Will mandated minimum nurse staffing ratios lead to better patient outcomes? *Med Care* 46(6):606–613, 2008.

Spetz J, Chapman S, Herrara C, et al: Assessing the impact of California's nurse staffing ratios on hospitals and patient care, *California Healthcare Foundation issue brief* (website), February 2009. www.chcf.org/publications/2009/02/assessing-the-impact-of-californias-nurse-staffing-ratios-on-hospitals-and-patient-care. Accessed February 25, 2012.

Strasen L: *Key business skills for nurse managers*, Philadelphia, 1987, JB Lippincott.

Swansburg R: *Budgeting and financial management for nurse managers*, Sudbury, Mass, 1997, Jones & Bartlett.

Unruh L: Licensed nurse staffing and adverse events in hospitals, *Med Care* 41(1):142–152, 2003.

Wan TT, Zhang NJ, Unruh L: Predictors of resident outcome improvement in nursing homes, *West J Med Res* 28(8):974–993, 2006.

Whelchel C: Executive exchange. Patients first when budgeting, *Nurs Manage* 35(3):16, 2004.

Yang KP: Relationships between nurse staffing and patient outcomes, *J Nurs Res* 11(3):149–158, 2003.

Revenue Budgeting

CHAPTER GOALS

The goals of this chapter are to:

- Discuss sources of revenues
- Explain the importance of prices and volume in revenue budgeting
- Clarify why revenues are often ignored in nursing budgets
- Discuss when revenues should be considered in nursing budgets

- Provide examples of revenue budget calculations
- Discuss revenues from managed care organizations
- Define *capitation*
- Explain the impact of capitation on risk
- Provide an example of how capitation rates can be calculated
- Define *risk-sharing pools* and discuss their use

✳ INTRODUCTION

The previous chapter discussed preparation of a nursing unit operating budget. However, it focused primarily on the expense side of that budget. Operating budgets consist of both revenues and expenses. This chapter focuses on issues related to revenues. Revenues are the amount the organization earns in exchange for the services it provides. Revenues are critical for every organization.

Revenues must be adequate to cover all the costs of providing services. In addition, revenues should be great enough to provide a profit. This is true whether the organization is a for-profit or not-for-profit organization. Profits are used to expand the type of services offered, expand the volume of services offered, and replace buildings and equipment. Both inflation and technological advances often cause new capital acquisitions (see Chapter 12 for a discussion of capital budgeting) to be more expensive than those they replace. Profits earned each year help the organization accumulate sufficient resources for replacements and expansion.

Many different sources of revenues are relevant to nurses. Typically, one thinks of patient revenues. These are amounts that are received directly either from patients or from third parties, such as insurance companies. They are payments for health care services provided. Buppert[1] explains some of the mechanisms for getting reimbursement directly for nursing services. However, in various nursing situations, there are a wide variety of other revenue sources as well. Swansburg[2] has listed some other sources of nursing revenue, as follows:

- Grants
- Continuing education
- Private practice
- Community visibility
- Health care students and staff
- Managed care organizations (MCOs)
- City health departments
- Industry
- Unions
- Professional corporations
- Nurse-managed centers

And this list is far from exhaustive.

In a growing number of situations, nurse managers and executives are required to prepare revenue budgets and are held accountable for revenue. This chapter begins with a discussion of some basic issues and addresses a number of questions related to revenues. What are they? How are they earned? Why are they often ignored in discussions about nursing budgets? When should they be considered? The chapter then moves on to a discussion of the calculation of revenues related to nursing.

The chapter concludes with a discussion of issues related to managed care revenues, with a particular emphasis on issues related to revenues from capitation arrangements. That section

---

[1]Buppert C. 2005. Third-party reimbursement for nurse practitioners' services on trauma teams: Working through a maze of issues. *J Trauma* 58(1):206-212.

[2]Swansburg R. 1997. *Budgeting and Financial Management for Nurse Managers.* Boston: Jones & Bartlett.

provides an introduction to managed care concepts, including risk. The role of risk pools in revenue budgeting is also addressed. An example of how capitation rates can be determined is provided.

✳ THE REVENUE BUDGET

The operating budget for any organization consists of a revenue budget and an expense budget. Often nurse managers and executives are responsible only for controlling spending and have no responsibility for revenues. But in many situations, nurses are accountable for revenues as well as expenses. For example, the director of the operating room traditionally has been charged with earning a profit based on having revenues that exceed costs. Units or departments that have responsibility for revenue as well as expense are called *revenue centers* in health care. Units or departments that do not have a revenue budget are called *cost centers* or *expense centers.*

Why Aren't All Nursing Units Revenue Centers?

In most industries, including health care, managers are generally responsible for only expenses. Think of the auto industry, for example. To make a car, there is an engine department, a bumper department, a door department, a steering wheel department, and other departments. Should each of those departments be revenue centers, assigned both revenues and expenses (as an outpatient surgery unit would be) or just be expense centers (as a typical medical-surgical nursing unit would be)? When you buy a car, you pay a set amount for the entire car. You do not think in terms of buying a separate engine, bumper, doors, and steering wheel. So what would be a reasonable way to allocate the price a car buyer pays for the car to each department of the car manufacturer? There is not any reasonable way. Any approach to the allocation would be arbitrary. As a result, the various departments are treated as expense centers and do not get any revenue assigned to them. Each department just has an expense budget based on what it should cost to efficiently manufacture the parts made by the department. As long as the total cost of all the parts is less than the price the car is sold for, the manufacturer is making a profit. This is fairly typical of most organizations. Revenue is not generally assigned to individual managers, departments, or units.

Similarly, in any health care organization (HCO) that receives a lump-sum payment for each patient (e.g., a Diagnosis Related Group payment), it makes sense to avoid setting up revenue centers. In many HCOs, nursing is similar to the engine department. It is critical to the final product. The car being manufactured cannot run without an engine. However, just as a car manufacturer cannot figure out a "correct" way to divide up the price of the car among the departments that made it, it is hard for an HCO to determine a fair or reasonable way to allocate the revenue from a lump-sum payment for a patient's care to the different departments that provided the care. As a result, revenue often is not allocated to departments in HCOs.

However, not all patients pay a flat amount for their care. There are still many situations in which patients are charged and pay for individual radiographs, laboratory tests, and pharmaceuticals. In those cases, revenue is often allocated to some of the departments providing those specific services. Often medical-surgical nursing units are not among those departments. Why not allocate revenue for nursing services? Because historically this was difficult to do. Exactly how much nursing care is consumed by each specific patient? It would be expensive to hire an accountant to follow each nurse and keep track of how much of the nurse's time was used to provide care to each patient.

Today, the health care industry is making rapid progress in the areas of computerization and information technologies. In some HCOs, nurses may scan their ID badge whenever they provide care to a patient, and the organization's information system may be able to track the different amount of nursing care received by different patients. So it is now becoming feasible to charge different patients different amounts for the nursing services they receive (see Chapter 9, Figure 9-7). Nevertheless, movement toward making nursing units revenue centers in hospitals has been slow. Finance officers have been resistant to change. However, there does finally seem to be some movement toward making the nursing portion of health care revenues more explicit. Both Maryland and Maine now have laws requiring separation of nursing on hospital bills.[3] This could be the beginning of a trend that would substantially extend the nurse manager's involvement and responsibility for revenues.

When Are Nurse Managers and Executives Responsible for a Revenue Budget?

Despite the slow movement to nursing revenue centers in hospitals, there are many situations in which nurse managers or executives are already responsible for developing revenue budgets, and these situations are likely to increase rapidly in the near future. In some cases, these opportunities may occur in hospitals, where nurses are already responsible for revenue budgets for the operating room, recovery room, labor and delivery, and other departments. However, hospitals should not be the sole focus. The past several decades have seen a clear shift away from hospital inpatient care to provision of care on an outpatient basis. This shift has created growing opportunities for nursing to have revenue responsibility.

In outpatient settings, nurse managers are often responsible for the revenue budgets of outpatient surgery units, clinics, community health centers, hospices, and home care agencies. In many cases, nurses need to prepare revenue budgets for their own clinical practice, consulting practice, or other type of venture. Nurse educators may be responsible for tuition revenues. Nurse researchers are responsible for grant revenues. The situations in which nurses must prepare and manage revenue budgets are extensive and growing.

---

[3]Ibid, p. 26.

The Elements of a Revenue Budget

The basic elements of a revenue budget are simple—price and volume. The revenue budget essentially consists of the price charged for each service provided by the unit, department, or organization multiplied by the number of units of service provided. The complications involved in a revenue budget are estimating the volume of services to be provided, deciding on the prices to charge, and estimating how much of the total amount charged will actually be collected.

Consider a simple example. Suppose that the Best Clinic treats patients on a cash basis. That is, patients pay for their treatment in cash as the treatment is provided by the clinic. If 10 patients are expected to be treated, the charge to each one is $100, and if all amounts are collected, the revenue will be:

$100/Patient × 10 Patients = $1,000 of Revenue

Even this simple first look at revenue is complicated. How did the organization decide to charge $100? How did it decide that 10 patients were likely? The following sections address the key elements of price and volume as they pertain to the revenue budgeting process.

Prices or Rates

A number of different types of prices are used in health care. Organizations set a price or charge for their services. However, some payers pay a percent of the charge that is less than 100% based on a contractual agreement. Other payers pay a flat amount per case regardless of the amount charged. Hospitals are sometimes paid on a per diem basis or a per discharge basis. The per discharge payment may be adjusted for diagnosis or might be a broad average payment regardless of patient type. Some payers just reimburse the organization for the costs that have been incurred in providing care. Home care can be reimbursed on a flat amount per visit or paid as a flat amount per patient regardless of the number of visits required. Under *capitation*, discussed later, the health care provider is paid a flat amount per member regardless of whether the member consumes any health care resources at all!

For some organizations, the finance department may provide the nurse manager with information about the prices (often called *rates*) that will be charged for each service. In such cases, the manager is primarily responsible for estimating the future number of each type of patient to be treated and for multiplying the volume of each service times the given prices to arrive at the revenue budget. The main difference between this and the $1,000 of revenue for Best Clinic discussed previously is the fact that there typically are many different kinds of patients with different prices, and the manager must be as accurate as possible in estimating the future volume of each type of patient.

In other cases, however, the nurse manager will be responsible for setting prices. This is often referred to as *rate setting*. Prices can be *market-based, cost-based, mark-up–based,* or *negotiated*. Market-based prices are those that are set based on a survey of what others in the community are charging for the same services. If one charges substantially more than others are charging, in some cases, customers may be lost. Some organizations intentionally set prices below the competition's in an effort to stimulate business. The success of strategies to undercut the competition or to charge above the market (and make more profit per patient) depends largely on how sensitive buyers are to price.

Many individuals shop around to buy a car, seeking the lowest price for what is essentially the exact same commodity. For example, if a specific model car from a specific manufacturer is sold by three different dealers in the area, the customer may shop for the best price from among the three dealers. What if a gallbladder operation can be obtained from three different surgeons at three different hospitals? The customer is less likely to view the sugeries as being identical. Shopping may be based more on the reputation of the surgeon or hospital than on the price.

Suppose that a nurse manager starts a home care agency in an area that already has two home care agencies. Will potential customers consider the service to be identical and therefore look for the lowest price? The nurse can decide to compete by charging less than the competition. Or the manager might decide to market the service directly to potential patients as being better in some way (e.g., higher-quality nurses, more caring attitude, longer visits). Or the manager might decide simply to charge the market price and then focus marketing efforts on hospital discharge planners, who are responsible for referring patients to home care agencies.

Alternatives to market-based prices are cost-based or mark-up–based prices. Cost-based refers to charging exactly what it costs to deliver care. By *cost*, we typically mean average cost. There are many instances in which laws or regulations require such prices. For example, a state might mandate that home care agencies charge Medicaid exactly the cost of providing care. Mark-up–based prices are those in which the manager determines the cost of care and sets the price a certain percentage above cost. For example, if a visit costs $40 to provide, an organization with a 20% mark-up would charge $48 for the visit (i.e., $40 + [20% × $40]).

It is also becoming more common for health care providers to use another strategy, negotiated rates, with insurance companies and other third-party payers. The negotiation can result in a variety of different payment approaches, such as flat fees, percent discounts, or payments per episode, which may vary by insurance company.

Suppose that the Best Clinic, using a market price strategy, sets its price at $100. Does that mean that the clinic will collect $100 for each patient? In reality, patients do not usually arrive with cash in hand. More often they have insurance. Some insurers will pay the full $100. But that is extremely rare. Many insurers only pay a specific amount for a particular service. Others demand a percentage discount. Often prices paid by insurers are the result of a protracted negotiation. A complete revenue budget must take into account the fact that health care providers do not usually collect the full amount charged.

For example, Blue Cross might say it will pay only $60 for services delivered at the Best Clinic. If the clinic wants to accept a Blue Cross patient, it can charge $100, but then it must give a $40 *contractual allowance* (i.e., a discount based on its contract with Blue Cross). The net charge, after subtracting the contractual allowance, is therefore $60. So, in preparing a revenue budget, it would be necessary to estimate the percent of patients who are insured by Blue Cross and calculate their net revenue as being $60 rather than $100. Another insurer might negotiate a percentage discount rather than a specific price for each service. Suppose that some of the clinic's patients are insured by Aetna and that the clinic's agreement with that insurer calls for it to pay 80% of charges. Best Clinic's revenue budget might look like Table 14–1. Total net revenue is $860, rather than the $1,000 revenue originally calculated for the 10 patients.

Some of the clinic's patients might be Medicare or Medicaid patients. Assume that Best Clinic has one of each. Suppose that Medicaid regulations call for it to pay the cost of care and that the cost of each visit is $55. The allowance or discount for the Medicaid patient is therefore $45. Suppose further that Medicare has a fee schedule that calls for it to pay $70 for this type of patient. The allowance for the Medicare patient is therefore $30. The revenue budget would now appear as shown in Table 14–2. Note that the total net revenue is $785.

At this point, it is clear that HCOs often collect substantially less than the amount they charge for services. One reason they charge so much for health care services is because so many customers receive discounts. This is exacerbated by the fact that some customers do not pay their charges at all! Some patients will not be able to pay for their care because they do not have the financial resources. Others may just not be willing to pay.

In the former case, the organization may decide to treat the patient as a charity case. In such instances, the organization will charge either a lower amount or nothing at all. Suppose that one of the patients treated has no insurance and is poor. Best Clinic decides to give the patient a 75% discount. In that case, the gross revenue from that patient will be only $25. We do not include care that is being given as charity as part of revenues. It is a gift, rather than a charge that is not collected. The cost of that care, however, will be included in the expense budget.

Some patients have the resources to pay for care but never pay. This occurs in two different ways. Some patients do not have insurance and simply fail to pay part or all of their bill. Many patients do have insurance but are required to pay a portion of the charge—perhaps 20% or 30%. That portion is called a *co-pay* or *co-payment*. If a patient fails to pay the co-pay portion, the insurance company often will not pay that amount either. When patients do not pay amounts that have been charged to them, the amounts not paid are referred to as *bad debts*. Bad debts may arise from self-insured patients who do not pay their bills or from the co-pay share of insured patients. Organizations should bill promptly, send monthly statements, and use collection agencies if necessary to collect as much of the money owed to them as possible.

Assume that Best Clinic has one *self-pay* (uninsured) patient whose bill is not paid. Table 14–3 shows the net revenue

✳ **TABLE 14–1** *Best Clinic Revenue Budget for the Year Ending December 31, 2014*

Patients by Payer	Gross Revenue	Contractual Allowances	Net Revenue
2 Blue Cross patients	$ 200	$ 80	$120
$100 × 2 = $200 gross revenue			
$100 − $60 = $40 allowance per patient			
$ 40 × 2 patients = $80 allowance			
3 Aetna patients	300	60	240
$100 × 3 = $300 gross revenue			
$100 × 20% = $20 allowance per patient			
$ 20 × 3 patients = $60 allowance			
5 Other patients	500	0	500
Total	$1,000	$140	$860

✳ **TABLE 14–2** *Best Clinic Revenue Budget for the Year Ending December 31, 2014*

Patients by Payer	Gross Revenue	Contractual Allowances	Net Revenue
2 Blue Cross patients	$ 200	$ 80	$120
$100 × 2 = $200 gross revenue			
$100 − $60 = $40 allowance per patient			
$ 40 × 2 patients = $80 allowance			
3 Aetna patients	300	60	240
$100 × 3 = $300 gross revenue			
$100 × 20% = $20 allowance per patient			
$ 20 × 3 patients = $60 allowance			
1 Medicaid patient	100	45	55
1 Medicare patient	100	30	70
3 Other patients	300	0	300
Total	$1,000	$215	$785

✳ **TABLE 14–3** *Best Clinic Revenue Budget for the Year Ending December 31, 2014*

Patients by Payer	Gross Revenue	Discounts and Contractual Allowances	Net Revenue
2 Blue Cross patients	$200	$ 80	$ 120
$100 × 2 = $200 gross revenue			
$100 − $60 = $40 allowance per patient			
$ 40 × 2 patients = $80 allowance			
3 Aetna patients	300	60	240
$100 × 3 = $300 gross revenue			
$100 × 20% = $20 allowance per patient			
$ 20 × 3 patients = $60 allowance			
1 Medicaid patient	100	45	55
1 Medicare patient	100	30	70
1 Charity self-pay patient (75% discount)	25	0	25
1 Bad debt self-pay patient	100	0	100
1 Other self-pay patient	100	0	100
Total	$925	$215	$ 710
Less bad debt			− 100
Net revenue less bad debts			$ 610

for the clinic. Note that bad debts are disclosed separately. Some organizations do a better job and some a worse job of collecting amounts owed to them. Seeing the bad debts as a separate item helps the reader get a sense of how well a particular organization has done in this area.

It is important to note that Best Clinic expects to collect only $610 for providing care to the 10 patients (see Table 14–3). Even though there were 10 patients who each received a $100 service, only $925 was charged in total (because of the charity care) rather than $1,000. The final amount collected was $610 because of allowances and bad debts. Unless the manager is careful to go through this computation, there may be a mistaken assumption that the organization has much more money available to spend on providing care than is actually the case. It is critical to estimate the actual amounts that will be collected for each patient as carefully as possible. This means spending time trying to determine the likely rate of bad debts (often from historical experience), reviewing contracts with insurers to determine payment rates, and even considering things such as discounts given to credit card companies for patients who charge their bills.[4]

Volume Estimates

Even if the amount collected per patient is meticulously considered, the revenue budget still depends heavily on estimates of volume. Volume can be estimated using the forecasting techniques discussed in Chapter 21. Note that it is not sufficient to estimate total patient volume. The volume of each type of patient or procedure for which there is a different charge must be estimated. This may entail estimation of home care visits by nurses versus aides. Or perhaps a manager will need

to estimate patients, patient days, treatments, hours, procedures, and tests. Some degree of flexibility is required to forecast based on type of patient or type of procedure or test, depending on the specific requirements of a particular situation.

In preparing the revenue budget, it is extremely important to consider all possible sources of revenue or support. In addition to patient charges for services, these sources might include ancillary sources such as gift shops or restaurants, endowment income, gifts, or grants. Clearly, the final revenue budget will be more complex than Table 14–3, showing revenues not only by type of payer but also by different types of patients or procedures and including information about other types of revenue. Table 14–4 presents a somewhat more sophisticated example for an outpatient organization that provides both same-day surgery and a variety of clinic services. However, even this example is simplified because it only breaks patients down into same-day surgery versus clinic groups as opposed to a more detailed breakdown by type of surgery, type of visit, procedure, or tests.

In Table 14–4, the first column on the left indicates the different revenue sources, listing the different types of patients by payer, and other revenue sources. The next column, column A, Quantity, indicates the forecast volume level for each revenue source. In this example, 1,000 same-day surgery patients with private insurance are expected. There are anticipated to be 7,000 purchases from the gift shop and 400 donations.

Moving to column B, Rate or Charge, the full charge on average for each type of service is indicated. For example, the average same-day surgery charge is expected to be $1,500. Obviously, a more realistic budget would show different types of surgery patients and different charges for each type. In column B, we also see that the average purchase at the gift shop is $17, and the average donation to the organization is $200.

Column C, the Gross Revenue, can be found by multiplying column A by column B. This represents the total of all charges by the organization to its patients, as well as gift shop charges and donations.

---

[4]If a patient charges a $100 bill for health care services on a credit card, the credit card company will typically pay the provider anywhere between $95 and $98. The difference between the $100 charge and the amount the credit card company pays is a fee to cover the costs and some of the profits of the credit card company.

✳ TABLE 14–4 *Surgery and Clinic Revenue Budget for the Year Ending June 30, 2015*

Revenue Source	(A) Quantity	(B) Rate or Charge	(C = A × B) Gross Revenue	(D) Average Net Charge	(E = C × D) Revenue Net of Discounts and Allowances
Same-day surgery					
Private insurance	1,000	$1,500	$1,500,000	75%	$1,125,000
Medicare	600	1,500	900,000	80%	720,000
Medicaid	400	1,500	600,000	60%	360,000
Self-pay	500	1,500	750,000	70%	525,000
Clinic patients					
Private insurance	3,000	250	750,000	75%	562,500
Medicare	1,800	250	450,000	80%	360,000
Medicaid	1,200	250	300,000	60%	180,000
Self-pay	1,500	250	375,000	85%	318,750
Gift shop	7,000	17	119,000	99%	117,810
Donations	400	200	80,000	100%	80,000
Subtotal			$5,824,000		$4,349,060
Less bad debt					−112,500
Net revenue less bad debts					$4,236,560

Column D, the average net charge, represents the average percent of the full charge that is collected. For example, if private insurance payments typically average 75% of the full charge, then column D shows 75%. Note that the percentage shown for self-pay patients in this column reflects contractual allowances but not bad debts, which appear later in the table.

The percentage shown for the gift shop reflects the fact that the organization provides a 10% discount for purchases by employees. If employees account for 10% of all purchases from the gift shop, that would result in an average discount of 1% across all gift shop sales (i.e., a 10% discount to employees who make up 10% of all purchases = 10% × 10% = 1% discount on all sales on average).

Column E is simply column C multiplied by column D. This represents the amount expected to be collected. At the bottom of this column, we see that bad debts are shown as $112,500. This represents 10% of all amounts charged to self-pay patients (i.e., [$750,000 same-day surgery + $375,000 clinic] × 10%). The 10% typically would be based on historical bad debt experience. Note in Table 14–4 that although Surgery and Clinic expects to have gross charges of $5,824,000, they expect to collect only $4,236,560 for the services provided for the year.

Environmental Scan

In predicting revenue for the coming year, managers should consider many issues. Managers need to be concerned not only with what they might want to do but also with other factors such as the economy, inflation, growth, employment, interest rates, competition, and so on. Managers should undertake a common-sense review of the likely impact of the economic environment on the organization. Just as an environmental scan is essential for budgeting in general, the information from the scan should be applied to the revenue budget.

Even a change in the proportion of patients covered by each type of insurer is a significant event. Consider what would happen to Surgery and Clinic in Table 14–4 if an economic downturn

forced a number of patients with private insurance to shift to Medicaid. In the table, Medicaid pays a much lower percent of charges than private insurance. Such a shift could have a dramatic impact on total revenues collected by the organization. Note that the number and types of patients would remain the same; therefore, the costs would remain the same. But a shift in payer mix can dramatically change both the revenues and overall fortunes of the organization, and managers must anticipate and consider the impact of such changes.

✳ REVENUES FROM MANAGED CARE

In an environment highly focused on controlling the costs of providing health care services, *managed care organizations* (MCOs) have flourished. An MCO is any organization that tries to control the use of health care services to provide cost-effective care. MCOs try to eliminate the provision of care that is not needed or is not cost-effective. The debate that often surrounds managed care relates to how we define care that is not cost effective.

Sometimes it is easy to spot cost-effective solutions. Suppose that a mother and her newborn are physically well and could be discharged from the hospital after 2 days. However, it is desirable to check the infant for jaundice on the third day. Should the mother and the infant be kept in the hospital for a third day, or should a neonatal nurse practitioner go to see the mother and the infant in their home on the third day? The cost of the home visit is substantially less than the additional day in the hospital. Assuming that clinical outcomes are equally good if the mother and infant are discharged after the second day, an MCO insurer will likely send them home after 2 days. The result is lower cost with no decline in outcomes.

However, many ethical problems arise from the definition that many MCOs use for cost-effective care. What if a test is needed to determine if a patient has a problem that is serious but highly unlikely? Perhaps the test costs $5,000 and would produce a positive result in only 1 of 1,000 people tested. That means that if the test were performed on 1,000 people, it would probably find one person with the illness. The 1,000 tests would cost a total of $5,000,000. Managed care would probably deem that test not to be cost-effective and would refuse to pay for it. In contrast, before the advent of managed care, if a physician ordered the test, many insurance companies would have paid for it. Is it right to deny payment for that test? That is a moral dilemma with no easy answer.

Capitation versus Fee-for-Service

Before managed care, almost all care was provided on a *fee-for-service* basis. Fee-for-service means that there is a charge for each type of service provided. Patients or their insurance companies paid based on the specific services they consumed. If patients had a lab test, they were charged for the lab test. If patients had a home care visit, they were charged for the visit. Patients consuming more services were therefore charged more than patients consuming fewer services. Managed care proponents argue that the fee-for-service system encouraged overprovision of services. That is, if the health care provider earned more money as more services were provided, why not provide a lot of services, whether needed or not?

Some might question whether the big insurance company should be the one to decide what services are needed and what services are not. But the reality is that some abuses likely did exist. Some patients probably did receive unnecessary lab tests, surgeries, or home visits. And to some extent, it is hard to determine what is really necessary and what is unnecessary. Would patients who receive home care visits once a day benefit if there were two visits a day instead? Probably. But how much would they benefit? Would the extra benefit be worth the extra cost of the additional visit? These are difficult questions to address. What we can say is that the assumption (correct or incorrect) that fee-for-service leads to some overprovision of services was one factor leading to the development of capitated payment. Nor is this just a moral dilemma or an issue of money. Overprovision of services can result in harm. For example, for every 1,000 unnecessary surgeries, some patients will have unfavorable outcomes because of risks such as anesthesia and infection.

Capitation is a flat payment per covered member (sometimes referred to as *per covered life*) regardless of the amount of care provided. Capitation agreements are contractual agreements between two parties for the provision of some defined set of health-related services in exchange for a flat periodic payment per patient. The purchaser of the services is the managed care company, and the seller is the health care provider. Although the most common capitated contracts are between MCOs and physicians or hospitals, such contracts can also be established with a variety of HCOs run by nurses, such as home care agencies or community health centers. Dunham-Taylor and colleagues[5] suggest that nurses can find opportunities in a capitated environment by marketing prevention-focused programs, safety programs, substance abuse programs, obesity and exercise programs, nutrition programs, family planning programs, independent clinics, home health care, and hospice.

A nurse practitioner could contract with an MCO to provide certain services to its members for a premium payment per member per month (PMPM). The MCO would provide a list of covered members and would pay a flat monthly amount regardless of how much care the members consume. In many months, the nurse practitioner will receive a payment for some members who do not consume any care at all, as well as for other patients that consume lots of care. One should not look at the profit or loss for any specific member. It is necessary to consider the total of the capitated payments received for the month for all members in contrast to the total amount of services provided to all covered members that month.

Many MCOs do not use capitation for all their contracts. Instead, they may negotiate a discount from normal fees. In those cases, revenue is still paid on a fee-for-service basis (although the fee may be discounted), and the discussion related to revenue earlier in the chapter applies. Capitation, however, is a dramatically different form of payment.

From the viewpoint of the MCO, capitation is beneficial because there is no incentive for providers to provide too much care to patients. If a home care patient receives extra visits, there is no extra payment received by the agency. So there is no reason to deliver unneeded care. From the perspective of the provider, capitation provides a predictable revenue stream. Daily ups and downs in the flow of patients have no impact on the regular monthly receipt of capitation payments. The provider gets paid whether the MCO members get sick or not.

It is also sometimes possible to negotiate payments in advance of the provision of services. A new nurse entrepreneur, just starting a business, who has many expenses, may work out an arrangement with payers to receive capitated payments at the beginning of each month. That money can be used to pay rent and salaries. It provides some revenue stability to the practice.

Capitated payment also has the potential to simplify paperwork. Each month, the provider gets a list of covered members. When a member comes for treatment, the provider often collects a minimal co-payment from the member (perhaps $10) on the spot. The only other payment is the monthly capitation.

The essence of the concept behind capitation is that it shifts risk to the provider of care. Under fee-for-service, the patient, employer, or insurance company is totally at risk. The more health care services the patient consumes, the more the patient or insurer pays. Capitation, however, puts the provider at risk. The more health care services consumed by a covered patient, the worse off the provider may become. This creates a situation in which the provider benefits from keeping the patient healthy. Preventive care is less costly to the provider than curative care, so providers may be more likely to provide services that keep patients healthy. Also, all providers have an incentive to use the lowest cost-efficacious treatment available. Rather than

---

[5]Dunham-Taylor R, Marquette P, Pinczuk J. 1996. Surviving capitation. *Am J Nurs* 96(3):28.

providing more care to existing patients, the way to increase revenue moves to having more covered members.

Money Flows under Capitation

In most capitated systems, the primary payment comes from the purchaser of health insurance. This is generally the employer and employee, who share the cost of the premium. The insurance company keeps part of the premium and uses the rest to pay for health care services. The two largest groups to receive payments are hospitals and physicians.

The key to revenues under capitation are the capitation rate and the number of capitated members. Suppose that a home care agency contracts with an MCO to provide all home care visits needed for $12 PMPM. If the MCO has 250 members who will be covered by the contract, the monthly revenue will be:

$$\text{\$12 PMPM} \times \text{250 Members} = \text{\$3,000}$$

The annual revenue will be:

$$\text{\$12 PMPM} \times \text{250 Members} \times \text{12 Months/Year} = \text{\$36,000}$$

The key to increasing revenue in a capitated environment is to get more covered members. This could either come from gaining a greater share of the members signed with one MCO or by signing additional contracts with other MCOs. Bear in mind that because fixed costs will not change (rent on physical facilities, salary for an office manager), volume of members (and therefore the total amount of capitated revenue) becomes critical to success. As long as the capitated payments exceed variable costs, more members lead to better financial outcomes.

Developing Capitated Rates

As a provider of health care services, setting the capitation rate is critical. Often a contract is signed committing the provider to accept the agreed-upon rate for at least 1 year. If the rate is set too low, the organization will lose money on patients throughout the year. Setting capitated rates is much more complicated than ordinary price setting. The reason is that capitated rates depend critically on utilization.

In a fee-for-service payment situation, one tries to compare the price of a particular service with the cost of providing that service. For example, suppose that the average cost of providing a home care visit is $38, and the fee charged is $45. One can therefore anticipate a profit on each visit. However, in a capitated situation, the payment is the PMPM, regardless of the number of visits for each patient. In negotiating a capitated rate, it is critical to evaluate the population covered and the likely utilization rate for that population. For example, an elderly population will obviously have far more home care visits than a younger population.

The starting point in determining a capitation rate is identification of the exact services to be covered by the contract. Next, the provider must obtain estimates of the utilization of each service offered. Utilization rates should be adjusted for actual population demographics. Costs should be estimated and converted to PMPM equivalents. It is helpful to set the marginal cost (i.e., incremental or additional cost) for the services to be provided as the lower limit and the fee-for-service charges as the upper limit for rate negotiations. Calculating the PMPM cost of each component on a charge, average cost, and marginal cost basis provides the manager with solid information to enter a negotiation. These elements for determining a capitation rate are discussed in the following paragraphs.

There is usually easy agreement over the services to be provided. The MCO wants to protect itself by having contracts to provide the services its members will need. So it will clearly specify what it wants to buy. In some cases, however, if there is great uncertainty about the cost of a service or the utilization of the service, there may be a *carve-out*. That is a service that would normally be provided but is excluded. For example, if liver and heart transplants are expected to be expensive and rare in a population, a provider of surgical services (e.g., a hospital) might exclude, or carve out, those two services from a contract to provide all hospital surgical care. If a patient needs a carved-out service, it would be provided on a fee-for-service basis.

Determination of expected utilization is more complex. A good place to start is with historical demand data. For example, assuming that a home health agency has already been providing services, it can use its own records to estimate the typical frequency of visits. Unfortunately, most providers can ascertain the visit frequency only for those patients who have at least one visit, treatment, admission, or other episode of care. What about all the members of the general population who do not seek any care during the year? Estimating utilization of capitated populations is difficult because the payment covers all members, whether they receive any care or not. Furthermore, the population covered by the managed care contract may be more or less likely to require care than the organization's historical patient base.

Although the MCO may offer its perspective on the amount of care needed for the population, one must consider that the managed care company has a vested interest in underestimating required care. The managed care company wants to pay the lowest rate it can. Often it is necessary to employ the services of an actuarial firm. Such a firm can examine the covered population, consider historical utilization rates for that population, adjust for utilization rates for the particular geographic region, and adjust for gender and age of the covered population.

After the services to be provided have been determined and the utilization rates have been estimated, the next element in the process is for the provider to determine the fee-for-service charges, average costs, and marginal costs for the services to be provided under the managed care contract. The charges are needed because that is the amount that the provider would ideally like the MCO to pay. If the agreed-upon capitation rate provides as much money as fee-for-service charges would have provided, the contract is bringing in additional patients and additional revenue at prices as good as those currently being earned.

Average cost represents a middle ground. In the short run, a rate based on average costs would make the provider better off. If some costs are fixed, as they undoubtedly are, the additional patients would improve the short-term profits of the provider. Marginal costs represent the minimum that should be accepted. If the capitated price provides less than the marginal cost, the provider will actually be financially worse off because of the contract with the MCO.

MCOs offer a price stated as a PMPM. This is because employers pay premiums on a monthly basis based on the number of insured employees for the month. As job turnover occurs, employers eliminate some individuals from health insurance coverage and add others. The MCO in turn eliminates some individuals from the payments made to the provider each month. Therefore, cost should be converted to PMPM equivalents.

Setting a Capitation Rate: An Example

Assume that you are the manager of a home care agency. You are currently negotiating a capitated rate with an MCO. Your charges for visits are currently $120 for a visit by a registered nurse (RN) and $50 for a visit by a nursing assistant (NA). Based on the history of the agency with noncapitated patients plus information provided by an actuary, you have the following expectations regarding utilization by members of the MCO[6]:

1.2 RN visits per member per year

3.0 NA visits per member per year

To provide the visits, you will need additional RNs and NAs. The number of RNs and NAs depends on productivity levels. Suppose you expect the following number of visits per employee:

1,400 patient visits per RN per year

1,000 patient visits per NA per year

and suppose further that the annual cost including benefits for a full-time equivalent (FTE) RN and NA is:

Annual compensation including benefits: $84,000 per FTE RN

Annual compensation including benefits: $20,000 per FTE NA

The direct labor cost for the visits can be calculated PMPM as follows:

RN Visits

$$\text{Average cost per visit} = \$84,000/1,400$$
$$= \$60.00 \text{ per visit}$$

$$\text{Per member per year} = \$60.00 \times 1.2 \text{ visits per year}$$
$$= \$72.00$$

$$\text{PMPM rate} = \$72.00 \div 12 \text{ months}$$
$$= \$6.00 \text{ PMPM}$$

NA Visits

$$\text{Average cost per visit} = \$20,000/1,000$$
$$= \$20.00 \text{ per visit}$$

$$\text{Per member per year} = \$20.00 \times 3 \text{ visits per year}$$
$$= \$60.00$$

$$\text{PMPM rate} = \$60.00 \div 12 \text{ months}$$
$$= \$5.00 \text{ PMPM}$$

Each visit also requires the use of some supplies. Assume that the supply cost per visit is $8. This can be converted to a supply cost per member per month as follows:

Supplies

$$\$8 \text{ per visit} \times 4.2 \text{ visits} = \$33.60$$

$$\$33.60 \div 12 \text{ months per year} = \$2.80 \text{ PMPM}$$

In addition, there will be support staff working for the agency. In some cases, such staff may be fixed, but in other cases, it may be variable. For example, the cost of the office manager will not vary with the number of visits. But other staff members are needed to schedule patient visits. The more patients, the more staff hours needed for such activities. Assume that the agency has found that it needs 0.1 FTE of a support staff member for each FTE RN or NA and that support staff members earn $20,000 on average. Such support staff will be considered to vary with the number of RNs and NAs and therefore with the number of members. Support staff that does not vary with the number of visits will be included in other overhead, as shown below.

Number of RNs per member
= 1.2 visits/1,400 visits per RN = 0.000857

Number of NAs per member
= 3.0 visits/1,000 visits per NA = 0.003000

Total RNs and NAs per member
= 0.000857 + 0.003000 = 0.003857

Support staff = 0.003857 × 0.1 support staff
per RN or NA
= 0.000386 support staff personnel
per member

Support staff cost = 0.000386 × $20,000
= $7.72 per member per year

Support staff cost PMPM = $7.72 ÷ 12 months
= $0.64 PMPM

Note how cumbersome the calculation becomes because of the small fractions. Utilization rates are often stated per 1,000 members to avoid dealing with small fractions. If the support staff calculation had alternatively been done per thousand members, it would appear as follows:

Number of RNs per 1,000 Members
= 1.2 Visits × 1,000 Members ÷ 1,400 Visits per RN
= 0.857 RNs per 1,000 Members

Number of NAs per 1,000 Members
= 3.0 visits × 1,000 Members ÷ 1,000 Visits per NA
= 3.000 NAs per 1,000 Members

Total RNs and NAs = 3.000 + 0.857
= 3.857 RNs and NAs per 1,000 Members

Support Staff Cost
= 3.857 × 0.1 Support Staff per RN or NA
= 0.386 Support Staff Personnel per 1,000 Members

---

[6]The data used in this example are hypothetical and do not reflect true utilization rates or costs for any home care agency.

Support Staff Cost
  = 0.386 × $20,000
  = $7,720 per 1,000 Members per Year

Support Staff Cost PMPM
  = $7,720 ÷ 1,000 Members ÷ 12 Months
  = $0.64 PMPM

Notice that whether the calculation is performed on a per member basis or per 1,000-member basis, the PMPM result is exactly the same. Assume that all other costs, such as fixed staff, rent, and electrical work, come out to $6 PMPM.

Using the previous information, a PMPM based on average costs can be calculated as follows:

PMPM

RNs	$ 6.00
NAs	5.00
Supplies	2.80
Support staff	0.64
Other overhead	6.00
Average cost PMPM	$20.44

It was noted earlier that the manager should calculate rates based on charges, average cost, and marginal cost. We have just calculated the average cost as being $20.44. Earlier it was noted that the charges for the agency are $120 for an RN visit and $50 for an NA visit. This can be converted to a PMPM as follows:

1.2 RN Visits per Member × $120 per Visit ÷ 12 Months
  = $12.00 PMPM

3.0 NA Visits per Member × $50 per Visit ÷ 12 Months
  = $12.50 PMPM

Total Charge for RN and NA Visits
  = $12.00 PMPM + $12.50 PMPM = $24.50 PMPM

The marginal cost of the visits can also be determined. The RNs, NAs, supplies, and support staff will all increase if the contract is signed. The other overhead is fixed and will be incurred in any event. Therefore, the marginal cost of providing the additional visits is $14.44 per member per month (i.e., $20.44 average cost – $6.00 other overhead). We can now compare the three measures:

	Charge	Average Cost	Marginal Cost
Per member per month	$24.50	$20.44	$14.36

This comparison provides the manager with critical information needed to enter PMPM capitation rate negotiations. The goal is to negotiate a revenue as close to the $24.50 PMPM charge as possible but in no case lower than the $14.44 marginal cost. After the rate has been agreed on, the revenue from the agreement is simply the capitation rate multiplied by the number of members covered by the agreement.

Incentive Risk Pools

Managed care contracts also often include incentive arrangements to minimize overall costs. For example, suppose that all providers are capitated except for hospitals. Assume that hospitals are paid on a discounted fee-for-service basis by the MCO. How can the MCO encourage providers to avoid unnecessary patient hospitalizations? A common arrangement is the use of inpatient services *risk pools*. Risk pools consist of some money that has been withheld from each provider. The withheld amount is eventually paid to the provider if utilization achieves certain targets.

For example, suppose that the home care agency discussed previously negotiates a $21 PMPM capitation rate from a managed care provider for 2,000 members. The agency is entitled to revenue of $42,000 per month ($21 PMPM × 2,000 members). However, the MCO is concerned about the incentives created by capitation. The agency might try to save money by not providing all the visits needed because it receives the same $21 PMPM regardless of the number of visits provided.

Failure to provide visits when needed might result in a patient's being rehospitalized. This is a poor outcome for the patient and costly for the MCO. To avoid this, the MCO might withhold 10% of the capitated payments until a year-end reconciliation is performed. That amount is combined with money withheld from other providers to create a risk pool. The agency would receive only $37,800 each month ($42,000 × 90%). At the end of the year, the agency would get back some or all of this 10% withheld amount based on actual hospital utilization versus an expected level of hospital utilization. If hospital utilization is unexpectedly high, the risk pool is used to pay the hospital, and there may be nothing left in the pool to pay the agency. The agency can lose the entire 10% that had been withheld. But if hospital costs are very high, the MCO will be liable for any costs that the risk pool cannot cover. So both the providers and the MCO are at risk to lose some money if utilization is higher than expected. This is referred to as *risk sharing*.

It should also be noted that in some cases, withholding arrangements may lead to poorer care. For example, to keep hospital utilization low, physicians or nurse practitioners might fail to admit patients who actually need hospital care. Some would argue that MCOs are not really worried about quality of care at all. From that perspective, risk pools are established solely to save money for the MCO by discouraging patient admissions and other costly forms of care. Nurse managers involved in managed care negotiations must always consider the implications of the contract for the quality of care to be provided to their patients.

✳ IMPLICATIONS FOR NURSE MANAGERS AND EXECUTIVES

Revenues are the amount the organization earns in exchange for the services it provides. Revenues are critical for every organization. Revenues must be adequate to cover all costs of providing services during the current year. In addition, revenues should be great enough to provide a profit. Profits are used to expand the type and volume of services offered and to replace capital equipment.

In some situations, nurse managers and executives are not given revenue responsibility because it is believed that nurses' actions and the care they deliver cannot affect the revenues of the organization. This would be the case in a situation in which all patients pay a fixed fee regardless of services received. More commonly, however, nurse managers and executives have not been given revenue responsibility because historically it was difficult to assess the amount of nursing resources consumed by different patients. Computer and information technologies are removing this barrier, and it is becoming more feasible to charge different patients for differing amounts of nursing care they may receive. Nurse managers and executives should continue to push for revenue responsibility.

The basic elements of a revenue budget are simple—price and volume. The revenue budget essentially consists of the price charged for each service provided by the unit, department, or organization multiplied by the number of units of service provided. The complications involved in a revenue budget are estimating the volume of services to be provided, deciding on the prices to charge, and estimating how much of the total amount charged will actually be collected. Nurse managers and executives who are responsible for the revenue of their unit, department, or organization should be actively involved in estimating or at least understanding these factors.

MCOs require special attention because of the way they pay for services. An MCO is any organization that tries to control the use of health care services to provide cost-effective care. In some cases, MCOs pay in much the same way as other payers, often negotiating a discount from standard fees or charges. In some cases, however, MCOs pay providers based on *capitation*.

Capitation refers to paying a set amount for each covered member, regardless of the amount of care consumed. From the viewpoint of the MCO, capitation is beneficial because there is no incentive for providers to overuse services provided to patients. From the perspective of the provider, capitation provides a predictable revenue stream. Nurse managers and executives need to understand their costs in order to negotiate effective capitation rates. They should also attempt to negotiate advance monthly payments if their organization frequently has trouble meeting its monthly expenses that must be paid in cash.

Nurse managers and executives should always be cautious when working on capitated arrangements. In such arrangements, the MCO shifts risk to the provider. If for whatever reason patients consume more resources than expected, it is the provider who will lose money as a result. Many providers buy insurance, called *stop-loss protection,* to protect themselves from severe losses resulting from unexpectedly high patient utilization rates.

The capitation payment, called the *PMPM rate,* must cover all costs and profits for the organization related to the covered members. The starting point in determining a capitation rate is identification of the exact services that are to be covered by the contract. Next, the provider must obtain estimates of the utilization of each service covered. Utilization rates are generally stated per 1,000 members. Utilization rates must be adjusted for actual population demographics, and costs must be converted to PMPM equivalents. It is helpful to use the marginal cost for the covered services as the lower limit and fee-for-service charges as the upper limit for rate negotiations.

After the PMPM has been determined, it can be multiplied by the number of covered members to determine the organization's revenue from the MCO. The key to increasing revenue in a capitated environment is to get more covered members. Special care should also be paid in negotiating risk pools. Risk pools represent portions of the PMPM rate that are held back and may not be paid if utilization rates or costs for specific types of care exceed a set amount.

✳ KEY CONCEPTS

Revenue centers   Organizational units or departments that have revenue budgets and are responsible for generating a budgeted amount of revenue are referred to as *revenue centers*. They are often called *profit centers* in other industries and generally have responsibility for expenses as well as revenues.

Cost or expense centers   Organizational units or departments that do not have revenue budgets and are not responsible for generating a budgeted amount of revenue are referred to as cost or expense centers because they are accountable only for controlling their expenses.

Elements of a revenue budget   Price and volume are the essential elements of a revenue budget, which essentially consists of the price charged for each service provided by the unit, department, or organization multiplied by the number of units of service provided.

Prices or rates   The prices or rates charged by a health care provider may be market-based, cost-based, mark-up–based, or negotiated:

- **Market based**   These are prices that are set based on a survey of what others in the community are charging for the same services.

- **Cost based**   These are charges that are exactly your cost. By *cost,* we typically mean average cost.

- **Mark-up–based**   These are prices that are a certain percentage above the cost of providing care.

- **Negotiated** As a result of negotiations, prices can result in a variety of different payment approaches, such as flat fees, percent discounts, or payments per episode.

Contractual allowance A discount that a payer is entitled to based on a contractual arrangement with the provider.

Charity care Care that is provided with no expectation of collecting payment or of attempting to collect payment. It is not included in the revenues of the organization.

Bad debts Amounts that the organization is legally entitled to collect for care, attempts to collect, but is ultimately unable to collect.

Co-pay or co-payment The portion of the charge for care that the patient is obligated to pay themselves even if they have insurance.

Self-pay Refers to uninsured patients who are obligated to pay the provider of care directly for health care services received.

Volume A critical factor in preparing a revenue budget is the volume of patients. Volume can be estimated using the forecasting techniques discussed in Chapter 21. Note that it is not sufficient to estimate total patient volume. The volume of each type of patient or procedure for which there is a different charge must be estimated. It is also extremely important to consider all possible sources of revenue or support.

Environmental scan Managers need to be concerned not only with what they might want to do but also with other factors such as the economy, inflation, growth, employment, interest rates, competition, and so on. Managers should undertake a common-sense review of the likely impact of the economic environment on the organization.

Managed care organization (MCO) Any organization that tries to control the use of health care services to provide cost-effective care.

Fee-for-service A charge for each type and unit of service provided. The predominant form of payment before MCOs. Managed care proponents argue that the fee-for-service system encourages overprovision of services. If the health care provider earns more money as more services are provided, why not provide a lot of services, whether needed or not?

Capitation A flat payment per covered member (sometimes referred to as *per covered life*) regardless of the amount of care provided. The purchaser of the services is the managed care company, and the seller is the health care provider.

Risk pools Money that has been withheld from the capitation payment that would normally be due to each provider. The withheld amount is eventually paid to the provider if utilization achieves certain targets. This provides an incentive to keep overall utilization of care low.

✳ SUGGESTED READINGS

Buppert C: Third-party reimbursement for nurse practitioners' services on trauma teams: working through a maze of issues, *J Trauma* 58(1):206–212, 2005.

Cleverley W, Cleverley J, Song P: *Essentials of health care finance*, ed 7, Sudbury, Mass, 2011, Jones & Bartlett.

Dacso S, Dacso C, editors: *Risk contracting and capitation answer book*, Gaithersburg, Maryland, 1999, Aspen Publishers.

Dunham-Taylor R, Marquette P, Pinczuk J: Surviving capitation, *Am J Nurs* 96(3):26–30, 1996.

Gapenski L, Pink G: *Understanding healthcare financial management*, ed 6, Chicago, 2011, Health Administration Press.

Hunstock L: Managed care and the world of capitated payment. In Flarey DL, et al: *Handbook of nursing case management: health care delivery in a world of managed care*, Gaithersburg, Maryland, 1996, Aspen Publishers, pp. 336–347.

Leeth L: Are you fiscally fit? Move your department from moneypit to money-maker by creating new—and capturing hidden—revenue, *Nurs Manage* 35(4):42–47, 2004.

Rapsilber L, Anderson E: Understanding the reimbursement process, *Nurse Pract* 25(5):36, 43, 46, 2000.

Swansburg R: *Budgeting and financial management for nurse managers*, Boston, 1997, Jones & Bartlett.

Tumolo J: Revving up revenue, *Adv Nurse Pract* 13(5):14, 2005.

Welton, J: Adjustment of inpatient care reimbursement for nursing intensity, *Policy Polit Nurs Pract* 7(4):270–280, 2006.

Wyld D: The capitation revolution in health care: implications for the field of nursing, *Nurs Adm Q* 20(2):1–12, 1996.

Zaumeyer C: Generating revenue, *Adv Nurse Pract* 12(12):16, 2004.

Zelman W, McCue M, Glick N: *Financial management of health care organizations: an introduction to fundamental tools, concepts, and applications*, ed 3, Hoboken, New Jersey, 2010, John Wiley & Sons.

Performance Budgeting

CHAPTER GOALS

The goals of this chapter are to:

- Introduce the concept of performance budgeting
- Identify weaknesses in traditional measures of performance
- Create an awareness of the importance of establishing goals and measuring their accomplishment

- Outline the specific steps in performance budgeting
- Identify potential measures for use by nursing in performance budgets

✳ INTRODUCTION

The extreme financial pressures faced by health care organizations (HCOs) in recent years have resulted in substantial budget cuts. Managers are being pressured to find ways to make do, and in some cases do more, with less. A major concern in today's cost-conscious health care environment is that the failure of HCOs to achieve certain outcomes means that the quality of patient care may suffer. It also means that the organization will pay the financial consequences. As noted in previous chapters of this book, there is a growing call for evaluation of the outcomes of HCOs and for linking quality of care with the payment for care delivered.

Traditionally, the budgeting process has focused on the resources used by a department or cost center. For example, there is detailed information on the number of nurses working on a unit and their pay rate. Supplies, educational seminars, and publication costs are also carefully considered. There are a couple of problems with this approach, however. First, all of these aforementioned elements of the budget are inputs. They are the resources the unit needs to achieve its objectives. Little attempt, if any, has traditionally been made to relate those inputs to the unit's achievement of its objectives or the degree to which objectives are or can be achieved. Instead, the achievement of outcomes is assumed.

Second, if budgets for patient care units are cut or inadequately increased to account for changes in patient acuity, nursing personnel wage increases, or other factors, there is often an expectation by top management that at least the same amount of work will be performed. This is often an unreasonable and unrealistic expectation. Although it is true that the number of patients cared for or the number of patient days incurred may

be covered with a smaller budget, the amount of care given may not be at the same level. The reality is that the care delivered and the outcomes achieved may deteriorate. Unfortunately, the linkage between the budget or amount spent and the amount of care provided is rarely considered beyond a simplistic measure such as the number of patient days.

To illustrate this point, consider a nursing unit that cares for 10,000 patient days in a year with a budget of $2,000,000. What happens if the budget is slashed to $1,750,000? If the unit still provides 10,000 patient days of care, traditional budgeting makes it appear that costs are down and output is unchanged. In reality, however, it is highly unlikely that outcomes are unchanged. Quality of patient care is likely to have declined along a number of dimensions—staffing may have decreased, nurses may have been forced to cut corners, leave patient care activities undone, or simply to do the best they could under the circumstances.

A traditional operating budget, focusing on the number of patient days, is unlikely to capture the actual changes in care delivery and patient outcomes that might have occurred. A different approach is needed to address important questions, such as: What are the goals of the unit? What is it trying to achieve? What is the expected cost of each achievement? Most cost centers use existing budget measures to answer these questions, which define goals only in the simplest terms, such as the number of visits, patient days, or procedures. Such measures are incapable of getting at issues such as quality of care per patient day or cost per unit of quality of care.

Today's pay-for-performance (or value-based purchasing) environment requires that HCOs reframe their thinking about how care is delivered and paid for, relative to certain quality outcomes. Because organizational reimbursements are becoming more closely tied to outcomes, organizations have an opportunity to consider their budgeting processes in light of quality. Also, because nursing care is front and center in an organization's ability to achieve quality, managers and executives need an approach that helps them focus on the results that their units, departments, and organizations achieve relative to the nursing inputs used. They also need an approach that considers outcomes beyond the simplistic measures described earlier. A process that can help to better align objectives and quality outcomes with the budgeting process, called *performance* or *outcomes budgeting,* is the topic of this chapter.

Performance budgeting is a technique that evaluates the activities of a cost center in terms of what the center accomplishes, as well as the costs of achieving its accomplishments. It is an approach to budgeting specifically designed to evaluate the multiple outcomes of cost centers rather than a single budgeted output, such as the number of home care visits. Performance budgeting provides a mechanism for gaining a better understanding of the relationships between financial resources and the level and quality of results. It also shifts the focus from the resources the unit plans to use to the various things it is trying to accomplish.

Performance budgeting can be used in any organization that has multiple goals and objectives. It allows the organization to define the various elements of performance that are important. Managers and departments can be assessed based on their accomplishments in terms of those elements. Departments can have their own unique set of performance or outcomes criteria that are relevant to the patients cared for or services delivered. Performance budgeting gives nurse managers and executives the ability to bring meaningful data about quality of care and its cost to engage nurses in the budgeting process and to help them see the value of their work.

This chapter first reviews the steps in the performance budgeting process, and then the technical aspects of performance budgeting are discussed. An example of the performance budgeting process is provided followed by a discussion of performance measures. In some cases, the use of multiple measures may be desired to gauge performance in one or more areas of a unit or departmental budget. Thus, a discussion about using multiple measures in the performance budgeting process is also provided.

✳ THE PERFORMANCE BUDGETING TECHNIQUE
Determining Key Performance Areas

Nurse managers and executives attempt to achieve a number of different objectives. One goal of nursing unit managers is to provide high-quality care. However, they also want to satisfy patient needs and desires. They want to control costs. If one does not clearly define the performance desired, success cannot be measured. The key is to develop a set of performance areas for measurement.

In developing performance areas, managers and executives should consider a variety of questions, such as: What are the important goals that should be measured? What elements of a unit's performance are within the control of the nurse manager, and what elements are not? How should the nurse manager most productively spend working time? How should the nursing staff most productively use their time? How can the performance of a nursing unit be evaluated?

In addressing these questions, it is necessary to categorize the major elements of the manager's and unit's jobs or functions. For example, consider the nurse manager of a 30-bed unit. Some of the manager's effort should go toward ensuring a high level of patient care. Some effort should go to staffing the unit, some to controlling unit expenses, some to improving productivity, some to improving patient and staff satisfaction, and some to innovation and long-range planning. These are some key performance areas for the manager and unit. There may well be other important outcome areas not listed here. Managers must establish performance areas based on their own unit or department's specific circumstances.

Technical Steps in Performance Budgeting

Identifying the performance areas for a cost center is the first step in performance budgeting. These can be developed from the unit's annual plans and goals that have been established and endorsed by the nursing division or higher levels in the organization. The second step is to identify the existing line item budget for the cost center being evaluated. In a nursing unit, this budget includes the cost of items such as the salary for the unit nurse manager, salaries for clinical staff, education costs, and supplies.

The next step is to define how much of the resources represented by each line item are to be devoted to each of the performance areas. This requires that the manager develop a resource allocation model. This process forces the manager to think about what elements of the job are really important and how important they are.

If, for instance, patient satisfaction is very important to the organization, the manager must consider whether an adequate amount of time and effort is being devoted to achieving patient satisfaction. The resource allocation for the performance budget explicitly notes the specific portion of the nurse manager's time, staff time, and other resources that should be spent on ensuring patient satisfaction.

It is up to the nurse manager to decide how to allocate resources among the various processes that are associated with the desired outcomes. How much of the resources should be focused on quality of care? How much on staffing? A percent of the total effort should be assigned to each of the performance areas. The manager's allocations will likely not be the same for management time, staff time, and other resources. Each resource is allocated based on differing needs. For example, unit nurse managers might allocate 5% of their own time, 35% of clinical staff time, and 90% of supplies to direct patient care. A chart or table should be developed that shows the performance areas and the percent of each line item cost being allocated to each performance area.

The allocation of resources to different performance areas should be based on explicit decisions related to organizational priorities. However, when a performance budget is first introduced, it is easier to make allocations based on historical information. This information can be gathered by having everyone keep a log of their time for several weeks or based on each individual's best estimate of how they use their time. After the performance budget is developed, more information will be available to the manager, and explicit choices can be made to reallocate resources in a more useful manner.

After the percent of each resource to be used to achieve each performance area has been decided, a calculation must be made to determine how much money has been budgeted for each performance area. This can be done by taking the percent of each line item allocated to each performance area and multiplying it by the total amount of money in the budget for that line item. For instance, if the nurse manager's salary is $80,000 and 10% of the manager's working time is spent on improving quality of care, then $8,000 is calculated ($80,000 × 10%) as being spent on quality. If the staff nurses for the unit earn $800,000 in total and they spend 5% of their efforts on improving quality, there is another $40,000 ($800,000 × 5%) being allocated to quality improvement. The nurse manager can total all the costs for each performance element. In this case, a total of $48,000 has been budgeted for improving quality of care.

The final step is to choose measures of performance for each performance area, budget a specific numerical objective for each area, and determine the budgeted cost per unit of each objective based on those measures. For instance, suppose that the nurse manager chooses to measure improvement in quality of care based on the number of medication errors. Suppose further that the performance budget calls for reducing the number of medication errors on the unit by 30 instances. Because $48,000 has been allocated to improve quality, it can be said that $1,600 has been budgeted per medication error eliminated. The next year the same amount of money might need to be budgeted just to maintain the level of care.

The performance budget specifies an amount of an outcome to be accomplished. For example, it might indicate that medication errors will be reduced by a specific number. The performance budget also specifies the inputs to be devoted to achieve that outcome. A certain amount of nurse time is budgeted to accomplish the reduction in medication errors. Thus goals are matched with resources needed for their accomplishment. We will use an example to clarify the process of performance budgeting.

✳ PERFORMANCE BUDGET EXAMPLE

The first step in developing a performance budget is to determine the performance areas that the nurse manager intends to use. The following is one possible set of performance areas:

- Provide direct and indirect care to patients
- Improve quality of care
- Provide staffing
- Control costs
- Increase productivity
- Improve patient satisfaction
- Improve staff satisfaction
- Introduce innovations and engage in long-range planning

The second step is to get the cost information for the unit from the operating budget. Converting operating budget information into a performance budget will give a clearer focus of how the unit spends the budgeted amount of money. The operating budget already gives information such as the number of full-time equivalents (FTEs) by skill level. However, those are inputs rather than outcomes. The performance budget will provide information about results rather than just inputs. Suppose, hypothetically, that the line item operating budget for a nursing unit is $1,000,000 for the coming year, as follows:

Nurse manager	$ 80,000
Clinical staff salaries	800,000
Education	20,000
Supplies	40,000
Overhead	60,000
Total	$1,000,000

The third step is to determine the percentage of operating budget resources allocated to performance areas. Not all employees on a patient care unit will have time devoted to each area. Allocation of the nurse manager's time to performance areas might be as follows[1]:

Improve quality of care	15%
Provide staffing	15%
Control costs	20%
Increase productivity	20%
Improve patient satisfaction	10%
Improve staff satisfaction	5%
Introduce innovations, engage in long-range planning	15%
Total	100%

By developing the allocation to areas of performance, a plan is provided for how the nurse manager's time should be spent and what areas are deemed to be either the most important or the most in need of the manager's efforts.

There is no reason to believe that all resources within a department or unit should necessarily be allocated in the same fashion. The time allocation for clinical staff might be as follows:

Provide direct patient care	30%
Provide indirect patient care[2]	30%
Improve quality of care	5%
Control costs	5%
Increase productivity	2%
Improve patient satisfaction	5%
Other	23%
Total	100%

The allocation of time for direct patient care seems low, but this is misleading. Because this budget is based on total unit costs, it includes non-worked time for sick leave, vacation, and holidays. It also includes worked time off the unit, such as education days. These items might account for most of the 23% "other" time. Furthermore, a substantial portion of time spent to improve quality of care and patient satisfaction may

---

[1] This simplified example treats the nurse manager's time as if it were all directly under the manager's control. A more realistic calculation might set aside an amount of time, such as 20%, for administrative mandated activities.

[2] For example, supervising staff or interacting with physicians.

in fact be additional direct patient care time with a specific focus on those two goals. Therefore, this allocation might imply that about half of nurses' time on the unit is spent on direct patient care.

To develop a full performance budget for the unit, it will also be necessary to determine how education, supplies, and overhead resources relate to the performance of the unit. Suppose that a reasonable expectation for the role of education in a given year is as follows:

Improve quality of care	20%
Control costs	20%
Increase productivity	20%
Improve patient satisfaction	10%
Improve staff satisfaction	10%
Introduce innovations, engage in long-range planning	20%
Total	100%

Supplies used by a nursing unit are primarily clinical supplies for direct patient care and, to a much lesser extent, administrative forms and other administrative supplies. Suppose that a reasonable expectation for the use of supplies is as follows:

Provide staffing	2%
Control costs	2%
Provide direct patient care	90%
Provide indirect patient care	5%
Other	1%
Total	100%

There is no uniquely correct way to allocate overhead, because much of it is assigned arbitrarily to a nursing unit. Ultimately, performance budget measures will be used to assess the cost of devoting resources to a particular activity, such as improving quality of care. Because overhead is not likely to vary based on how much effort the manager and clinical staff devote to improving quality of care on the unit, it is reasonable to assign the unit's overhead completely to direct patient care. However, this is an arbitrary allocation, and alternative approaches are possible.

Provide direct patient care	100%

The above percentage allocations are summarized in Table 15–1. Every line item category within the original operating budget has a percentage assigned to the individual performance areas.

The original operating budget can now be assigned to performance areas, as seen in Table 15–2. This table takes the total cost for each line item in the operating budget and multiplies it by the percentages in Table 15–1 to determine the budgeted cost for each performance area for each line item. For example, Staff Salary is budgeted at a total of $800,000 (Table 15–2, Totals column). Of this amount, 5% is allocated to improve quality of care (Table 15–1, Quality column, Staff Salary row). As a result, 5% of $800,000, or $40,000, is allocated to improve quality of care (Table 15–2, Quality column, Staff Salary row).

The total budgeted cost of each of the performance areas can be assessed. It is expected that the nursing unit will spend $56,000 in total on quality improvement efforts (Table 15–2, Quality column, Totals row), $12,800 on staffing, $60,800 on cost control, and so on. In Table 15–2, compare the *bottom row*, which gives the total for each key performance area, with the *Totals column*, which gives the total by line item from the original operating budget. The original operating budget appears to be primarily a fixed budget over which the unit has little control. It shows only the amount to be spent on each input resource consumed. However, the bottom row shows that implicit choices are being made about the allocation of the operating budget resources to different priority areas. Each column in Table 15–2 tells the amount of money budgeted for each performance area. The manager does in fact have at least some ability to modify how these resources are spent. It could be decided that relatively greater efforts should be made in one particular area and less in another. Knowing that $56,000 is budgeted for improving quality, $50,000 for improving patient satisfaction, and $336,000 for providing direct patient care is much more valuable information than knowing that $800,000 is budgeted for staff salaries. The focus has shifted from inputs to performance.

Note, however, that a performance budget has still not been fully developed. The allocation of operating budget to performance areas (Table 15–2) is a valuable plan that provides an indication of whether the unit is planning to proceed in the most appropriate manner. It does not go far enough, however. It is not specific in terms of quantifying the goals for each performance area.

Table 15–3 presents the next step—the actual performance budget. In Table 15–3, the performance areas have been moved from the top row to the left side of the table. For each area, the difficult task of choosing a performance measure and quantifying the budgeted level for each performance area must be addressed.

HCOs try to produce improved health for patients to whom they provide care. Because this cannot be measured directly, in most cases proxies such as the number of patient days of care are used. Performance budgets add additional proxies to assess the accomplishment of the organization's goals. In Table 15–3, it is seen that a budget can be developed that gives information about such items as the budgeted cost to attain a reduction in patient care planning errors. In this example, the budgeted cost is $5,600 for each 1% drop in the rate of failure to comply with patient care plan procedures (Table 15–3, Average Cost column, Quality Improvement row). The next section addresses the issue of developing proxies for performance measurement.

✳ DEVELOPING PERFORMANCE AREA MEASURES

To be able to create a performance budget that will be as useful as possible, there must be specific ways to measure accomplishments in each performance area. Some of the measures developed for the different performance areas will appear to be crude proxies at best. However, patient days is itself a crude proxy for the process of providing health care, which in turn is a proxy for improved health. Yet patient days is a very useful measure. Over time, performance budgeting will improve as better proxies are suggested and incorporated into the technique. What are some

✳ TABLE 15–1 *Summary of Percentage Allocation to Performance Areas*

					Performance Areas						
Cost Item	**Quality**	**Staffing**	**Cost Control**	**Productivity**	**Patient Satisfaction**	**Staff Satisfaction**	**Innovation and Planning**	**Direct Care**	**Indirect Care**	**Other**	**Totals**
Nurse manager	15%	15%	20%	20%	10%	5%	15%	0%	0%	0%	100%
Staff salary	5%	0%	5%	2%	5%	0%	0%	30%	30%	23%	100%
Education	20%	0%	20%	20%	10%	10%	20%	0%	0%	0%	100%
Supplies	0%	2%	2%	0%	0%	0%	0%	90%	5%	1%	100%
Overhead	0%	0%	0%	0%	0%	0%	0%	100%	0%	0%	100%

✳ TABLE 15–2 *Allocation of Operating Budget to Performance Areas*

					Performance Areas						
Cost Item	**Totals**	**Quality**	**Staffing**	**Cost Control**	**Productivity**	**Patient Satisfaction**	**Staff Satisfaction**	**Innovation and Planning**	**Direct Care**	**Indirect Care**	**Other**
Nurse manager	$ 80,000	$12,000	$12,000	$16,000	$16,000	$ 8,000	$4,000	$12,000	$ 0	$ 0	$ 0
Staff salary	800,000	40,000	0	40,000	16,000	40,000	0	0	240,000	240,000	184,000
Education	20,000	4,000	0	4,000	4,000	2,000	2,000	4,000	0	0	0
Supplies	40,000	0	800	800	0	0	0	0	36,000	2,000	400
Overhead	60,000	0	0	0	0	0	0	0	60,000	0	0
Totals	$1,000,000	$56,000	$12,800	$60,800	$36,000	$50,000	$6,000	$16,000	$336,000	$242,000	$184,400

✳ TABLE 15–3 *Performance Budget*

Performance Areas	Activity	Description of Output Measure	Amount of Output Budgeted	Total Cost of Activity	Average Cost
Improve quality	Prevention of pressure ulcers	Number of patients who develop stage III and IV pressure ulcers	10% reduction in pressure ulcer rate	$ 56,000	$5,600 per percent drop in Stage III and IV pressure ulcer rate
Provide staffing	Daily staff calculations	Number of daily calculations Reduction in paid hours per patient day	365 daily calculations 0.20 hour paid per patient day	12,800	$35.07 per daily calculation $6,400 per 0.1 hour reduction
Control cost	Reduce cost	Reduction in cost per patient day	$8.33 per patient day	60,800	$7,299 per $1 reduction
Increase productivity	Revise procedures Work more efficiently	Reduction in total unit cost per direct care hour	$3 reduction per direct care hour	36,000	$12,000 per $ reduction
Increase patient satisfaction	Respond to needs	Complaints	10% reduction in complaints	50,000	$5,000 per 1% reduction in complaints
Increase staff satisfaction	Respond to needs	Turnover	5% reduction in staff turnover	6,000	$1,200 per 1% reduction in turnover
Innovation and planning	Planning sessions	Number of meetings	12 meetings	16,000	$1,333 per meeting
Direct care	Direct patient care	Hours of care	10,000 hours	336,000	$33.60 per direct care hour
Indirect care	Patient charting	Number of patient days	7,300 patient days	242,000	$33.15 per patient day
Other				184,400	
Total				$1,000,000	

potential output measures for evaluating the results of a nursing unit? Each of the performance areas likely has some associated key activities that can be budgeted and measured.[3]

It will take a fair amount of thought to come up with a good set of performance areas and measures of performance. For example, are patient complaints an appropriate measure of patient satisfaction with the nursing unit? If the patients complain about nurses, is it because the quality of care or attention to patients is not what it should be or simply that the patients are reflecting their general mood related to their illness? However, *increases* in the rate of complaints may well be a meaningful performance measurement.

Quality of Care

The quality of care measure will be addressed first because quality always presents a particular measurement challenge. Earlier, the use of medication variances was suggested as one possible measure for the change in quality of care. Another possible approach is to focus on a patient care quality indicator, such as the number of patients who develop pressure ulcers on

a general medical unit.[4] If staff nurses are not actively engaged in activities to reduce the occurrence of pressure ulcers among unit patients, patient care and quality may suffer, and ultimately, organizational reimbursements will be affected. Although nurses on the unit may already engage in activities aimed at preventing the development of pressure ulcers for patients admitted to the unit, their efforts may not be factored into the budget and linked to this important quality outcome indicator. Therefore, it is possible to assess the quality of nursing care delivered to patients by evaluating how well the unit performs in terms of its patients who develop pressure ulcers. Outcome measurement can be based on the *percent* reduction in the number (or incidence) of stage III and IV pressure ulcers or based on the *number* (or incidence) of stage III and IV pressure ulcers developed by patients on the unit. Many patient care units already measure the quality of care delivered to their patients, including an evaluation of pressure ulcers developed by patients admitted to the unit. However, with performance

---

[3] The measures described are a mix of both process and outcome measures. They also overlap to some extent. Eventually, performance budgeting may be refined to a point where such problems can be overcome.

[4] Stage III and IV pressure ulcers have been identified as a hospital-acquired condition by the Centers for Medicare and Medicaid Services, and hospitals are subject to payment denial based on their performance on this quality indicator. Also, stage III and IV pressure ulcers have been identified as a patient safety indicator by Agency for Healthcare Research and Quality and a nurse-sensitive indicator by the American Nurses' Association and the National Quality Forum.

budgeting, not only is the quality-relevant outcome measured, but the measurement is also associated with the expected cost of improving the outcome.

In the first row of Table 15–3, it can be seen that Improve Quality is one performance area being budgeted. The measure used for this performance area will be the percent reduction in stage III and IV pressure ulcers. A 10% reduction is budgeted. As Table 15–2 showed, $56,000 is devoted to this area of the budget. Therefore, it is expected that each percent reduction in stage III and IV pressure ulcer rates will cost $5,600. This represents the total $56,000 to be spent in this area divided by the volume of output expected—in this case, $56,000 divided by a 10% reduction equals $5,600 per percent.

This approach recognizes that improvements in performance cost money. It is insufficient to simply dictate that a patient care unit must improve pressure ulcer rates by, for example, changing care delivery processes to focus on the prevention of pressure ulcers without providing additional resources to measure, monitor, and accomplish this end. Can this unit lower its pressure ulcer rate even more? Yes, it probably can. However, the performance budget provides explicit information that improved patient care to prevent the development of pressure ulcers in patients on the unit requires more attention from the nursing staff. Such additional attention may require real additional resources in terms of increased staffing (e.g., the devotion of time by a wound care nurse or training a nurse on the unit to become an expert in the area). If additional staffing is not provided, the only way to improve patient pressure ulcer rates is to devote a greater percent of staff time to compliance in this area (unless productivity can be increased). However, this will mean devoting less time to other areas.

It is possible that a unit already performs well with regard to its pressure ulcer rates. The nurse manager of the unit may not believe that it is worth additional effort and cost to further improve this care outcome. However, even maintaining a given level of quality requires staff attention. Thus, the performance budget might show a goal of no change in the number of patients who develop pressure ulcers on the unit. An explicit portion of the performance budget would still be allocated to the quality area to achieve that steady state. Alternatively, the budget could show the cost of not allowing the rate to increase. For example, it could reflect $16,800 being spent to avoid a 3% increase in the rate of pressure ulcers from the current rate.

What happens if the overall budget for the nursing unit is cut? The performance budget allows determination of areas in which resources should be cut. If a choice is made to cut resources in an area that affects quality, it would not be surprising to detect later that the number of patients who develop pressure ulcers increases. The performance budget would show how the cuts to the unit are expected to affect the various performance areas. Budget cuts must be explicitly assigned to the performance areas to be cut. Rather than expecting no impact of budget cuts, explicit choices are made, and the unit can demonstrate what outcomes are likely to deteriorate as a result of the budget cut.

Staffing

A nursing unit manager must make many staffing decisions throughout the year, as well as manage vacations, holidays, sick leave, and busy and slow periods. In Table 15–3, it is assumed that daily calculations are made for staff adjustments. This requires some managerial time each and every day.

Calculations by the unit manager to adjust unit staffing could be made weekly or just once a month. If staffing were only adjusted monthly, extra staff might be assigned all month long to ensure adequate staff for busy days. Less frequent work on staffing would save managerial time but would likely result in higher staffing costs. Monthly calculations might only require the unit to devote about $250 of management resources to staffing annually instead of the $12,800 annual cost when staffing is adjusted daily. However, the cost of extra nursing staff might offset the savings. The performance budget serves a useful function by making explicit the costs of daily calculations.

The performance budget can also show the benefits of daily calculations. Suppose that it is expected that by adjusting staffing daily, 7 days a week, to the desired staffing level for the actual workload, it is possible to reduce the overall average paid hours per patient day for staff by 0.2 hour (12 minutes) per patient day. Presumably, by monitoring staffing needs very closely, it is possible to avert unneeded overtime, excessive use of agency nurses, or periods of overstaffing. If the 0.2 hour per patient day reduction is achieved by calculating staffing daily, $12,800 of the departmental budget will be devoted to staffing calculations. However, if the nursing unit has an average census of 20 patients, there would be a savings, on average, of 4 paid nursing hours per day (20 patients × 0.2 hour per patient day), or 1,460 nursing hours per year. The cost of 1,460 nursing hours would far outweigh the $12,800 investment in daily calculations to adjust staffing.

For example, suppose that the average nurse wage on the unit is $30 per hour. The total wage savings is $43,800. A return on investment can be calculated by dividing the savings of $43,800 by the cost of $12,800, or 3.42. In other words, $3.42 is saved for every dollar spent by doing staffing adjustments daily.

Cost Control

The purpose of cost control is to reduce or restrain increases in the organization's costs. For health care providers paid under a prospective payment system, such as capitation on Diagnosis Related Groups, reduced costs per patient directly improve the organization's financial health. The performance measure for cost control in Table 15–3 focuses on a reduction in the cost per patient day. The activity—reduce cost—really represents a goal rather than a specific description of how the nurses on the unit are to go about accomplishing the goal. However, the budget shows a clear commitment in this area: $60,800 is allocated specifically to accomplishing this end. Referring to Table 15–2, it is possible to see how much of the cost control effort is expected to come from the nurse manager's time, how much from the staff, how much from formal education, and so forth. In this example, each staff nurse is expected to spend 5% of the time, or about 2 hours per week, specifically focusing on cost reduction. This could mean spending 8 hours at a continuing education program once per month to learn about new approaches that may help the unit deliver care more efficiently. It does not necessarily mean that each nurse will spend 2 hours each week specifically on cost control.

In Table 15–3, it can be seen that the performance budget calls for a cost reduction per patient day of $8.33. The costs of the efforts in this area are budgeted to be $60,800. Most of this comes from requiring the staff to make a specific effort to find ways to contain costs. When the $60,800 budgeted cost for cost control is compared with the budgeted cost reduction of $8.33 per patient day, for each dollar saved in cost per patient day, it will cost the unit $7,299.[5] That seems rather high. Perhaps the unit is spending more on this activity than it is worth. In some cases, the performance budget may make explicit the fact that the unit is spending more to accomplish some end than it is worth.

However, care must be exercised in interpreting the performance budget. If $7,299 is spent to save a dollar per patient day, there must be a consideration of how many patient days there are likely to be. If the unit's average census is 20, there will be 7,300 patient days during the year (20 patients per day × 365 days in a year), and the savings at $1 per patient day would be $7,300, or only $1 more than the $7,299 cost. If the census is 28, the savings would be substantial. If the census is 14, the efforts to save money are costing more than they are saving.

Cost control is a general goal. Although the cost per patient day is a rough proxy intended to measure success with respect to that goal, the cost control efforts may also save money by getting patients discharged sooner. The shorter length of stay decreases overall costs. To determine the true payback for cost control efforts, it would be necessary to combine the savings from the reduced cost per patient day with the savings from the shorter length of stay. The same $60,800 effort for cost control will be working toward both of those ends. For this reason, although it is more complicated, it is often worth using several different measures of performance to more completely assess the unit and its accomplishments. This is discussed later in the Multiple Measures section of this chapter.

Increased Productivity

The desired productivity outcome is for the unit to accomplish more with the same or fewer resources. Procedures may need to be revised to help the staff accomplish this. Although it is difficult to specify exactly how this can be accomplished, it is not difficult to establish how to measure success. Assume that the organization is concerned about the cost of direct hours of care per patient day. If the total budgeted cost for the department is divided by the total direct patient care hours, a cost per direct care hour can be determined. It will probably be necessary to do occasional special studies to measure, on average, how many direct patient care hours are being provided.

Performance can then be assessed by the reduction in the overall unit cost per direct patient care hour. Such a reduction would indicate either a reduction in total costs or an increase in direct care hours. This approach has a big advantage over simply looking at the cost per patient day. If the cost per patient day declines, this could mean that patients are getting less care during each day. With this measure, cost of care is directly linked to the number of hours of direct care.

Patient and Staff Satisfaction

The key approach to satisfaction is to be responsive to the needs of individuals. Most hospitals use a formal instrument for collecting data on patient satisfaction. That would be a good measure to use for performance budgeting. However, other HCOs may not formally collect patient satisfaction data or may not have the resources to spend on data collection that using a formal instrument would require. In this case, performance budgeting can still be useful. One simply needs to be a bit more creative in establishing the measurement proxies.

For example, to measure patient satisfaction, the number of complaints could be counted. It may be true that some complaints are unreasonable or are about things that are not controllable. Many dissatisfied patients may not complain. However, some reduction in the number of complaints may be a way to go about measuring improvement in patient satisfaction. As with other areas, it must be determined how much improved patient satisfaction it is hoped can be generated, and whether the cost of the improvement is acceptable relative to the expected level of improvement.

Many organizations also measure staff satisfaction using a nursing-specific satisfaction measure (e.g., the nurse satisfaction measure included in the National Database of Nursing Quality Indicators, or other national nurse satisfaction surveys), or a general employee opinion survey. If an organization does not have the resources to engage in such an effort, staff satisfaction might also be measured in terms of complaints by the nursing staff. However, turnover rates for different members of the nursing staff might be a better indicator. If the hypothetical numbers in the example were correct, then taking actions to increase staff satisfaction that require $6,000 of total cost would be worthwhile because it would cost only $1,200 for each 1% reduction in staff turnover on the unit. This is a small cost compared with the cost of staff turnover described in Chapter 10.

Innovation and Planning

Sometimes it is difficult to measure performance. Innovative activity is one example. Proxies for performance in this area tend to be particularly weak. On the other hand, one of the most important things that a manager can do is to be innovative and to foster innovation. By making innovative activity an explicit part of the performance budget, the necessity of devoting energies to this area can be recognized even if the proxies available to measure performance are weak.

One measure of innovative activity and accomplishment is the number of practice changes introduced based on recently published research. Another is the number of meetings held

---

[5] Typically, we find the cost per unit, such as the cost per percent reduction in turnover, or the cost per percent reduction in the incidence of pressure ulcers. This is similar to finding the cost per patient day or the cost per discharge.

related to the implementation of a practice change. The fact that meetings are taking place is probably an indicator that activity is going on in this area. Are the meetings themselves the end goal? No. Do more meetings necessarily mean that more is being accomplished? No. They do, however, provide some sense of the degree of innovative activity.

Meetings are also important for managers, executives, and staff to engage in developing long-range plans for the unit, division, and organization. Again, the number of meetings held for long-range planning can be considered as an indicator that managers and staff are actually engaging in activities to think strategically in planning for the future, brainstorm opportunities for future growth, discuss new services to be added or discontinued, and consider how the unit will direct its future efforts.

It is also beneficial to see how expensive meetings are (see Table 15–3). When managers and staff are aware of the cost per meeting, there is likely to be more serious work done, in less time, with fewer meetings.

Although the number of meetings is used in Table 15–3, it is clearly a measure of process rather than of actual innovation or planning. The number of useful innovative ideas generated or new initiatives undertaken might be a better measure. The degree to which innovations are sustained over time may be another good measure. Certainly some formal system that rewards employees and provides incentives for generating innovative ideas and working to sustain organizational innovations will foster positive results in this area.

Direct Care

The measure suggested for performance evaluation in this area is the direct care cost per direct care hour. Lowering the cost per direct care hour can be achieved either by increasing the number of hours produced for the same cost or by lowering the costs for a given number of direct care hours. This is not the total unit cost per direct care hour. Rather, it considers the total cost for only the hours of direct care provided, divided by the hours of direct care. This will generate information on the cost per hour of the direct care. If this cost can be lowered, it often implies that less overtime or fewer agency nurses are being used. Another common way to achieve this goal is to substitute less skilled caregivers (e.g., unlicensed assistive personnel) for registered nurses (RNs) or to substitute less expensive RNs for more experienced and more expensive RNs. Although these approaches may decrease costs, they may also adversely affect patient outcomes.

Indirect Care

Indirect care is more difficult to measure than direct care because it comprises a wide variety of activities, such as documenting care delivered and communication with physicians. One approach is to measure the cost per patient day for these indirect activities. Reducing the cost per patient day for indirect activities is likely to indicate improved efficiency unless the quality of the activities deteriorates. However, if there is a series of quality performance measures, such as patient care planning, adverse patient events, and other checks on quality, such deterioration would probably not go unnoticed.

Other

Some activities do not lend themselves to quantification and analysis. It is preferable to reduce the portion of the budget used for "other" purposes by as much as possible. However, to the extent that it exists, there is no simple way to measure performance with respect to the use of resources devoted to these activities.

This discussion is not meant to be comprehensive. Rather, it presents some examples of how specific measures can be associated with various performance areas. It is necessary for the nurse manager to closely manage staff to ensure that they follow the performance budget as closely as possible. If staff members are included in the process of preparing performance budgets, they are more likely to strive to achieve the budgeted targets. One indication of the success of the performance budget approach is the extent to which the unit achieves its performance budget goals.

✳ MULTIPLE MEASURES

In most of the cases previously mentioned, one measurement was used for each of the various performance areas. This is not always an optimal approach. For example, the percent of patients who develop a pressure ulcer is not the only measure of quality nursing care on patient care units. Adverse events such as medication errors or the number of patient falls could also be measured. As performance budgets become more sophisticated, it would not be unreasonable for the $56,000 allocated for quality to be subdivided. Perhaps half of the quality efforts will be related to pressure ulcer prevention and surveillance, one-quarter to reducing patient falls, and one-quarter to reducing the number of medication variances. In that case, the $56,000 in the performance budget would be subdivided into $28,000 for reducing pressure ulcer rates, $14,000 for reducing patient falls, and $14,000 for reducing medication variances. The budgeted cost per fall prevented and the budgeted cost per medication variance avoided could be calculated in the same way as the budgeted cost for reducing pressure ulcers was calculated earlier.

This multiple measure approach is clearly superior to use of one measure for each performance area. Because it is likely that the nurse manager will be trying to improve quality in many areas, assigning all $56,000 to one area is likely an overstatement of the cost per unit of performance in that area. It also ignores other important activities. Some quality improvement activities, such as providing evidence-based care, may improve several areas of quality, but other approaches, such as a staff development program on decreasing medication errors, is specific to one area.

Suppose that the quality outcome area is subdivided, and it is determined that 10 medication variances can be eliminated by focusing specific attention in that area. Suppose further that it would cost $14,000 to do this. The cost per medication variance eliminated would be $1,400. Is this too much to spend on this problem? Perhaps it is so low that even more should be spent to try to eliminate additional medication variances. The key is that this approach allows the manager to quantify the financial impact of many activities that are done now without any specific measurement of cost effectiveness. With performance budgeting, it is possible to assess whether the results in a given area warrant the resource investment in that area.

In some cases, rather than allocating the cost to several different areas, it simply makes sense to aggregate the benefits yielded by the unit's efforts. For example, in the case of cost control, there may be efforts to reduce the cost per direct care hour, reduce supply costs, and reduce the average length of stay. In real-life situations, it is probably hard to determine how much staff effort goes to reduce length of stay and how much effort goes to reduce direct hours per day. One solution is to calculate the benefits from both shorter length of stay and reduced direct hours per patient day and combine them. Thus, the total benefits can be compared with the total costs.

❋ SUMMARY OF THE PERFORMANCE BUDGETING PROCESS

Performance budgeting involves a different series of steps than the traditional budgeting process. The first step in performance budgeting is to define the objectives, goals, or areas of accomplishment for the unit or department. These are called *performance areas*. Some examples of performance areas are quality of care, nursing satisfaction, patient satisfaction, productivity, and innovation. The second step is to identify the operating budget costs for the cost center being evaluated. In a nursing unit, these costs include items such as the salary for the unit nurse manager, salaries for clinical staff, education costs, and supplies. The third step is to determine what percentage of available resources should be used for each performance area. The fourth step is to assign the budgeted costs for the center to the individual performance areas on the basis of those percentages. The fifth and final step is to choose measures of performance for each performance area and to determine the cost per unit of workload based on those measures. This means that measures must exist to evaluate performance in the area so that the manager can determine that an improvement has been made or that high-level performance has been maintained. Along every step in the process, the manager should engage staff to determine any changes that may be needed to improve or maintain performance, and to involve them in these important activities that affect budgeting and resource allocation.

❋ IMPLICATIONS FOR NURSE MANAGERS AND EXECUTIVES

A wealth of information can be gained from performance budgeting. It is a tool that is likely to substantially improve both the planning and control processes in HCOs. Performance budgeting also represents a proactive approach to management. This approach follows a basic concept of budgeting: Managers and executives prepare a *plan* and attempt to manage according to that plan.

The starting point in performance budgeting is to determine the key performance areas. Next the operating budget is used to determine available resources. There is no conflict between the operating budget and the performance budget. They should work together. The operating budget focuses primarily on input resources. How much is going to be spent on RNs, how much on aides, and how much on supplies? The performance budget focuses on both processes and outcomes. How much is being budgeted to improve quality, how much to provide direct patient care, and how much to innovate?

As HCOs move forward in managerial sophistication, they must move beyond the focus on inputs and begin to focus on performance. Financial pressure to be more efficient can easily lead to deterioration in the quality of care provided. However, cuts in resources do not have to affect performance in a random or arbitrary manner. Performance budgeting can show where resources are being used. Movement toward a measurement focus on the cost of the goals of the nursing unit can allow the manager to make choices and to allocate scarce resources wisely among alternative possible uses.

It should be noted that performance budgeting may force units and organizations to consider how they will address suboptimal performance. Does suboptimal performance mean that care delivered has been deficient? Maybe or maybe not; only an evaluation of the measures can help to make this determination. If care is found to be deficient, how will deficiencies be addressed? Do the measures provide any insights into how the problem or deficit might be addressed? Will there be additional resources devoted to correcting the problem? Because improvements sometimes cost money, these questions are important to consider. This process, however, may help managers, executives, and staff to envision how care processes may be changed to provide better care at the same, and in some cases, lower cost.

Performance budgeting requires that data are used to determine financial impact. This approach fosters the linking of data with the budget as well as with practice. Engaging nurses at all levels in the process of performance budgeting is a way to help nurses, in general, come to understand the human and financial resources required to provide high-quality patient care. Having the structures and processes in place to bring meaningful data to nurse managers, executives, and staff is essential in this process. As Lessard notes, "When nurses are educated about performance and quality measures, engaged in identifying outcomes and collecting meaningful data, actively participate in disseminating quality reports, and are able to recognize the value of these activities, then data become one with practice."[6]

Performance budgeting is time-consuming and challenging. In some cases, the allocation of money to goal achievement will be inexact or arbitrary. However, it has tremendous potential value in HCOs, especially with the shift to a pay-for-performance environment. Performance budgets can allow for an indication of the level of quality of care expected in a planned budget. They can *explicitly* show quality decreases that are likely if budgets are cut without corresponding reduction in patient days. Given current national concerns about quality of care and national efforts underway to base health care reimbursements on quality outcomes, it is likely that as part of the evolution in budgeting, this is an approach that will gain wider use.

---

[6] Deborah Lessard, RN, BSN, MA, JD, CPHRM, personal communication from her review of the third edition of this book, to assist us in preparation for this new edition.

❋ KEY CONCEPTS

Performance budgeting   Technique that evaluates the activities of a cost center in terms of what the center accomplishes and the costs of that accomplishment. It is an approach to budgeting specifically designed to evaluate the performance of cost centers in terms of a variety of goals rather than a single budgeted output, such as the number of home care visits.

Performance areas   Objectives or areas of accomplishment for the unit or department.

Determining key performance areas   In developing performance areas, a variety of questions should be considered, such as:

- What are the important goals?
- What elements of a unit's performance are within the control of the nurse manager, and what elements are not?
- How should nurse managers most productively spend their time?
- How should the nursing staff most productively use their time?
- How can the performance of a nursing unit be measured?

Technical steps in performance budgeting   The process for developing a performance budget is to:

- Identify key performance areas.
- Identify line item budget costs for the cost center.
- Define how much of the resources represented by each line item are to be devoted to each of the performance areas.
- Calculate the dollars budgeted for each performance area. This can be done by taking the percent of each line item allocated to each performance area and multiplying it by the total amount of money in the traditional operating budget for that line item.
- Choose measures of performance for each performance area, budget a specific numerical objective for each area, and determine the budgeted cost per unit of each objective based on those measures.

Multiple measures   Selection of more than one basis for measurement of performance in each performance area.

❋ SUGGESTED READINGS

Bridglall B: Improving patient flow, patient satisfaction, and productivity with performance budgeting: a case study, *Hosp Cost Manag Account* 9(1):1–8, 1997.

Domino E: Nurses are what nurses do—are you where you want to be? *AORN J* 81(1):187–190, 193–201, 2005.

Finkler S, McHugh M: *Budgeting concepts for nurse managers*, ed 4, Philadelphia, 2007, WB Saunders.

Herzlinger R, Nitterhouse D: *Financial accounting and managerial control for nonprofit organizations*, Cincinnati, Ohio, 1994, South-Western Publishing.

Kalb K, Cherry N, Kauzloric J, et al: A competency-based approach to public health nursing performance appraisal, *Public Health Nurs* 23(2):115–138, 2006.

Lee R Jr, Johnson R, Joyce P: *Public budgeting systems*, ed 7, Boston, 2003, Jones & Bartlett.

Rave N, Geyer M, Reeder B, et al: Radical systems change. Innovative strategies to improve patient satisfaction, *J Ambul Care Manage* 26(2):159–174, 2003.

Schwendimann R, Buhler H, DeGeest S, Milisen K: Falls and consequent injuries in hospitalized patients: effects of an interdisciplinary fall prevention program, *BMC Health Serv Res* 6(1):69, 2006.

Simpson R: Who's minding our profession? Assessing the quality of nursing performance, part 1. *Nurs Manage* 35(4):20–21, 2004.

Simpson R: Who's minding our profession? Assessing the quality of nursing performance, part 2. *Nurs Manage* 35(6):20–21, 2004.

Van der Helm J, Goossens A, Bossuyt P: When implementation fails: the case of a nursing guideline for fall prevention, *J Comm J Qual Patient Saf* 32(3):152–160, 2006.

Zelman W, McCue M, Milikan A, Glick N: *Financial management of health care organizations: an introduction to fundamental tools, concepts, and applications*, ed 3, Cambridge, Mass, 2009, Wiley-Blackwell.

Controlling Operating Results

CHAPTER GOALS

The goals of this chapter are to:

- Introduce the concept of management control systems
- Explain the role of employee motivation in control
- Explore alternative incentive systems, including their strengths and weaknesses
- Consider the negative implications of unrealistic expectations
- Discuss the role of communication in the control process
- Clarify the importance of interim evaluation
- Define *variance analysis* and explain the reasons for doing variance analysis
- Distinguish between the concept of an "unfavorable" variance and a bad outcome

- Discuss traditional unit or department line-item variances
- Outline some possible causes of variances
- Explain flexible budgeting
- Introduce flexible budget variance analysis notation
- Define *volume*, *quantity*, and *price variances*
- Provide variance analysis tools and examples
- Provide insight into the problems encountered when variance information is aggregated
- Introduce the concept of exception reports and explain their benefits
- Discuss revenue variances

✳ INTRODUCTION

Organizations exercise control over operations through the use of a *management control system*. Such a system is a complete set of policies and procedures designed to keep operations going according to plan. Furthermore, a management control system detects any variations from plan and provides managers and executives with information needed to take corrective actions when necessary.

The focus of health care management control systems is on *responsibility accounting*. Responsibility accounting is the assignment of the responsibility for keeping to the plan and carrying out the elements of the management control system. Such responsibility is generally assigned to managers of cost centers. This chapter discusses a variety of elements of the management control system.

✳ THE BUDGET AS A TOOL FOR MOTIVATION

The budgeting process primarily concerns individuals, not numbers. If the employees of an organization do not work to make the organization succeed, the numbers constituting a budget will have little relevance. Motivation of staff and managers cannot be overemphasized. If *people* are not motivated to carry out the budget, it is likely to fail. That is why budgets arbitrarily imposed from above without fair consideration of input from those expected to carry them out tend to do so

poorly. It is why managers and executives feel such a sense of frustration when they are denied the needed authority to go along with their responsibility. It is why budget flexibility is needed in the face of changing realities. Motivation is the critical underlying key to budget success.

Control is complicated by the fact that individuals act in their own self-interest. The primary goal of the nursing staff may be to help patients. However, they have other goals as well. It is the basic nature of individuals for their own personal goals to be different from the goals of the organization for which they work. This does not mean that human nature is bad but only that there is such a thing as human nature, and it would be foolish to refuse to recognize it.

For example, other things being equal, most employees of a hospital would prefer a salary substantially larger than they are receiving. There is nothing particularly wrong in their wanting more money. In fact, ambition is probably a desirable trait in staff. However, all organizations must make choices concerning how to spend their limited resources. Health care organizations (HCOs) will not provide employees with 100% raises because they lack the revenues to pay for those raises. Although the nursing staff is not wrong to desire the raises, the organization is not wrong to deny them.

Thus, the fact must be faced that even when morale is generally excellent and is not considered a problem, an underlying tension will naturally exist. Even though the employees may want to achieve the mission of the organization in providing care, their personal desires will be for things the organization will choose not to provide. This is referred to as *goal divergence* (Figure 16–1).

The organization must bring together the interests of the individual and its own interests so they can work together. In the budgeting process, there must be some motivation for the people involved to want to control costs. Bringing the individual's and the organization's wants and desires together is referred to as *goal congruence* (Figure 16–2). To be sure that the employees will in fact want to control organizational costs, managers need to make sure that it is somehow in their direct best interests for costs to be controlled. Organizations generally achieve such congruence by setting up a system of incentives that make employees want to work toward the best interests of the organization.

❋ MOTIVATION AND INCENTIVES

Although nurses are motivated by factors other than money, it would be foolish to ignore the potential of monetary rewards to influence behavior. As HCOs search for the proper mix of incentives that will motivate managers and staff to control costs, financial incentives are frequently used. The most basic financial incentives are the ability to retain a job and to get a good raise.

Another motivating tool is a bonus system. Because managers and executives have many desires that relate to spending more money (e.g., larger offices, fancier furniture, larger staffs), formalized approaches need to be developed that will provide incentives to spend less money. For example, the HCO chief financial officer can tell a nurse manager that last year the manager's department spent $2,000,000 and that next year its budget is $2,080,000 (a 4% increase). However, for any amount that the department spends below $2,080,000, the manager and the staff can keep 10% of the savings. If spending is below the budgeted $2,080,000, the nurses and the organization benefit. In this case, goal congruence is likely to be achieved.

Many HCOs have added bonus systems. Such systems have both positives and negatives. The positives relate primarily to the strong motivation employees have to reduce costs. The

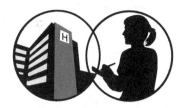

CONVERGENT GOALS

Organization   Individual

INCENTIVE EFFECT

FIGURE 16–2. Congruent goals.

negatives relate to the potential detriment to quality of patient care and to the potential negative effect on employee morale.

When an incentive is given to accomplish one end, sometimes the responses to that incentive are unexpected. Bonus systems may give a nurse manager an incentive to provide less staff nurse time per patient day. HCOs must be concerned about the impact their incentives will have on the quality of patient care. A strong internal quality assurance program is essential.

Furthermore, bonuses are not necessarily the solution to all motivational problems. If everyone gets a bonus, no one feels that individual actions have much impact. As long as everyone else holds costs in check, all individuals may believe they do not have to work particularly hard to reap the benefits of the bonus. On the other hand, giving bonuses to only some employees may generate jealousy and discontent. This may create a competitive environment in a situation in which teamwork is needed to provide high-quality care.

There are alternatives to using bonuses as an incentive. For example, one underused managerial tool is a letter from a supervisor to an employee that either recognizes the employee for introducing important cost-saving practices or points out areas for needed improvement. Also, all individuals responsible for controlling costs should be explicitly evaluated with respect to how well they do in fact control costs. That evaluation should be communicated in writing. Such approaches, which make use of both the carrot and the stick, cost little to implement but can have a dramatic impact.

Telling managers if they did or did not do a good job acknowledges that their boss is aware of a job well done, or that they should try to improve their efforts in the next year. In the real world, praise is both cheap and, in many cases, effective. On the other hand, criticism, especially in writing, can have a stinging effect that managers and staff will work hard to avoid in the future.

❋ MOTIVATION AND UNREALISTIC EXPECTATIONS

Although motivational devices can work wonders at getting an organization's staff to work hard for the organization and its goals, they can also backfire and have negative results. This occurs primarily when expectations are set at unreasonably high levels.

A target that requires hard work and stretching but is achievable can be a useful motivating tool. If the target is reached, there might be a bonus or there should be at least

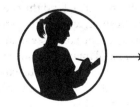

DIVERGENT GOALS

Organization   Individual

Low salaries   High salaries
Small staff   Large staff
Small offices   Large offices

FIGURE 16–1. Divergent goals.

some formal recognition of the achievement, such as a letter. At a minimum, the worker will have the self-satisfaction of having worked hard and reached the target.

But all those positive outcomes can occur only if the target is reachable. Some HCOs have adopted the philosophy that if a high target makes people work hard, a higher target will make them work even harder. It may seem as if the organization is short-changing itself whenever someone achieves a target. The manager may think, "We set the target too low. Perhaps if the target were higher, this person would have achieved even more. Because the target we set was achieved, we have not yet realized all of the employee's potential." There are risks associated with that logic.

If people fail to meet a target because they are not competent or because they do not work very hard, a signal of failure is warranted. In fact, repeated failure may be grounds for replacement of that individual in that job. But if an employee is both competent and hard-working, failure is not a message that should be sent. Even though it is desirable to encourage the individual to achieve even more, the signal of failure will be discouraging. When people work extremely hard and fail, they often question why they bothered to work so hard. If hard work results in failure to achieve the target, then why not ease off? Failure is failure—why kill yourself if you will have a poor evaluation no matter what? Managers must be extremely judicious to ensure that all goals assigned are reasonable, and that employees are supported in their efforts to achieve them.

✳ COMMUNICATION AND CONTROL

Communication is an essential part of a management control system. Communication should be an ongoing process. When a manager has a once-a-year meeting with the staff concerning the budget, it is quickly forgotten. To reinforce that meeting, a short weekly or monthly meeting should be held to discuss the budget. It is adequate to discuss just one or several items, such as bandage tape, diapers, chest tubes, disposable gloves, or sponges, at each meeting. It does not even have to be a separate meeting; it can be 2 minutes of any regularly scheduled meeting. The key is to make the staff aware of specific, definite, attainable goals that they can work toward. Furthermore, by mentioning the budget often, awareness is created, and it becomes second nature to conserve the organization's resources.

If the manager does not mention the budget until after a month of excessive use, a strong admonition at that time will tend to create budget antagonism rather than cost control. When a nurse manager routinely conveys specific, measurable goals, cost control can become a routine part of the way nurses function.

✳ USING BUDGETS FOR INTERIM EVALUATION

Interim evaluations are of particular importance in controlling operational results. If the manager simply prepares a budget, tells everyone what it is, and then puts it in a drawer until it is needed to help prepare next year's budget, an important element of motivation and control is lost. The budget has not been used to evaluate how well the unit, staff, and manager are doing and where improvements are needed. The role of evaluation should be primarily to focus on learning from past results to improve future outcomes.

Each month there should be comparisons between what was expected and what has been accomplished. First, this will allow the manager to give feedback to the staff nurses and to the manager's supervisor as to whether the budget's goals are being attained. Telling the staff the unit's goals without giving timely reports on whether they are being attained will weaken their motivation. In fact, failure to give this type of feedback is a common frustration among staff. Second, these monthly evaluations help to bring any unanticipated results to the manager's attention. Then the manager may be able to adjust staffing or take other corrective actions so that the budget will be met in future months.

Monthly information also allows a manager to provide early notice to a superior if a problem outside the manager's control exists. If the problem is controllable elsewhere in the organization (e.g., by the purchasing department), appropriate action can be taken. In evaluating any individual in an organization, one primary rule must be followed: *Responsibility should equal control.* If managers are held accountable for things over which they have no control, the organization will reward and punish the wrong individuals. The result is invariably demoralization of managers and staff. Using budgets for control can help locate the cause of inefficiency and help prevent waste. In addition, in the hands of a skilled manager, budgeting can help establish a defense for not meeting the budget (i.e., if there are valid reasons for spending in excess of budget, such as increases in noncontrollable costs).

We now turn our attention to the topic of variance analysis, one of the most widely used tools for interim evaluation.

✳ VARIANCE ANALYSIS

Variance analysis is the aspect of budgeting in which actual results are compared with budgeted expectations. The difference between the actual results and the planned results represents a *variance,* that is, the amount by which the results *vary* from the budget. Variances are calculated for three principal reasons. One reason is to aid in preparing the budget for the coming year. By understanding why results were not as expected, the budget process can be improved and become more accurate in future planning. The second reason is to aid in controlling results throughout the current year. By understanding why variances are occurring, actions can be taken to eliminate some of the undesirable variances over the coming months. The third reason for variance analysis is to evaluate the performance of units or departments and their managers.

For variance reports to be an effective tool, managers must be able to understand the causes of the variances. This requires investigation, which in turn requires the knowledge, judgment, and experience of nurse managers. Variances can be calculated by financial managers. However, finance personnel do not have the specific knowledge to explain why the variances are occurring. Without such explanation, the reports are not useful managerial aids.

Variance reports are given by finance to nurse managers for *justification.* The word "justification," which is often used, is unduly confrontational. It focuses attention on the evaluation role of variance analysis instead of on the planning and control roles. The goal of the investigation process is to obtain an explanation of why the variances arose. In a majority of cases, the variance report is used to understand what is happening and to control future results to the greatest extent possible. The focus should not be on a defensive justification of what was spent.

If variances arise as a result of inefficiency (e.g., duplicating work due to poor information flow), the process of providing cost-effective care is out of control. By discovering the inefficiency, actions can be taken to eliminate it and to bring the process back under control. In this case, future costs will be lower because of the investigation of the variance. The improvement comes, however, not from placing blame on who failed to control past results but on using the information to improve control of future results. It is important to realize that variance analysis provides its greatest benefits when it is used as a tool to improve future outcomes rather than as a way to assign blame for past results.

It would be naive, however, not to realize that in many cases HCOs do use variances to assign blame for the organization's failures. Therefore, this chapter and Chapter 17 provide tools to aid nurse managers and executives not only in explaining variances but also in deflecting blame for any variances that arise because of factors outside their control.

In many cases, variances are in fact caused by factors outside the control of nursing units or the nursing department. For example, increases in the average level of patient acuity may well cause staffing costs to rise. External price increases may cause more spending on clinical supplies than had been budgeted.

Although these factors are out of the control of nurse managers and should be explained as such, their impact on total costs should not be ignored. Competent nurse managers should be aware of the fact that even variances beyond their control may require responsive actions to be taken. Spending in excess of the budget in one area often results in a need to restrict spending in another. Adjustments to the entire budget must be considered and either made or rejected in the overall context of the organization and its financial situation.

On the other hand, if spending increases are the result of an increase in the number of patients, more revenue is likely being received by the organization as well. In that case, there should be less pressure to restrict costs. It therefore becomes critical to understand why variances are occurring. Are they controllable or not? If they are controllable, can actions be taken to reduce or eliminate the variances? If they are not controllable, is their nature such that responsive actions are required or not?

✳ TRADITIONAL VARIANCE ANALYSIS

At the end of a given time period, the organization will compare its actual results with the budget. Suppose that the organization does this monthly. Several weeks after each month ends, the accountants gather all the cost information and report the actual totals for the month.[1]

---

[1] One sign of the quality of a finance department is how quickly it provides department and unit managers with variance reports. If a finance department the reports in 2 weeks or less, it is doing an excellent job. Three weeks is acceptable performance but is not excellent. Longer than 3 weeks indicates a need for improvement.

The simplest approach is to compare the total costs that the entire organization has incurred with the budgeted costs for the entire organization. For example, suppose that Wagner Hospital had a total budget for the month of March of $4,800,000. The actual costs were $5,200,000. Wagner spent $400,000 more than they had budgeted. The difference between the amount budgeted and the amount actually incurred is the total hospital variance. This variance is referred to as an *unfavorable variance* because the organization spent more than had been budgeted. Accountants use the term *favorable variance* to indicate spending less than expected.

Assuming that the Wagner Hospital begins its year on January 1, its variance could appear in a format somewhat like the following:

This Month

Actual	Budget	Variance
$5,200,000	$4,800,000	$400,000 U

Year-to-Date

Actual	Budget	Variance
$15,150,000	$14,176,000	$974,000 U

In HCOs, nurse managers and executives are generally provided with cumulative information for the year to date as well as information for the current month. However, for simplicity, in the remaining examples in this chapter, we generally focus on just the results for the most recent month.

The capital U after the variance refers to the fact that the variance is unfavorable. That is, we actually spent more money than had been budgeted. If the variance had been favorable, it would be followed by a capital F. An alternative presentation to using U and F is to use a negative number for an unfavorable variance and a positive number for a favorable variance. Alternatively, parentheses can be placed around unfavorable variances and no parentheses around favorable variances. Parentheses indicate a negative number. The interpretation of variance notation should be approached with caution. Any systematic approach can be used to indicate favorable versus unfavorable variances. It would not be wrong to use negative numbers for favorable variances and positive numbers for unfavorable variances as long as the use is consistent throughout the organization. There is no consistent approach followed by all organizations in the health care industry.

Why did Wagner have a $400,000 unfavorable variance for the month of March? If variance analysis is to be used to evaluate results, it is necessary to be able to determine not simply that the organization was $400,000 over budget but also why that occurred. Given just this total information for the entire organization, the chief executive officer (CEO) has no idea of what caused the variance. The CEO does not even know which managers to ask about the variance because all that is known is a total for the entire organization.

One solution would be to have organization-wide *line-item* totals—that is, the total amount budgeted for salaries for the entire organization could be compared with actual total salary costs. The total amount budgeted for surgical supplies could be compared with the actual total amount spent on surgical supplies. However, there would still be no way to determine what caused the variances. All departments have salaries. A number of departments use surgical supplies. Who should be asked about the variances?

To use budgets for control, it must be possible to assign responsibility for variances to individual managers. Those managers can investigate the causes of the variances and attempt to eliminate the variances in the future. The key is that it must be possible to hold individual managers accountable for the variance. This leads to the necessity for determining variances by unit and department. Although the following example uses a hospital, all variance analysis techniques discussed in this book apply equally to all types of HCOs.

Unit and Department Variances

The overall Wagner variance of $400,000 is an aggregation of variances from a number of departments. Focus on the results for the nursing department.

THE WAGNER HOSPITAL
Department of Nursing Services
March Variance Report

Actual	Budget	Variance
$2,400,000	$2,200,000	$200,000 U

Apparently, half of the variance for the Wagner Hospital for March occurred in the nursing services area. Previously, it was known that there was an excess expenditure of $400,000, but it was not known how that excess came about. Now it is known that half of it occurred in the nursing area. The chief nurse executive (CNE) can be asked to explain why the $200,000 variance occurred.

Unfortunately, at this point, the CNE has not been given much to go on. The CNE simply knows that there was $200,000 spent that was not budgeted. Most hospitals would take this total cost for the nursing department and break it down into the various nursing units. Each nursing unit that has a nurse manager who is responsible for running that unit should have both a budget for the unit and a variance report that shows the unit's performance compared with the budget.

The variance for one particular nursing unit might appear as follows:

THE WAGNER HOSPITAL
Department of Nursing Services
Medical-Surgical 6th Floor West
March Variance Report

Actual	Budget	Variance
$120,000	$110,000	$10,000 U

Line-Item Variances

Even after the total nursing department variance has been divided among the various nursing units, more information is still needed as a guide. Is the variance the result of

unexpectedly high costs for nursing salaries? Does it relate to use of supplies? There is no way to know based on a total variance for the unit or department. More detailed information is needed.

To have any real chance to control costs, there must be variance information for individual line items within a unit or department. The CNE must know how much of the nursing total went to salaries and how much to supplies. Nurse managers must have similar information for their own units. For example:

THE WAGNER HOSPITAL
Department of Nursing Services
Medical-Surgical 6th Floor West
March Variance Report

	Actual	Budget	Variance
Salary	$108,000	$100,000	$ 8,000 U
Supplies	12,000	10,000	2,000 U
Total	$120,000	$110,000	$10,000 U

This is obviously a great simplification. There should be line items for employee benefit costs. There should be separate line items for each type of employee. Licensed practical nurses (LPNs) would be separate from registered nurses (RNs). Each major type of other-than-personnel services (OTPS) cost could be a separate line item (e.g., Table 16–1). The more detailed the line items are, the more information that is available. Variance reports with detailed line-item results for each unit and department are generally available in HCOs today.

Understanding Variances

The objective in doing variance analysis is to determine why the variances arose. Nothing can be done with respect to the goal of controlling costs until the nurse manager or executive knows where the unit or department is deviating from the plan and why. The more detailed the line-item information, the easier it will be to identify specific areas where variances are occurring.

After the variance for each line item for each unit has been calculated, it must be determined whether or not to investigate the variance. Minor variances can be ignored. Variances that are significant in amount must be investigated. (The issue of how to determine if a variance is significant enough to warrant investigation is discussed in Chapter 17 under the heading Investigation and Control of Variances.) By dividing variances into nursing units, each unit manager can be assigned the responsibility of determining the causes of the variances for the unit. The manager of 6th Floor West must explain the causes of the $10,000 total unfavorable unit variance.

By dividing the variances into line items, the unit manager can begin the investigation. In the previous example, $8,000 of the variance is the result of labor costs, and $2,000 is the result of spending more on supplies than the budget allowed.

✳ **TABLE 16–1** *Sample Variance Report—March 2013*
Cost Center: 6th Floor West Medical-Surgical

This Month				Year to Date		
Actual	Budget	Variance	Account No./Description	Actual	Budget	Variance
$ 58,951	$ 53,431	$ 5,520	010 Salaries—RNs	$164,245	$160,296	$3,949
32,110	31,098	1,012	011 Salaries—LPNs	94,930	93,294	1,636
14,124	13,256	868	012 Salaries—NAs	41,569	39,768	1,801
4,581	4,088	493	020 FICA	13,742	12,263	1,479
1,081	1,014	67	021 Unemployment tax	3,241	3,041	201
351	313	38	022 Disability tax	1,051	938	113
209	200	9	050 Life insurance	627	600	27
343	350	(7)	060 Other fringes	1,029	1,050	(21)
$111,750	$103,750	$ 8,000	**(a) Personnel cost**	$320,435	$311,429	$9,185
$ 4,970	$ 3,000	$ 1,970	300 Patient care supplies	$ 8,950	$ 9,000	($ 50)
828	800	28	400 Office supplies and forms	2,484	2,400	84
650	650	0	500 Seminars and meetings	1,950	1,950	0
750	750	0	600 Noncapital equipment	2,250	2,250	0
425	400	25	700 Maintenance and repair	1,275	1,200	75
45	50	(5)	800 Miscellaneous	135	150	(15)
582	600	(18)	900 Interdepartmental	1,746	1,800	(54)
$ 8,250	$ 6,250	$ 2,000	**(b) OTPS**	$ 18,790	$ 18,750	$ 40
$120,000	$110,000	$10,000	**(c) Total unit costs (c = a+b)**	$339,225	$329,999	$9,225

Note: In this table, unfavorable variances are positive numbers and favorable variances are negative numbers.
OTPS, other-than-personnel services.
Adapted from Finkler SA: *Budgeting concepts for nurse managers,* ed 3, Philadelphia, 2001, Saunders.

Note that although the $8,000 labor variance is much larger than the supplies variance in absolute dollar terms, the labor variance is 8% over budget, and the supply variance is 20% over budget. Both of these variances should be investigated and their causes determined. When possible, corrective action should be instituted to avoid similar variances in future months.

Traditional variance analysis requires that the nurse manager proceed to use the unit line-item variance information to attempt to discover the underlying causes of the variances. Consider the $8,000 variance for salaries. Why was $8,000 more than budgeted spent on salaries? No matter how narrowly defined the line items for salaries (e.g., separating RNs from LPNs from Nursing Assistants [NAs]), the question still arises: Why was $8,000 more than budgeted spent on salaries?

In the absence of supporting evidence, the 6th Floor West unit manager and nurses may be told that they did not do a good job of controlling the use of staff. This is an unwarranted conclusion. Expenditure for staff in excess of the budgeted amount could have a number of possible causes. Investigation may disclose which potential cause was in fact responsible in a given instance.

It is correct that one potential cause of the $8,000 salary variance is that the unit manager just did not do a good job in controlling the usage of staff. As a result, more hours of nursing care per patient were paid for than had been expected. However, another possibility is that the patients were sicker than anticipated, and the higher average acuity level caused more nursing hours to be used per patient. Another possible cause is that the hourly rate for nurses increased. Nurse managers may have no direct control over base salaries. On the other hand, the higher cost could have been because of increased overtime.

Still another possible cause of the variance is that there were more patients, and the additional patients caused more consumption of nursing hours. The most serious problem with traditional variance analysis is that it compares the predicted cost for a predicted workload level (e.g., volume of patient days adjusted for acuity) with the actual cost for the actual workload level.[2] Unless the actual workload is exactly as predicted, there is little chance that a unit will achieve exactly the budgeted expectations.

Essentially, with traditional variance analysis, an attempt is being made to match actual costs to a budget that is relevant for a given workload level. But that workload level is usually not the actual workload that occurs. If a nursing unit has more or fewer patients, the original budget is no longer relevant. If costs fall by 5%, under traditional variance analysis, there is a temptation to praise the manager for coming in under budget. However, if patient volume falls by 20% and costs fall by only 5%, it does not make sense to offer that

---

[2] The general term *workload* is used here because there is no one unique measure of workload that will always be relevant for budgeting. Sometimes we will use the technocratic term *output* interchangeably with *workload*. If we are dealing with a home health agency, workload is measured by the number of visits. For the radiology department, the workload measure is likely to be the number of radiographs. For a nursing unit, workload would generally be the number of patient days adjusted for acuity. For an operating room, it might be the number of procedures or hours of surgical procedures, and so on.

praise. Such a large patient decline might have warranted a bigger decrease in costs.

Similarly, if patient workload increases by 20% and costs rise by only 5%, it makes little sense to have a variance analysis system that is oriented toward criticizing the unit and manager for having gone over the original budget. The problem with traditional variance analysis is that it is overly focused on the original budget. A *flexible budget* approach allows for more sophisticated analysis.

✳ FLEXIBLE OR VARIABLE BUDGETS

Flexible or *variable budgeting* takes into consideration the fact that the actual output level often differs from expectations. Managers must have some way of controlling operations in light of varying levels of activity.

Preparing a budget requires many assumptions and predictions. One of the most prominent of these concerns the workload level. If the volume of services, cost of services, and revenues related to services all rose and fell in equal proportions, this might not create a significant problem. However, that is generally not the case. Revenues may change in a sharply different proportion than costs. Managers need to be able to anticipate such variations, and a flexible budget is a tool to aid managers in this area.

A flexible budget is an operating budget for varying workload levels. For example, suppose that the Best Clinic expects 4,000 visits and had the following operating budget for the coming month:

Best Clinic
Budget for Next Month

Revenues	
Patient Care	$165,000
Expenses	
Salaries	$115,000
Supplies	30,000
Rent	12,000
Other	6,000
Total Expense	$163,000
Surplus	$ 2,000

This budget provides Best Clinic with information that a modest surplus of $2,000 is projected. But what will happen if the number of visits is greater or fewer than expected?

Assume that revenue changes in direct proportion to the number of visits. However, some of the expenses are fixed costs (see Chapter 8 for a discussion of fixed and variable costs). They will not change as the volume of visits changes. For example, rent on the clinic building is a flat monthly amount regardless of visits. For most organizations, however, some costs are also variable. They vary as the volume of visits goes up or down. Best Clinic will have to buy more supplies if it gets very busy. Or the clinic can buy fewer supplies if it has fewer patients.

A flexible budget takes the basic operating budget and adjusts it for the impact of possible workload changes. Assume that revenues and supplies are the only items that vary with the number of visits. For this simple example, we will assume that the clinic's staffing is fixed for any likely range of activity. Consider a flexible budget for Best Clinic, assuming that 3,600 or 4,400 visits, a 10% decrease or increase, respectively, occurs next month:

Best Clinic
Flexible Budget for Next Month

	Volume of Clinic Visits		
	3,600	4,000	4,400
Revenues			
Patient Revenue	$148,500	$165,000	$181,500
Expenses			
Salaries	115,000	115,000	115,000
Supplies	27,000	30,000	33,000
Rent	12,000	12,000	12,000
Other	6,000	6,000	6,000
Total Expense	$160,000	$163,000	$166,000
Surplus/(Deficit)	($ 11,500)	$ 2,000	$ 15,500

This flexible budget shows that if the number of visits increases by just 10% from 4,000 to 4,400, a surplus or profit of $15,500 will occur. But a 10% fall in visits will result in a loss of $11,500. This information can serve as a warning to the managers in the planning stage. They need to be aware of the potential for losses if volume does not meet expectations, as well as the possible benefits from extra visits.

During the month, if managers see that visits are fewer than expected, they can anticipate the likely financial shortfall without waiting until the end of the month or later to find out. Actions can be taken to increase fund-raising efforts or to find ways to cut costs. Decisions can be made regarding whether the clinic can sustain a financial loss. If it cannot, it may have to find ways to cut costs.

Flexible or variable budgets focus on volume. Nursing units in hospitals have patient days. Home care agencies provide visits. Operating rooms have procedures. In each case, some measure of volume is needed to prepare a flexible budget.

The key to preparing a flexible budget is identification of fixed and variable costs. As volume varies up or down, which numbers in the budget are likely to change, and which are likely to remain the same? Will the costs change in direct proportion to volume changes, or will their change be more or less than proportional? Managers must work to understand revenue and cost structures enough to be able to anticipate the changes caused by volume variations.

Flexible budgets not only are useful for planning but also serve a critical role in variance analysis. By understanding flexible budgets, the manager is able to interpret more accurately why variances occur and to take any required actions as a result of variances.

✳ FLEXIBLE BUDGET VARIANCE ANALYSIS

Flexible budget variance analysis is a system that requires a little more work than traditional variance analysis but can provide nurse managers with substantially more information. The information provided can help managers understand the causes of variances so that they can be controlled. It can also demonstrate that certain unfavorable variances are not the fault of a manager's unit or department but were caused by factors outside of the unit or department's control.

Suppose that the following was the variance report for nursing department salaries for the month of March:

THE WAGNER HOSPITAL
Department of Nursing Services
March Variance Report

	Actual	Budget	Variance
Salary	$1,000,000	$1,000,000	$0

It looks like the department came in right on budget. The department's managers likely would be feeling pretty good about this line item for March. Suppose, however, that the budget of $1,000,000 for nursing salaries was based on an assumption of 25,000 patient days, but there were actually only 20,000 patient days. One would expect that the lower patient-day volume should have allowed for reduction in overtime and elimination of some temporary agency nurse time. The department should have spent less than $1,000,000.

When used for variance analysis, the flexible budget is a restatement of the budget based on the volume actually attained. Basically, the flexible budget shows what we would have expected a line item to cost given the workload level that actually occurred.

In variance analysis, the flexible budget is prepared after the fact. The actual volume must be known in order to prepare the flexible budget for that specific volume.[3] Keep in mind that because some costs are fixed and some are variable, total costs do not change in direct proportion with volume. One would normally expect that a 10% increase in patient days would be accompanied by *less* than a 10% increase in costs because only some costs are variable and increase as census does. On the other hand, a 10% reduction in workload would only be expected to be accompanied by a *less* than 10% reduction in cost because the fixed costs would not decline.

Using the flexible budget technique allows the variance for any line item to be subdivided to get additional information. Essentially, the variance already calculated (i.e., the difference between the budgeted amount and the actual result) will be divided into three parts: a *volume variance,* a *quantity variance,* and a *price variance.*

The Volume Variance

The *volume variance* is the amount of the variance in any line item that is caused simply by the fact that the workload level has changed. For example, if the budget calls for 25,000 patient days when there were actually 30,000 patient days, it would be expected that it would be necessary to spend more. Variable costs would undoubtedly rise. The cost of the resources needed for an extra 5,000 patient days constitutes a volume variance.

A substantial number of unfavorable unit line-item variances may result simply from the fact that workload increased above expectations. Such an increase is generally outside of the

control of the nurse manager. For many HCOs, an increase in workload is a good thing. Higher hospital occupancy may mean that there are more patients sharing the fixed overhead of the institution. Similarly, with home health agencies, more visits mean more patients to share the fixed costs of the agency.

Higher volume demands higher cost. The flexible budget approach allows for specific identification of how much of the variance for any line item is attributable to changes in the workload volume versus other causes. If the higher volume was not budgeted for, there will be spending in excess of budget. Note that revenue will likely be higher than budget as well. More often than not, however, nurse managers are held responsible for controlling costs, but they do not receive any benefit from increases in revenues.

The Quantity, or Use, Variance

The second general type of variance under the flexible budgeting scheme is the *quantity,* or *use, variance.* This is the portion of the overall variance for a particular line item that results from using more of a resource than was expected for a given workload level. For example, if more supplies were used per patient day than expected, this would give rise to a quantity variance, because the quantity of supplies that were used per patient day exceeded expectations.

This variance is also frequently referred to as a *use variance* because it focuses on how much of the resource has been used. For example, if one-half roll of bandage tape was used per patient day but the expected usage was only one-quarter roll, there would be a use variance. The terms *quantity* and *use* are often used interchangeably.

The Price, or Rate, Variance

The *price,* or *rate, variance* is the portion of the total variance for any line item caused by spending more per unit of some resource than had been anticipated. For example, if the average wage rate for nurses is more per hour than had been expected, this would give rise to this type of variance. When the variance is used to measure labor resources, it is generally called a *rate variance* because the average hourly rate has varied from expectations. When considering the price of supplies, such as the cost per package of sutures, it is called a *price variance* because it is the purchase price that has varied. The terms *price* and *rate* are often used interchangeably in practice.

If a unit manager expected to pay $1.00 per roll for bandage tape but actually paid $1.10 per roll, this would give rise to a price variance. Or suppose there is a line item for nurses hired on a temporary basis from an outside agency. If the unit manager expected to pay the agency $45.00 per hour but actually paid an average of $48.00 per hour, this would give rise to a rate variance.

The price, or rate, variance may or may not be under the control of the nurse manager. If the purchasing department predicts all prices used for supplies and then winds up paying a higher price than predicted, it should be possible to measure the price variance so that the responsibility can be placed with the purchasing department. If the nursing department bears the responsibility for price variances on supplies, the purchasing department will have no incentive to find the best

---

[3] As part of the budget preparation process, some organizations prospectively prepare flexible budgets. This provides the organization with a sense of what costs are likely to be at differing levels of workload.

prices. On the other hand, if the nurse manager hires temporary nurses directly from the agency, then the responsibility for the rate variance may rest with the nurse manager. Were overqualified people hired? Was an attempt made to seek out an agency that would give the best rate? The manager who can exercise some control over the outcome should be the manager held accountable for the outcome.

❋ DETERMINATION OF THE CAUSES OF VARIANCES

Before discussing how these different flexible budget variances can be calculated, there is another critical issue to be considered first. The volume, price, and quantity variances will be used to find out more information about why the budget differs from the actual results. Using these variances, it will be possible to find out how much of the variance was caused simply by a change in the workload volume, how much by a change in prices, and how much by changes in the amount of each resource consumed for a given level of workload.

What the nurse manager will not get from this analysis is the ultimate explanation of causes of the variances. The nurse manager will still have to investigate *why* these variances have occurred. The analysis provides significant new information by pointing a finger in a specific direction instead of waving a hand in a vague direction.

For instance, if twice as many surgical supplies were used per patient day as expected, the nurse manager knows exactly what to investigate. The analysis does not tell why there was a variance, but it does tell where. Rather than simply saying that the operating room is over budget, it is known that the line item for surgical supplies is over budget. Furthermore, rather than simply noting that too much was spent on surgical supplies, it has been determined that the problem was not caused by extra procedures, and it was not caused by the price of surgical supplies going up. It is specifically known that the problem lay in using more surgical supplies per procedure than had been budgeted. Managers must take over at this point and investigate why this occurred. Why were more surgical supplies used per procedure than expected? Was it sloppy use? Clear-cut waste? Pilferage? A change in surgeons' practices? The hiring of a new surgeon? Was there a major disaster that did not increase the number of procedures considerably but did bring in patients requiring a great amount of surgical supplies? Is the budget wrong, and thus it is not really possible to get by with the budgeted amount of surgical supplies per procedure?

If answers to these questions were not needed, the variance process could get by with a lot more accountants and computers and a lot fewer nurse managers. Accountants and computers, however, cannot answer questions. Ultimately, the nurse manager or executive must find out the actual underlying cause of the variance.

❋ THE MECHANICS OF FLEXIBLE BUDGET VARIANCE ANALYSIS

The first step in flexible budgeting is to establish the flexible budget for the actual workload level. Given the actual cost for a particular line item and the original budgeted amount, it must be determined what it would have been expected to cost for that line item given the workload level that actually occurred.

For example, consider the supplies budgeted for and used by the Medical-Surgical 6th Floor West nursing unit at the Wagner Hospital in March:

THE WAGNER HOSPITAL
Department of Nursing Services
Medical-Surgical 6th Floor West
March Variance Report

	Actual	Budget	Variance
Supplies	$12,000	$10,000	$2,000 U

The actual consumption was $12,000. The budgeted consumption was $10,000. Suppose that the budget assumed that there would be 500 patient days for this unit for March, but there actually turned out to be 600 patient days. (For the time being, ignore the acuity level of the patients. Using acuity in the variance model is explicitly addressed in Chapter 17.) Assuming that the consumption of supplies would normally be expected to vary in direct proportion to patient days, the planned consumption was $20 per patient day. This is calculated by dividing the $10,000 budget by the 500 expected patient days.

For 600 patient days at $20 per patient day, $12,000 (i.e., 600 × $20) would have been budgeted for supplies. This is the flexible budget. It is the amount the department would have expected to spend had the actual number of patient days been known. Notice that in this case, the flexible budget and the actual amount spent are identical:

THE WAGNER HOSPITAL
Department of Nursing Services
Medical-Surgical 6th Floor West
March Variance Report

	Actual	Flexible Budget	Original Budget
Supplies	$12,000	$12,000	$10,000

The difference between the original budget and the actual amount spent is the total variance. This is still $2,000 U:

Original Budget	$10,000
−Actual	−12,000
Total Variance	$ 2,000 U

The difference between the original budget and the new flexible budget is the volume variance. In this case, the difference is $2,000 U.

Original Budget	$10,000
−Flexible Budget	−12,000
Volume Variance	$ 2,000 U

The entire variance that we see in the total variance was caused by the difference between the budgeted and the actual volumes. Note that this volume variance is considered unfavorable, because the flexible budget requires more spending than was expected. The increased workload may well have been a favorable event for the organization if it brought in more revenues and profit, but the accountant always refers to cost in excess of the original budget as being an unfavorable variance. The word unfavorable does not automatically denote a bad outcome when it is used in variance analysis.

What about the nursing salaries for the unit? Recall the variance report for nursing salaries:

THE WAGNER HOSPITAL
Department of Nursing Services
Medical-Surgical 6th Floor West
March Variance Report

	Actual	Budget	Variance
Salary	$108,000	$100,000	$8,000 U

To keep the discussion relatively simple at this point, assume that nursing salary costs should vary in direct proportion to the number of patient days. In other words, assume that nursing salary costs are variable. A more realistic example is discussed in Chapter 17 after flexible budget mechanics have been fully developed.

Nursing salaries had been budgeted at $100,000, with an expectation of 500 patient days. This is a cost of $200 per patient day ($100,000 ÷ 500 patient days = $200 per patient day). Assuming nursing salary costs are variable, had it been known that there would be 600 patient days, $120,000 would have been budgeted ($200 × 600 = $120,000). The variance report can be restated as follows:

THE WAGNER HOSPITAL
Department of Nursing Services
Medical-Surgical 6th Floor West
March Variance Report

	Actual	Flexible Budget	Original Budget
Salary	$108,000	$120,000	$100,000

The difference between the original budget and the flexible budget is the volume variance. It is found to be $20,000 U.

Original Budget	$100,000
−Flexible Budget	−120,000
Volume Variance	$ 20,000 U

It is unfavorable because the greater number of patients required more labor. When the flexible budget is compared with the actual cost, it turns out that there is a remaining variance of $12,000 F. We can call that a flexible budget variance. It represents the causes of the total variance aside from changes in volume.

Flexible Budget	$120,000
−Actual	−108,000
Flexible Budget Variance	$ 12,000 F

Note that the volume variance is unfavorable, because the extra patients require more spending. However, the actual amount spent was less than the flexible budget, resulting in a favorable flexible budget variance. We actually spent less than we would have expected to for that number of patients.

If the volume and flexible budget variances for salaries are combined, there is an unfavorable total variance of $8,000. Note that if both variances were favorable, they could be added together, and the result would be $32,000 F. If they were both unfavorable, they could be added, and the result would be $32,000 U. Because one of the variances is favorable and one is unfavorable, the smaller one must be subtracted from the larger one to get a combined total variance. The total variance will have the same label (i.e., favorable or unfavorable) as the larger of the two variances. Hence, $20,000 U − $12,000 F = $8,000 U.

At this point in the analysis, there is not yet sufficient information to determine the causes of the flexible budget variance. Suppose that the CNE of the organization had come to the unit manager in the middle of April and complained about a total lack of cost control on the unit. The unit had a $2,000 unfavorable supplies variance and an $8,000 unfavorable salary variance. Based on traditional variances (without using a flexible budget), there would be no way the unit manager could determine the cause of the problem.

Certainly, the unit manager is aware of increased patient volume and would argue that extra patient days were a major factor. But how major? By using a flexible budget, it is possible to find out exactly what dollar impact the extra patient days should have had. In the example, flexible budgeting has shown that the entire variance in supplies is attributable to the extra patient days. Furthermore, the volume variance was $20,000 U for salaries. Based on that variance, the department manager should have expected to spend $20,000 more on nursing salaries than was in the original budget. In fact, only $8,000 was spent above the original salary budget. Rather than being blamed for having gone over budget, the unit manager can now show that given the actual number of patient days, the unit actually spent $12,000 less than should have been expected!

Data for Flexible Budget Analysis

To compute volume, quantity, and price variances, we need to know the budgeted and actual values for three different variables. First, we need to know the workload: number of patients (or other volume measure, such as patient days, procedures, or other unit of service). Next we need to know the amount of resources needed per patient (or patient day, procedure, or other unit of service). Finally, we need to know the hourly wages for the staff and the prices of supplies. That is, we need to know the:

- Budgeted number of patients, procedures, or other units of service
- Actual number of patients, procedures, or other units of service
- Budgeted resources needed per patient, procedure, or other unit of service
- Actual resources used per patient, procedure, or other unit of service
- Budgeted price per unit of resource needed
- Actual price per unit of resource used

For example, to use this method to compute labor variances for a nursing unit, we would need to know the budgeted and actual number of patient days for the unit, the budgeted and actual hours of nursing care per patient day, and the budgeted and actual nursing pay rates per hour.

An Example of Volume, Price, and Quantity Variances

Suppose that Wagner Hospital had the following line item in its variance report for a nursing unit for the month that just ended:

	Actual	Budget	Variance
Nursing Labor	$50,220	$42,000	$8,220 U

The unit manager wants to find out what caused the variance, so the following information is gathered:

- Budgeted number of patient days: 400
- Actual number of patient days: 450
- Budgeted nursing hours per patient day (HPPD): 3.0
- Actual nursing HPPD: 3.1
- Budgeted average nursing pay rate per hour: $35
- Actual average nursing pay rate per hour: $36

Before proceeding to use these data, consider what is involved in obtaining the information. Information is worthwhile only if it is more valuable than the cost to collect it. All three of the budgeted items are already known. It would not have been possible to prepare an operating budget without a forecast of patient days, the budgeted nursing HPPD (or at least the total budgeted time, which can be divided by the expected patient days to get the budgeted HPPD), and the average pay rate for nurses. What about the actual results? The actual number of patient days is readily available. The actual wage rate and the actual total amount of paid nursing hours are available from the payroll department. Given the actual total nursing hours and the actual number of patient days, one can divide to get the actual average nursing HPPD. Therefore, all of the data needed for flexible budget variance analysis are readily available.

The first step in using these data to compute variances is to use them to calculate the original budget. The original budget is simply the expected number of nursing HPPD multiplied by the hourly pay rate for the nurses multiplied by the expected number of patient days. In this case, the expectation is that we will need 3.0 nursing care HPPD at a rate of $35 per hour for 400 patient days. Therefore, the budget is $42,000 as follows:

Original Budget
Budgeted Quantity × Budgeted Price × Budgeted Volume
3.0 × $35 × 400 = $42,000

In other words, you find the original budget by multiplying the budgeted values for these variables. Notice that we are using "budgeted quantity" to refer to the budgeted number of nursing care HPPD. We can use budgeted quantity more generally to refer to the budgeted amount of any resource that is needed for each patient, patient day, procedure, or other unit of service. We are using "budgeted price" to refer to the budgeted hourly nursing wage rate. We can use budgeted price more generally to refer to any budgeted price for a particular supply item or wage rate. Finally, we are using "budgeted

volume" to refer to the budgeted number of patients on this unit. We can use budgeted volume more generally to refer to the budgeted number of patients, patient days, procedures, or other units of service. If these three numbers are multiplied together, the result is the originally budgeted cost for nursing labor.

The next step is to find the flexible budget. Keep in mind that the flexible budget is the amount one would have expected to spend if the actual number of patient days had been known in advance. It is therefore computed by using the budgeted quantity (i.e., amount of nursing HPPD) by the budgeted price (i.e., the nursing wage rate per hour) by the actual volume (i.e., the actual number of patient days). The only change from the original $42,000 budget computed above is that instead of using the budgeted 400 patient days, the computation uses the actual 450 patient days. The flexible budget can be calculated as follows:

Flexible Budget
Budgeted Quantity × Budgeted Price × Actual Volume
3.0 × $35 × 450 = $47,250

Note that the difference between the original budget and the flexible budget is caused by a difference in the number of patient days. Other than that, the calculations are the same. The originally budgeted amount of $42,000 can be compared with the flexible budget amount of $47,250 to determine the volume variance of $5,250 U (i.e., $42,000 − $47,250 = $5,250 U). Because patient days are higher than expected, cost would be expected to exceed the original budget. This will give rise to an unfavorable variance. The comparison between the original budget and the flexible budget can be shown as follows:

Original Budget vs. Flexible Budget
Budgeted Quantity × Budgeted Price × **Budgeted Volume**
−Budgeted Quantity × Budgeted Price × **Actual Volume**

3.0 × $35 × **400** = $42,000
−3.0 × $35 × **450** = −47,250
Volume Variance = $ 5,250 U

The next step is to create a value that is referred to as the *subcategory*. The subcategory has no specific intuitive meaning. It is simply a device to allow us to compute the price and quantity variances. The subcategory is defined as the actual quantity multiplied by the budgeted price times the actual volume. The subcategory can be calculated as follows:

Subcategory
Actual Quantity × Budgeted Price × Actual Volume
3.1 × $35 × 450 = $48,825

This flexible budget can be compared with the subcategory to generate the quantity variance, as follows:

Flexible Budget vs. Subcategory
Budgeted Quantity × Budgeted Price × Actual Volume
− **Actual Quantity** × Budgeted Price × Actual Volume

3.0 × $35 × 450 = $47,250
−3.1 × $35 × 450 = −48,825
Quantity or Use Variance = $ 1,575 U

Note that for both the subcategory and the flexible budget, we are using the budgeted price of $35 per hour for nursing time and the actual volume of 450 patient days. The only variable that differs between the subcategory and the flexible budget is the quantity. The subcategory uses the actual quantity, and the flexible budget uses the budgeted quantity. Because that is the only variable that differs in the two computations, the $1,575 difference between the subcategory and the flexible budget must be the result of the quantity of nursing hours used per patient day. Therefore, this variance is called the *quantity* or *use variance*. It is unfavorable because we used 3.1 HPPD even though we had only expected to need to use 3.0 hours.

How did that happen? The quantity variance of $1,575 U can be explained in a number of ways. It is possible that because of the substantial increase in patient days above expectations, many part-time nurses were hired. These nurses were unfamiliar with the institution and therefore were not as efficient as the regular nurses. Another possibility is that the population was sicker than anticipated and required more care per patient day. Of course, there is also the possibility that supervision was lax and that time was simply being wasted. Variance information can only point out the direction; the manager must investigate and then make the final determination regarding why the variance occurred and how to avoid it in the future.

Next we need to compute the actual amount spent. The actual spending is based on the actual quantity of resource used per patient multiplied by the actual price paid per hour for the resource multiplied by the actual patient volume. In this case, the 3.1 actual nursing HPPD is multiplied by the actual $36 hourly rate that was paid to the nurses multiplied by the actual 450 patient days. It should not be surprising that to find the actual amount spent, we have to use the actual value for each of the variables. The computation is as follows.

Actual Cost
Actual Quantity × Actual Price × Actual Volume
3.1 × $36 × 450 = $50,220

If we compare the subcategory to the actual cost, we can compute the price variance:

Subcategory vs. Actual Cost
Actual Quantity × **Budgeted Price** × Actual Volume
− Actual Quantity × **Actual Price** × Actual Volume

$$3.1 \times \$35 \times 450 = \$48,825$$
$$- 3.1 \times \$36 \times 450 = \underline{-50,220}$$
$$\textbf{Price or Rate Variance} = \underline{\$\ 1,395\ U}$$

Notice in this computation that the actual quantity, 3.1 hours of nursing time, and the actual volume, 450 patient days, are used for both the actual cost and the subcategory. The only difference between the actual and the subcategory is that the actual uses the $36 actual nursing hourly rate, and the subcategory uses the budgeted $35 per hour nursing rate. Therefore, the $1,395 difference between the actual and the subcategory must be caused by the difference between the actual and the hourly rates. It is therefore referred to as a *rate* or *price variance*.

Why did the rate variance occur? The actual $36 hourly rate instead of the budgeted $35 rate may have occurred because of poor scheduling, resulting in unnecessary overtime. On the other hand, perhaps it resulted from a larger raise for nursing personnel than the nurse manager had been told to put into the budget by the personnel department. Then again, look at the volume variance. Whenever there is a large unfavorable volume variance, it means that the workload was much greater than expected. Such unanticipated increases in workload put a great strain on nursing time, frequently requiring overtime or the addition of high-priced agency nurses. All of these possibilities should be investigated by the nurse manager.

To use flexible budgeting, managers should have an idea of how the pieces fit together. If we were using more traditional budgeting, we would just compare the budget with the amount actually spent to find the variance for each line item. For example, for nursing labor, we would have a total unfavorable variance of $8,220:

Original Budget vs. Actual Cost
Budgeted Quantity × Budgeted Price × Budgeted Volume
− Actual Quantity × Actual Price × Actual Volume

$$3.0 \times \$35 \times 400 = \$42,000$$
$$- 3.1 \times \$36 \times 450 = \underline{-50,220}$$
$$\textbf{Total Variance} = \underline{\$\ 8,220\ U}$$

Why did this variance occur? We do not know. It has something to do with our nursing labor cost, but that is all we know from the above computation. However, using the flexible budget variance analysis approach, we have computed a volume, price, and quantity variance. These variances were:

$$\text{Volume Variance} = \$5,250\ U$$
$$\text{Quantity or Use Variance} = 1,575\ U$$
$$\text{Price or Rate Variance} = \underline{1,395\ U}$$
$$\text{Total Variance} = \underline{\$8,220\ U}$$

Notice that the total of the volume, quantity, and price variances add up to the same $8,220 that we find when we compare the actual with the budget. We are not creating new variances. We are subdividing the total $8,220 variances into its components so that the manager can more easily investigate the variances and see what is causing them. This will improve our chances of taking corrective actions to eliminate or at least reduce undesired variances in future periods.

Using the variance analysis of this chapter, it is possible to determine that of this total $8,220 variance, $5,250 was caused by the increase in patient days. It is now also known that $1,395 of the variance was caused by having paid a higher average rate to the nurses than was anticipated and that $1,575 of the variance was caused by consuming more nursing hours per patient day than had been anticipated. Why these specific variances occurred is not known, but there is a much better focus on where the problem areas are. The nurse manager can now begin the investigation with more specific direction about where the variances are arising.

A generic model for computing flexible budgeting variances is shown in Exhibit 16–1. In looking at the model in this table, several things should be kept in mind. First of all, recall that basically all the necessary data are generally readily available. Second, the

✳ EXHIBIT 16–1 *Volume, Quantity, and Price Variances*

Volume Variance:
Budgeted Quantity × Budgeted Price × **Budgeted Volume**
− Budgeted Quantity × Budgeted Price × **Actual Volume**

Quantity or Use Variance:
Budgeted Quantity × Budgeted Price × Actual Volume
− **Actual Quantity** × Budgeted Price × Actual Volume

Price or Rate Variance:
Actual Quantity × **Budgeted Price** × Actual Volume
− Actual Quantity × **Actual Price** × Actual Volume

Total Variance:
Volume Variance
+ Quantity or Use Variance
+ Price or Rate Variance
= **Total Variance**

accounting and information systems departments generally calculate variances when they do monthly variance reports and provide that variance information to nurse managers for investigation and analysis. So, generally, nurse managers do not have to compute all of these variances. Their primary managerial role is in investigation of these variances, determination of why they occurred, and then developing and implementing an action plan to prevent undesired controllable variances from occurring in the future.

It sometimes is not obvious whether a variance is favorable or unfavorable. However, you can determine this as follows: Whenever something happens that causes us to spend more than expected, that results in an unfavorable variance, and vice versa. If we spend less than expected, the result is a favorable variance. So if we have more patients than expected, it would result in an unfavorable volume variance. If we use more of a resource than expected, it would result in an unfavorable quantity variance. And if we pay a higher rate or price for our resource than expected, it would result in an unfavorable price variance. Note, however, that the words *unfavorable* and *favorable* have limited meaning. Unfavorable does not necessarily mean that this was bad for the organization, and favorable does not necessarily mean something good happened. This will be explained in the next chapter.

✳ REVENUE VARIANCES

The nurse manager's primary variance analysis effort focuses on expenses. This is predominantly because managers of HCOs have a greater degree of control over expenses than they do over revenues. However, the information that can be yielded from revenue variance analysis is also important. For example, changes in revenue that result from changes in patient volume may be outside the control of the organization and its managers. Such changes, however, may require management actions or reactions to protect the organization's financial position.

Revenue variance methodology follows the same pattern as expense methodology. A traditional variance focuses on the difference between the total revenue expected and actually achieved for a unit or department. A flexible budget methodology helps to identify the various underlying causes of variances. The total revenue variance for a unit, department, or organization can be broken down into a *volume variance*, a *mix variance*, and a *price variance*.

Consider an outpatient surgery department that has budgeted revenues of $1 million for the month just ended. Actual revenues were $850,000. Traditional variance analysis identifies a $150,000 unfavorable revenue variance ($1,000,000 − $850,000 = $150,000). What caused the $150,000 shortfall? We can get a better insight if we break down that total variance into several components.

The first step for flexible budget revenue variance analysis would be to identify the original revenue budget. The budget for revenue will depend on the number of patients, the mix of patients, and the price we expect to collect for each type of patient. Suppose that 800 patients were expected for the month. Further assume that we expected half of them to be patient type A with a price of $1,000 and half of them to be patient type B with a price of $1,500. In that case the total budgeted revenue would be $1,000,000 calculated as follows:

Original Budget
Budgeted Mix × Budgeted Volume × Budgeted Price
A: 50% × 800 × $1,000 = $ 400,000
B: 50% × 800 × $1,500 =   600,000
$1,000,000

The type A patients are expected to generate $400,000 of revenue, and the type B patients are expected to generate $600,000 of revenue. Of course, there could be many more different types of patients in a real situation, but just types A and B are sufficient to show how the variance analysis would work.

If there were actually only 750 patients, a flexible budget for revenue of $937,500 could be calculated as follows:

Flexible Budget
Budgeted Mix × Actual Volume × Budgeted Price
A: 50% × 750 × $1,000 = $ 375,000
B: 50% × 750 × $1,500 =   562,500
$ 937,500

The revenue flexible budget indicates the amount of revenue that would have been budgeted if the number of patients had been forecast exactly correctly. The difference between the original budget for 800 patients and the flexible budget for 750 actual patients is an unfavorable volume variance of $62,500, computed as follows:

Original Budget vs. Flexible Budget
Original Budget = $1,000,000
− Flexible Budget = − 937,500
Volume Variance = $ 62,500 U

The volume variance is considered to be unfavorable because the lower volume of patients would be expected to generate less revenue than expected.

The next calculation concerns the mix of patients. Not only is the total number of patients not likely to turn out to be exactly as budgeted, but the actual mix of patients will also likely vary from the budget. Suppose that it turns out that actually 60% of our patients were type A and only 40% were type B. In that case, we can compute a subcategory as follows:

Subcategory
Actual Mix × Actual Volume × Budgeted Price
A: 60% × 750 × $1,000 = $450,000
B: 40% × 750 × $1,500 = $\underline{450,000}$
$900,000

Not only are there fewer patients than expected, but the mix of patients has changed as well. Fewer than half of the patients are the more highly priced type B patients. Based on the actual number of patients and the actual mix, revenues would be expected to be $900,000. If we compare the flexible budget of $937,500 (what revenue would have been expected to be for 750 patients) to this new "subcategory" value based on the actual mix, the difference is $37,500. This is the mix variance, which is unfavorable. The variance is unfavorable because there is a greater proportion of lower-revenue patients. The mix variance can be computed as follows:

Flexible Budget vs. Subcategory
Flexible Budget = $937,500
− Subcategory   = $\underline{-900,000}$
Mix Variance = $\underline{\underline{\$37,500\ U}}$

Next we can compute a price variance. A price variance would arise if the amount we collect for each type of patient differs from our budget. We expected to collect $1,000 for each type A patient and $1,500 for each type B patient. However, suppose that because of negotiated rates with insurance companies, the average price for type B patients was only $1,333.33. In that case, actual revenue would be $850,000 calculated as follows:

Actual
Actual Mix × Actual Volume × Actual Price
A: 60% × 750 × $1,000.00 = $450,000
B: 40% × 750 × $1,333.33 = $\underline{400,000}$
$850,000

The $50,000 difference between the $900,000 from the mix calculation and the actual revenue is an unfavorable price variance. It is unfavorable because the price was less than budgeted. This price variance can be computed as follows:

Subcategory vs. Actual
Subcategory   = $900,000
− Actual   = $\underline{-850,000}$
Price Variance = $\underline{\underline{\$50,000\ U}}$

The manager is now in a better position to investigate the revenue variances. In sum, the three revenue variances are:

Volume Variance = $$$ 62,500 U
Mix Variance = 37,500 U
Price Variance = $\underline{50,000\ U}$
Total Variance = $\underline{\underline{\$150,000\ U}}$

The $150,000 total variance matches the amount that we initially calculated by computing the overall budgeted revenue of $1,000,000 with the actual revenue of $850,000. But now the manager can better focus the investigation based on knowing how much of that variance was caused by the number of patients, how much by the mix of patients, and how much by the price we collected per patient.

Often revenue variances are calculated based on the contribution margin (Price − Variable cost) rather than the price. The price we collect per patient places too great a focus on the total charge for different types of patients rather than on the profit implications of each type patient. A patient with high price could have even greater expenses and cause losses. Another patient with only a modest prices could be quite profitable. Managers do not just need information about changes in the amount we collect per patient. Rather, they need to know whether the revenue changes are in profitable or unprofitable areas. It is possible, therefore, to use the budgeted contribution margin, rather than the amount collected per patient, in all the calculations just discussed.

Knowing whether variances are caused by changes in prices, the mix of patients, or the volume of patients is important information that managers can use in taking actions to respond to increases or decreases in revenues. For example, if the number of patients is falling, steps should be taken to find out why and to make sure that there are corresponding reductions in organizational expenses. If the mix of patients is changing, it may be necessary to shift resources within the organization. If prices differed from budget, an effort must be made to understand why the variance occurred and its overall implications for the organization's finances.

❋ IMPLICATIONS FOR NURSE MANAGERS AND EXECUTIVES

Budgeting is a process of planning and controlling. If a budget is prepared but is not used to control results, a substantial part of the potential benefit of budgeting is lost. The key issue to remember, however, is that organizations do not control costs; people do. Organizations need to take steps to ensure that their employees are motivated to accomplish the organizations' objectives.

The difference between the budget and what actually occurs is called a *variance*. Comparing actual results with budgeted expectations and analyzing the resulting variances should be done monthly. This can allow for midstream corrections that will improve the year-end results. It also provides information for preparing the coming year's budget and for evaluating units, departments, and managers' performance.

Many HCOs prepare variance reports by comparing the information in the original budget with the actual results. There are several problems with that type of comparison. First, it does not tell as much about the cause of the variance as one would like to know; for instance, traditional variance analysis does not indicate whether a variance is caused by more resource use per patient or by higher prices for resources used. Second, traditional variance analysis ignores the fact that resource consumption would be expected to vary with workload volume. One can compare the budgeted cost for an expected patient volume with the actual cost for the actual patient volume. Part of the variance, therefore, will just be the result of changes in workload levels, rather than being related to efficiency.

This has caused many HCOs to start using a method called *flexible budgeting* and *flexible budget variance analysis*. Flexible budgeting establishes an after-the-fact budget (i.e., what it would have been expected to cost had the actual workload been known in advance). Using flexible budgets, it is possible to break a unit or department's line-item expense variances down into components caused by (1) changes in prices or salary rates from those expected; (2) changes in the amount of input used per unit of workload or output, such as the amount of nursing time per patient day; and (3) changes in the workload volume itself. It is also possible to divide revenue variances into the portion caused by volume, mix, or price changes.

Managerial expertise and judgment are still needed to investigate and evaluate the variances that are determined by using flexible budget variance analysis. Ultimately, this technique can make the manager's job easier by segregating the variance into its component parts. This allows the manager to spend more time understanding and explaining why the variance occurred. However, input from the nursing manager or executive is essential in trying to understand the ultimate causes of variances.

✳ KEY CONCEPTS

Management control system A complete set of policies and procedures that an organization uses to make sure that it achieves its plans to the greatest extent possible.

Responsibility accounting System of assigning responsibility for keeping to the organization's plan and carrying out the elements of the management control system. Responsibility is generally assigned to managers of cost centers.

Motivation The role of motivation of staff and managers in controlling operating results cannot be overemphasized. If people are not motivated to carry out the budget, it is not likely to be achieved. A variety of incentives, such as bonuses, can be used to help motivate staff and managers. If targets are set unrealistically high, the negative motivational implications are likely to offset any hoped-for benefits.

Communication Both the budget and actual results compared with the budget must be communicated throughout the organization. This is an essential element of control and should be an ongoing process.

Responsibility should equal control If managers are held responsible for things they have no control over, the organization will reward and punish the wrong individuals. The result will invariably be demoralization of managers and staff.

Interim evaluations These are of particular importance in controlling operational results. Each month, there should be comparisons between what was expected and what has been accomplished.

Variance analysis Aspect of budgeting in which actual results are compared with budgeted expectations. Variances are used to improve future planning, allow for corrective actions to better control results in coming periods, and evaluate the performance of units or departments and their managers.

Traditional variance analysis Compares the budget with actual results for the most recent month and year-to-date for each line item in each cost center.

Flexible or variable budgeting Takes into consideration the fact that the actual output level often differs from expectations.

Flexible budget variance analysis Expands upon traditional variance analysis by dividing the total variance into price, quantity, and volume variances.

Price or rate variance Part of the total difference between the budget and actual amount spent or revenue earned that results from a higher or lower hourly rate or price than budgeted.

Quantity or use variance Part of the total difference between the budget and actual amount spent that results from the use of more or less resources per patient than budgeted.

Volume variance Part of the total difference between the budget and actual amount spent or revenue earned that results from a different volume of patients than budgeted.

Revenue variances Can be calculated using either prices or contribution margin to identify volume, mix, and price variances.

✳ SUGGESTED READINGS

Cavouras C, McKinley J: Variable budgeting for staffing analysis and evaluation, *Nurs Manage* 28(5):34–36, 39, 1997.

Dunham-Taylor J, Pinczuk J: *Health care financial management for nurse managers,* ed 2, Sudbury, Mass, 2010, Jones & Bartlett.

Felteau A: Budget variance analysis and justification, *Nurs Manage* 23(2):40–41, 1992.

Finkler S, McHugh M: *Budgeting concepts for nurse managers,* ed 4, St. Louis, 2008, Saunders.

Finkler S, Ward D, Baker J: *Essentials of cost accounting for health care organizations,* ed 3, Sudbury, Mass, 2007, Jones & Bartlett Publishers.

Horngren C, Datar S, Rajan M: *Cost accounting: a managerial emphasis*, ed 14, Englewood Cliffs, New Jersey, 2011, Prentice-Hall.

Maitland D: Flexible budgeting and variance analysis: why leave staff nurses in the dark? *Hosp Cost Manag Account* 5(9):1-8, 1993.

Swansburg R: *Budgeting and financial management for nurse managers,* Boston, 1997, Jones & Bartlett.

Wilburn D: Budget response to volume variability, *Nurs Manage* 23(2):42–45, 1992.

Variance Analysis: Examples, Extensions, and Caveats

CHAPTER GOALS

The goals of this chapter are to:

- Provide additional variance analysis examples
- Provide insight into the problems encountered when variance information is aggregated
- Introduce the concept of exception reports and explain their benefits
- Explore further the interpretation of variances
- Explain how flexible budgeting can be used even if staffing patterns are rigid

- Provide a tool for determining the variance caused by changes in patient acuity
- Discuss causes of variances
- Discuss when a variance is large enough to warrant managerial attention and investigation
- Discuss variance analysis as related to performance budgeting

✻ INTRODUCTION

Chapter 16 presented the basic mechanics of flexible budgeting. This chapter provides several exercises to help readers become more familiar with the notation and process of flexible budget variance analysis. Flexible budgets differ from original budgets because some costs are variable. Those costs should be expected to change as workload levels change. Therefore, one may have questions regarding how to integrate flexible budgets with fairly rigid staffing patterns. Integration of acuity measures into flexible budgeting will be of interest to many as well. These extensions are discussed in this chapter. Finally, issues concerning fixed versus variable costs, the causes of variances, variance investigation and control, and variance analysis of performance budgets are addressed in the last part of this chapter.

✻ AGGREGATION PROBLEMS

The Nearby Hospital had the following results for labor costs for the past month:

Salary	Actual	Original Budget	Variance
All departments	$518,800	$519,000	$200 F

Should the hospital administrator investigate this variance? Is more information about the variance required? Your immediate

reaction is probably to leave well enough alone. The total amount of the variance is small—and favorable at that. Why worry about a $200 variance?

The problem with these results is that when variances are combined, there is a tendency to lose information. There could be large favorable (F) and unfavorable (U) variances that offset each other. The net result may be small, and the two large variances cannot be observed. For example, assume that the departmental breakdown of the $200 variance was as follows:

Salary	Actual	Original Budget	Variance
Operating Room	$150,000	$125,000	$25,000 U
Dietary	100,000	125,000	25,000 F
Nursing	144,000	144,000	0
Lab	124,800	125,000	200 F
Totals	$518,800	$519,000	$ 200 F

Given this extra information, it becomes apparent that it would be a mistake not to investigate further. In this case, which departments need to be investigated? It is fairly obvious that one should be especially concerned with the operating room. And even though the dietary variance is favorable, it would probably be wise to find out what is happening in that department as well.

However, focus attention on the nursing department even though there is no variance. Suppose that the following information for the nursing department is available[1]:

- Budgeted number of patient days: 1,500
- Actual number of patient days: 1,250
- Budgeted nursing hours per patient day (HPPD): 3.0
- Actual nursing HPPD: 3.6
- Budgeted average nursing pay rate per hour: $32
- Actual average nursing pay rate per hour: $32

It would appear that everything is fine because there is no variance. However, let's calculate the volume, quantity, and price variances anyway.

To calculate a volume variance, we need to know the original and flexible budgets. The original budget is the budgeted quantity of resource per unit of workload (in this case, per patient day) multiplied by the budgeted price of the resource (in this case, the nursing labor hourly rate) multiplied by the budgeted volume (in this case, the number of patient days). Information about all of these variables is available, so we can derive the original budget:

Original Budget
Budgeted Quantity × Budgeted Price × Budgeted Volume
3.0 × $32 × 1,500 = $144,000

Next we need the flexible budget (i.e., the amount that would have been budgeted if the actual workload level had been predicted accurately). The flexible budget is the budgeted quantity of resource per unit of workload (in this case, per patient day) multiplied by the budgeted price per unit of the resource (in this case, the nursing labor hourly rate) multiplied by the actual volume (in this case, the number of patient days). The flexible budget can be calculated as follows:

Flexible Budget
Budgeted Quantity × Budgeted Price × Actual Volume
3.0 × $32 × 1,250 = $120,000

Using the original and flexible budgets, we can calculate the volume variance:

Original Budget vs. Flexible Budget
Budgeted Quantity × Budgeted Price × **Budgeted Volume**
−Budgeted Quantity × Budgeted Price × **Actual Volume**

$$3.0 \times \$32 \times \mathbf{1,500} = \$\ 144,000$$
$$-3.0 \times \$32 \times \mathbf{1,250} = -120,000$$
$$\text{Volume Variance} = \$\ \underline{24,000}\ F$$

The volume variance is a favorable $24,000. Given the $0 variance for nursing that we saw earlier, this is a dramatic turn of events. This favorable volume variance means that the workload

was down substantially. If it is assumed that nursing staff costs are variable (this assumption will be relaxed later in the chapter), then a volume variance should be accompanied by reduced spending. For most hospitals, a reduction in patient days from the expected level would often be an *unfavorable* event. It probably means that admissions and revenues are down substantially. It is called a *favorable* variance because treating fewer patients implies that less money would be spent. However, that does not mean that something *good* has happened. It is important for managers and executives to be aware of favorable volume variances as early as possible so that adjustments can be made to staffing if necessary.

To calculate quantity and price variances, it is necessary to be able to calculate the subcategory value. This requires multiplying the actual quantity of resource per unit of workload by the budgeted price by the actual volume of patients. The subcategory can be calculated as follows:

Subcategory
Actual Quantity × Budgeted Price × Actual Volume
3.6 × $32 × 1,250 = $144,000

The flexible budget can be compared with the subcategory to generate the quantity variance as follows:

Flexible Budget vs. Subcategory
Budgeted Quantity × Budgeted Price × Actual Volume
−**Actual Quantity** × Budgeted Price × Actual Volume

$$3.0 \times \$32 \times 1,250 = \$\ 120,000$$
$$-3.6 \times \$32 \times 1,250 = -144,000$$
$$\text{Quantity or Use Variance} = \$\ \underline{24,000}\ U$$

This variance is unfavorable. Although we do not know what caused this variance, it is quite possible that the reduced patient load was not accompanied by reduced staffing. If staffing was kept virtually the same, the amount of nursing time available per patient day would rise, and an unfavorable quantity variance would occur. This means that workload and possibly revenue are falling but that costs are not decreasing. This would mean financial losses would occur.

If we compare the subcategory value to the actual spending, we can determine the price variance. The actual spending was:

Actual Cost
Actual Quantity × Actual Price × Actual Volume
3.6 × $32 × 1,250 = $144,000

Comparing the subcategory to this actual, we find:

Subcategory vs. Actual Cost
Actual Quantity × **Budgeted Price** × Actual Volume
−Actual Quantity × **Actual Price** × Actual Volume

$$3.6 \times \mathbf{\$32} \times 1,250 = \$\ 144,000$$
$$-3.6 \times \mathbf{\$32} \times 1,250 = -144,000$$
$$\text{Price or Rate Variance} = \$\ \underline{\quad 0\quad}$$

As you can see, there was no rate variance. So it turns out that there was a $24,000 favorable volume variance and an offsetting $24,000 unfavorable quantity variance. Although we do not

---

[1] Recall from Chapter 16 that to calculate volume, quantity, and price variances, we need the following pieces of information:
- Budgeted number of patients, procedures, or other units of service
- Actual number of patients, procedures, or other units of service
- Budgeted resources needed per patient, procedure, or other unit of service
- Actual resources used per patient, procedure, or other unit of service
- Budgeted price per unit of resource needed
- Actual price per unit of resource used

know for sure, the most likely problem is that as patient volume decreases, the nursing unit did not appropriately respond by reducing nurse staffing. Although the overall variance looked like there was no problem, this was quite deceiving. Ultimately, the revenue decline from the reduced patient volume would have a dramatic negative impact on the organization because it did not find a way to reduce spending.

The point of this example is to get a good understanding of how problems may get buried when variances are aggregated and evaluated in total. When the overall variance for the hospital is examined, the offsetting variances in the operating room and dietary departments are not apparent. Variance information for each department separately is needed. The manager would certainly want to investigate the large unfavorable variance in the operating room, and even though it is favorable, determine what caused the large favorable variance in the dietary department as well.

However, even looking at each department's variance would not reveal the problem within the nursing department. It is possible that different units in the nursing department might have variances that would offset each other. So it is really necessary to look at variances for each unit. And then, within an individual nursing unit, it is possible that an unfavorable salary variance could be offset by a favorable supply variance. Managers must look at each line item of each unit.

In this example, falling patient volume was offset by a quantity variance. A manager who simply examined the line-item variance for nursing salaries in a particular nursing unit would not be aware of that problem. Only by using flexible budget variance analysis to generate volume, quantity, and price variances for each line item can the manager get more information about what is going on within a line item. After managers have such information, they can investigate the variances. In this example, the flexible budget variance might have been the result of a failure to reduce staffing as workload decreased. But it might have been the result of a change in patient mix or some other issue causing the paid staff HPPD to rise. The expertise of the manager is needed to make the final determination. However, the ability of managers to use their knowledge and expertise is substantially enhanced if price, quantity, and volume variances are calculated for each line item for each unit.

✳ EXCEPTION REPORTING

Aggregation problems create substantial difficulty. The only way to be sure that one variance is not being offset by another variance is by examining every single price, quantity, and volume variance of every single line item of every single unit of every single department of the organization. This creates a potentially unmanageable burden. Should the chief executive officer (CEO) of the organization examine every individual variance for the entire organization? Should the chief nurse executive (CNE) have to examine every individual variance for all units of the nursing department? The time required would be enormous. A solution to this problem is the use of *exception reports*.

Assuming a computer prepares all the variances for each cost element, it is a simple process to have the computer prepare a list for the CEO of only those individual variances throughout the entire organization that exceed a certain limit. This is called an *exception report*. It only lists the variances that are large. How large depends on the desires of the individual CEO. When tight, centralized control is desired, smaller variances are of interest. For example, although some CEOs might be interested only in monthly or year-to-date variances that are greater than 25% of the budget or $50,000, a CEO running a more centralized operation might be interested in variances greater than 20% or $20,000.

This does not mean that variances less than $20,000 go unnoticed. The CNE would get a report for Nursing at a more detailed level, perhaps 15% or $10,000. Continuing the process, mid-level nurse managers would receive detailed exception reports for the variances in units under their supervision. These might indicate all variances greater than 10% or $5,000. Ultimately, the unit nurse manager would want to review all variances for that unit. In all cases, if a nurse manager feels that a particular variance indicates a problem that is likely to grow worse in future months, the higher levels of nursing administration should be alerted to the problem, rather than waiting until the variance is great enough to appear on the mid-level nurse manager's or CNE's exception reports.

✳ INTERPRETATION OF VARIANCES

Assume that you are the nursing administrator for a medical group practice. This may be either a fee-for-service organization or a prepaid-group practice. Suppose that the organization is expecting a severe outbreak of the Hoboken flu this winter, so it has hired extra agency nurses to treat the patients and administer flu shots. The budgeted expectation was that 1,000 hours of part-time services would be needed at $40.00 per hour for a total cost of $40,000. It was also expected that the part-time nurses would average a half hour for each of 2,000 patients. The results at the end of the flu season were as follows:

Salary	Actual	Original Budget	Variance
Part-time nurses	$50,000	$40,000	$10,000

Would this be considered a favorable or an unfavorable variance? On the surface, more was spent than was expected; therefore, it would be recorded as an unfavorable variance from an accounting viewpoint. The physician director of the medical group may well be complaining about the total lack of budget control exhibited by the unexpected $10,000 excess cost. At this stage, however, there is more to the variance than simply what was expected to be spent and what was actually spent.

Consider how much work was done for the $50,000 actually spent. Suppose that 2,600 patients were actually treated by the part-time nurses, who worked a total of 1,200 hours. What are the variances that can be calculated from this information? The original budget was $40,000, and the actual cost was $50,000. The number of patients actually treated was 2,600; the budgeted time per patient was one-half hour; and the budgeted hourly rate was $40.00. Therefore, the flexible budget would be $52,000 ($\frac{1}{2} \times \$40 \times 2,600$). If we compare the original budget of $40,000 to the flexible budget of $52,000, we have a $12,000 unfavorable volume variance ($40,000 − $52,000 = $12,000 U).

The subcategory would compare the actual quantity of hours to treat each patient, at the budgeted hourly rate of $40, for the actual number of patients. The actual time taken to treat the actual number of patients has been given as 1,200 hours. For 2,600 actual patients to be treated in 1,200 hours, an average of 0.46154 hours must have been used per patient (1,200 hours ÷ 2,600 patients = 0.46154 hours per patient). Therefore, the subcategory is $48,000 (0.46154 hours per patient × $40 per hour × 2,600 patients). If we compare the flexible budget of $52,000 with the subcategory value of $48,000, we get a $4,000 favorable quantity variance ($52,000 − $48,000 = $4,000 F).

The actual costs were given as being $50,000. If we compare the subcategory value of $48,000 with the actual costs of $50,000, we get a $2,000 unfavorable price variance ($48,000 - $50,000 = $2,000 U).

Let's discuss the volume variance first because it is the largest. That variance is attributable to the fact that there were 2,600 patients instead of the expected 2,000 patients. Is this result good or bad for the organization? What is the likely effect of these extra patients on revenues? If the medical group practice is a *prepaid-group plan,* such as a health maintenance organization (HMO) or other managed care organization (MCO), the volume variance is bad news. It means that the number of patients treated has gone up substantially without any increase in revenue. On the other hand, if it is a *fee-for-service* organization, the extra cost will be associated with increased billings. The number of patients treated is 30% greater than expected, and so is the revenue. Therefore, even if the actual costs were $12,000 more than the budgeted $40,000 (i.e., the unfavorable volume variance of $12,000), the organization would still be better off because of the increased revenues. In any case, a clear argument can be made that the portion of the unfavorable variance caused by increased patient flow is beyond the control and therefore beyond the responsibility of the nurse administrator.

What about the two remaining variances—the $2,000 unfavorable price or rate variance and the $4,000 favorable quantity variance? Certainly, one can come up with several possible scenarios. For instance, because more part-time hours were needed than had been expected, some experienced RNs were hired rather than just new graduates (i.e., there were not enough new graduates available to fill the need). The experienced registered nurses (RNs), however, were so skillful that their higher wage rate (resulting in the unfavorable rate variance) was more than offset by the speedy efficiency with which they worked (resulting in the favorable quantity variance). If this was in fact the case, the organization should learn for the future that it may be more cost-effective to use experienced RNs.

An alternative scenario would be that the rate variance was simply the result of overtime wages. When the patients started coming, there was not enough time to hire anyone else, so the organization just worked the agency nurses it had for longer hours, resulting in an overtime premium. However, the rate variance resulting from the overtime premium was more than offset by the fact that there were so many patients that the nurses never had idle time. Because some idle time had been built into the budget, the favorable quantity variance resulted.

This can also tell something about the future. Perhaps the nurses were thrilled that they did not have to sit around bored. In this case, next time fewer nurses should be hired, and they should be kept relatively busy. On the other hand, a possible implication of a favorable quantity variance is a reduced level of quality of care, with each patient receiving less time and attention. Reduced quality of care will normally show up as a favorable quantity variance. If quality of care suffered, one would want to avoid that situation in the future. Another possibility is that the nurses worked hard and fast (the patients were lined up right out into the hall, so it was continuous work), but they are so mad at being overworked that they will never work for the organization again. A "favorable" quantity variance does not always mean favorable things for the organization.

Nothing can be concluded for certain about the rate and quantity variances for the medical group practice because the reader was not actually there and knows little about the organization. A really useful variance report can be developed only by someone with knowledge of the specific situation. The value of flexible budgeting, however, should be reasonably clear. The methodology does help to separate out the elements that are totally beyond the unit or manager's control, such as the number of patients. It is then possible to see clearly the magnitude of the rate and quantity variances. If they are substantial, the manager can turn attention to finding out why they occurred. This information is needed for two reasons: (1) so the organization can be managed more efficiently in the future and (2) so the manager can reasonably defend the way the department or unit was run.

❋ **EXHIBIT 17-1** *Hoboken Flu Example Variances*

Original Budget
Budgeted Quantity × Budgeted Price × Budgeted Volume: .5 hour × $40 × 2,000 patients   = $40,000

Flexible Budget
Budgeted Quantity × Budgeted Price × Actual Volume: .5 hour × $40 × 2,600 patients   = $52,000

Subcategory
Actual Quantity × Budgeted Price × Actual Volume: 1,200/2,600 hour × $40 × 2,600 patients = $48,000

Actual Cost
Actual Quantity × Actual Price × Actual Volume: 1,200/2,600 hour × $41.667 × 2,600 patients = $50,000

Continued

✳ **EXHIBIT 17-1** *Hoboken Flu Example Variances—cont'd*

Original Budget vs. Flexible Budget

Budgeted Quantity × Budgeted Price × Budgeted Volume: .5 × $40 × 2,000	= $ 40,000
− Budgeted Quantity × Budgeted Price × Actual Volume: −.5 × $40 × 2,600	= −52,000
Volume Variance	= $ 12,000U

Flexible Budget vs. Subcategory

Budgeted Quantity × Budgeted Price × Actual Volume: .5 × $40 × 2,600	= $ 52,000
− Actual Quantity × Budgeted Price × Actual Volume: −.461 × $40 × 2,600	= −48,000
Quantity or Use Variance	= $ 4,000F

Subcategory vs. Actual Cost

Actual Quantity × Budgeted Price × Actual Volume: .461 × $40 × 2,600	= $ 48,000
− Actual Quantity × Actual Price × Actual Volume: −.461 × $41.67 × 2,600	= −50,000
Price or Rate Variance	= $ 2,000U
Total Variance	$ 10,000U

✳ RIGID STAFFING PATTERNS

The medical group practice example presents an extreme in that nurses were hired by the hour. Flexible budgeting makes the assumption that if one more patient is treated, it is possible to consume just one more tongue depressor, one-quarter roll more of bandage tape, or one-half hour more of nursing time. This may be true in the case of tongue depressors and bandage tape, but it implies a lot more flexibility of nurse staffing than most organizations have.

Health care organizations often have some flexibility to transfer nurses from one shift to another or from a unit with a temporarily low occupancy to one with a higher occupancy. In some cases, however, such flexibility may be limited. This is particularly the case at unionized organizations with strong work rules, or in small practices or clinics with few staff and limited resources to hire agency staff. The key to flexible budgeting is that if the workload (e.g., patient days) increases or decreases, costs should increase or decrease as well. But nursing costs cannot be reduced if patient days are just one or two fewer than expected. Nurse staffing tends to be variable only if there are more substantial workload changes.

Suppose that a department has rigid work rules. No nurses can be shifted into or out of the department. Either new nurses are hired or nurses are let go if the patient volume changes significantly. Obviously, for small changes in workload, a manager will not change staffing levels. However, flexible budget variance analysis can still be used.

For simplicity's sake, this example considers variances for an entire year, using annual full-time equivalents (FTEs) and annual salaries. In practice, the nurse manager would want to find the variances on a monthly basis. Suppose that the staffing pattern in this department is as follows:

Staffing Guide

FTEs (RNs)	Patient Days
4	0– 6,000
5	6,001– 7,000
6	7,001– 8,000
7	8,001– 9,000
8	9,001–10,000

Further, assume the same for the year just past:

	Actual	Original Budget	Variance
Nurses salaries	$481,000	$560,000	$79,000 F

Also assume for this same year that:

Expected patient days	= 10,000
Expected salary per FTE	= $70,000
Actual patient days	= 7,750
Actual salary	= $74,000
Actual FTEs	= 6.5

Although the variance is listed as $79,000 favorable, one can readily see from the Staffing Guide that for the actual workload of 7,750 patient days, staffing should have been 6 FTEs, but we paid for 6.5 FTEs. The so-called favorable variance may largely stem from a volume variance, and there may be underlying price and quantity variances that would warrant investigation.

With a rigid staffing guide, there is no need to find both the quantity of resource used per patient and the number of patients and then multiply them to find the total amount of resources budgeted. The staffing guide can be used to simplify this process.

The original budget is concerned solely with budgeted amounts. At a volume of 10,000 patient days, the staffing guide calls for 8 FTEs. If that number is multiplied by the $70,000 budgeted price per FTE, the result is the original budgeted $560,000. That is, with a rigid staffing pattern, we can calculate the original budget as:

Original Budget
Budgeted Price per FTE × Budgeted Total Number of FTEs
$70,000 × 8 = $560,000

The actual results are based on the actual quantity amounts. In this example, the actual total quantity of nursing consumed is 6.5 FTEs. If that is multiplied by the actual $74,000 price per FTE, the result is the actual $481,000 that was spent, as follows:

Actual Cost
Actual Price per FTE × Actual Total Number of FTEs
$74,000 × 6.5 = $481,000

Comparing the original budget with the actual cost, we find that the total variance is $79,000 favorable, as follows:

Original Budget vs. Actual Cost
Budgeted Price per FTE × Budgeted Total Number of FTEs
−Actual Price per FTE × Actual Total Number of FTEs

$70,000 × 8 = $560,000
−$74,000 × 6.5 = −481,000
Total Variance = $ 79,000 F

The flexible budget is what would have been budgeted had the actual workload level been known. In this case, patient days were actually 7,750. According to the staffing guide, 6 FTEs should have been used for that number of patient days. The flexible budget is the 6 FTEs that we would have expected to consume for 7,750 patient days multiplied by the budgeted pay rate of $70,000. That comes out to be $420,000, as follows:

Flexible Budget
Budgeted Price per FTE × Budgeted Total Number of FTEs for Actual Patient Volume
$70,000 × 6 = $420,000

If we compare the original budget of $560,000 with the flexible budget of $420,000, we get a $140,000 favorable volume variance, as follows:

Original Budget vs. Flexible Budget
Budgeted Price per FTE × Budgeted Total Number of FTEs
−Budgeted Price per FTE × Budgeted Total Number of FTEs for Actual Patient Volume

$70,000 × 8 = $ 560,000
−$70,000 × 6 = −420,000
Volume Variance = $ 140,000 F

Although that is a large favorable variance, we have to realize that such a large decrease in patient volume may well be bad for the organization.

To calculate the quantity and rate variances, we will need a subcategory. This will consist of the budgeted price for each FTE multiplied by the actual number of FTEs. That is, if we take the $70,000 budgeted price multiplied by the 6.5 actual FTEs, we find the subcategory of $455,000 as follows:

Subcategory
Budgeted Price per FTE × Actual Number of FTEs
$70,000 × 6.5 = $455,000

If we compare the flexible budget with the subcategory, we can calculate our quantity variance as follows:

Flexible Budget vs. Subcategory
Budgeted Price per FTE × Budgeted Total Number of FTEs for Actual Patient Volume
−Budgeted Price per FTE × Actual Number of FTEs

$70,000 × 6 = $ 420,000
−$70,000 × 6.5 = −455,000
Quantity Variance = $ 35,000 U

What caused this $35,000 unfavorable quantity variance? Staff RNs are budgeted at $70,000 per FTE per year. Because we used 6.5 FTEs for a number of patients that our staffing guide indicates would require 6 FTEs, we should not be surprised to see that the extra half FTE we used caused us to incur an extra cost of $35,000, or half of the cost of a full FTE.

Comparing the subcategory value with the actual cost will give us the information to calculate the rate or price variance. We can see that as follows:

Subcategory vs. Actual Cost
Budgeted Price per FTE × Actual Number of FTEs
−Actual Price per FTE × Actual Total Number of FTEs

$70,000 × 6.5 = $ 455,000
−$74,000 × 6.5 = −481,000
Rate Variance = $ 26,000 U

We can see that the higher FTE average cost of $74,000 versus the budgeted $70,000 rate has resulted in an unfavorable price variance of $26,000.

The largest variance is the volume variance. This is a favorable variance only in the sense that the unit expected to need 8 FTEs for 10,000 patient days. In fact, the unit should have needed only 6 FTEs for 7,750 patient days. If the manager had reacted immediately, $140,000 less would have been spent. The way accounting records variances, spending less results in a favorable variance even if the workload decline is bad for the organization.

Now the results can be evaluated in the same way as if nurses could be moved around by the hour, but one must be cognizant of the implications of the staffing pattern. The volume variance is not of much interest if it is outside the manager's control. This may not always be the case. There are situations in which poor management can keep beds empty when there are patients waiting to fill them. In such cases, the volume variance may be at least partly a nursing responsibility.

The quantity variance is of some concern. Did the nurse manager of this unit do a good or bad job in controlling staffing costs? Despite the large unfavorable variance, there is strong reason to believe that the manager did a reasonably good job. To come down from the budgeted 8 FTEs to the appropriate staffing level of 6 FTEs, a full 25% of the unit's staffing had to be either laid off or permanently reassigned elsewhere. Given the high costs associated with attracting, training, and retaining qualified nurses, a manager must be reluctant to let a nurse go unless there is evidence that a downturn in patient days is not merely a passing aberration but rather a permanent trend. Finishing the year with additional consumption of only 0.5 FTE would appear to indicate that the manager sized up the situation well and acted reasonably quickly.

What about the rate variance? Certainly, if it is the result of overtime or unexpected shift-differential increases, that might indicate poor scheduling control in light of the decrease in patient days. A much more plausible explanation is that the two nurses who were released had the least seniority and the lowest pay rate. The six nurses who were retained are likely to have been earning a higher rate. This would raise the average rate thereby causing the price variance.

Thus, even when staffing patterns are relatively rigid, managers and executives can still benefit from flexible budget variance analysis.

❋ CAUSES OF VARIANCES

Throughout the last several chapters, there have been numerous examples of variances and suppositions as to what might have caused them. It is important to be aware that variance analysis is only a tool to point toward the right direction. The nurse manager or executive must make the investigation and final determination of what caused a variance to arise and what, if anything, should be done about it.

Common internal causes of variances include shifts in quality of care provided, changes in technology being used, changes in the efficiency of the nurses, changes in organization policy, or simply incorrect standards. Variance analysis can highlight a quantity variance, but it cannot indicate whether quality of care is improving or if poor communication is causing bottlenecks in the flow of patients through the system. Both might show up as an unfavorable quantity variance. Poor staff scheduling may be resulting in undue overtime, or pay raises may have increased labor costs. Both would show up as an unfavorable rate variance.

External causes of variances commonly include price changes for supplies, volume changes in workload, and unexpected shifts in the availability of staff. Flexible budgeting is somewhat more helpful in these cases than with the internally caused variances. Shifts in workload can be isolated in the volume variance. Going over budget on supplies can be isolated in the price variance if the problem is in the purchasing department, as opposed to lax nursing control over the quantity of supplies used.

In any event, flexible budget variance analysis can greatly ease the problem of determining the cause of a department's overall variance. It can even simplify the problem of determining the cause of the variance in any one specific line item. However, the final responsibility for determining the cause of the variance and actions to address the variance ultimately rests on the shoulders of nurse managers and executives.

❋ INVESTIGATION AND CONTROL OF VARIANCES

Probably the most difficult aspect of variance analysis is determining when a variance is large enough to warrant investigation. As has been shown in this chapter, even a small variance can be hiding significant problems when variances are aggregated. But suppose that variances have not been aggregated and information is available on each individual price, quantity, and volume variance for each cost element. Should a manager investigate $5, $50, $100, or $1,000 variances? How big a variance is too big to tolerate without investigation?

It must be kept in mind that budgets are "guesstimates" of the future. They cannot be expected to come out exactly on target. Generally, small variances are assumed to be the result of uncontrollable, random events. A manager would not spend much time investigating a $40 variance. Only variances that are either large in dollar amount or as a percentage of the budgeted amount are investigated. Determination of whether an amount is large enough to warrant investigation requires both skill and judgment, and no easy rules of thumb exist.

One solution favored by the authors is as follows: When a manager looks at a variance, it should be assumed that it will occur in the same amount month after month until the end of the year. For instance, suppose that a $500 unfavorable variance was found for January for nursing assistants' salaries. If that variance occurred every month, it would total $6,000 for the year. If $6,000 is an unreasonably high variance, the $500 January variance should be investigated as soon as possible.

Suppose that the January variance was only $100 and that $1,200 is a variance that would be acceptable for the year. No immediate investigation would likely take place. In February, the variance might be $200, but perhaps the unit can live with a $2,400 variance as well. If the variance is $300 in March, the manager must be concerned even if $3,600 would be an acceptable level. The monthly increase in the variance indicates a growing problem. At this point, the manager would probably investigate the variance to make sure that it does not continue to grow even further out of control.

Some organizations use *control charts* to determine when investigation of variances is needed.[2] Control charts plot actual results over time against the budget, with limits above and below the budgeted amount. If the limits are exceeded, the variance must be investigated. For example, Figure 17–1 presents an example of a control chart for variance analysis, showing annual nurse staffing costs by month. The chart shows both budgeted and actual costs for each month.

The key to a control chart is that a determination is made of how far actual costs can vary from the budget before we are concerned and believe investigation is necessary. In this chart, we have used plus or minus 15%, but that range is up to the manager and organization. Statistical measures such as standard deviations can be used to determine the limits, or they can be simple dollar or percent amounts. The upper and lower limits are plotted on the chart. Each month, nurse managers and executives review the charts to see if spending has gone beyond the limits. In the months that actual results are either above the upper limit or below the lower limit, that indicates to the nurse manager that the variation is great enough to require investigation.

In Figure 17–1, we see that in May, actual spending dipped slightly below the lower limit. Even though spending was less

---

[2]Readers of this book may also be familiar with the use of control charts to examine outcomes on a monthly or quarterly basis for quality improvement purposes. Although we use control charts to examine actual expenditures against budget expectations, the principles are the same.

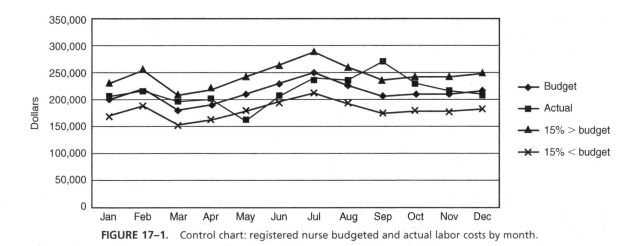

FIGURE 17–1. Control chart: registered nurse budgeted and actual labor costs by month.

than budgeted, this should still be investigated. If spending is so far from budget because there is something wrong, we need to know about it. If there is nothing wrong, then we want to understand the variance so we can learn how to duplicate that lower spending. From May to September, spending steadily increased and in September it exceeded the upper limit and required investigation. Often, only the person who has supervised a department has enough actual knowledge of that department to effectively determine why it spent more or less than expected. As a result, finance officers often generate variance reports, but each nurse manager or executive would need to prepare an analysis of why variances occurred in their department. The key to controlling variances is to be timely, to correct behavior if necessary, and to use the information from variances to correct rates promptly. If variances are not investigated promptly after each month's variance report is received, then the budget will only serve as a planning tool and not a tool that helps the organization control its operations. Information about last month's performance should be used to improve the performance for the remaining months of the year.

Such improvement will likely depend on taking actions to correct behavior when necessary. This may mean meeting to discuss areas of waste, tightening rules on communication flows, the personal use of supplies, and so forth. For the most part, the key to improvement is simply a heightened awareness of the budget throughout the year. Everyone is enthusiastic about meeting the budget for the first month or two, but then they gradually slip back into old, sometimes wasteful, habits. By bringing budget variances to the attention of relevant employees whenever the variances start to get out of line, the manager can reinforce the beneficial motivating aspects of the budget that were prominent right after the budget was adopted. If necessary, more forceful means should be used to modify behavior when budget variances are the result of employees not doing their jobs properly.

Finally, in some cases, it will be found that the variances are simply out of the unit's or the manager's control. A shortage of a key raw material may drive up the price of supplies. If there appears to be a protracted change that is outside the control of the manager and that will result in continuing unfavorable

variances, it is important to bring this to the attention of the organization's rate-setting personnel. The sooner this is known and the rates are corrected upward, the better it is for the financial stability of the organization.

✳ PERFORMANCE BUDGETS AND VARIANCE ANALYSIS

Performance budgeting was the topic of Chapter 15. In a sense, most of this chapter on variance analysis revolves around performance budgeting. Flexible budgets are an attempt to match actual costs incurred with the costs that should have been incurred based on the actual workload. By looking at the actual workload rather than the original budgeted expectations, variances are being calculated with at least some measure of performance being taken into account. However, in developing performance budgets, Chapter 15 went beyond the flexible budget. Performance budgets were established based on a variety of key performance areas.

In the example in Chapter 15, it was suggested that a percentage of the cost of each line item could be allocated to each key performance area. For example, 15% of the nurse manager's time might be devoted to quality improvement (see Table 15–1). Based on these percentage allocations, a cost could be budgeted for each key performance area. For example, $56,000 might be budgeted for quality improvement (see Table 15–2). A budgeted cost could then be determined for each unit of output in each key performance area. For example, the budgeted cost might be $5,600 per 1% drop in the rate of Stage III and IV pressure ulcers (see Table 15–3). How can these performance budget calculations be compared with actual results and variances between budget and actual determined?

The first step is to assess how much output was actually accomplished in each key performance area. In establishing the performance budget, output measures that are quantifiable are chosen. For example, at the end of the month or year, the percent reduction in pressure ulcers can be determined and compared with the budgeted reduction. Similar measures are used for the other key performance areas. For example, the number of patient complaints can be compared with the budgeted number of complaints; the nurse turnover rate can be compared with the budgeted turnover rate. Thus, getting a variance in terms of volume of output achieved is readily possible.

The next step would be to compare the actual cost per unit of work accomplished with the budgeted cost. For instance, suppose $56,000 was budgeted for reducing pressure ulcers, with a budgeted goal of a 10% reduction in the rate of Stage III and IV pressure ulcers (a budgeted cost of $5,600 per 1% drop in the failure rate). Suppose that the actual results were that the failure rate fell by 12%. If the total actual cost for this quality improvement is divided by 12, the actual cost per 1% drop can be determined and compared with the budgeted cost of $5,600.

Unfortunately, it is difficult to calculate the actual amount that was spent on quality improvement. This amount consists of a percentage of the cost of each line item. The actual costs for each line item will be known. This cost information is used in the traditional and flexible budget variance analyses discussed earlier. However, there is no ready mechanism for determining the exact percentage of each line item that was actually devoted to each key performance area.

Consider the following information, abstracted from the tables in Chapter 15. It includes the budgeted percent effort (just for the quality improvement key performance area) for each line item (see Table 15–1), the budgeted cost for each line item, and the budgeted cost for quality improvement (see Table 15–2). A total of $56,000 was included in the performance budget for quality improvement.

Line Item	Line Item Total Cost	Percent Effort Devoted to Quality Improvement		Cost Budgeted for Quality Improvement
Nurse Manager	$ 80,000	×	15%	= $12,000
Staff	800,000	×	5	= 40,000
Education	20,000	×	20	= 4,000
Supplies	40,000	×	0	= 0
Overhead	60,000	×	0	= 0
Total				$56,000
Divided by budgeted outcome (% reduction in Stage III and IV pressure ulcers)				÷10
Budgeted cost per percent reduction in failures				$ 5,600

In the example, the nurse manager was budgeted to devote 15% of her total effort to quality improvement. Did she in fact devote 20% or perhaps only 10%? In most organizations (if not all), the data collection systems are not nearly sophisticated enough to capture such information. Therefore, it is generally necessary to estimate the actual percentage allocations.

Suppose that the nurse manager's salary was budgeted to cost $80,000 but that because of a change in fringe benefit rates, the actual salary cost was $81,000. Also suppose that the manager makes an ex post allocation of her total time and estimates that 16% of her effort was devoted to quality improvement. In that case, instead of the budgeted $12,000 of manager cost for quality improvement, the actual manager cost for quality improvement was $12,960 (total nurse manager cost of $81,000 × 16% effort on the quality area).

Assume that the actual results for each line item in the quality improvement area were as follows:

Line Item	Line Item Total Cost	Percent Effort Devoted to Quality Improvement		Actual Cost for Quality Improvement
Nurse Manager	$ 81,000	×	16%	= $12,960
Staff	823,000	×	6	= 49,380
Education	19,000	×	15	= 2,850
Supplies	38,000	×	0	= 0
Overhead	64,000	×	0	= 0
Total				$65,190
Divided by actual outcome (% reduction in Stage III and IV pressure ulcers)				÷12
Actual cost per percent reduction in failures				$ 5,433

The actual cost information would come from the unit's regular variance reports. The percentages of actual effort would be based on estimates by the unit manager and the unit's staff. The budgeted cost for quality improvement was $56,000, and the actual cost was $65,190. The difference between these two numbers represents a $9,190 unfavorable variance. However, this variance does not consider actual work accomplished.

Just as with the flexible variance analysis discussed earlier, it is necessary to consider more than simply the absolute amount of money spent. In terms of accomplishing the goal of reducing the rate of pressure ulcers, the budgeted cost was $5,600 per 1% reduction in the failure rate. The actual result was a cost of $5,433 per percent reduction in the failure rate. The cost per percent dropped because even though total costs for quality improvement were over budget, the failure rate dropped by 12% rather than 10%.

Had one anticipated the 12% reduction, the budgeted cost would have been $67,200 ($5,600 × 12). Although there is a total variance of $9,190 unfavorable, the volume variance was $11,200 unfavorable ($56,000 budgeted − $67,200 flexible budget for a 12% reduction). The $65,190 actual cost for the actual volume was less than the $67,200 that would have been expected for that volume.

In analyzing performance budget results, it is also interesting to look at each line item. In this case, staff salaries of $49,380 were devoted to quality improvement. In the original budget, the amount was $40,000. This greater effort has apparently led to a greater reduction in the failure rate. Even though the cost per percent reduction was less than budgeted, this result would require careful scrutiny by the nurse manager. If greater efforts were being made in this area, where were efforts less than budgeted? Depending on where we cut back, this may not be considered to be a favorable use of time. On the other hand, if the reduction in effort elsewhere was in the area of indirect time, rather than direct patient care time, this may represent a favorable outcome.

As with all areas of variance analysis, the calculations provide raw information about what has occurred. The judgment and experience of competent managers and executives are needed to interpret the variances and determine both their underlying causes and whether they represent favorable or unfavorable events for the unit and organization.

✳ IMPLICATIONS FOR NURSE MANAGERS AND EXECUTIVES

Flexible budget variance analysis is a useful but complex tool. Care must be taken to make sure the analysis helps the manager. For example, aggregation of variances can hide serious problems. Offsetting variances are quite common. If variances are aggregated, offsetting variances may go undetected. Exception reports are particularly useful to keep large variances from going unnoticed.

Flexible budgeting assumes that costs are variable. With fixed costs, there will be no volume variance, because fixed costs by definition do not vary with volume. However, nursing labor costs, even with rigid staffing patterns, can be evaluated using flexible budget analysis.

Variances are generally caused by internal changes in efficiency, technology, or quality of care or by externally caused changes in workload volume or prices. Whatever the causes, efficient management requires investigation and evaluation of variances on a timely basis followed by corrective action whenever possible.

✳ KEY CONCEPTS

Aggregation of variances   Managers and executives should be careful to identify all individual variances, because favorable variances and unfavorable variances offset each other when added together. Such aggregation can hide serious problems.

Exception reports   Can be used to identify critical variances. An exception report is based on computerized examination of all variances and lists only individual variances that exceed a certain limit. This allows the higher level managers and executives to focus only on large variances. However, lower levels of management should view all variances, not just those listed on the exception report.

Investigation and control of variances   Variances should be investigated promptly on a monthly basis in order for variance analysis to be an effective control tool.

✳ SUGGESTED READINGS

Dunham-Taylor J, Pinczuk J: *Financial management for nurse managers*, ed 2, Sudbury, Mass, 2009, Jones & Bartlett.

Finkler S, Ward D, Baker J: *Essentials of cost accounting for health care organizations*, ed 3, Sudbury, Mass, 2007, Jones & Bartlett.

Horngren C, Datar S, Rajan M: *Cost accounting: a managerial emphasis*, ed 14, Englewood Cliffs, New Jersey, 2011, Prentice Hall.

Benchmarking, Productivity, and Cost-Benefit and Cost-Effectiveness Analysis

CHAPTER GOALS

The goals of this chapter are to:

- Define *benchmarking*
- Explain the benchmarking technique and the critical steps in the benchmarking process
- Define *productivity* and *productivity measurement*
- Provide tools for productivity analysis
- Discuss productivity standards
- Introduce the concept of unit costing
- Explain the relationship between productivity standards and unit costing

- Explore the notion of productivity improvement
- Define the concepts of cost-benefit analysis and cost-effectiveness analysis
- Explain the principles of cost-benefit analysis and cost-effectiveness analysis
- Define comparative effectiveness research

✳ INTRODUCTION

Budgeting is not simply about preparing a plan for the organization to do what it has always done the way it has always done it. Rather, budgeting should help the organization to constantly get better—to be more effective and efficient in providing its services. Benchmarking, productivity measurement, and cost-benefit analysis (CBA) and cost-effectiveness analysis (CEA) are approaches that organizations use to become better at what they do.

Benchmarking is a technique aimed at finding the best practices of other organizations and incorporating them into an organization. Benchmarking is the first major topic covered in this chapter.

Many health care organizations (HCOs) today are also concerned with *productivity*. As financial resources become more constrained, improvements in productivity represent one way of "cutting the fat." The area of productivity measurement, however, remains somewhat of a mystery in many industries, not just health care. In health care, the difficulties are compounded by problems related to quality and outcomes measurement.

As an organization works to improve productivity in health care, one must always guard against the motivation to sacrifice mission to achieve productivity increases. It is possible to reduce the number of hours of care per patient day. Many health care providers consider such a reduction to be a sign of increased productivity. However, if the reduction is accompanied by a decrease in the quality of patient care,

then productivity has not really improved. True productivity improvements are those that enable the organization to use fewer resources for each unit of service provided without decreasing the quality of the services provided.

In recent years, there has been a trend to reorient the focus of nursing productivity measurement from hours per patient day (HPPD) or full-time equivalents (FTEs) per adjusted occupied bed[1] toward the cost per unit of service provided. The essence of this *unit costing* is that if we can lower the dollar cost of providing a unit of a specific service, we do not need to worry about things such as the number of care hours used to provide the service. Unit costing is discussed in the productivity section of the chapter.

The chapter concludes with a discussion of CBA and CEA, and an introduction to comparative effectiveness research (CER). The techniques of CBA and CEA are important tools for managers to understand and use as they attempt to improve the productivity of their departments. CER, on the other hand, holds promise for helping to evaluate the usefulness of different treatment options. This approach can help health care providers better understand what treatments work, the populations and patient groups for whom the treatments work, and the conditions and settings within which they work. These techniques are defined and their basic principles are discussed.

---

[1]Adjusted occupied beds is a measure that combines both inpatient days and outpatient care by using a formula for the number of outpatient visits considered to be the equivalent of one inpatient day.

❋ BENCHMARKING

One of the roles of budgeting is to help the organization continuously improve over time. The budget should incorporate changes that will allow it to provide services more efficiently. Ultimately, such constant improvement helps the organization to better accomplish its mission while providing it with an edge over its competitors. Benchmarking is a technique that many organizations use to help set the direction for change. Simply stated, *benchmarking* is a technique that organizations use to find best practices and to incorporate those practices within the organization.

Benchmarking is linked closely with a variety of process improvement and quality management techniques such as total quality management (TQM) and continuous quality improvement (CQI) (discussed in Chapter 11). However, those techniques may be used with a totally internal focus on an organization's processes. The essence of benchmarking is examination of what others are doing. By forcing the organization to look beyond itself, many useful approaches developed elsewhere can be used to benefit the organization. This means that an organization may benefit from rare insights or the costly trials and errors of others. It allows the organization to avoid spending substantial resources to reinvent the wheel every time it needs to improve in some area.

Benefits of Benchmarking

There are a number of different ways that benchmarking leads to improved organizational results. Some of the most prominent focuses of benchmarking studies are in the areas of meeting customer requirements, developing accurate measures of productivity, and improving competitiveness.

As health care becomes increasingly competitive, it becomes more important than ever to concentrate on the customer. The knowledge of the services that other organizations are providing to customers is incredibly valuable. To remain competitive, organizations must be aware of what the competition is doing. If it can be determined that elsewhere in the country a service is provided that is not offered by any local competitors, then the organization can gain insights on how to provide its customers with even more than they expect. The most successful organizations are those that are proactive rather than reactive. The organization that introduces new services first has an edge over those that follow. Because the health care industry is largely localized, it is not necessary to invent all new services. Rather, organizations should strive to keep abreast of innovations around the country and to have the flexibility to be "the first ones on the block" to offer those services.

One of the greatest difficulties in assessing productivity is trying to determine the right level of productivity. How long *should* it take to do a certain procedure? We can measure productivity in terms of improvement over time. However, some would argue that the organization cannot be productive unless it has some optimum standard for comparison. Benchmarking evaluates the level of productivity of other organizations. This allows the organization to compare itself to the best organizations, creating productivity targets that are challenging yet attainable. Productivity is discussed later in this chapter.

Rates of change within organizations are highly variable. Some organizations change rapidly. Others tend to maintain what they believe is a good way of providing care. It is surprising that despite the rapid change in clinical techniques, health care management techniques often tend to be stagnant. It is difficult to spend a great deal of time being innovative while at the same time trying to complete the day's work. Benchmarking helps by allowing organizations to change without having to invent all the changes. This not only reduces the amount of effort required to find changes that truly result in improvements but also allows the organization to leapfrog over competing organizations. Benchmarking is also beneficial because it gives clinicians, managers, and policymakers a tool by which to take advantage of evidence-based approaches to improve care.[2]

Benchmarking Approaches

The three primary approaches to benchmarking are competitive benchmarking, cooperative benchmarking, and collaborative benchmarking.[3] *Competitive benchmarking* refers to finding specific information about individual organizations providing the same services as a particular organization. *Cooperative benchmarking* refers to seeking information from organizations in other industries that can be adapted to the health care industry to improve health care practices (i.e., to improve quality or reduce cost). *Collaborative benchmarking* refers to finding information within a particular industry but based on industry-wide statistics.

When people think of benchmarking, they often focus their thoughts on competitive benchmarking. Hospital managers may want to determine how a specific function is done at the hospital recognized to perform that function the best. A visiting nurse agency may want to know the best practices related to supplies inventory at other home care agencies. These are the hardest type of benchmarking data to obtain. Naturally, organizations are reluctant to share their secrets with the direct competition. For this reason, it is often easier to fly across the country and observe several organizations that are not in direct competition with the organization than to observe the practices of direct competitors in the same area as the organization. It is not unusual for exchanges to be worked out in which organizations that are similar but in different markets allow visitors to examine their procedures.

Sometimes competitive benchmarking is done without direct permission. This can occur through informal observation or by using a variety of publicly available information. Health care providers generally issue many reports to the public and government that can be useful in assessing their approaches. Consultants have access to many organizations and are often willing to share the best practices that they have observed. As Pavlock notes, "The goal is to find out what the competitors are doing, how, and how well in order to compare their practices

---

[2]Donaldson N, Brown D, Aydin C, et al. 2005. Leveraging nurse-related dashboard benchmarks to expedite performance improvement and document excellence. *J Nurs Adm* 35(4):163-172.

[3]Info-Line, Understanding Benchmarking. July 1992. *The Search for Best Practice*. Alexandria, VA: American Society for Training and Development, Issue 9207, pp. 5-6.

with the benchmarker's operations."[4] There are many ways to get that information. For example, agency nurses often work for many different providers. They can be an invaluable source of information on how other organizations do things. Newly hired and experienced nurses can also bring a wealth of knowledge from the other HCOs where they have worked previously.

Cooperative benchmarking takes a substantially different approach. Rather than focusing on specific competitors, it looks at organizations in totally different industries. Although this might seem odd at first, it actually has great merit. Suppose that a health care provider finds that it consistently ranks low in customer satisfaction. A cooperative benchmarking approach would be to select an organization that is known for its great customer service. For example, the Nordstrom department store over the years has had such a reputation. Spending some time visiting Nordstrom and learning its philosophy and how it operationalizes that philosophy and maintains high customer satisfaction might be enlightening. Why should Nordstrom agree to let someone do this? First, everyone loves flattery. And seeking to learn from any organization certainly flatters that organization. Second, many organizations view helping health care providers to be an act of public service. Finally, the time may come when you will have some information that might benefit Nordstrom.

It is important to bear in mind that as long as benchmarking is limited to the benchmarker's own industry, it is not possible to become the leader. The organization doing the benchmarking is always following someone else in the industry. By going outside of the industry, an organization gains the possibility of becoming the industry leader.

Some organizations actually make a business of allowing themselves to be used for benchmarking purposes. Disney offers a formal program called "The Disney Approach to Quality Service for Healthcare Professionals." In a three and a half day program costing about $3,500 per participant, Disney offers "A Unique Benchmarking Opportunity." In the program, Disney provides not only information about how Disney does things but also linkages to how its approaches can be used in the health care industry.

Collaborative benchmarking is a process whereby a number of organizations in the same industry pool data so that all members of the pool can determine where they stand relative to the best members of the pool. Generally, there is confidentiality, with members of the pool being anonymous. Each organization sees its own data and where it stands relative to everyone else but does not know who has better or worse ratings. An example of collaborative benchmarking is the University HealthSystem Consortium (UHC), a partnership between academic health systems that provides members with aggregated data with which to benchmark and compare organizational performance to peer organizations and target improvements and innovations.[5]

The collaborative approach is more of a *how much* approach rather than a *how* approach. With competitive or cooperative benchmarking, the benchmarker tries to learn as much about the best practice process to make it easy to adopt that practice. Collaborative benchmarking does not allow for an understanding of process. On the other hand, if collaborative benchmarking is used, it can help highlight weaknesses. The organization can then move aggressively into one of the other approaches of benchmarking to find ways to convert that weakness into an area of competitive strength.

The Benchmarking Process

The process for benchmarking has been summarized by Camp[6] as having 10 steps:

1. Decide what to benchmark.
2. Identify organizations with best practices.
3. Collect data for comparison.
4. Assess the gap between best practice and your performance.
5. Project likely improvement in best practices over the next 3 to 5 years.
6. Communicate findings.
7. Establish goals.
8. Create specific plans for improvement.
9. Implement plans.
10. Reestablish benchmarks as they change over time.

Every organization does too many things to be able to benchmark fruitfully all processes. Benchmarking usually focuses on problem areas. The organization must first decide where it is most in need of outside comparison (step 1). A study team should be formed. The team should first focus on identifying areas for which a difference in performance will lead to a difference in achievement of mission. In other words, one must select areas where change might result in a meaningful impact. There is a difficult chicken-and-egg problem. How do you know where you fall short until you benchmark? But how do you know what you want to benchmark until you know where you fall short? Collaborative benchmarking can be used to highlight where some significant opportunities for improvement are likely to exist, and they can become the focus of competitive benchmarking. However, ultimately, managers must thoroughly understand their own processes. It can be especially beneficial to focus efforts on areas that are costly (because they have the most potential for cost savings) and areas that are creating morale problems.

Next, the study team should select organizations with best practices (step 2). This requires a fair amount of investigation. Reading publications, asking around, talking to consultants, and general networking are essential to this step. Pavlock suggests that you "talk with industry experts, the firm's employees, customers, suppliers and others knowledgeable about the areas or business practices being targeted. Ask whose products, services or business practices are similar in some way to the benchmarking firm. A benchmarking consultant may be

---

[4]Pavlock E. 1994. *Financial Management for Medical Groups.* Englewood, CO: Center for Research in Ambulatory Health Care Administration, p. 588.

[5]University HealthSystem Consortium. Retrieved March 2, 2012, at https://www.uhc.edu/12443.htm.

[6]Camp R. 1989. *Benchmarking: The Search for Industry Best Practices That Lead to Superior Performance.* Milwaukee, WI: American Society for Quality Control, pp. 9-12.

helpful."[7] The more you have to offer in return to benchmarking partners, the more likely they are to allow you to review their organizations. So part of the selection process must include consideration of what you have to offer in exchange and who would be likely to want it.

Step 3 concerns data collection. The data collection process involves not only data but also people. In collecting data about your own organization and the comparison organization, it is critical to involve the right people on the study team. That includes the managers most familiar with the existing processes at both organizations, as well as the person responsible for implementing any changes. To the extent possible, the staff members who ultimately will have to make any changes succeed should be involved in the process. If they do not view the changes as their changes, they will not have a vested interest in having them succeed. The data to be collected must be usable. So, before collecting data, one should question what types of changes might be needed. Although this cannot be answered fully before data are collected, it will help formulate the measurement instruments so that data are collected in a usable form.

Change is often difficult and costly. If the gap between best practice and your performance is not great, it may not be worthwhile trying to implement change. So it is important to assess the gap between current and best practices (step 4). If the measurement tools are well designed and a sizable gap is evident, the benchmarker will be able to see where change is needed.

Knowledge of the gap allows the organization to set targets for improvement. However, the targets should not necessarily be set at the level that exists in the best practices organization now. That organization is likely to make improvements during the period the benchmarker is implementing changes. Therefore, the benchmark established needs to be set at the level that will likely exist at the best practices organization several years in the future (step 5).

It is critical that the findings of the benchmarking process are widely communicated (step 6). There will undoubtedly be ripple effects resulting from any change. The more support developed for changes, the more likely they are to succeed. But support is not possible without clear communication of what has been found and why the findings dictate that changes would be beneficial.

Step 7 is the establishment of goals. These goals should be those that the study team believes are appropriate in order to maximize the benefit gained from adopting the best practices. These goals should be developed with a careful eye toward both the existing gap and the estimation of where the best practices organization will be in several years, as discussed earlier.

The goals must be translated into objectives that form the basis for specific plans for improvement (step 8). To the extent possible, all persons who will be involved in the implementation of the changes should be involved in designing the plans for change.

Next comes the actual implementation of the plans (step 9). Assuming that the new benchmarks are well communicated and the action plans well designed, the organization should start to make progress fairly quickly. If progress is not visible in a short time, staff may become discouraged and fall into old patterns of behavior. Although the process of gathering the benchmarking data can be challenging and time-consuming, one cannot relax after the data have been collected. Unless the actual implementation is supervised carefully, all of the preceding efforts may turn out to have been wasted.

The final step is to reestablish benchmarks as they change over time (step 10). One of the fundamental principles on which benchmarking is based is that change is essential. There is no one correct way to do things. It is not as simple as getting all aspects of the organization to reach the correct plateau. Rather, processes need to be improved continuously. Even if the organization achieves the status of an industry leader that everyone wants to evaluate for its benchmarking efforts, continued improvement is essential.

Requirements for Successful Benchmarking

One thing that should be clear from the current discussion is that benchmarking is a big deal. It is not a brief activity undertaken at little cost. Rather, it is an ongoing process that involves the time of many managers over substantial periods of time. Benchmarking is unlikely to work unless there is a strong management commitment to the process. Managers in the organization must study their current processes. It is difficult to change to something else unless you first know where you are now. There must also be a willingness to change. Such willingness is much harder to obtain than we often think. Change has been described as being similar in some respects to heaven: Everyone extols its virtues, but most people are not actually in much of a rush to get there.

✳ PRODUCTIVITY

Contrary to popular belief, productivity is not focused primarily on getting people to work harder. The concern, rather, is to have employees' efforts be more productive. What is meant by productivity? The most common productivity measure is the amount of output produced by each unit of input. This can be calculated as follows:

$$\text{Productivity} = \frac{\text{Total outputs}}{\text{Total inputs}}$$

For example, suppose that a nurse practitioner can see 250 patients during a month when 100 hours are devoted to seeing patients. The productivity measure would be:

$$= \frac{250 \text{ Patients}}{100 \text{ Hours}} = 2.5 \text{ Patients per Hour}$$

If activities can be altered to allow the nurse to see more patients per hour, productivity would improve, assuming that the care provided remains the same. For example, suppose that the nurse practitioner currently records everything manually in the patient chart after the visit. However, an electronic charting system with a touch screen function would allow for

[7]Pavlock, *Op. cit.*, p. 589.

faster data entry and chart updating. Because less time is spent charting, more patients could be scheduled. Suppose that after the implementation of the electronic charting system, the nurse can now see 270 patients in the same 100 hours. Productivity has improved to:

$$= \frac{270 \text{ Patients}}{100 \text{ Hours}} = 2.7 \text{ Patients per Hour}$$

If the cost of each hour is the same and visits per hour rise from 2.5 to 2.7, the practice is more productive. Assuming that the extra visits per hour generate more revenue, it is more profitable as well. (Note that we have not yet considered the cost of the electronic charting system and the computer hardware requirements. That will be addressed later in this chapter.)

Productivity Standards

In the previous example, it was hypothesized that a nurse practitioner used electronic charting to improve productivity from 2.5 patients per hour to 2.7 patients per hour. One problem with such a measure of productivity is that the only comparison is over time. Often managers would prefer to also have a benchmark or standard for comparison. Standards can be based on broad industry average experience, on best industry practice, or simply on the organization's budget.

For example, suppose that the nurse practitioner believes that an ideally functioning practice would see three patients per hour. The nurse practitioner has determined this after reading many articles about similar practices and from talking to peers around the country. Productivity can be measured by comparing actual results of this practice with that standard. For example, the practice productivity was originally 2.5 patients an hour. Compared with the standard, this represents an 83% productivity rate calculated as follows:

$$\frac{\text{Actual Productivity}}{\text{Standard Productivity}} \times 100\% = \text{Productivity Percent}$$

$$\frac{2.5 \text{ Patients per Hour}}{3.0 \text{ Patients per Hour}} \times 100\% = 83\%$$

After the innovation with the computer charting, the practice productivity rose to 90%.

$$\frac{2.7 \text{ Patients per Hour}}{3.0 \text{ Patients per Hour}} \times 100\% = 90\%$$

If an industry standard cannot be found, the productivity percent can be calculated as a percent of the budget or of some perceived ideal. It should be noted, however, that the resulting percentage must be interpreted differently based on the type of standard used. If the budget is used as the value for the denominator of the fraction, then the goal should be to attain 100% productivity or better. That would imply that the organization is achieving or exceeding its budget. In contrast, what if the denominator of the fraction is based on a perceived ideal? It is highly unlikely that an ideal result can ever be attained. Therefore, the manager must bear in mind that we would always expect productivity to be less than 100%, and

performance should be assessed based on how close we come to 100%.

Unit Costing

In the previous example, productivity rose from 83% to 90% after the electronic charting system was introduced. However, we must still question whether that productivity change is an improvement. More and more managers are choosing to stop looking at productivity simply in terms of inputs and outputs and to make sure that the cost per unit of service is considered in the calculation. This approach is called *unit costing*.

For example, hospitals have long used HPPD as a productivity measure. This is actually an inversion of the typical productivity measure. Consider a nursing department that consumed 10,000 hours of nurses' time in a month when it provided 2,500 patient days of care. The standard productivity measure would be outputs divided by inputs to find the amount of output per unit of input. For the nursing department the calculation would be:

$$= \frac{2,500 \text{ Patients Days}}{10,000 \text{ Hours}} = 0.25 \text{ Patient Days per Hour}$$

The result here is cumbersome because each unit of output (i.e., a patient day) requires more than one unit of input (an hour of care). One-quarter of a patient day of care is generated by each hour of nursing care. By inverting the fraction, we can measure the HPPD:

$$= \frac{10,000 \text{ Hours}}{2,500 \text{ Patient Days}} = 4 \text{ HPPD}$$

This is a common hospital productivity measure. However, in today's environment of tight financial resources, this measure fails to indicate the cost of care, which is critical. If we replaced all licensed practical nurses (LPNs) with registered nurses (RNs), it is possible that we could reduce the HPPD. But would that make the organization more productive? That is a complicated question. An RN can do activities that an LPN cannot do. But the cost per hour for an RN is also higher than it is for an LPN. Consider the following example. Suppose that an RN earns $49 per hour, including benefits, and an LPN earns $35 per hour, including benefits. Suppose further that an LPN requires 20% more time to accomplish activities than an RN would require for the same activities (this is because some activities can only be performed by an RN). Assume that currently we have 100 hours of RN time and 120 hours of LPN time, and we have an output of 50 patient days. The HPPD under the current staffing would be:

$$\frac{100 \text{ RN Hours} + 120 \text{ LPN Hours}}{50 \text{ Patient Days}} = 4.4 \text{ HPPD}$$

and the cost per unit of service would be:

100 RN Hours × $49	=	$4,900
120 LPN Hours × $35	=	+4,200
Total Cost	=	$9,100
Patient Days		÷ 50
Cost per Patient Day		$ 182

If we shifted to an all-RN staff, we could replace the 120 LPN hours with 100 RN hours. The HPPD would then be:

$$\frac{100 \text{ RN Hours} + 100 \text{ RN Hours}}{50 \text{ Patient Days}} = 4.0 \text{ HPPD}$$

The HPPD have fallen from 4.4 to 4.0. But is the unit more productive? What has happened to the cost of care provided:

200 RN Hours × $49	= $9,800
Patient Days	÷ 50
Cost per Patient Day	$ 196

Productivity is difficult to assess in absolute terms. Shifting from a staff with RNs and LPNs to an all-RN staff resulted in fewer required hours of care for each patient day in the previous example. But the cost per patient day rose from $182 to $196. Clearly, simply measuring productivity based on HPPD does not make sense. HPPD can fall while cost per patient rises. We cannot say this makes us more productive. On the other hand, productivity measures should take quality of care into consideration. Shifting to the all-RN staff did raise the cost per unit of service, but it may have also raised the level of quality of care. So we cannot say clearly that the increased cost per patient day reduced productivity.

On the other hand, we could identify an acceptable level of quality of care. As long as that level of quality is maintained, reductions in the cost per unit of service would be considered to be productivity increases. In the previous example, if the care being provided by 100 RN hours and 120 LPN hours was of acceptable quality, then the shift to an all-RN staff would reduce productivity because it increases the cost per patient day. We cannot let traditional productivity measures such as the reduction in HPPD from 4.4 to 4.0 lead us to believe productivity is improving when the cost per patient day is increasing. Financial resources are too limited for us to focus solely on measures such as HPPD. The productivity measure provided by cost per unit of service is much more meaningful to managers who are trying to make the best use of their limited financial resources.

Therefore, at least one author has called on HCOs to shift their measures of productivity toward the cost per unit of service, or unit costing. This calls for replacing measures of input with measures of cost.[8] Rather than thinking about the HPPD, we could consider the cost per patient day. Similarly, in various situations, we could measure productivity in terms of the cost per patient, cost per procedure, or cost per visit.

For example, consider the case of the nurse practitioner and the rise in productivity percent from 83% to 90% after purchase of an electronic charting system. Did productivity really rise or fall? Maybe the cost of the system—including both the hardware and software—was greater than the benefit. Suppose that the total costs of the practice for the month

(including the salary of the nurse practitioner) without the electronic charting system were $8,000. The new system is leased for $300 per month (for all hardware and software). The cost of the practice rose from $8,000 to $8,300. What happened to the cost per unit of service? Originally it was:

$$\frac{\$8,000 \text{ Cost}}{250 \text{ Patients}} = \$32.00$$

After the electronic charting system implementation, the cost per unit of service was:

$$\frac{\$8,300 \text{ Cost}}{270 \text{ Patients}} = \$30.74$$

It turns out that productivity has indeed improved as a result of the computer, because the cost per visit, even including the cost of the computer, fell from $32.00 to $30.74.

Notice also that the cost per unit of service approach does not require us to measure the amount of different resources used. In the example as initially stated, it was assumed that the nurse practitioner worked 100 hours in both situations. Most likely, the number of hours spent seeing patients would vary from month to month. However, we can calculate productivity of the practice from month to month without having to track the number of hours worked or the amount of other resources used. All that is needed is the total cost for the services provided each month and the number of units of service provided.

For example, an operating room department or outpatient surgery unit can simply divide its total costs by the number of hours of surgery to get a cost per hour or cost per minute. If the cost per hour of surgery falls from month to month, then productivity is improving, assuming that case mix is constant. Similarly, a home care agency could calculate the cost per home care visit by dividing total costs by the total number of visits. Such measures can be tracked either over time or compared with some budget or standard, as discussed previously.

The problem with this approach is that you must be willing to accept some averaging. For instance, if a home care agency provides visits by nursing assistants (NAs), LPNs, and RNs, the average cost per visit may be misleading. What if the number of visits by RNs is falling and the number of visits by NAs is rising? It is likely that the cost per visit will fall. But that may not be indicative of true productivity improvement. This is especially so if the profit of RN visits is greater than the profit on visits by NAs. This is further complicated by the fact that RN visits will typically be much shorter than NA visits, which could last up to 12 hours.

One way to handle such a situation is to divide the costs of the health care unit or organization into separate categories and measure productivity for each category. We could measure the costs of RN visits, costs of LPN visits, and costs of NA visits and then divide those costs by the number of visits of each type to assess productivity. For example, suppose that the costs for the agency for the month were $240,000 and there were 4,000 visits. One productivity measure would be:

$$\frac{\$240,000 \text{ Cost}}{4,000 \text{ Visits}} = \$60 \text{ Cost per Visit}$$

---

[8]Barren J. 1994. Productivity and cost per unit of service. In Spitzer-Lehmann R, editor. *Nursing Management Desk Reference*. Philadelphia: WB Saunders, pp. 260-277.

However, a more sophisticated approach would be to determine the volume and cost by type of visit and calculate productivity as:

$$\frac{\$100,000 \text{ Cost of RN Visits}}{1,000 \text{ RN Visits}} = \$100 \text{ Cost per RN Visit}$$

$$\frac{\$60,000 \text{ Cost of LPN Visits}}{1,000 \text{ LPN Visits}} = \$60 \text{ Cost per LPN Visit}$$

$$\frac{\$80,000 \text{ Cost of NA Visits}}{2,000 \text{ NA Visits}} = \$40 \text{ Cost per NA Visit}$$

Over time, we could track changing productivity for each type of visit.

The difficulty of such productivity measurement is assigning costs to each group. Clearly, the cost of RN visits would include the cost of RNs, the supplies they use, and their travel and charting costs. The problem is determining what share of rent, supervision, billing, and other costs to assign to one group versus the other groups. There is no simple rule for such allocations. Overhead costs can be allocated based on the number of visits (if half of the visits are by NAs, assign half of the overhead to NAs), based on the revenue from visits (if half of the revenue comes from RN visits, assign half of the overhead to them), or based on a number of other approaches. No one approach is more valid or correct than any other.

Although many organizations use arbitrary ways to allocate overhead or indirect costs, an alternative approach is to ignore overhead costs. Productivity could be measured based on just the direct costs per unit of service. This approach will help assess productivity improvement or declines related to direct costs. Unfortunately, it does not provide information about changes in productivity in overhead areas of the organization, such as the billing department. This is especially important if changes in RN productivity are associated with changes in overhead departments. However, we could separately measure productivity for overhead by measuring things such as the cost per bill issued.

Current nursing productivity measures such as HPPD generally do not account adequately for inputs that pertain to nurses' intellectual or human capital—that is, the knowledge, skills, and abilities they bring to their work—and how that important input contributes to productivity and quality of care.[9] Hall[10] presents a framework for examining nursing productivity that includes nurses' intellectual capital, as well as aspects of the nursing work environment that may also impact productivity, such as organizational trust and commitment, job satisfaction, nursing turnover, absenteeism, and replacement costs (including orientation and training). This is where a knowledgeable manager's perspective can make an important contribution in evaluating nursing productivity.

As you can see, productivity measurement is complex. Managers cannot simply apply productivity formulas blindly. Thought must go into deciding how to measure productivity and how to interpret productivity measures. Nevertheless, unit costing is feasible. We must define the unit (e.g., patient day, RN visit, or nurse practitioner treatment) and divide the number of units of service into the cost of providing that service. We can have broad average costs or more specifically measured costs.

Barron nicely summarizes the issue related to productivity measurement as follows:

Managers cannot be held to both dollar and hour limits. Either they manage the hours and watch what happens to the dollars, as is the common practice, or they manage the dollars and watch what happens to the hours. Past practice has led to tightly controlled hours and escalating dollars. A dollars per unit of service system tightly controls dollars while allowing flexible hours.[11]

Barron's point is important because it focuses on the fact that productivity is unlikely to improve in HCOs until management changes its thinking. If there is a goal to control costs, finance should not persist in holding managers accountable for measures such as HPPD. That thinking stifles innovation instead of encouraging it. Executives who say that they support innovation and creativity but then evaluate employees based on adherence to a measure such as HPPD clearly are not putting their money where their mouth is. They are forgetting that people respond well to the incentives that the organization provides. If the goal is to control spending per visit, per treatment, or per patient, then the productivity measurement and evaluation must be based on those units of service as well.

Unit Costing and Productivity Standards

If unit costing is used to assess productivity, we can still use productivity benchmarks or standards. For instance, in the home care agency example described previously, we could assess the cost of each visit versus a benchmark. If we believe the ideal cost per RN visit is $220, then we could divide the actual $250 cost (see previous calculation) into the ideal $220 cost, as follows:

$$\frac{\$220 \text{ Ideal Cost}}{\$250 \text{ Actual Cost}} \times 100\% = 88\% \text{ Productivity}$$

As the actual cost per visit declines, we would get closer to 100% productivity. Such measures require careful thought about what should go in the numerator and the denominator to get a meaningful indicator.

Productivity Improvement

For most HCOs, the focus on productivity does not exist simply for the purpose of measuring the level of productivity. Rather, we are concerned with improving productivity. Such improvements can be accomplished by forcing staff to work harder. Generally,

[9]Moody R. 2004. Nurse productivity measures for the 21st century. *Health Care Manage Rev* 29(2):98-106.

[10]Hall L. 2003. Nursing intellectual capital: A theoretical approach for analyzing nursing productivity. *Nurs Econ* 21(1):14-19.

[11]Barron J. 1994. Productivity and cost per unit of service. In Spitzer-Lehmann R, editor: *Nursing Management Desk Reference*. Philadelphia: WB Saunders, p. 271.

however, such efforts are self-defeating. They result in declining morale. Although short-term improvements may be possible as a result of such strategies, in the longer term, declines in productivity may occur as a result of the pressures placed on employees. Furthermore, the quality of care provided may decline as a result of the pressure on employees.

Working smarter, not harder, is the key to improving productivity. Productivity measurement should be used to generate information to follow the progress of serious process improvement efforts. Learning how to do things more efficiently is likely to result in permanent productivity gains and should not require increased and often unsustainable individual efforts by employees.

The key to working smarter, not harder, lies in changing processes. Benchmarking, discussed earlier in this chapter, is one approach to improve productivity. Adopting the best practices of others is likely to change processes in a way that increases productivity. Reengineering, TQM, CQI, and value-added approaches similarly are aimed at improving underlying processes. The essence, however, lies not in the use of a specific technique such as TQM or CQI but rather in a review of the way the organization provides its services.

Managers must be given the time and support necessary to promote change. Productivity improvement is unlikely to occur without change. The organization must foster an environment that encourages change. Managers must know that innovation is expected from them. If the message given to managers is that they are overseers of an existing operation, they will simply oversee that static provision of care. Improvement is likely to occur only when innovation is actively supported, encouraged, and rewarded.

Productivity improvements also require an understanding of why resources are consumed. We must know first why an organizational unit exists. What is the mission of the unit or department? Next, the unit must be examined to determine if all the resources it consumes are really necessary to accomplish that mission. This is not to say that some resources are simply wasted. Rather, one must take a cost-benefit perspective. Are the benefits of each of the unit's activities great enough to justify the cost of those activities? Some longstanding practices may need to be eliminated because their costs have risen so high over the years that they can no longer be justified.

For example, for each activity of the organizational unit, one might ask:

- When is it performed?
- How often is it performed?
- Where is it performed?
- Who is performing it?
- Is it necessary to perform it at all?[12]
- Is the activity performed in a manner consistent with the available evidence?

The answers to these questions may provide the information needed to make changes that will result in productivity increases without substantial reduction in services provided. We might find that a function always handled by one department has been superseded by an activity now done with new technology for a lower cost in another department. The old activity not only may be duplicative but also may be providing inferior information to that already available in the other department.

Over time, space needs change as well. Productivity relates to all resources consumed, not just to labor. If the organization is not using space wisely, it is possible that money is being wasted. Organizations often grow haphazardly. Space is allocated based on immediate necessity rather than careful planning. It may be worth an organization's time to have a space planner examine operations and reallocate space. It is possible that space savings will occur that might allow the organization to rent less outside space, thus saving money.

For example, there has been substantial movement in hospitals from inpatient care to outpatient care. While new outpatient facilities have been built, what has happened to the excess space formerly needed for inpatients? It is possible that much of that space is being used in a suboptimal fashion. Spending some money for redesign and even remodeling could result in substantial reductions in the cost of space and could even make provision of care more efficient, resulting in reduced labor costs, and safer, resulting in higher quality of care.[13]

At this point, we have questioned the need for the organization to exist and have evaluated its activities to see if they could be eliminated or performed differently. The facilities used by the organization have also been considered. Finally, productivity improvement requires careful evaluation of the staff and supplies used. It is often difficult to assess whether staffing patterns are appropriate. Collaborative benchmarking, as discussed earlier, can be helpful. By considering issues such as the number of visits per home care worker at other home care agencies, one can get a sense of the organization's productivity in the use of staff. This information can be a starting point in at least getting a sense of where an organization is on a continuum of resource consumption.

However, it is critical to keep in mind that collaborative benchmarking results in "how much" information rather than "how" information. Many consulting firms tell health care providers that they can provide their services with fewer staff because others do so, but they do not provide the "how" piece of information. It may be that there are unique factors related to the organization's physical structure, patient mix, or even culture that make such productivity standards impossible.

For example, suppose that abortions are relatively inexpensive to perform compared with other obstetric procedures. Hospitals that do more abortions in its labor and delivery department will need fewer RNs per 1,000 patients than hospitals that perform fewer abortions. Suppose that a hospital performing many abortions has a ratio of 2 RNs per 1,000 obstetric procedures. Suppose further that the average hospital that does some abortions uses 2.5 RNs per 1,000. A consultant tells a

---

[12]Pavlock, *Op. cit.*, p. 595.

[13]Hendrich A, Fay J, Sorrells A. 2004. Effects of acuity-adaptable rooms on flow of patients and delivery of care. *Am J Crit Care* 3(1):35-45.

Catholic hospital that does no abortions that best practice for obstetrics calls for the use of 2 RNs per 1,000. The Catholic hospital currently has a ratio of 2.7 RNs per 1,000. How useful is that information? Not very. And it may be destructive if top management blindly calls for departments to use benchmarked data without an understanding of how the numbers were achieved. Productivity improvement requires careful analysis and consideration of mission, vision, and cultural aspects, rather than simplistic pursuit of targets that are not well understood.

Finally, supplies and equipment should also be considered when an organization is trying to assess productivity improvement. For example, a thorough review of the process related to supplies may find that the HCO does not get the best buy on supplies. Or it may show that it did get a good price but purchased too much and then had to dispose of some supplies that reached their expiration date. Or it may show that the hospital buys the correct amount but has trouble distributing the supplies to where they are needed, when they are needed, creating bottlenecks that delay patient treatment. Often productivity improvement requires nothing more than a careful examination of how the organization does things, a determination of where problems are occurring, and then development and implementation of solutions to avoid the problems in the future.

Where do we often find room for productivity improvement? Pavlock notes that, "Scheduling modifications for patients, staff and physicians are probably the most important way to improve the overall productivity."[14] This requires a delicate balance. Patients do not like to wait for care. However, if caregivers have to wait for patients to arrive, they are being paid for time when they are not productive. Inefficiencies in health care delivery have made waiting a "necessary evil" for patients and an unrealistic but acceptable behavior for providers, such that it may take changing both patient and provider expectations to bring about real "patient-centered" change. This problem is exacerbated by the fact that it takes different amounts of time to treat different patients, and the time needed for any one specific patient cannot be anticipated accurately in advance.

✳ COST-BENEFIT AND COST-EFFECTIVENESS ANALYSIS

CBA and CEA are methods used to consider the advantages and disadvantages of decisions. These techniques are often used in assessing the implementation of best practices based on a benchmarking study or other changes designed to improve productivity. They are used in a variety of other situations as well.

CBA is a method that compares the benefits related to a decision about a new project or other change to the costs of that decision. The method holds that the decision makes sense if the benefits related to the decision will exceed the costs. In terms of numbers, we create a ratio by dividing benefits by costs. If:

$$\frac{\text{Benefits}}{\text{Costs}} > 1$$

then the project is said to have a positive benefit-cost ratio and adds value. That is, the only way the benefits divided by the costs results in a number greater than 1 is if the benefits are greater than the costs. To determine the ratio, it is necessary to assign values to both the costs and the benefits in monetary terms. In practice, it is often very difficult to assign monetary values to health care outcomes. We have trouble measuring the value of a life and even more difficulty measuring the difference in health outcomes that do not involve life or death.

CEA is not as ambitious as CBA in that it does not require a measurement of the value of the benefits. Rather, it relies on using comparisons. One considers whether a project is cost-effective in comparison with some outcome or alternative approach. An approach that achieves a specific desired outcome for the least possible cost is considered to be cost-effective.

Cost-Benefit Analysis

Cost-benefit analysis, as its name implies, compares the costs and benefits of an action or program. CBA has been defined as being an:

> . . . *analytical technique that compares the social costs and benefits of proposed programs or policy actions. All losses and gains experienced by society are included and measured in dollar terms. The net benefits created by an action are calculated by subtracting the losses incurred by some sectors of society from the gains that accrue to others. Alternative actions are compared, so as to choose one or more that yield the greatest net benefits, or ratio of benefits to costs. The inclusion of all gains and losses to society in cost-benefit analysis distinguishes it from cost-effectiveness analysis, which is a more limited view of costs and benefits.*[15]

In the minds of many people, CBA is associated with large-scale public projects, such as the building of a dam. However, the technique can be extremely useful even for evaluating small purchases such as a personal computer. Health care policymakers will be likely to include the impact on society in their CBAs. Health care managers are more likely to focus specifically on the impact of a decision on their organization.

All organizations attempt to determine if the benefits from spending money will exceed the cost. If the benefits do outweigh the costs, it makes sense to spend the money; otherwise it does not. Careful measurement of costs and benefits provides the information needed to support a spending decision.

There are several key elements in performing a CBA:
- Determine project goals.
- Estimate project benefits.
- Estimate project costs.
- Discount cost and benefit flows at an appropriate rate.
- Complete the decision analysis.

[14]*Ibid.*, p. 597.

[15]Mikesell J. 1995. *Fiscal Administration: Analysis and Application for the Public Sector,* 4th edition. Fort Worth, TX: Harcourt Brace College Publishers, pp. 559-560.

Determine Project Goals

To determine the benefits, it is first necessary to understand what the organization hopes the project will accomplish. So identification of goals and objectives is essential. Suppose that a home care agency is trying to decide if it should acquire a van that would drop off nurses and NAs at patient homes. The first question is why it believes that it would be better off with a van. The goals may be few or numerous, depending on the specific situation. Perhaps staff members currently have difficulty parking, or they spend a lot of time searching for parking and often incur parking tickets for illegal parking because there are no legal spaces available. The agency may wish to reduce the cost of parking and parking tickets and to save the time staff spends searching for parking.

Estimate Project Benefits

After the goals have been identified, the specific amount of the benefits must be estimated. The benefits should include only the incremental benefits that result from the project. For instance, the manager would not include the benefit of providing existing services to existing customers because the services are already provided. However, if freeing up staff time allows for more patients to be cared for, then the revenue from that extra service should be included in the analysis. Benefits may also arise from cost reductions. All additional benefits should be considered, estimated, and included in the cost-benefit calculation.

In the home care agency example, it is likely that the manager will be able to calculate the benefits fairly directly. For example, the agency may have logs showing travel time separately from visit time. It can use that information to calculate the labor cost of time spent by staff members searching for parking. It certainly knows the amount it currently pays for parking lots and parking tickets. Measurement of other benefits is more complicated. If more patients can be seen, the benefit would really be the profit from those additional patients rather than their entire revenue.

Estimate Project Costs

Projects have costs as well as benefits, and those costs must also be estimated as part of the CBA. In the case of the van, the primary costs relate to the acquisition of the van and the labor cost for the driver. However, care should be exercised to include all costs, such as the cost of gasoline and maintaining the vehicle. Some consideration is also needed for coverage when the driver is sick or on vacation. In CBA, it is also critical to consider *opportunity costs*. Opportunity cost refers to the fact that when a decision is made to do something, other alternatives are sacrificed. In the case of buying a van, the agency buys the van with cash that might have been used to pay rent on a new office location in an adjoining community. Perhaps the money in that alternative use would generate many more patients and great amounts of additional revenues and profits.

Discount Cost and Benefit Flows

Often project benefits and costs accrue over a period of years. This creates a calculation problem, because money has a different value at different times. Money is more valuable today than the same amount of money in the future. If one pays $40,000 for a van today and receives $15,000 of net benefits per year over the 4-year life of the van, one cannot compare the $40,000 with the sum of $15,000 for 4 years. At a minimum, the agency could have invested the $40,000 and earned interest each year.

This creates a problem in comparing benefits and costs. They cannot simply be totaled for the life of the project and then compared to see if the benefits exceed the costs. The timing is critical. This is especially true because projects often have higher costs in early years and higher benefits in later years. Simple addition of total benefits and total costs could lead to improper decisions. The approach to deal with the problem is referred to as *discounting cash flows*. This approach uses an interest rate, referred to as the discount rate, to convert all costs and benefits to their value at the present time. See the discussion of the time value of money in the Appendix to Chapter 12 for additional discussion related to discounting of future cash flows.

Complete the Decision Analysis

After all of the relevant costs and benefits of a project have been estimated and adjusted in a discounting process, they can be compared with each other in the form of a ratio. Generally, benefits are divided by costs. If the result is greater than 1, it means that the benefits exceed the costs, and the project is desirable. The greater the benefit-to-cost ratio, the more desirable the project.

Cost-Effectiveness Analysis

As noted earlier, an approach that achieves a specific desired outcome for the least possible cost is considered to be cost-effective. If we do not have a comparison, we run into difficulties. Consider, for example, a project that will save lives. If we know that we can save lives at a cost of $50 per life, would we consider that to be cost-effective? Certainly. However, in drawing such a conclusion, we are implicitly placing at least a minimum value on a human life by saying it is worth more than $50. This creates a difficulty in trying to establish a cutoff point. Is a project that saves lives at a cost of $10,000 per life cost effective? How about $1 million? How about $1 billion?

Some might argue that many alternative options could save lives for less than $1 billion per life saved. Therefore, the project that costs $1 billion per life is not cost-effective. In comparison with other alternatives, the $1 billion per life project costs more to accomplish the outcome of saving lives than alternatives cost. The problem with assuming that $50 per life saved is cost-effective is that it puts a value on the benefit rather than simply holding the benefit constant. A CEA-oriented approach and the cost effective alternative would consider different approaches to saving a life and find out which one costs the least.

Therefore, to operationalize CEA, one must compare alternatives that generate similar outcomes. For example, suppose that an HCO has been treating a certain type of patient using a particular approach. Now an alternative approach is suggested. Is the new approach cost-effective? The first step is to establish that the clinical outcomes are equal. Then it must be shown that the new approach costs less money than the old approach.

If a new approach generates the exact same outcome or a better outcome for less money than the old approach, it is cost-effective.

Note how CEA avoids the problem of measuring the value of the benefits. Because the benefits are held constant, any approach that costs less must inherently be superior to other approaches. In reality, however, it is often difficult to find different techniques that yield the exact same or better health care outcomes.

As a result, researchers have developed a variety of techniques to enable the comparison of outcomes across interventions, conditions, and diseases. Researchers have been able to model the long-term effects of clinical treatments on patients. With this ability, CEA can now go beyond simple comparisons of the cost per life saved to more precise comparisons of cost per life years saved (LYS), cost per quality-adjusted life years (QALYS), and cost per disability-adjusted life years (DALYS). The latter two outcome measures (QALYS and DALYS) assume that a life year in a fully functional state is different (more valuable) than a life year in an impaired state.

Will this approach work in all cases? No. It is possible for an alternative to yield an improved health benefit but to cost more. Will that approach be deemed cost-effective? No. Even though improved health may be worth the extra cost, it is not considered cost-effective, because it costs more. CEA is limited to evaluating less costly alternatives with at least the same outcome. It cannot comment on the advisability of more costly alternatives that provide better outcomes. This requires the skills of a well-informed manager to distinguish whether a more costly alternative is worth the investment.

Finally, many managed care programs are looking at CEA as a guide for deciding what treatments will be covered. CEA provides information to assist in decision making. It does not provide the answer. Although strictly allocating resources based on the results of CEAs may be problematic politically or ethically, CEA at least brings information to the table to inform the decision-making process. If an alternative is shown to be cost-effective, we know that it is a superior alternative because we get at least as good a result for a lower cost.

✳ COMPARATIVE EFFECTIVENESS RESEARCH

In recent years, a new approach has been developed called *comparative effectiveness research* (CER). This approach has been defined by the Institute of Medicine as "the generation and synthesis of evidence that compares the benefits and harms of alternative methods to prevent, diagnose, treat, and monitor a clinical condition or to improve the delivery of care. The purpose of CER is to assist consumers, clinicians, purchasers, and policy makers to make informed decisions that will improve health care at both the individual and population levels."[16] The essence of CER is to compare at least two alternative treatments to assess which provides the best outcomes for patients and which alternatives pose the greatest benefits and harms.

CER emphasizes measurement of effectiveness over efficacy. That is, the focus is not on whether or not the treatment works but on how effective it is. When CER considers costs, it goes beyond CEA, because it will sometimes favor a more expensive treatment if the extra value of that treatment exceeds its extra cost.[17] Because it measures both benefits and harms, CER represents a sophisticated approach to CBA.

Comparative effectiveness research does not consist of one specific research method. Rather, CER encompasses any or all of *nonexperimental studies* (observational settings), *experiments* (randomized and cluster randomized, as well as nonrandomized, controlled trials), and *synthesis* of existing studies (systematic reviews and meta-analysis, technology assessments, and decision analysis) in its effort to determine the most effective among alternative possible treatments. This approach holds great promise for nurse managers and executives because it can help them to make more informed decisions about what treatments work, the patients and populations for whom they work, and the settings or situations in which they work.

✳ IMPLICATIONS FOR NURSE MANAGERS AND EXECUTIVES

Budgeting in the 21st century requires a lot more than simply "minding the store." Nurse managers and executives must find ways to improve the performance of their units proactively. To do this, they need to understand productivity and productivity measurement and use the techniques of benchmarking, CBA, and CEA. They must consider CER to help make better decisions.

How does an HCO get to be outstanding? It must foster and facilitate innovation and improvement. Unless there is an environment that is supportive and even encouraging of change, progress is likely to be hampered severely. Many organizations like to say that they believe in innovation, but the culture they create stifles rather than rewards change. Suggestions for change are viewed as criticism of the way top management is doing its job. Often, such criticism is not welcomed. Staff quickly learns that it is wiser to be quiet and allow the waste and inefficiency they observe to continue. It should not be surprising that the most significant changes in organizations occur only after the top management has been replaced. At those times, the new top management can admit openly to problems and the need for change. After all, the existing problems can be attributed to those who have just left.

For change to occur, it is critically important for nurse managers and executives to assess their current situation. The better that existing processes are understood, the easier it is for the manager to be willing to take the risk of replacing some of them. Benchmarking is an invaluable aid, especially for organizations that are looking to make quick, significant improvement. The task of undertaking a benchmarking study is involved and can be costly. Most organizations are well advised to use benchmarking (at least competitive and cooperative

[16]Committee on Comparative Effectiveness Research Prioritization, Institute of Medicine. 2009. *Comparative Effectiveness Research*. Washington, DC: National Academic Press, p. 29.

[17]*Ibid.*, p. 34.

benchmarking) only when they believe there is potential room for significant improvement.

The true benefit of benchmarking does not come from knowing *how much* the benchmarking organization differs from the best practices organization that it studies. Rather, the benefit comes from understanding *how* it differs. Knowing that another organization has a lower cost does not really motivate managers to match that cost. It frustrates them because they have no idea how to match the cost. Clear efforts must be made to ensure that benchmarking is not just a tool for leverage to try to make staff work harder. Benchmarking should be used to show the way to true improvements in productivity.

Productivity assesses the amounts of inputs needed to produce an organization's outputs. HCOs need to work constantly on reducing the resources needed to provide high-quality patient care. Such improvements may come about from implementation of technological change or from low-tech changes in procedures. Nurse managers must develop an approach to measuring productivity so that changes in productivity can be monitored. The measure should also be meaningful. As discussed in this chapter, measures such as HPPD may be inadequate. If the real goal of improved productivity is to decrease the cost per patient, that goal must be incorporated into the measurement. One approach is to focus on unit costing. Ultimately, however, it is not measurement alone but rather improvement in productivity that is essential for healthy organizations.

Two techniques that are sometimes used by managers to help assess whether changes are likely to improve productivity are CBA and CEA. CBA is a technique that compares the benefits of a change with its costs. If the benefits are greater than the costs, the change is worthwhile. Often, however, managers will not be able to measure benefits. Benefits are particularly hard to value when human life is involved. What is a life really worth?

CEA has an appeal because it requires only that the manager estimate costs. In the cost-effectiveness approach, an alternative is evaluated to see if it produces at least as good a benefit as another alternative but for a lower cost. Nurse managers and executives may frequently find themselves faced with whether or not to make a change in the way a unit or organization does something. CEA is helpful because if the change will keep results as good as they currently are or better, the analysis needs to focus only on whether the change will cost less.

Another technique, CER, is a relatively new approach that compares least two alternative treatments to assess which provides the best outcomes for patients and which alternatives pose the greatest benefits and harms. Nurse managers and executives should consider published reports of CER as they make decisions, because CER can help them consider the practical implications of their decisions, including whether a treatment might work, the patients and populations for whom it might work, and the settings or situations in which it would work.

✳ KEY CONCEPTS

Benchmarking   A technique aimed at finding the best practices of other organizations and incorporating them into an organization.

Competitive benchmarking   Finding specific information about individual organizations providing the same services as your organization. Sometimes competitive benchmarking is done without direct permission.

Cooperative benchmarking   Seeking information from organizations in other industries that can be adapted to the health care industry to improve health care practices (e.g., to improve quality or reduce cost).

Collaborative benchmarking   Finding information within your industry but based on industry-wide statistics. In collaborative benchmarking, a number of organizations pool data so that all members of the pool can determine where they stand relative to the best members of the pool.

The benchmarking process   The process for benchmarking has been summarized by Camp as having 10 steps:

1. Decide what to benchmark.

2. Identify organizations with best practices.

3. Collect data for comparison.

4. Assess the gap between best practice and your performance.

5. Project likely improvement in best practices over the next 3 to 5 years.

6. Communicate findings.

7. Establish goals.

8. Create specific plans for improvement.

9. Implement plans.

10. Reestablish benchmarks as they change over time.

Productivity   The most common productivity measure is the amount of output produced by each unit of input.

$$\text{Productivity} = \frac{\text{Total outputs}}{\text{Total inputs}}$$

Productivity standards   Can be based on broad industry average experience, best industry practice, or simply the organization's budget. If an industry standard cannot be found, the productivity can be calculated as a percentage of the budget or of some perceived ideal.

Unit costing   More and more managers are choosing to stop looking at productivity simply in terms of inputs and outputs and to make sure that the cost per unit of service is considered in the calculation. The essence of this *unit costing* is that if we can lower the dollar cost of providing a unit of a specific service, we do not need to worry about things such as the number of care hours used to provide the service.

Productivity improvement   Working smarter, not harder, is the key to improving productivity. Learning how to do things more efficiently is likely to result in permanent productivity gains and should not require increased and often unsustainable individual efforts by employees.

Cost-benefit analysis (CBA) and cost-effectiveness analysis (CEA)   Methods that are used to consider the advantages and disadvantages of projected changes:

Cost-benefit analysis (CBA)   A method that compares the benefits related to a decision about a new project or other change to the costs of that decision. The method holds that the decision makes sense if the benefits related to the decision will exceed the costs. The key elements in performing a CBA are:

- Determining project goals
- Estimating project benefits
- Estimating project costs
- Discounting cost and benefit flows at an appropriate rate
- Completing the decision analysis

Cost-effectiveness analysis (CEA)   Argues that an approach that achieves a specific outcome for the least possible cost is cost-effective. Researchers have developed a variety of techniques to enable the comparison of outcomes across interventions, conditions, and diseases. With this ability, CEA can now go beyond simple comparisons of the cost per life saved to more precise comparisons of cost per life years saved (LYS), cost per quality-adjusted life years (QALYS), and cost per disability-adjusted life years (DALYS). The latter two outcome measures (QALYS and DALYS) assume that a life year in a fully functional state is different (more valuable) than a life year in an impaired state.

Comparative effectiveness research (CER)   "The generation and synthesis of evidence that compares the benefits and harms of alternative methods to prevent, diagnose, treat, and monitor a clinical condition or to improve the delivery of care. The purpose of CER is to assist consumers, clinicians, purchasers, and policy makers to make informed decisions that will improve health care at both the individual and population levels."[18]

---

[18]*Ibid.*, p. 29.

✳ SUGGESTED READINGS

Allred C, Arford P, Mauldin P, Goodwin L: Cost-effectiveness analysis in the nursing literature, 1992–1996, *Image J Nurs Sch* 30(3):235–242, 1998.

Boardman A, Greenberg D, Vining A, Weimer D: *Cost benefit analysis: concepts and practice*, ed 4, Upper Saddle River, New Jersey, 2011, Prentice Hall.

Buerhaus P: Milton Weinstein's insights on the development, use, and methodologic problems in cost-effectiveness analysis, *Image J Nurs Sch* 30(3): 223–227, 1998.

Camp R: *Benchmarking: the search for industry best practices that lead to superior performance*, Milwaukee, Wis, 1989, American Society for Quality Control.

Chatburn R, Ford R: Procedure to normalize data for benchmarking, *Respir Care* 51(2):145–157, 2006.

Chenoweth D, Garrett J: Cost-effectiveness analysis of a worksite clinic: is it worth the cost? *AAOHN J* 54(2):84–91, 2006.

Donaldson N, Brown D, Aydin C, et al: Leveraging nurse-related dashboard benchmarks to expedite performance improvement and document excellence, *J Nurs Adm* 35(4):163–172, 2005.

Folland S, Goodman A, Stano M: *The economics of health and health care*, ed 6, Upper Saddle River, NJ, 2010, Prentice Hall.

For best results, critically examine process behind benchmarking data, *Healthc Benchmarks* 5(3):29–32, 1998.

Gold M, Siegel J, Russell L, Weintein M: *Cost-effectiveness in health and medicine*, New York, 1996, Oxford University Press.

Hall L: Nursing intellectual capital: a theoretical approach for analyzing nursing productivity, *Nurs Econ* 21(1):14–19, 2003.

Hendrich A, Fay J, Sorrells A: Effects of acuity-adaptable rooms on flow of patients and delivery of care, *Am J Crit Care* 3(1):35–45, 2004.

Horngren C, Foster G, Datar S, et al: *Cost accounting*, ed 13, Englewood Cliffs, New Jersey, 2008, Prentice Hall.

Info-Line: Understanding benchmarking: the search for best practice, *Am Soc Train Dev* 92(7):5–6, 1992.

Kobs A: Getting started on benchmarking, *Outcomes Manag Nurs Pract* 2(1): 45–48, 1998.

McIntosh E, Donaldson C, Ryan M: Recent advances in the methods of cost-benefit analysis in healthcare. Matching the art to the science, *Pharmacoeconomics* 15(4): 357–367, 1999.

Mikesell J: *Fiscal administration*, ed 8, Boston, 2011, Wadsworth.

Moody R: Nurse productivity measures for the 21st century, *Health Care Manage Rev* 29(2):98–106, 2004.

Muennig P: *Cost-effectiveness analysis in health: a practical approach*, San Francisco, 2008, Jossey-Bass.

Ozcan Y: *Health care benchmarking and performance evaluation*, New York, 2008, Springer.

Pink G, Brown A, Daniel I, et al: Financial benchmarks for Ontario hospitals, *Healthc Q* 9(1):40–45, 2006.

Productivity standards can help forecast cuts in staffing, *Hosp Mater Manage* 14(7):10, 1989.

Rhoads J, Ferguson LA, Langford CA: Measuring nurse practitioner productivity, *Dermatol Nurs* 18(1):32–34, 37–38, 2006.

Ried W: QALYs versus HYEs—what's right and what's wrong. A review of the controversy, *J Health Econ* 17(5): 607–625, 1998.

Saul J: *Benchmarking for nonprofits: how to measure*, manage, and improve performance, St. Paul, 2004, Amherst H. Wilder Foundation.

Siegel J: Cost-effectiveness analysis and nursing research—is there a fit? *Image J Nurs Sch* 30(3):221–222, 1998.

Stapenhurst T: *The benchmarking book: a how-to guide to best practice for managers and practitioners*, Oxford, UK, 2009, Butterworth-Heinemann.

Stone P: Methods for conducting and reporting cost-effectiveness analysis in nursing, *Image J Nurs Sch* 30(3):229–234, 1998.

Warner K, Luce B: *Cost-benefit and cost-effectiveness analysis in health care: principles*, practice, and potential, Ann Arbor, Mich, 1982, Health Administration Press.

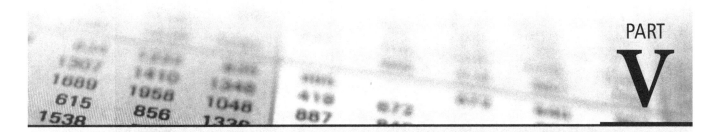

✳ MANAGING FINANCIAL RESOURCES

All managers of health care organizations (HCOs) manage resources. Determining which personnel and other resources to use and how to use them is a managerial function. Financial resources also represent a subset of organizational resources. To the same extent that clinical and human resources must be used carefully, financial resources must be managed efficiently.

Decisions concerning where and how to get financial resources is a key management concern for nurse managers and executives. Some resources in for-profit HCOs come from investments owners make in the organization. In not-for-profit HCOs, a common source of financial resources is charitable donations. Profits are a potential source of financial resources for all types of HCOs. It is also common for HCOs to borrow money to finance their operations.

When an organization has financial resources, it must manage them efficiently. Decisions must be made concerning how much cash to have on hand. Management techniques must ensure that cash is received as promptly as possible. Managers must ensure that cash is available when needed for purposes such as employee payrolls and loan repayments. This requirement to have control over the inflow and outflow of cash necessitates management of other assets and liabilities that directly affect cash. As a result, receivables, inventories, marketable securities, payables, and leases fall under the heading of management of financial resources.

Although some managers may perceive the management of financial resources as the strict domain of financial managers, that way of thinking is short-sighted. For example, a financial manager can do little to control inventory levels. Nurse managers and executives are in a much better position to make determinations regarding necessary inventory levels and to enforce policies established to prevent unnecessary stockpiling of inventory. The current health care environment requires that nurse and financial managers work together in the management of financial resources to arrive at an optimal outcome for the organization.

In addition, nurse managers and executives should be aware of even those aspects of the management of financial resources that do not bear directly on their day-to-day activities. For example, organizational decisions to borrow money or invest it may seem to have little direct bearing on the nurse manager's

daily work. However, the reality is that the organizational decisions such as these concerning the allocation of resources to various cost centers is essential to unit operations; the ability of the nurse manager or executive to acquire the supplies, personnel, and related resources needed to care for patients; and the success of the organization. Therefore, it is beneficial for nurse managers and executives to be aware of the "bigger picture" of organizational resources, and the factors involved in the management of financial resources.

This part of the book is divided into two chapters. Chapter 19 focuses directly on the management of the short-term financial resources of an organization. Chapter 20 is concerned with the long-term financing of HCOs.

Short-term financial resources appear in the current asset and current liability sections of the balance sheet. Such resources generally provide or require cash within a relatively short period, usually less than 1 year. These short-term resources and short-term sources of resources are referred to as the organization's *working capital*.

Long-term financing relates to the alternatives the organization has for acquiring financial resources that will not have to be repaid within less than 1 year. To be able to acquire capital assets—buildings and equipment—the organization must know that it can acquire money that does not have to be repaid in a short time. The choices it makes regarding such long-term financing can have dramatic effects on the ability of the organization to provide health care services and to compete in the health care marketplace.

Given the changes in health care financing that will result from health care reform efforts and a constantly changing economic climate, managers must be prepared now and in the future to act in response to those changes and to proactively manage resources in ways that position their organizations favorably for the future. Many organizations are faced with reducing the number of personnel, reducing or eliminating equipment purchases, and cutting their overall budgets. Nurse managers and executives need knowledge of both short- and long-term financing to understand how they can best manage nursing and patient care resources in the most efficient and effective manner possible and, in turn, help position their organizations to thrive in a constantly changing health care environment.

Short-Term Financial Resources

CHAPTER GOALS

The goals of this chapter are to:

- Define *working capital* and *working capital management*
- Describe the role of cash in the organization
- Explain techniques for cash management
- Distinguish between cash flows and revenues and expenses
- Describe the cash budgeting process

- Provide a description of the elements of accounts receivable management
- Discuss factors related to efficient inventory management
- Define trade credit terms related to accounts payable
- Discuss elements of working capital management for other current liabilities

✳ INTRODUCTION

Working capital is the organization's current assets and current liabilities. *Net working capital* is the current assets less the current liabilities. The term *working capital management* refers to the management of the organization's current assets and current liabilities. (A basic discussion of current assets and current liabilities is provided in Chapter 6.)

Working capital is sometimes referred to as *cash register money*. When a store opens for business, there must be some money in the cash register to make change for the first customer who makes a purchase. In addition, some customers may charge their purchases. In those cases, the store will not receive any cash immediately, but it still must pay its suppliers for the items it has acquired for sale, and it also has to pay its employees. There must be adequate cash for the store to use during the lag time between when it must pay for its resources and when it receives cash from its customers.

The cash resources of an organization are of concern to all of its managers. Why should a nurse manager or executive be concerned with issues such as cash flow and inventory levels? All organizations have limited resources. If intensive care unit nurses stockpile certain supplies, the organization will pay out more cash now for inventory than is otherwise necessary. This in turn could mean that medical-surgical nurses will be told that there is no cash available to buy their needed supplies. Nurses sometimes cope with this situation by stockpiling supplies so they will have the supplies needed to care for patients. This creates a vicious cycle. Because all nurses try to keep high levels of inventory to protect their patients, the overall inventories are maintained at levels that are higher than needed. This

means that money has been spent to support higher-than-needed inventories rather than deposited in a bank and earning interest. The lost interest means that there is less total money available to purchase supplies. A cooperative working relationship is needed throughout the organization to allow inventory levels to be maintained at adequate levels and money to be available for purchases when needed without wasting resources by keeping unduly high inventory levels.

One can envision a working capital cycle (Figure 19–1) in which cash is used to buy inventory items such as clinical supplies. Then patients are treated, consuming inventory items and using employees' services. Then the organization bills patients and waits to collect payment. Finally, cash is received, and the cycle starts again.

Working capital management is the role of the manager to ensure that there is adequate cash on hand to meet the organization's needs and minimize the cost of those resources. To do this, the manager must carefully control cash inflows and outflows. To be efficient, cash must not lie idle, so there should not be too much cash on hand. Cash not immediately needed should be invested, earning a return for the organization. Similarly, excess inventory should not be kept by the organization. The money spent to pay for inventory that is not needed can be used by the organization for some other purpose. Receivables from customers should be collected promptly so that the organization will have that cash available for its use.

By the same token, current liabilities must be managed carefully. The organization desires to have sufficient cash to pay its obligations when they are due. However, if the organization pays its bills before they are due, it will lose the interest it could

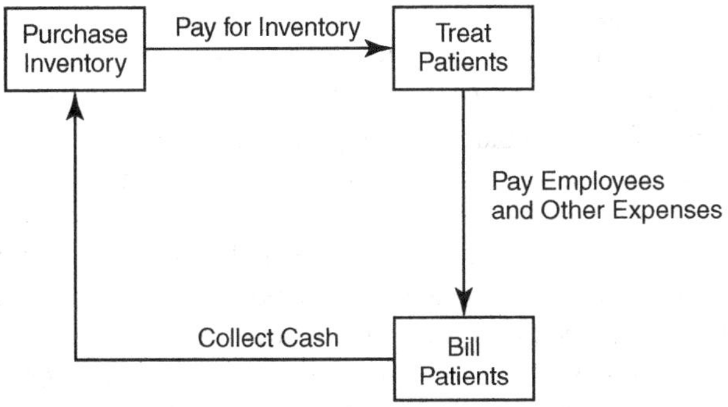

FIGURE 19–1. Working capital cycle.

have earned if it had invested its cash for a little longer rather than paying the obligation.

This chapter focuses on the management of all elements of working capital. The discussion begins with current assets. Then we will turn our attention to issues related to current liabilities.

✳ CURRENT ASSETS

A number of current assets require careful management, but the most essential financial resource is cash. Cash is generally defined as both currency and balances available in bank accounts for withdrawal upon demand (e.g., checking accounts). Organizations must have cash to pay obligations as they come due.

Other current assets that require careful management include marketable securities, accounts receivable, and inventory. Marketable securities provide managers with an outlet to invest idle resources while maintaining access to the resources when needed. Accounts receivable often constitute the largest single element of working capital. Inventories also receive a great amount of attention because historically, managers have had difficulty in managing them.

Cash and Marketable Securities

Organizations have cash requirements for three main purposes:

- Transactions
- Safety
- Investments

Cash must be available for transactions—that is, the day-to-day normal operating expenses of the organization such as staff payroll and supplies and services from vendors. A health care organization (HCO) cannot wait to receive patient payments before paying many of the organization's obligations; cash is needed for that purpose.

Safety is the second reason for holding cash. Managers are unable to anticipate all of the organization's needs. Emergencies may require immediate, unexpected cash outlays. In some situations, managers may anticipate the likelihood of the event but not know exactly when it will occur. In other cases, the event may be totally unanticipated. Experience has proved that it is wise for an organization to have immediate access to cash just in case an unexpected need arises.

The third purpose for holding cash is to have cash available if a desirable investment opportunity arises. Such an opportunity may be the possibility of earning an attractive profit, or it may relate to the possibility of providing services to the community.

Given these reasons to hold cash, managers might desire to keep large amounts available just to be safe. However, that is not necessarily an optimal approach. Cash does not generate a return for the organization. Often it sits in a non–interest-bearing checking account. Even if it is kept in a savings account, the rate of return is likely to be minimal. If the organization wants to maximize the benefits from all its resources, it must minimize the extent to which it has unproductive assets.

Therefore, there is a conflict in cash management. The more cash on hand, the safer the organization but the lower its return on the money it has invested in its buildings, equipment, investments, and other assets, and also the less health care services it can provide to the community. The less cash the organization chooses to keep on hand, the better its financial profits and the more health care services provided but the higher the risk. There is less protection against unexpected cash needs. Managers must walk a fine line, attempting to determine a reasonable cash balance and keeping neither too much nor too little cash.

In a well-run organization, cash is actively managed. An initial projection is made regarding the timing of cash receipts from philanthropy, investments, patients, the government, and insurance companies. A projection of the organization's required payments must also be prepared. The cash excess or shortfall is calculated for each period of time.

If a shortfall is anticipated, it may be possible to go to a bank and arrange for a line of credit to be available at the time cash is projected to be needed. Before such a loan is secured, however, other approaches should be considered. Can the financial managers take actions to process patient billings more quickly so that payments will be received sooner? Will the extra cost of speedier invoicing be offset by the interest saved by borrowing less money from the bank? What if payments to the organization's vendors are delayed by 30 days to avoid borrowing money? How angry will that make the organization's vendors?

If a cash surplus is forecast, it can be invested to earn interest, used to repay loans, or used to provide more health care services. Financial managers must ensure that the organization always has enough cash to meet obligations, but they should also be careful to ensure that the organization is not missing opportunities to provide additional health services because it is keeping too much cash in the bank. Either too little or too much cash leaves the organization in a less than optimal situation.

Short-Term Cash Investment

Cash should rarely if ever be kept in non–interest-bearing accounts. In fact, even after checks are written, it is possible to invest the money in the interim period until the check is cashed. That period is called the *float*. Many banks have arrangements that allow money to be automatically transferred into a checking account as checks are presented for payment. Until that point, the money can remain in an interest-bearing savings account. However, with the advent of electronic funds transfers and the conversion of checks to electronic payments, use of the float by organizations is becoming more and more limited.

Managers should make great efforts to ensure that cash is deposited into interest-bearing accounts as quickly as possible and withdrawn only when actually needed. All organizations should have specific policies that result in cash and check receipts being processed and deposited promptly.

Interest-bearing bank accounts pay relatively low rates of interest. Many alternatives are available for health care managers to invest cash at a higher rate of return. In most cases, however, this requires reducing the organization's ability to get immediate access to the cash. Short-term investments include treasury bills, certificates of deposit (CDs), and repurchase agreements. Treasury bills are issued for 1 year or less, with current maturities of 4 weeks, 13 weeks, and 26 weeks. However, they are traded actively, making it easy to convert them into cash when necessary. CDs generally tie up the organization's money for at least 1 month. However, CDs often pay interest rates higher than treasury bills. Repurchase agreements are flexible bank-related financial instruments. They can be for periods as short as 1 day. However, their interest rates are generally lower than those of treasury bills.

It is also possible for HCOs to invest in other types of marketable securities such as corporate stocks and bonds. However, managers must exercise care in making such investments because they are subject to market rate fluctuations; that is, their value might fall while they are invested. In a particularly volatile market, or one in which stock prices fluctuate greatly, this can be especially risky. Although a reduction in investment value may be recovered if the securities are held for a period of time, the organization may well suffer a loss if it must liquidate the investment to get the cash. In general, risk and return represent a tradeoff in investments. To earn a higher return on invested money, one must be willing to take a greater risk with the initial principal investment.

Cash Flow versus Revenue and Expense

Cash management concentrates on the inflows and outflows of cash. This is in contrast to the operating budget focus on revenues and expenses. Operating budgets consider overall profitability, but they do not consider when payments are made. Therefore, the manager cannot use them to determine whether adequate cash will be available at any given point in time for the organization's needs.

At times cash management may cause the organization to make decisions that directly affect nurse managers and that seem to make no sense. For example, consider a request by the nursing department to buy bedside computers for several nursing units at a total cost of $200,000. The computers are expected to have a useful lifetime of 10 years and will improve the quality of documentation. This will result in improved care and will decrease overtime required for charting by $40,000 per year. The $400,000 of reduced overtime over the 10-year period is enough to make the initial investment of $200,000 financially sensible. Yet the financial officers may say that the organization cannot afford the computers. How can that decision make any sense?

Even though the computers would save more money than their cost, it is not clear that the organization can afford to purchase them. The entire price of $200,000 for the computers will have to be paid in cash this year even though the overtime savings are expected to be only $40,000 this year. Where will the cash for the initial $200,000 purchase come from?

The potential for reduced costs or for increased profits does not by itself provide the cash needed to make the investment. It might be wise to lease the asset rather than pay all the cash up front, especially in light of rapid changes in health care information technologies and the costs of maintaining and upgrading both software and hardware. Maybe the organization can borrow the money from a bank. Perhaps it can raise the money through contributions. Although the organization's managers should try to pursue various ways to get the cash for worthwhile investments—whether they are worthwhile because they are profitable or simply because they are good for patients—there is a responsibility to the well-being of the organization not to spend the money until it is first determined that there will be sufficient cash available to spend.

Financial officers must carefully consider the cash implications of the operating and capital budgets before they are approved. In effect, various departments submit their operating and capital budget requests. A cash budget is developed based on those requests. One reason that departmental budgets may be rejected is that the cash budget may show that the organization will simply run out of cash if it makes all the requested payments. If an organization finds itself without cash to meet its obligations, it may be forced into bankruptcy. Even if the organization is making a profit, without careful management, it may run out of cash and get into financial difficulty.

Cash Budgets

Given the importance of cash balances, HCOs generally prepare a cash budget for the entire coming year on a monthly basis. The format of cash budgets is fairly standard. Each month begins with a starting cash balance. The expected cash receipts for the month are added to this. These receipts may be broken down into categories such as inpatient, outpatient, other operating, and non-operating or by payer (e.g., Medicare, Medicaid, Blue Cross, other insurers, self-pay patients, donations, and cafeteria sales). The starting cash balance is added to the total receipts to get a subtotal of available cash. Then expected cash payments are subtracted (see Chapter 12).

Accurate cash budgeting requires managers to estimate how much cash will be received by type of payer. Different types of payers have different bad debt rates and pay on different schedules. For example, one insurance company might pay an organization more promptly than Medicare but less promptly than other private insurance companies. Payer mix information, combined with knowledge about the lag time in payment by each type of payer, can be used to project cash receipts for each month.

For example, suppose that an HCO had revenues of $500,000 in January and that the payer mix is as shown in Table 19–1. The payment lag times represent averages. Especially with respect to self-pay patients, there is likely to be a mix of faster and slower paying patients. Assuming that there are no bad debts, when will the $500,000 in revenue from January be received in cash?

❋ TABLE 19–1 *Payment Lag by Payer*

Payer	Percentage of Patients	Payment Lag Time (months)
Medicare	30	3
Medicaid	20	4
MCOs	25	2
Other insurers	10	1
Self-pay	15	3

MCOs, managed care organizations.

The timing of these receipts is shown in Table 19–2. The payers with a 1-month lag will pay in February, those with a 2-month lag in March, those with a 3-month lag in April, and those with a 4-month lag in May. For example, a total of $225,000 from January revenues would be collected in April, because in this example, both Medicare and self-pay patients pay with a 3-month lag.

If the expected cash balance for any month exceeds the minimum desired balance, the excess can be invested. This is true even if a surplus one month is followed by an expected shortfall the next. It may pay to invest the extra cash in a very short-term investment, such as a money market fund. In that way, the excess cash from one month can earn some interest and still be available to meet the shortage the next month. Borrowing can thus be avoided or minimized.

Maintaining Security over Cash

Of all the assets the organization has, cash requires the greatest care to ensure that it is not misappropriated. Systems must be put into place that have checks and balances. Individuals who handle cash should be different from those who reconcile cash receipts. Controls should exist for both cash receipts and cash disbursements.

Disbursements are often easier to protect. Whenever possible, payments should be made by check. Large checks should require two signatures. All checks should be numbered. All checks should require an authorization by someone other than the one involved in drawing the checks.

Cash receipts should be handled by individuals who are bonded, reliable and take vacations. Bonding is an insurance procedure that protects the organization from cash theft by the insured individual. The organization must have trustworthy individuals working in the cash area. Even with trustworthy individuals, it is a good practice to require individuals to take

vacations. Knowing that someone else will be handling the function while they are on vacation makes individuals less likely to do anything inappropriate that might be discovered in their absence.

Accounts Receivable

When an organization's customers do not pay for goods or services at the time they are provided, they are said to be buying the services "on account." An account is set up by both the buyer and the seller to keep track of the amount owed. Providers of the service expect to ultimately receive payment, so they call the money owed them an *account receivable*. Buyers will ultimately pay the amount owed, so they have an *account payable*.

Management of accounts receivable focuses on speed, accuracy, and communication. Managers must try to minimize the time between provision of care and ultimate receipt of payment. Accounts receivable earn no return for the organization. The sooner cash is collected, the sooner the organization can use that cash for its operations or invest it. Also, efforts to collect cash quickly tend to reduce bad debts. For accounts to be collected on a timely basis, all documentation must be accurate and complete. Also, there should be great efforts to keep the lines of communication open between the organization and the payers.

The process of managing accounts receivable should start before a patient is admitted to an HCO. Preadmission data collection is one of the most important activities an organization can undertake to ensure efficient collection of its accounts. Another essential feature is the establishment of credit policies. Which patients is the organization willing to treat, and under what circumstances? During a patient's course of treatment, there should be ongoing data collection. When a patient is discharged, there should be a review to ensure comprehensive inclusion of charges, and a bill should be issued. Receivables management does not stop at this point. Receivables should be monitored while outstanding using an aging schedule. If necessary, the organization should use a collection agency to collect delinquent accounts. When cash does arrive, there should be specific procedures to safeguard it until its ultimate deposit in the bank. These elements are discussed next.

Preadmission Data Collection

The process of managing accounts receivable should start before a patient is admitted to a health care institution. Many organizations have a conference with the patient to determine the sources of payment for the patient's care. Patients may have Medicare, Medicaid, or other insurance coverage. If that is

❋ TABLE 19–2 *Timing of Cash Receipt for January Revenues*

Payer	Percentage of Patients		Total Revenue		Revenue Share	Month Collected
Medicare	30	×	$500,000	=	$150,000	April
Medicaid	20	×	500,000	=	100,000	May
MCOs	25	×	500,000	=	125,000	March
Other insurers	10	×	500,000	=	50,000	February
Self-pay	15	×	500,000	=	75,000	April

MCOs, managed care organizations.

the case, all pertinent information should be recorded so that upon discharge, a bill can be processed expeditiously. All forms should be completed, signatures obtained, and insurance companies called to verify coverage and obtain all necessary preadmission approvals. Many managed care organizations (MCOs) deny coverage if the patient was admitted without prenotification to the company.

In some cases, it may be determined that the patient is eligible for Medicaid but has not enrolled. Many HCOs have specific policies regarding helping patients enroll for Medicaid. In fact, some hospitals actually have state Medicaid employees working in the hospital to enroll patients. Enrolling an eligible patient often represents the difference between a substantial payment for the care provided to that patient and receiving little payment, if any at all.

If the patient has no insurance coverage, financial planning for payment can take place at the preadmission conference. In some cases, this means establishing a payment schedule so that patients can pay what they can afford over an extended period. In some cases, it is determined that patients have no capacity to pay, and they will be classified as indigent for medical purposes. In that case, their care will be considered charity care. Some states provide financial assistance to HCOs to reimburse some part of the charity care provided. However, careful documentation is required so that a claim can be filed properly. It is now common for patient bills to be sent electronically, decreasing the time from billing to payment.

Credit Policies

Some medical care is true emergency care, and standards in the United States require that such care be provided regardless of the patient's ability to pay. This certainly is justified on moral and ethical grounds. Other care, however, is elective. Health care providers have greater ethical and legal latitude in deciding what non-emergency care to provide to whom. At the opposite extreme from emergency care are procedures that are desired by individuals for personal reasons but are not indicated for health reasons, such as cosmetic surgery. Few would blame an HCO that refused to provide cosmetic surgery to an indigent patient.

Health care organizations must establish clear rules that guide their decisions on whether to offer credit to patients. These rules must reflect both the financial and the medical condition of the patient. There should be a clear policy on when patients are treated regardless of their ability to pay and when they are not. Some organizations are more permissive than others for a variety of reasons. For example, one organization may have a better financial position than another and be better able to afford to provide charity care. Other organizations may have a mission to provide care to patients who cannot pay.

To carry out the organization's credit policy, preadmission data collection is essential. In addition to providing the information needed for prompt, accurate billing, it provides information the organization needs to make decisions about when to provide care. Although it is distasteful to have to deny any care to anyone, it is a reality of the health care system. Organizations have credit policies to protect the organization so it can remain in business and continue to provide essential care to all.

Ongoing Data Collection

During a patient's course of treatment, there should be continuous collection of data. The organization must track the services that the patient is consuming so that they may be properly included in the patient's bill.

If data collection is postponed until discharge or shortly thereafter, there is the risk that some charges will be overlooked. The number of patient days, radiographs, and laboratory tests must all be accumulated on an ongoing basis.

Nursing has always had a responsibility to participate in this ongoing data collection in a number of ways. Inventory items used are recorded on the patient chart. Charge slips for various procedures are also often placed in the chart by the nursing staff. In organizations with sophisticated health care information systems in place, this charge may be generated electronically when nursing care is charted or a supply is retrieved. In organizations with less sophisticated information systems, this type of charge must be made manually. Although it may seem cumbersome to have to place a charge slip for a catheter on the patient's chart, without that step, the patient will not be billed for the item. In that case, the organization will lose that money and have fewer resources available for the provision of patient care. Even if charges are made at negotiated rates for MCOs and other payers, this step remains important. Often the negotiated rate is a percent discount from full rates. Collecting 70% of the charge is better than collecting 0%. Also, it is easier to negotiate rates if management has a good knowledge of what resources patients consume.

This role is likely to grow in the future as variable billing for nursing services becomes more widely used. Specifically, to charge for nursing services, it is necessary to have information on patients' consumption of nursing resources. This is generally obtained from the patient classification system. Although most acute care hospitals have such systems, they may not actively use them. To charge patients for nursing, information on their daily classification level must be accumulated on an ongoing basis.

Discharge Review and Billing

At discharge, a number of activities must take place in short order. The original patient payment information must be reviewed to ensure that it is complete. Something as minor as a missing zip code in the patient address could lead to a payment delay of several months or more.

The diagnosis of the patient must be firmly and clearly established at discharge. Medicare Diagnosis Related Group (DRG) payments for inpatients rely on the DRG assignment. That assignment in turn relies on a number of factors recorded in the medical report, such as principal and secondary diagnoses, surgical procedures, and age. If any of those elements is missing, a DRG cannot properly be assigned, and payment will be delayed. When a patient bill is "kicked out" of the system, a payment delay of at least several months is the rule rather than the exception.

When the record has been reviewed and found to be complete with respect to both payer information and clinical information, a bill should be promptly issued. This information may even be transmitted electronically, eliminating the entire time that a bill would normally be in transit. Many large payers now accept electronic billing, rather than requiring paper bills. Some payers require electronic submission of bills.

Even a savings of 2 or 3 days can have a significant impact. For any one bill, it does not seem to matter if there are a few delays. However, when all bills are considered, the impact of prompt billing is significant. For example, suppose that a large hospital issues $200 million in patient billings each year. Also assume that the hospital has outstanding loans from banks at a 10% interest rate. If electronic processing of bills directly to payers means that each bill is collected 3 days sooner than it otherwise would be, and the money is used to pay down the outstanding loans, the interest savings would be more than $164,000 a year! ($200 million × 10% ÷ 365 = $54,800 interest per day; $54,800 × 3 days is approximately $164,000 per year.)

Electronic processing is only one element. Consider a hospital that processes laboratory charges only once a month. Bills for patients discharged in January could not be issued until laboratory charges are processed for January. That might not be completed until February 5. Then all the laboratory charges would have to be posted to the individual patient accounts. That might take another week. It is conceivable that in a totally manual system, it might well be February 15 until any bills are issued for patients discharged any time in January. On average, it would be a month after discharge until a patient bill was issued.

Delaying billing by a month delays receipt of cash by a month. In a hospital with $200 million in net patient revenues, such a delay could cost over $1.5 million per year. It should be no surprise that most HCOs have automated data entry and billing systems. Every day earlier that bills can be issued saves a significant amount of money.

Aging of Receivables

After bills have been issued, it is important for the organization to monitor receivables and to follow up on unpaid bills. This is true not only for self-pay patients, who are viewed as bad debt risks, but also for the government and insurers. Often the large third-party payers will not pay a bill if they find any problem with it. The HCO must be on top of receivables to ensure that any problems preventing specific bills from being paid are resolved.

A tool used to keep track of potential accounts receivable problems is an *aging schedule*. An aging schedule shows how long a receivable has been outstanding since a bill was issued. For example, at the end of June, a summary aging schedule might look like the example in Table 19–3.

The aging schedule allows managers to monitor outstanding receivables. In Table 19–3, we notice that only 53.4% of the receivables outstanding are outstanding for less than 1 month. Almost half the receivables are outstanding more than 30 days since the date the bills were issued. On the other hand, a relatively small 3% of outstanding receivables are more than 90 days old.

If large payers constitute a significant portion of the organization's revenue, the organization should attempt to arrange for periodic interim payments (PIPs). In a PIP arrangement, the payer makes payments in advance of the receipt and processing of specific bills. For instance, in the example in Table 19–3, the hospital might find that every month, it bills MCOs for about $700,000. Rather than wait for the billings, each month, the MCOs might issue a payment of perhaps $500,000 for care to patients during the current month. The balance to be paid for each month's care would wait until the specific bills are received. This PIP practice allows the HCO to receive its revenues in cash sooner than would otherwise be the case. Unfortunately, in recent years, payers, also under financial pressure, have been reluctant to make PIPs.

The over-90-days category in the aging schedule is a particular concern even though it is a small part of the total. These accounts probably reflect problems encountered in processing the bills by third-party payers or inability or unwillingness to pay by self-pay

✳ **TABLE 19–3** *Sample Aging Schedule: June 30 Aging Report*

Payer	1–30 Days	31–60 Days	61–90 Days	>90 Days	Total
By Total Dollars					
Medicare	$ 802,054	$ 795,633	$402,330	$ 52,050	$2,052,067
Medicaid	325,020	342,943	85,346	28,345	781,654
MCOs	682,285	114,583	14,354	4,364	815,541
Other insurers	437,899	46,722	8,563	7,773	500,957
Self-pay	174,799	103,295	67,322	43,588	389,004
Total	$2,422,057	$1,403,131	$577,915	$136,120	$4,539,223
By Percent					
Medicare	17.7%	17.5%	8.9%	1.1%	45.2%
Medicaid	7.2	7.6	1.9	0.6	17.2
MCOs	15.0	2.5	0.3	0.1	18.0
Other insurers	9.6	1.0	0.2	0.2	11.0
Self-pay	3.9	2.3	1.5	1.0	8.6
Total	53.4%	30.9%	12.7%	3.0%	100.0%

MCOs, managed care organizations.

patients. The HCO should have specific follow-up procedures, which should include sending monthly statements and making phone calls to determine why payment has not been made.

Some of this process can be avoided if indigent patients are clearly identified in advance. Although the HCO will want to pursue individuals who can pay for the care they receive, it is a costly waste of effort to spend resources trying to collect payment from truly indigent patients.

In some cases, it is necessary to use a collection agency if other efforts have failed and it is believed that the patient can afford to make payments. This is a costly approach, because collection agencies retain as much as half of all amounts they are successful in collecting.

Cash Receipt and Lock Boxes

When cash arrives, there should be specific procedures to safeguard it. One common approach is to direct all payments to a lock box. This is generally a post office box that is emptied directly by the bank. The bank removes the payments and processes them directly to the organization's account. The paperwork associated with the payment is then forwarded to the organization.

There are two key advantages to this approach. First, because the bank empties the boxes at least once a day, the receipts are deposited to interest-bearing accounts immediately, rather than sitting in a business office for several days or weeks until they are deposited. Second, there is a substantially decreased risk that receipts will be lost or stolen. Maintaining security over cash resources is a key element of working capital management.

Inventory

The last major current asset category is inventory. This is the category with which nurses are often directly involved. HCOs tend to have a wide variety of inventory items, such as clinical supplies, drugs, office supplies, food, and housekeeping supplies. The cost of inventory in HCOs is generally much smaller than the amount of accounts receivable. Nevertheless, careful inventory management can result in significant savings. A general rule of thumb is that inventory levels should be kept as low as possible, consistent with patient needs. The less inventory on hand, the less money tied up in inventory.

The major problem HCOs face with respect to inventory is the unpredictability of patient flow and patient needs. If the organization runs out of an item, its unavailability could mean the difference between life and death. However, that fact is sometimes used to justify excessive stockpiles of a wide variety of inventory items that do not have life-and-death implications. Management needs to develop a system that ensures that inventory is available when needed but also that it is used efficiently and that levels are kept as low as possible.

Inventory should be ordered and stored in a central area whenever possible. Although ready access to supplies justifies maintaining some items in a number of different areas, the amount in each area should be the bare minimum, with restocking from one central point. Otherwise, each area will have a large inventory, and resources will needlessly be tied up in inventory that may not be used for weeks or even months. This

is an area that is sometimes difficult for staff nurses. Nurses do not like to run out of supplies. Although electronic inventory systems can help with the management of inventory and limit stockpiling, use of such systems may still not eliminate it completely. The nurse manager must balance staff nurse needs for immediate access to supplies with the organization's needs to control inventory costs.

Perpetual Inventory

One approach that can be helpful is maintenance of a perpetual inventory of high-cost items. With a perpetual inventory, each use of an item is recorded (usually electronically) and a running balance maintained. This allows the organization to know how much it has of each item at any point in time. Reordering can take place when inventory falls below a certain level.

Generally, less inventory is required when a perpetual system is used. There is less need to hold a large safety stock because the manager always knows how much inventory is available. Reordering can take place whenever inventory of an item is low. Without a perpetual system, it is necessary to take a physical count of inventory to determine how much is available. That is a costly, time-consuming process that is not frequently undertaken.

Perpetual inventory systems are costly and time-consuming as well. However, automated systems have reduced the cost of such perpetual systems substantially. Some hospitals, for example, use uniform price codes (bar codes) to automatically update their perpetual inventory records as each item is used. If inventory is maintained on an automated perpetual system, managers have greater control over their stock and therefore can get by with less of each item.

Economic Order Quantity

Inventory not only entails a cash outlay when it is acquired but is associated with other, less well-recognized costs: It must be stored. That requires physical storage space. Over time, inventory may become damaged or obsolete or its expiration date may pass. There are costs related to placing an order and having it shipped. There are potentially high costs of running out of an item. These many factors can be balanced using a method called the *economic order quantity (EOQ)*.

EOQ is a quantitative technique that weighs all the pros and cons of ordering large amounts of inventory infrequently versus ordering small amounts more frequently. The result of an EOQ calculation is the optimal number of units that should be ordered each time an item is restocked and how frequently orders should be made. Horngren and Foster[1] describe five categories of costs associated with supplies: (1) cost of the product, (2) ordering costs, (3) carrying costs, (4) stockout costs, and (5) quality costs. *Cost of the product*— that is, what the organization must pay for the product—can be affected by quantity discounts and timing of payment. *Ordering costs* include costs associated with placing the order,

---

[1] Horngren C, Foster G. 1990. *Cost Accounting: A Managerial Emphasis*, 7th edition. Englewood Cliffs, NJ: Prentice Hall, p. 741.

such as clerk time for preparation of a purchase order. *Carrying costs* are often called *opportunity costs* and are costs of having money tied up in inventory rather than in a revenue-producing endeavor such as an interest-bearing bank account. They also include other costs such as insurance on the inventory and rent of the space where it is stored. *Stockout costs* are costs incurred when inventory is not available but is needed. If this is a supply item that the nurse must have for patient care, often the supply must be purchased at a higher price from a local vendor when the unit runs out of stock. Finally, *quality costs* are costs incurred to ensure that the product is of the required quality. These may include costs such as inspection or replacement costs and the costs associated with patient harm done because a low-quality item was used.

Nurse managers are most often concerned with stockouts. Because many of the supplies used have a direct impact on the quality of patient care provided, nurse managers are particularly sensitive to this issue. In some cases, supplies are not readily available from other sources. Patient care may then suffer, or a patient may need to be transferred to another institution and revenues will be lost. Although the manager cannot predict with certainty what supplies will be needed, previous experience and expectations about future patient care needs can be used to estimate supply needs.

At the unit level, the nurse manager is usually concerned with balancing the space required to store supplies with the goal of avoiding a stockout. The following example shows how to calculate the reorder point for catheter kits. Suppose that the nurse manager knows that the unit usually uses about 0.2 catheter kits per patient day.

Identify the average daily census on the unit: 25
Identify average catheter kits/patient day: 0.2
Calculate daily usage = Census × Usage per patient day
    = 25 × 0.2
    = 5 kits needed per day

Identify safe level of supply on unit: 10
Identify lead time to order supplies: 2 days
Reorder point = (Lead time × Average daily use) + Safe level
    = (2 × 5) + 10 = 20

Assuming that the census remains at about 25, catheter kits should be reordered when there are 20 remaining. This simple approach to determine inventory supplies, however, does not tell the manager how much to order. The amount ordered is based on a calculation that takes into account the carrying costs or the ordering costs.

EOQ is an approach to determine the balance between ordering costs and carrying costs. The goal of inventory control is to minimize costs while avoiding a stockout. The manager estimates the optimal quantity of supplies to order and lead time necessary to place that order. For example, suppose that based on historical use, the nurse manager on a medical-surgical unit knows that when the unit has 25 patients, the staff uses 5,000 syringes per year. It takes 2 days from the time the request is made to the time the supplies reach the floor. Preparing a central supply request costs $5 of a clerk's time. The central accounting office has determined that the organization currently borrows money at a rate of 10% to pay some of its bills and that it costs the organization $0.50 per unit of inventory for insurance, storage, and other carrying costs per year. This $0.50 includes 10% interest on the average inventory level.

Table 19–4 shows an example of the calculations that can be used to estimate the balance between ordering costs and carrying costs. **A** is defined as the demand for the supply for the year. **E** is the size of each order. Therefore, the average inventory on hand is **E ÷ 2**. There is one purchase order for each order, so the total number of purchase orders per year will be **A ÷ E**. The cost of placing orders is the cost per purchase order (**P**) multiplied by the number of orders (**A ÷ E**). The total cost of carrying inventory is the cost to carry one unit for 1 year (**S**) multiplied by the average inventory level (**E ÷ 2**). The total inventory costs, **C**, in addition to the purchase price of the units, is the order cost **P × (A ÷ E)** plus the carrying costs **S × (E ÷ 2)**. The nurse manager has estimated that the demand (**A**) for syringes is about 5,000 per year (or about 14 per day). In the example shown, each column represents a different possible order size (**E**): 50, 316, and 5,000.

The easiest approach might appear to be the third alternative: order once per year. If you need 5,000 units for the year and you order 5,000 at one time, you only need to place one order a year. In that case, the total ordering cost would be $5. However, the average inventory on hand would be 2,500 syringes. That would result in high carrying costs of $1,250. The total cost for ordering and carrying the inventory is $1,255. This does not include the cost of the syringes, which will be the same for all of the alternatives. At the other extreme, an order of 50 syringes is sufficient stock for the unit. The costs to the organization of that alternative are $513.

Both the first and the third alternatives are substantially more expensive than the EOQ, which is 316 (cost = $159). Ordering a little more than once per month (16 times per year) will minimize the costs of inventory. The EOQ of 316 is calculated with the following formula:

$$EOQ = \sqrt{\frac{2AP}{S}}$$

$$= \sqrt{\frac{2 \times 5,000 \times \$5}{\$0.50}}$$

$$= 316$$

❋ **TABLE 19–4** *Economic Order Quantity for Purchase of Syringes*

A	Demand	5,000	5,000	5,000
E	Order size	50	316	5,000
E ÷ 2	Average inventory	25	158	2,500
A ÷ E	Number of purchase orders	100	16	1
P × (A ÷ E)	Annual ordering costs @ $5.00	$500	$ 80	$ 5
S × (E ÷ 2)	Annual carrying costs @ $0.50	13	79	1,250
C	Total annual relevant cost	$513	$159	$1,255

This formula does not take into account that there are sometimes discounts for quantity. The manager should consider what discounts are available and calculate the higher carrying costs associated with larger orders to determine if it is worth taking the discount.

For example, suppose in this problem that there was a $250 discount in purchase price for five orders of 1,000 units each as opposed to 16 smaller orders. To order 1,000 units at a time, there would be five orders at a cost of $5 each. Therefore, the order cost would be $25. The carrying cost would be S × (E ÷ 2), or $0.50 × (1,000 ÷ 2) = $250. The total costs would be $275. This is $116 higher than the EOQ cost of $159. If we can reduce the purchase cost of the inventory units by $250, the savings will more than offset the $116 increase in inventory management costs. Five orders per year instead of 16 will be justified.

Even if the nurse manager is not responsible for inventory control, an appreciation of the costs incurred in inventory may make the manager and the staff more sensitive to the issues. It is common for nurses to stockpile supplies. Because nurses believe they cannot provide care without certain supplies and because they have run out of supplies in the past, often extra supplies are hidden for future use. Organizations incur costs associated with inventory. The use of organizational resources can be optimized by efficient inventory control.

❋ CURRENT LIABILITIES

Management of current liabilities often receives less attention than current asset management, but it is also important. Careful planning and management of short-term obligations can save the organization significant amounts of money.

The typical current liabilities that most organizations have and that must be managed as part of working capital are *accounts payable*, *payroll payable*, *notes payable*, and *taxes payable*. Accounts payable represent amounts that are owed to suppliers. Payroll payable relates to obligations to employees. Notes payable represent short-term debt, usually loans from banks. Taxes payable include not only income taxes for proprietary organizations but also a variety of payroll taxes for all organizations.

The basic approach to management of current liabilities is deferral of payment and avoidance of borrowing to the extent possible. The longer the organization waits to make payments, the longer the cash will remain in the organization's interest-bearing accounts. This allows it to earn a return that can be used to provide more services. The less money the organization borrows and the later it borrows it, the less interest it must pay.

Accounts Payable

Accounts payable are often referred to as *trade credit*. Trade credit is generally free for a short time. After a purchase is made, the organization usually has several weeks to 1 month to pay the bill. After that time, some suppliers charge interest; others do not. A more common practice than charging interest for late payments is to offer a discount for prompt payment.

Discount terms are often stated as 2/10 N/30 (read as "two ten net thirty"). That means a 2% discount is given for payments received within 10 days of the invoice date. Otherwise, the full amount, referred to as the net (N) amount, is due 30 days from the invoice date. Sometimes only a 1% discount is offered, in which case it would be referred to as 1/10 N/30. Some vendors use terms based on the end of the month (EOM). For example, 2/10 EOM means that the buyer can take a 2% discount for payments made by 10 days after the end of the month in which the invoice is issued. In general, trade credit is offered only to trustworthy buyers. In some cases, when the supplier has not had a long-term relationship with the buyer, goods will be sold cash on delivery (COD).

Does it pay to take the discount when it is offered? In most cases, it clearly does make sense to take the discount. A formula can be used to determine the annual interest rate implicit in trade credit discounts:

$$\text{Implicit Interest Rate} = \frac{\text{Discount}}{\text{Discounted Price}} \times \frac{365 \text{ Days}}{\text{Days Early}} \times 100\%$$

For example, suppose that your organization purchased $1,000 worth of goods and was offered terms of 2/10 N/30. A 2% discount on a $1,000 purchase is $20. This means that if the discount is taken, only $980 will have to be paid. If the discount is taken, payment is due on the 10th day rather than the 30th day. This means that payment is made 20 days earlier than would otherwise be the case.

$$\text{Implicit Interest Rate} = \frac{\$20}{\$980} \times \frac{365 \text{ Days}}{20 \text{ Days}} \times 100\%$$
$$= 37.2\%$$

Although the discount appears to be a very small percentage, on an annualized basis, the rate is actually 37.2%! Effectively, one can think of this as if the organization has an obligation of $980 due on the 10th day. If it waits an extra 20 days to make payment, the interest charge is $20. Twenty dollars of interest on a $980 loan for 20 days represents a 37% annual interest rate. Clearly, if the organization takes the discount, it is avoiding a high charge for deferring payment by a few weeks.

What if the organization does not have enough cash to take all discounts? In that case, it makes sense to incur short-term debt, that is, to borrow the money from the bank to get the money to pay the bill on the 10th day, as long as the bank charges a rate less than 37%.

However, this strategy assumes that the organization will in fact pay the bill on the due date if it does not take the discount. What if a hospital is in financial difficulty and is paying its bills after 150 days? That is an undesirable position to be in, as suppliers may stop making future sales. Nevertheless, it is not uncommon to find some HCOs paying bills 90 days, 120 days, or even 150 days late. If a hospital would normally pay a bill after 150 days, then taking the discount on the tenth day means that payment is made 140 days sooner than it otherwise would be.

$$\text{Implicit Interest Rate} = \frac{\$20}{\$980} \times \frac{365 \text{ Days}}{140 \text{ Days}} \times 100\%$$
$$= 5.3\%$$

In this situation, the implicit interest rate is much lower. Any hospital paying after 150 days probably has a cash shortage. It is unlikely that this hospital could borrow from a bank for a rate as low as 5.3%. Therefore, in this situation, it is not financially advantageous to take the discount. The decision to take or not take a discount is not automatic. It depends on both the amount of the discount and the implications for how much sooner payment must be made.

Payroll Payable

Payroll payables are generally very short term. At the end of each payroll period, salaries and wages are paid and the obligation is eliminated. This does not mean, however, that management has no ability to manage in this area.

First, policy decisions must be made regarding when and how often employees are paid. Paying some employees monthly instead of every 2 weeks effectively defers payment of half their salary by 2 weeks. Over the course of the year, that adds up to a significant amount of savings for the organization. Similar savings accrue from paying employees every 2 weeks instead of every week. In addition, less frequent payments mean less paperwork and other administrative costs.

Second, there is the issue of how long the delay is from the end of the payroll period until payment. If the payroll period ends on Friday and payroll is paid on the following Thursday, the organization has gained the use of the money for nearly an extra week.

On the other side of the ledger, one must give consideration to the organization's relationship with its employees. Although it will require some time to process the amounts that are due to employees (and to print checks if that method of payment is still used), a good relationship between employer and employees calls for payment of payroll as promptly as possible.

Notes Payable

The most common type of short-term debt owed by HCOs is unsecured notes payable to banks. Many HCOs also borrow money from financing and factoring companies using their accounts receivable as collateral. In addition, some HCOs issue commercial paper.

Unsecured notes are loans that do not have any collateral. Collateral is a specific asset pledged to the lender. If the borrower defaults on the loan, the lender can sell the collateral to recover its money. In the case of an unsecured note, if the organization fails to repay the money, the lender has no specific claim on an asset owned by the organization. Rather, it would be a general creditor and would share the assets of the organization with all the other general creditors. This makes lending money more risky and drives up the interest charged.

An alternative available to HCOs is to put up accounts receivable as security or collateral for the loan. This is called *financing accounts receivable*. It is also possible to directly sell receivables. This is called *factoring*. The buyer of the receivables, called the *factor* or the *factoring agent,* takes on the risk that patients or third-party payers may not pay. Factoring tends to be an expensive alternative because of the risk that the factor takes. Financing is less expensive. The HCO borrows money, and the receivables are simply security in case the organization fails to repay the loan. Because much of the receivables are due from the government (Medicare and Medicaid), they are seen as reasonably good collateral. This may make borrowing with receivables as collateral less costly than an unsecured bank loan.

A last alternative is commercial paper. This is a form of borrowing in which the borrower issues a financial security that can be traded by the lender to someone else. This is an uncommon approach for any organization other than large, for-profit chains. Although the commercial paper is referred to as a *security*, it is generally unsecured.

In general, short-term debt bears a higher interest rate than long-term debt. This is because whereas short-term debt is typically unsecured, long-term debt is often secured by specific assets. Also, transaction costs are related to the borrowing and repaying of loans. These costs are more substantial for short-term loans because they cannot be spread out over a long lifetime of a loan. Therefore, if an organization needs an amount of money for a long time, it usually borrows on a long-term basis. Long-term borrowing is discussed in Chapter 20. Short-term debt is generally used only for short-term needs.

Taxes Payable

Even not-for-profit organizations get involved with taxes. For the most part, these relate to FICA (Social Security taxes) and employee income tax withholding. FICA is paid by both the employee and the employer. The organization must withhold an amount for FICA from its employees and then make payments to the government for both its share and the employees' share. The organization must also withhold a portion of each employee's wages and pay it to the government for the employee's income taxes. Generally, specific rules determine when these tax payments are due. Aside from not paying the taxes before they are due, there is relatively little management can do in this area. However, these taxes must be paid on time or the organization is subject to financial penalties.

Other Payables Made on Behalf of Employees

Most HCOs also withhold portions of employees' wages for purposes other than taxes. Defined contribution retirement accounts (e.g., 401(k) or 403(b) contributions) are probably the most common example. In these cases, the organization will withhold retirement contributions made by employees and periodically make payments to the administrators of the retirement plan. Organizations may also withhold other funds on behalf of employees (e.g., medical, dental or other insurance premiums) that also require periodic payments to be made by the organization. Managers must budget for and manage these obligations paid on behalf of employees. Failure to do so may not only put the employer at risk but also jeopardize the health and financial well-being of employees.

✳ IMPLICATIONS FOR NURSE MANAGERS AND EXECUTIVES

Some nurse managers and executives may question the importance of this chapter. Except for a minority of them, readers of this book are unlikely to be in charge of decisions concerning collection of accounts receivable and payment to suppliers. However, understanding the principles of working capital management is important for all nurse managers and executives because they manage nurses who are themselves organizational resources and who also have the potential to impact the use of the organization's resources.

Nurse managers and executives do not just manage their cost centers; they also manage a part of the larger organization. Because of this, it is essential that they understand the financial workings of the organization. In many instances, the actions of nurse managers and executives have an effect on working capital. Decisions made about working capital also affect nurse managers and executives by way of the resources available to their cost centers or departments.

There was a time when nurse managers and executives were restricted primarily to clinical management. This is no longer the case. Their role has changed, and continues to change, because nurse managers and executives control the largest share of resources in most health care institutions. Therefore the financial management of the entire organization should be a concern of nurse managers and executives. Inefficient use of working capital invariably has an impact on the resources available for patient care.

The impact nurse managers can have on working capital should not be understated. The most obvious area in which nurses can have an impact is inventory management. Efficient control of inventory resources is one working capital ingredient. Another is payroll liabilities. Nurse managers, through their staffing decisions, do have an impact on that current liability. Decisions to purchase inventory and equipment come into play as well. The timing of such purchases should be made in light of their implications for working capital.

On the other hand, although delaying purchases of equipment until the equipment is actually needed makes sense, delaying purchases may reduce quality of care. Understanding working capital management can help nurse managers and executives understand why a financial manager might want to delay an acquisition as long as possible. That understanding should help the nurse manager or executive engage in meaningful dialogue with financial management over the acquisition of purchases. Mutually beneficial solutions are more likely to be achieved when both parties understand the needs and concerns of their areas of responsibility.

✳ KEY CONCEPTS

Working capital   Organization's current assets and current liabilities.

Working capital management   Management of the current assets and current liabilities of the organization to ensure that there is adequate cash on hand to meet the organization's needs and to minimize the cost of short-term resources.

Cash requirements   Cash is needed by organizations for three main purposes: transactions, safety, and investments.

Cash management   Management of inflows and outflows of cash.

Cash budgets   Starting cash balance plus expected cash receipts less expected cash payments.

Management of accounts receivable   Minimization of the time between provision of care and receipt of payment. Accounts receivable earn no return for the organization. The sooner cash is collected, the sooner the organization can use that cash for its operations or invest it.

Aging schedule   Tool used to keep track of potential accounts receivable problems by showing how long each receivable has been outstanding since a bill was issued.

Inventory management   Refers to the appropriate ordering and storage of supplies, considering the product cost, *ordering costs*, *stockout costs*, *carrying costs*, and *quality costs*.

Economic order quantity (EOQ)   Approach to determine the optimal quantity for each order. It is based on creating a balance between *ordering costs* and *carrying costs*.

Ordering costs   The costs associated with placing the order, such as clerk time for preparation of a purchase order.

Carrying costs   The costs of having money tied up in inventory rather than in a revenue-producing endeavor such as an interest-bearing bank account, plus costs such as storage and insurance.

Stockout costs   The costs incurred when inventory is not available but is needed.

Quality costs   The costs incurred to ensure that the product is of the required quality. These may include costs such as inspection or replacement or patient harm done by using a low-quality item.

Management of current liabilities   Process of deferring payment and avoiding borrowing to the extent possible. The longer the organization waits to pay, the longer the cash is in the organization's interest-bearing accounts, earning a return that can be used to provide more services. The less the organization borrows and the later it borrows, the less interest it must pay.

Accounts payable   Often subject to credit terms such as 2/1 N/30. The implicit interest rate contained in such terms may be calculated as follows:

$$\text{Implicit Interest Rate} = \frac{\text{Discount}}{\text{Discounted Price}} \times \frac{\text{365 Days}}{\text{Days Earlier}} \times 100\%$$

Short-term debt   Unsecured short-term loans.

✳ SUGGESTED READINGS

Cleverley W, Cleverley J, Song P: *Essentials of health care finance*, ed 7, Sudbury, Mass, 2011, Jones & Bartlett.

Emery D, Finnerty J, Stowe J: *Principles of financial management*, Upper Saddle River, New Jersey, 1998, Prentice Hall.

Finkler S: *Finance & accounting for nonfinancial managers*, ed 4, Chicago, 2011, CCH.

Finkler S, Ward D: *Accounting fundamentals for health care management*, ed 2, Sudbury, Mass, 2012, Jones & Bartlett.

Gapenski L: *Healthcare finance: an introduction to accounting and financial management*, ed 4, Chicago, 2007, Health Administration Press.

Horngren C, Datar S, Foster G: *Cost accounting: a managerial emphasis*, ed 12, Upper Saddle River, New Jersey, 2005, Prentice Hall.

Keown A, Martin J, Petty J: *Foundations of finance*, ed 7, Upper Saddle River, New Jersey, 2010, Prentice Hall.

McLean R: *Financial management in health care organizations*, ed 2, Albany, New York, 2002, Delmar.

Zelman W, McCue M, Milikan A, Glick N: *Financial management of health care organizations: an introduction to fundamental tools, concepts, and applications*, ed 3, Cambridge, Mass, 2009, Wiley-Blackwell.

Long-Term Financial Resources

CHAPTER GOALS

The goals of this chapter are to:

- Describe the sources of long-term financing for health care organizations
- Explain the relative merits of equity financing versus debt financing
- Distinguish among the different equity sources of financing
- Consider the changing roles of equity sources of financing

- Explain the types of debt financing and the trade-offs of each type
- Introduce bond ratings and bond insurance
- Explain what bond refinancing is and why it takes place
- Explain the purpose of and methods used for feasibility studies
- Consider the future of long-term financing for health care organizations

✳ INTRODUCTION

Chapter 19 covered a number of sources of short-term financing for health care organizations (HCOs). We now turn to sources of *long-term financing*. Long-term financing represents sources of money that the organization can use for longer than 1 year. In many cases, these sources are critical to the existence of the organization.

Most, if not all, buildings and equipment are financed on a long-term basis. It would probably be impossible to find a lender willing to make a 90-day or 6-month loan to acquire a building. It is unreasonable to expect that enough profits could be earned within a short period to repay the entire cost of a building. It is more likely that at the maturity, or due date, of the short-term loan, a new loan would be required to get the money to repay the old loan. If a new loan cannot be obtained, the organization would likely have to default on its old loan. The lender would consider the risk of not being repaid too high.

As a result, long-term assets are generally acquired with money that the organization knows it can keep and use for a long time. The two principal sources of long-term money are *debt* and *equity*. Debt represents borrowed money. Interest must be paid during the period of the loan, and the original amount borrowed must be repaid. Equity represents ownership. In some cases, equity represents money that outsiders have given the organization in exchange for owning it and having a claim on its profits. In other cases, equity represents money that the organization itself owns.

Although nurse managers and executives may not deal with issues that pertain to organizational debt and equity on a daily basis, knowledge of the organization's long-term resources are necessary because they will likely be involved in decisions that may affect or be affected by the availability of these resources. Knowledge of these issues will also help them better understand how and why certain decisions are made within organizations. This chapter therefore presents issues that pertain to long-term financing, including the sources of organizational debt and equity, so that nurse managers and executives are prepared to contribute to related discussions and decision making in HCOs.

✳ EQUITY SOURCES OF FINANCING

The four principal sources of equity financing for HCOs are philanthropy, corporate stock issuance, government grants, and retained earnings.

The main advantage of equity financing is that there is no legal requirement to make annual payments. This is in contrast to debt, which generally calls for at least annual payments of interest. Even if an HCO has a bad year, it is legally required to make interest payments on its debt. If it does not have enough cash to make those interest payments, it might have to go out of business. That risk is not associated with equity sources of financing.

If a for-profit HCO has a bad year, it can skip dividend payments to its stockholders. The usual form of stock, called *common stock,* has no requirements that dividends of any amount be paid even if the organization is making a profit. A special form of stock called *preferred stock* requires a specific dividend each year, but in hard economic times, payments can be deferred to future years or in some cases skipped entirely.

Other forms of equity such as retained earnings and philanthropic funds do not have required payments of any type. This freedom from interest payments relates to a concept called *leverage*. The greater the extent to which an organization uses debt financing, as opposed to equity, the more highly leveraged it is considered. The benefit of leverage is that high leverage implies a low amount of required equity investment. The detriment of leverage is that it creates risk because of the need to make interest payments.

Philanthropy

Philanthropy represents gifts to the organization. These gifts may be small, or they may come in the form of multimillion dollar endowments. There may be costs related to generating the gifts, but after being received, they do not require interest or dividend payments, and the amount of the gift need never be repaid to someone outside the HCO. Philanthropy has been a declining percentage of long-term financing for HCOs.

The decline in philanthropy is probably caused by a number of factors, most of which are outside the control of any specific HCO. These include changes in the tax rates, the introduction of Medicare and Medicaid, the proliferation of for-profit HCOs, increased competition from non–health care charities, cuts in federal support of social welfare, and the rising costs of generating philanthropic donations. In addition, the existence of other sources for financing has made health care managers less aggressive in pursuing philanthropy.

Tax changes in the 1980s made it less advantageous to donate money to charitable organizations. Before that time, many philanthropists were in a 70% federal income tax bracket. A donation of $1 resulted in a 70¢ tax savings. Considering the tax implications, it cost a person in that bracket only 30¢ to make a $1 contribution. With state income taxes added on, the effect was even more extreme. With the current lower marginal tax rates, each dollar contributed costs the donor more on an after-tax basis. For example, a gift of $1 million in 1980 might have cost a rich benefactor only $250,000 after considering the savings in federal and state taxes. That same contribution today, after the tax changes, might cost the donor $650,000 or more.

Before the introduction of Medicare and Medicaid, many philanthropists believed that they had a mission to help provide for the health care of elderly adults and people with lower socioeconomic status. With the government role that was created by Medicare and Medicaid, many philanthropists no longer believe that the same degree of need still exists. Although it is true that many people are still uninsured or underinsured, the mere existence of a major role for the government in payment for health care possibly has made many people believe that the need for charity has disappeared from the health care industry.

At one time, hospitals were viewed as community benefit organizations whose mission was to serve the people in the community. In many cases, especially in large cities, this is no longer true. Thus, people in the community do not have the same sense of responsibility to the hospital.

This is probably reinforced by the fact that HCOs view themselves more and more as businesses rather than charities. Although running HCOs in a financially sound, business-like manner does not eliminate their charitable mission, it does change the way people perceive the industry. The proliferation of for-profit HCOs tends to make the entire industry appear more similar to a business. And many people believe that the last place they would donate money to is a business.

At the same time that HCOs have lost some of their allure as charities, there has been tremendous growth in the non–health care not-for-profit sector. More charities today are competing for dollars, and they are learning how to do it better. This increased volume of charities and improved fundraising skills has occurred at the same time as a government cutback in social services. The federal government has increasingly pushed more of its social welfare function back to localities. The result has been numerous cuts in social services because the localities are themselves strapped for resources to provide even the most basic of local services, such as fire protection and emergency services. Many charitable organizations have, over time, stepped in to try to restore some services. That has created an additional, highly visible outlet for philanthropic giving.

Another problem with philanthropy for HCOs has been the rising cost of generating philanthropic donations. As competition for philanthropy has grown, organizations have had to develop more sophisticated and expensive approaches to generating gifts. Expensive advertising campaigns join the more traditional dinners as a way to raise money. Full-time personnel must be hired to work at the task of "development" (i.e., gift generation).

Most, if not all, of these factors contributing to the decreasing role of philanthropy cannot be greatly influenced by managers and executives of an organization. Nevertheless, many not-for-profit HCOs have dropped the ball with respect to raising philanthropic funds. Not only have philanthropists started to view health care as a business, but many health care managers have as well. There is a need to distinguish between running the organization in a businesslike manner and being a for-profit corporation.

Many health care managers believe that among Medicare, Medicaid, Blue Cross, private insurers, managed care organizations (MCOs), and other payers, there should be enough revenue to run a health care business. The error in that perception is that in the case of not-for-profit organizations, health care is not a business. The mission is not centered on making money but on providing service to the community. Not-for-profit organizations inherently undertake some activities at a loss because of their mission. One way to offset those losses is to earn high profits on other services. Most HCOs try to accomplish that. However, another way to offset those losses is to actively solicit donations from a wide variety of sources, including past patients and community leaders.

Realistically, however, although efforts to receive donations should continue and perhaps even be stepped up, philanthropy can no longer be viewed as a major source for long-term financing. The costs of the health care industry have grown too high. New buildings are so expensive that in most cases, their cost has gone beyond the reach of the best philanthropic efforts.

Corporate Stock Issuance

A major growth area in health care financing has been the *issuance of corporate stock*. In direct contrast to philanthropy, this approach says that health care can in fact be a business. Individuals can give money to HCOs in exchange for stock. The stock makes the individuals part owners of the business. As the business earns profits, it distributes part of them to the owners in the form of dividends. The owners can sell the stock to someone else as a way of getting back their original investment, perhaps with a profit. The new owner of the stock can then receive the future dividends from the business's profits.

Owning stock of health care providers is not always the route to riches. For example, an organization's stock price may drop substantially because of poor financial performance. At the turn of the 21st century, large for-profit hospital chains faced difficult financial conditions and saw their stock prices plunge. Some stock prices have recovered, some hospital chains were acquired or merged with other HCOs, and some hospitals closed. Despite uncertainty, the for-profit sector is still seen as potentially profitable, but the rapid rate of growth in the for-profit hospital sector has slowed. Many new HCOs, including those that develop or provide new health information technologies, home health services, or temporary staffing or are part of the globalization of health care services, are getting their start by issuing stock to get a considerable portion of their initial financial resources.

Stock issuance is only available to for-profit organizations. It is unlikely that many not-for-profit HCOs will switch to being for-profit simply to access this form of financing. Such a step would likely have wide ramifications for the organization. On the other hand, organizations that are already for-profit must decide how much equity financing of this form they want. It is possible to issue enough stock to raise all the necessary long-term financing for an organization. However, that may not be an optimal strategy.

When stock is issued, a major benefit to the owners who invest money in the business is the dividend flow. Dividends are a distribution of profits. They are paid after taxes have been calculated on profits. Interest, on the other hand, is a tax-deductible expense. By issuing some stock and some debt, some of the payments for financing become tax deductible, therefore lowering the taxes paid to the government. That is one reason that most for-profit organizations have a mixture of stock and debt.

Government Grants

Government grants were a common financing mechanism at one time, especially for hospitals. Hill-Burton funds were available in the 1950s for the construction of new hospital buildings. In recent years, there has been a growing reluctance by the government to create more capacity in the health care system. Studies have demonstrated that increased capacity tends to create higher levels of utilization. Furthermore, there is an excess of capacity for health care services in many areas of the country. As a result, government grants are no longer a significant source of financing for HCOs. They are available, however, for programs such as the development of primary care clinics. One such exception has come through the American Recovery and Reinvestment Act of 2009, which has contributed significantly to the development and expansion of the health information system in the United States.

Retained Earnings

The last significant source of equity financing is *retained earnings*. Each year that an HCO makes a profit, that profit is either paid to owners in the form of a dividend or retained in the organization. Money retained can be used for short-term operations or to finance long-term assets.

Retaining earnings is a critical factor in the long-term survival of HCOs. To stay viable, it is necessary to replace plant and equipment as they physically deteriorate or become technologically obsolete. In addition, organizations must add new services and technologies to remain current as health care changes. The combination of inflation, technological change, and expanding community needs often drives the cost of replacement buildings and equipment well above the cost of the original items. It would not be surprising for an old hospital building that cost $100 million to build 60 years ago to be replaced now for $500 million or more. If profits have been earned, retained, and invested, the organization will have some of the money needed for the new facility.

Even on a less grand scale, retained earnings are essential. Suppose that a home health agency wishes to buy a new patient monitor for $25,000. If it goes to a bank to borrow the money, the bank probably will want the home health agency to make a down payment of 20% or more. The reason for this is discussed later in the "Mortgages and Long-Term Notes" section. If there is adequate philanthropy or cash from stock issuances, the home health agency will be able to buy the equipment. If not, it is likely that it will only be able to acquire the equipment if it has enough money for the down payment available from earnings that have been retained and have not yet been used for another purpose. Retained earnings represent a source of equity financing that is of growing importance to HCOs.

✳ DEBT SOURCES OF FINANCING

Relatively few HCOs are entirely free from debt. The need to raise large amounts of long-term financing causes many, if not most, HCOs to borrow money. There are a number of different approaches to borrowing. Depending on the specific circumstances for which money is needed, at times, some approaches will be superior, and at other times, other approaches will be more suitable.

The major forms of *long-term debt* are mortgages, long-term notes, leases, and bonds. Mortgages and long-term notes generally represent money that a bank lends to the organization. However, it is possible to have a mortgage or note with a non-bank. For instance, some equipment manufacturers will lend the buyer money to acquire equipment from them. Leases are arrangements to rent equipment or facilities under a contract.

Bonds are formal borrowing arrangements in which the debt is transferrable. The issuer of the bonds receives money and owes the buyer. The buyer in turn can sell the bond to another party, to whom the issuer is then obligated.

Mortgages and Long-Term Notes

Mortgages and *long-term notes* are referred to as *conventional debt*. A long-term note is a loan. It is sometimes secured by collateral and sometimes it is unsecured. If secured, the collateral is often in the form of financial securities rather than physical property. The obligation to repay the loan is generally evidenced by a formal legal document, called a *note*, that is signed by the borrower. When a note is secured by a specific piece of physical property such as a building, piece of equipment, or land, it is referred to as a *mortgage*. If the borrower fails to repay a mortgage, the lender can foreclose on the property, sell it, and pay the borrower only the amount realized from the sale that exceeds the outstanding loan balance.

Mortgages and long-term notes are common, can be issued with little delay, and require relatively little paperwork. They tend to be more expensive than bonds but less expensive than leasing.

Mortgages are often used to finance a specific acquisition. Usually lenders require that the borrower make a down payment of anywhere from 20% to 50% of the purchase price of the asset. This protects the lender in case there is a payment default, and the asset cannot be sold for its full original cost. Mortgages generally call for monthly payments of a constant amount. The payments consist of interest on the balance of the loan that was outstanding during the previous month plus a repayment of a portion of the original loan. Over time, the amount of interest in each payment declines, and the amount of loan repayment in each payment rises. At the end of the term of the mortgage, the loan has been fully repaid. In contrast, notes generally call for monthly payments of interest only. At the maturity date of the loan, the full amount of the original loan is repaid.

For example, suppose that an MCO wanted to purchase equipment for a new group practice office. The total cost of the equipment needed is $500,000. The MCO plans to invest $100,000 of its own funds and borrow $400,000. Suppose that if it borrowed on a 10-year unsecured long-term note, the interest rate would be 8%. If it took a mortgage for 10 years, using the equipment as collateral, the interest rate would be 6%. The collateral lessens the lender's risk, so a lower interest rate is available. Assume for this example that payments are only made once a year. What are the annual payments under the two alternatives?

The long-term note has annual payments of $32,000 (8% of $400,000), as seen in Table 20–1. The loan balance of $400,000 remains constant over the 10-year life of the loan. At the end of the loan, there is an interest payment, plus a payment for the full $400,000.

The annual mortgage payments on a $400,000 loan are $54,347.[1] Note that this is a higher amount than the annual $32,000 payment on the long-term note even though the interest rate on the mortgage is only 6% and the rate on the note is 8%. This is because the mortgage payments include not only interest but also repayment of a portion of the original loan. These mortgage payments are shown in Table 20–2.

Note that in the early years, most of each mortgage payment is interest. However, because there is some repayment of the original loan, each year a smaller amount is owed. Because less money is owed, there is less interest. The annual payments are a constant amount. If the amount of interest decreases each year, the amount of the annual payment available for repaying the loan increases. Thus, in the later years, most of each payment is loan repayment rather than interest. By the end of 10 years, the loan is fully paid off.

Note that in total the mortgage payments came to $543,472 and the note payments came to $720,000. The reason is that there is more interest on the note. This is partly because of the higher interest rate and partly because the full $400,000 for the note is owed during the entire 10 years, but the mortgage obligation declined over the 10 years.

---

[1]The $54,347 constant annual payment is exactly the amount of money that is needed to provide for a 6% interest payment on the outstanding balance of the loan plus repayment of the loan so that there is no remaining balance at the end of 10 years. That number can be calculated using the time-value-of-money techniques discussed in the Appendix to Chapter 12. In this case, the number of compounding periods is 10, the interest rate is 6%, the present value of the loan is $400,000, and the annual payment is being sought.

✳ **TABLE 20–1** *Payment Schedule for a Long-Term Note*

Year	Loan Balance Start of Year	Interest Payment	Loan Repayment	Total Payment	Loan Balance End of Year
1	$400,000	$32,000	$ 0	$ 32,000	$400,000
2	400,000	32,000	0	32,000	400,000
3	400,000	32,000	0	32,000	400,000
4	400,000	32,000	0	32,000	400,000
5	400,000	32,000	0	32,000	400,000
6	400,000	32,000	0	32,000	400,000
7	400,000	32,000	0	32,000	400,000
8	400,000	32,000	0	32,000	400,000
9	400,000	32,000	0	32,000	400,000
10	400,000	32,000	400,000	432,000	0
				$720,000	

✳ TABLE 20–2 *Payment Schedule for a Mortgage**

Year	Loan Balance Start of Year (A)	Interest Payment (B)	Loan Repayment (C)	Total Payment (D)	Loan Balance End of Year (E)
1	$400,000	$24,000	$30,347	$ 54,347	$369,653
2	369,653	22,179	32,168	54,347	337,485
3	337,485	20,249	34,098	54,347	303,387
4	303,387	18,203	36,144	54,347	267,243
5	267,243	16,035	38,313	54,347	228,930
6	228,930	13,736	40,611	54,347	188,319
7	188,319	11,299	43,048	54,347	145,271
8	145,271	8,716	45,631	54,347	99,640
9	99,640	5,978	48,369	54,347	51,271
10	51,271	3,076	51,271	54,347	0
				$543,472	

(A) Loan balance at the start of the year is the original loan balance in the first year. In subsequent years, it is the ending balance from column E for the previous year.

(B) 6% interest rate multiplied by loan balance in column A.

(C) = (D) − (B).

(D) = Annual payment calculated using time-value-of-money techniques. See Chapter 12 appendix.

(E) = (A) − (C).

*Note: Some numbers may vary slightly because of rounding.

Leases

Leases are rental agreements made under a contract referred to as a lease. The lessee rents a building or equipment from the lessor. Unless otherwise agreed, at the expiration of a lease, the lessor continues to own the property. It is possible, however, to design the lease to transfer the property to the lessee at the end of its term. It is also possible to design the lease to give the lessee the option to purchase the property at the end of the lease for a specified price. Leases usually call for equal payments payable at the beginning of each month.

Lease payments generally have three components, although the lessee is only told the total monthly payment. The first component pays for part of the cost of the property being leased. This is equivalent to the principal portion of a mortgage payment. The second component is an interest charge equivalent to the interest portion of a mortgage payment. The last component is profit for the lessor.

In many ways, leases are simply an alternative to mortgages. In both cases, the organization wishes to have the use of an asset, but it does not have the cash to go out and buy the asset. It needs to use cash from someone else, either the mortgage lender or the lessor. Leases in effect obligate the lessee to make monthly lease payments for a number of years into the future in the same way that the user of the equipment would be obligated to make monthly mortgage payments had the property been purchased with a mortgage. It is because of the long-term obligation to make payments on a lease that accountants treat long-term noncancelable leases as long-term debt.

Other things being equal, leases are more costly than mortgages. In either case, the user of the property must ultimately pay the cost of the property, and the user of the property must pay interest for the use of the money needed to buy the property. That interest includes a profit for the lender. In the case of a lease, however, the lessor has generally borrowed the money to buy the property. Suppose that the lessor borrows from a bank to finance the asset purchased. The bank and its depositors must receive interest, and the lessor must also earn a profit. This extra party to the transaction, the lessor, adds the need for additional profits and therefore creates additional costs to the lessee. The bank and its depositors and the lessor earn a profit. With a mortgage, only the bank and its depositors need earn a profit.

Then why would one lease rather than buying a property and taking a mortgage? For one thing, leases do not require a down payment. If the organization does not have the 20% to 50% of the asset cost needed for a down payment, the lease may be viewed as advantageous even if it is more expensive. Another advantage of leasing is that the leasing company may be better able to sell the used property than the user of the property.

Consider a home health agency that provides cars to its nursing staff for making home visits. At the end of 3 or 4 years, the agency may wish to replace the cars. The agency probably cannot get a high value for the cars when it sells them because it is not an expert in the used car market. On the other hand, if the cars are leased, the leasing company can probably sell the cars for a reasonable price because it is an expert. By sharing the extra amount received on the ultimate sale with the lessee, the lease may become attractive.

Another potential advantage of leasing is that in some leases the lessee can call for the equipment to be replaced if it becomes obsolete. This removes some risk that HCOs take when they buy equipment. On the other hand, the leasing company will probably charge a higher monthly amount to pay it for taking that risk.

The total rate being charged to cover interest and profits on a lease can usually be estimated using the time-value-of-money techniques. Suppose that a nursing home is considering buying some equipment for $200,000 or leasing it for $5,000 per month for 5 years. If it purchases the equipment, there will be an immediate down payment of $50,000 plus monthly mortgage payments based on a 12% interest rate for 5 years. If it leases the equipment, it will have 60 monthly payments of $5,000. If the number of months equals 60, the payment each month is $5,000, and the present value of the equipment is $200,000, then the annual interest rate on the lease is approximately 18%.[2] This is substantially higher than the bank rate of 12%. On the other hand, the nursing home would need only $5,000 at the start for the first month as opposed to $50,000 for a down payment.

Bonds

Bonds are formal certificates of indebtedness. The certificate indicates a promise to pay interest, usually semiannually, and the face value of the bond at a specified maturity date. Bonds are financial obligations that can be traded from one party to another. For example, Mr. Smith can lend money to the HCO (i.e., he can buy a bond) in exchange for a promise that interest plus the original loan will be repaid. That promise is evidenced by the bond certificate. In turn, Mr. Smith can sell the bond certificate to someone else, and the borrower will then owe the money to the new owner of the bond instead of to Mr. Smith. Bonds are issued by the borrower. Sometimes it is said that the borrower sells the bonds or floats a bond.

Bonds are an advantageous way of obtaining debt for several reasons. First, the borrower obtains the money directly from the ultimate lender. Second, bonds tend to disperse risk.

In the case of a bank loan, the borrower gets money from a bank, which in turn gets money from depositors. The depositors must make a profit, and the bank must make a profit. With a bond, the money is borrowed directly from individuals, who might otherwise put their money in a bank. By eliminating the middleman bank, the depositors can be paid more than the bank would pay them, and the borrower can pay less than would be paid to a bank. Both the borrower and the ultimate lender are better off if they can eliminate the bank's role.

The second major advantage is that there is dispersal of risk. If a bank were to lend $500 million for a hospital expansion, it would take on a tremendous amount of risk. If the hospital were to default, the bank would be faced with a huge potential loss. Bonds, however, are often divided into hundreds or thousands or even hundreds of thousands of relatively small loans. For a $500 million total debt, each lender may lend as little as $5,000. Thus, no one single person or organization takes on the full risk of one organization's defaulting on a loan.

With mutual funds, investors may effectively disperse their risk even further. An individual could invest $5,000 in a mutual fund that has combined the investments of thousands of individuals to buy hundreds of different bonds. Thus, an individual's risk from any one hospital's defaulting might be several hundred dollars or less. By lowering risk, the borrower lowers the interest rate that must be paid to adequately reimburse the lender for the risks taken.

Bonds are also advantageous because they do not require down payments for projects, and they may have extremely long maturity periods. Forty-year bonds are not uncommon. These factors can be very important to an HCO borrowing money to construct a new building. The organization can have the full depreciation period of the building to accumulate the money needed to pay for its construction.

Usually bonds pay interest semiannually. Every 6 months, a payment is made based on a stated interest rate and the face value of the bond. Bonds are generally issued in denominations of $5,000 and multiples of $5,000, such as $10,000, $25,000, and $100,000. The total amount issued by the borrower is generally large, often more than $100 million. At the due date or maturity of the bond, the original face amount must be repaid.

Although bond interest is paid at the stated rate and the face value is repaid at maturity, the bonds may actually be issued for a greater or lesser amount than the face value. This is because interest rates fluctuate in the financial marketplace. Bond certificates may be printed indicating a promise to pay a 10% interest rate. If the issuer finds that market conditions have changed and no one is willing to lend money unless it is possible to earn a 10.1% return on the money, then a discount will have to be offered to get anyone to buy the bonds.

Consider a $10,000, 20-year, 10% bond paying interest semiannually that is issued when interest rates on similar bonds are 10.1%. No one will give the issuer the full $10,000 for a 10% bond if they could get 10.1% elsewhere. So the issuer might accept payment of $9,915 for the bond. In exchange for the $9,915, the borrower will make payments of $500 twice a year for 20 years (i.e., the $10,000 face × 10% a year, ÷ two payments per year), plus a payment of $10,000 at the end of 20 years. The borrower received $9,915 but repays $10,000. The extra amount converts the 10% stated interest rate to the 10.1% market interest rate, so lenders will do just as well buying this bond as another.

If interest rates fall, the bond will be issued at a premium. If interest rates in the marketplace are only 9.8% and the bond offers 10% based on a face value of $10,000, investors will be willing to pay more than $10,000 to get the bond.

A number of decisions must be made before bonds are issued. These decisions can have a dramatic impact on the interest rate that must be paid on the outstanding bond obligations. Bonds may be issued in either taxable or tax-free form. The issuer can request to have the bond rated. The issuer can also purchase insurance that guarantees the payments of bond interest and principal. Another decision concerns whether to make interest payments or let the interest accrue and pay both the interest and face value at the maturity date. That is called a *zero-coupon bond*. After bonds have been issued, another question that sometimes arises is whether the bonds should be refinanced. These issues are discussed below.

Taxable versus Tax-Free Bonds

A taxable bond is one on which the lender of the money (also called the buyer of the bond) must pay income tax on the interest received. Under certain conditions, it is possible to offer

---

[2]Using the methods from the Appendix to Chapter 12, i = ?% per month, N = 60 months, the present value is $200,000, and the monthly payments = $5,000. Note that with a lease, payments are made in advance of each period rather than at the end of each period.

bonds free of federal income tax and free of state and local income taxes in the state or locality issued. The advantage of a tax-free bond is that people are willing to lend money in exchange for a lower interest rate if they can avoid paying income taxes on the interest payments they receive.

Suppose that a hospital wanted to borrow money and found that with a taxable bond, it would have to pay 12% interest. However, there are a number of potential lenders from the state where the hospital is located. Many of these lenders are in a combined federal and state income tax bracket of 33%. That means that they will have to pay one-third of any interest received in taxes. If they could earn the interest free of taxes, it would save a lot of money. In fact, if the hospital paid just two-thirds as much interest, or 8% interest on a tax-free bond, the lenders would still have just as much money after taxes!

Not all lenders are necessarily in such a high tax bracket. Also, some lenders may be from another state, which will tax the bond interest. As a result, it is likely that the hospital can issue the bond for a rate somewhere between 8% and 12%. If the bond is issued at 10%, that can still mean a savings of millions of dollars per year to the hospital.

Issuing a tax-free bond, however, requires compliance with a number of federal and state regulations. Generally, an HCO itself cannot issue a tax-free security. That is a privilege reserved for governmental bodies. For that reason, tax-free bonds are usually referred to as *municipal bonds*. Most states have governmental bond-issuing authorities. They act as a link allowing not-for-profit HCOs to issue tax-free securities. However, they usually assume no liability for repayment.

Given the possibility of avoiding taxes, why would taxable bonds ever be issued? There are several reasons. First, for-profit organizations are generally not given access to the tax-free market. Second, laws govern the total amount of bonds that can be issued on a tax-free basis. If that ceiling has been exceeded, only a taxable bond offering may be possible. The most common reason for issuing taxable bonds, however, is because it is possible to have lower expenses related to the issuance of the bond. Municipal bonds add to the complexity and regulatory compliance costs of issuing bonds.

A number of costs are related to the issuance of bonds, such as legal fees and placement fees. Bonds tend to require a great deal of sophisticated legal work to properly protect all parties. There is legal counsel for the issuer, counsel for the investors, and counsel for the investment firm that finds the buyers. In addition, substantial amounts of money are paid to the investment firm, called the *underwriter* of the bond. The underwriter is generally an investment banking company that places the bonds with investors. An HCO does not typically have direct access to the thousands of potential investors necessary to issue a bond successfully. Investment bankers have that large client base and are expert at finding buyers for bonds.

Despite the high legal and placement costs, it is worthwhile to issue bonds. Even a 1% savings in the interest rate compared with conventional debt would save $5 million per year on a $500 million bond flotation. To borrow that much money for 40 years, issuance costs of $3 or $4 million may be considered reasonable.

However, for a smaller bond such as $5 to $20 million or a shorter term bond such as 10 years or less, the issuance costs may be too much. Taxable bonds do not require that the organization go through nearly so great a legal and regulatory process as tax-exempt bonds do. Furthermore, if the bond is issued to a small group of investors rather than to the public at large, both legal and placement costs can be reduced even further. In such a case, it may be worthwhile to pay the higher interest rate on a taxable bond. Consider that a 2% interest difference on a $7 million, 3-year bond would amount to only about $400,000. If the costs of a tax-exempt issuance always exceeded $1 million, the taxable approach would make sense. Why not just borrow $7 million for 3 years from a bank? The bank would probably charge a higher interest rate than even a taxable bond. Recall that the bank represents an extra middleman that must make a profit.

Bond Ratings and Insurance

A primary reason for issuing bonds rather than using conventional debt is to get a lower interest rate. One of the most important determinants of interest rates is risk. If investors perceive an investment to be risky, they require a higher return. The way they get a higher return on money they lend is by charging a higher interest rate. The purpose of bond ratings and bond insurance is to reduce perceived or actual risk levels in order to lower the interest rate that must be paid on a bond.

The dominant bond-rating agencies in this country are Standard and Poor's (S&P) and Moody's Investor Services, followed by the Fitch Group. For a fee, these agencies evaluate the issuer of a bond and assign a rating to the quality of the bond. Quality is a measurement of the likelihood that the borrower will make all payments required by the bond. The highest rating is triple A, indicated by AAA (S&P and Fitch) or Aaa (Moody's). The ratings then decline to AA, A, BBB, BB, B, CCC, CC, C, and D (S&P and Fitch) or Aa, A, Baa, Ba, B, Caa, Ca, and C (Moody's). Anything below BBB or Baa is considered a risky, speculative investment.

Triple A bond ratings are reserved for only the safest investments. Extremely few, if any, HCOs can merit a triple A rating on the basis of their financial condition. Even double A ratings tend to be reserved for the most elite of HCOs. Ratings of single A and below are common in health care. The specific rating assigned to an organization's bonds will have a significant bearing on the interest rate it must pay.

There is no requirement that an organization have its bonds rated. The organization can avoid paying a fee to the rating agency and simply issue "nonrated" bonds. The fee for rating a bond is high because the bond rater must continue to follow the organization's financial condition over the life of the bond so that it can change its rating if the financial circumstances of the organization change. Failure to have a bond rated is not an indication that the bonds are a safe or unsafe investment. It may simply mean that the bond offering is too small to warrant the expense of a rating. However, many investors are reluctant to invest in such bonds.

Another alternative to rating is bond insurance. However, the premium for bond insurance is even more costly than obtaining a rating. The borrower pays a company to insure its obligations under the bond. Prior to 2007, four major organizations insured tax-exempt bonds. At the time this text was written, only one significant bond insurer (Assured Guaranty Corporation—formerly FSA) remained in the municipal bond insurance industry. As a result of defaults during the financial crisis of 2007 and the Great Recession that followed, some bond insurance companies went out of business, some were acquired and all lost their AAA bond ratings, rendering the value of their insurance nearly worthless to municipal issuers.

Bond insurers such as Assured Guaranty Corporation undertake a study of the financial situation of the bond issuer to assure themselves that the chance of default is extremely low. If they are satisfied, they issue the insurance. However, given turmoil in the financial markets in 2007 and the years that followed, combined with the extremely low interest rate environment which makes bond insurance less attractive, it is likely that far fewer HCOs have insured their new bond issues in recent years. Furthermore, some investors worry that if a serious financial crisis occurs that causes widespread bankruptcies among state and local governments or not-for-profit organizations, these insurers might not be financially capable of paying all insurance claims.

An insured municipal bond will have the same rating as that of the insurance company that insured it. Those ratings vary with the financial strength of each of the insurance companies.

Zero-Coupon Bonds

Typical bonds pay interest semiannually. Another type of bond, called a *zero-coupon bond* or simply a *zero,* does not make periodic interest payments. Instead, the interest is calculated every 6 months and is added onto the outstanding loan balance. At the maturity date, the payment consists of the original loan plus all the accrued interest. Note that every 6 months, the accumulated obligation grows, and in future periods, interest accrues on prior interest as well as on the original principal amount. In other words, because interest is not paid out every 6 months, compound interest applies to all amounts owed the lender.

Zero-coupon bonds are issued at deep discounts, and the interest is built into the face value of the bond. For example, a $10,000, 10%, 20-year-maturity, zero-coupon bond might be issued for $1,420. The $10,000 payment at maturity would cover both the original $1,420 loan as well as the interest from the entire life of the loan.

Zeroes have a great advantage in that they do not require any payments of interest until the maturity date. At the same time, there is also an increased risk. Lenders generally receive at least interest over the life of a loan. If they have to wait until the very end of a loan before they receive any payment at all, they are likely to demand a higher rate of interest to compensate them for that increased risk.

Zero-coupon bonds get their name from an era when bond certificates had a coupon attached for each interest payment. The lender would clip a coupon every 6 months and present it for payment. At that time bonds were often issued in bearer form. When a bond was sold by one party to another, the borrower was not informed. Whoever presented the coupons for payment was assumed to be the owner. For reasons of safety (to avoid loss or theft) and for tax purposes (to avoid people not paying taxes on taxable bonds), bonds are no longer issued in bearer form. They are all registered. The borrower maintains a record of the owner of the bond. The interest payments are automatically made without presentation of a coupon. In fact, paper certificates are no longer used. Instead everything is done with electronic record-keeping. Zero-coupon bonds were so called because they had no coupons attached since there were no periodic interest payments.

Debt Refinancing

From time to time, organizations review their bond obligations and consider whether it would be advantageous to refinance the debt. Generally, refinancing means that the organization pays off outstanding debt with high interest rates and substitutes new debt with a lower interest rate.

Interest rates in the financial markets tend to rise and fall with the economy. When there are recessions, interest rates fall. This is largely because there is not much business demand for money. In the Great Recession and the years that followed, the Federal government intentionally kept interest rates low for an extended period to help stimulate the economy by making it inexpensive for businesses to borrow money. When the economy is strong and there is a great demand for loans, the price (i.e., the interest rate) rises.

Sometimes an HCO borrows money despite relatively high interest rates because there is a pressing need for the assets that will be bought with the money. The economy's cycles take a long time. It might be 5 years, 10 years, or even longer before interest rates decline. When the rates do decline, however, the organization must consider whether it pays to refinance the outstanding bonds.

Refinancing is not automatic for a number of reasons. First, there are all the costs related to a new bond issuance. These costs are high but make sense when spread over a long period. If the bonds are refinanced every 5 years, the issuance costs could overwhelm much, if not all, of the interest rate benefit. Second, when bonds are issued, assurances are given to the lenders (i.e., the buyers of the bonds) that they will earn the stated interest rate. Often a penalty is charged to the issuer of the bond for early repayment of the bonds. The borrower may have to pay not only the face value of the bonds but also an extra amount.

The amount of the penalty, if any, depends on the *call provisions* of the bond. Call provisions are the conditions in the bond agreement that specify the rights the borrower has to call in the bond early and pay it off. If the call provisions are easy on the borrower, the original interest rate will be high. If the call provisions make it difficult to call in and pay off the bond, the interest rate is somewhat lower. When the bond is first issued, a tradeoff must be made as the call provisions are established.

So far, we have considered refinancing from the point of view of calling in and paying off an outstanding bond at its face value. A related element of refinancing is the purchase of the organization's own bonds on the open financial market. However, unlike the refinancing done when interest rates fall, purchase refinancing is likely to occur when interest rates rise. If interest rates climb, the market price of bonds drops. Why would anyone want a bond that pays 10% when new bonds pay 12% or 13%?

If interest rates have risen and bond prices have fallen and if the organization has some cash available, it can buy its own bonds at the market price. The advantage of this is that the price is less than the organization will have to pay if it waits for the maturity of the bond.

Frequently, organizations establish a *sinking fund* when they have an outstanding bond liability. A sinking fund is a pool of money accumulated for a specific purpose. The purpose of a bond sinking fund is to accumulate money to eventually pay the bond face value at maturity.

If interest rates have risen and the bonds are selling below their face value, money from the sinking fund can be used to buy the bonds and retire them early. By retiring the bonds, the interest payments for those specific bonds purchased no longer have to be paid. And by buying them below face value, the organization saves the difference between the price paid and the face value that would eventually have had to be paid. On the other hand, the money is no longer in the sinking fund, earning interest at the relatively high current rate.

✳ FEASIBILITY STUDIES

When large amounts of money are borrowed on a long-term basis, the lenders often require that the borrower undertake a *feasibility study* to demonstrate the organization's capacity to repay the loan. The organization will generally hire an outside consultant such as a certified public accounting firm to perform the study. Feasibility studies evaluate all the financial implications of the proposed investment. They show expected revenues and expenses over a long period, usually 5 to 10 years.

A feasibility study will not only show the expected profitability of a particular investment or venture but will also project pro forma financial statements for the entire organization.[3] In addition, feasibility studies include ratio analysis showing the capacity of the organization to cover the interest charges and principal payments on its total debt, including the proposed borrowing.

One of the most telling elements of the feasibility study is the ratio that relates to interest coverage.[4] If the organization cannot make interest payments when due, it risks having to seek protection of the bankruptcy laws and possibly even closure. Therefore, lenders are interested in how much cushion is anticipated for coverage of such payments.

Another element of feasibility studies that is considered fairly important relates to the attitude of the staff in the organization. If the majority of people in the organization believe in a project and are committed to its success, that does not guarantee success. But when the majority are opposed to, disinterested in, or not committed to a project, there is a strong likelihood of failure.

If a commissioned feasibility study raises serious questions about the success of an expansion or new venture, the organization should seriously consider the weaknesses that have been raised. Not only will there be a question about whether financing can be obtained; there is also the more important question about whether the organization is making a mistake by undertaking the project.

✳ THE FUTURE OF HEALTH CARE FINANCING

To thrive, an organization must be able to maintain its major facilities. Buildings must be modernized and eventually replaced. Equipment must be kept up to date. This all requires major capital investments, which in turn require cash resources.

The sources of financing for health care have changed quite a bit over time, and it is likely that this change will continue. Before the 1960s, philanthropy was a major source of cash for long-term investments by HCOs. Then the government became the major supplier of cash resources. Most recently, long-term debt has become the single largest element for new construction.

However, the continued availability of debt is not assured. There are movements to eliminate tax-free bonds. That would severely hurt HCOs, particularly hospitals. Even with the continued existence of tax-free bonds, there is cause for concern. The Affordable Care Act (ACA) of 2010 is expected to create pressure on hospitals and other HCOs to become more efficient in the provision of health care services. It is possible that HCOs that are unable to do this may go out of business. This risk will increase the scrutiny of lenders and may make it more difficult for some HCOs to issue bonds. The basic ability of the organization to issue bonds depends on its actual and perceived risk as an investment.

Whether the ACA will close off a major source of financing for some HCOs or simply make it more expensive cannot be determined at this time. On the other hand, the more successful health care providers may find it easier to issue debt.

Where will the resources come from in the future? Some have suggested that as the government tries to control the amount it pays to health care providers, corporations will have to get together to generate the monies needed. In effect, that proposal is a return to philanthropy but at the corporate level because individuals do not have the vast sums necessary for modern health care facility construction.

Another view of the future is that the government will completely take over the health care system (the so-called "single-payer" option) similar to the approaches of England and Canada. In that view, the government will decide what facilities are needed and will build them using tax dollars.

Yet another view is that many HCOs will go out of business, reducing excess capacity. The remaining organizations will be financially healthy and will continue to have access to the major debt markets.

We have no special insight regarding a solution. We do, however, clearly see a problem. Nationwide, and particularly in certain regions such as the Northeast, the severe financial distress of HCOs such as hospitals and nursing homes has prevented some of them from replacing or even adequately maintaining their facilities. Given this situation and the state of the economy at

---

[3]Pro forma financial statements are discussed in the section on business plans in Chapter 22.

[4]A discussion of ratios is included in Chapter 7.

large, concerns about health care financing are likely to continue well into the future.

✳ IMPLICATIONS FOR NURSE MANAGERS AND EXECUTIVES

The highest levels of nurse managers and executives in any HCO must be involved in the specific long-term financing decisions. Other nurse managers also have an important role in the financing process.

The decision to finance using conventional debt, tax-free bonds, or leasing will have a dramatic impact on the financial well-being of the institution. This decision should not be left solely to financial managers, because they may lack vision about the organization. They have greater financial expertise than nurse managers, but they generally do not have a strong understanding of the clinical aspects of the organization.

This fact is evidenced by the interest that lenders, bond raters, and bond insurers all have in the attitude and thoughts of the staff of an HCO. If the physicians are unhappy, they will not admit patients. If the nurses are unhappy, patients will not want to come to the institution. Financing should be done for investments that will make the HCO as a whole work better. The nursing staff can provide critical input in this area.

Bear in mind that major long-term financing such as a bond issuance is not an area of expertise of anyone in most HCOs. Except for the larger academic medical centers, bond flotation may be something that occurs just once in the career of a chief executive officer, chief financial officer, or chief nurse executive. The input of all areas of the institution can help the organization make the correct decisions.

Some other types of long-term financing are more common. Mortgages and leases are used with great frequency. However, the choice of a mortgage or a lease is not strictly financial. Rather than having financial managers make such decisions on their own, nurse managers should provide input into the process. From a departmental or unit point of view, what are the advantages of a lease or the advantages of ownership compared with a lease? Does the lessor provide some essential support service that is otherwise not readily available? Perhaps the equipment is subject to repeated breakdown. A lease arrangement may provide cheaper service than ownership plus a service contract.

Nurse managers and executives should not assume that the financing of the organization is something outside their management sphere of activity or expertise. A participatory team attitude and approach between nursing and finance are more likely to result in financing decisions that will benefit the entire organization, including nursing services.

✳ KEY CONCEPTS

Long-term financing   Sources of money that the organization can use for longer than 1 year.

Debt   Borrowed money. Interest is generally paid on the debt.

Equity   Represents ownership sources of financing. In some cases, equity represents money that outsiders have given the organization in exchange for an ownership interest. In other cases, equity represents money that the organization itself owns. The four principal sources of equity for HCOs are philanthropy, issuance of corporate stock, government grants, and retained earnings.

   Philanthropy   Gifts to the organization.

   Issuance of corporate stock   Sale of ownership interests in the organization; only available to for-profit organizations.

   Government grants   Direct payments to HCOs, often to finance construction.

   Retained earnings   Profits earned by the organization and retained in the organization to finance asset acquisitions.

Long-term debt   Represents borrowed sources of financing where repayment will be more than one year after the money is borrowed. This includes mortgages, long-term notes, leases, and bonds.

   Mortgages and long-term notes   Conventional loans to the organization. Notes are sometimes secured by collateral and are sometimes unsecured. A note secured by a specific piece of physical property such as a building, piece of equipment, or land is referred to as a *mortgage*.

   Leases   Rental agreements evidenced by a contract referred to as a *lease*. Considered long-term debt because they obligate the organization to making payments over a period of years.

   Bonds   Formal certificates of indebtedness. The certificate indicates a promise to pay interest, usually semiannually, and the face value of the bond at a future specified maturity date. Bonds are now recorded electronically, rather than with the issuance of a physical paper certificate.

Call provisions   Elements of the loan agreement between a bond issuer and a bond purchaser indicating the rights of the bond issuer to call in and pay off the bonds early and specifying penalties that must be paid if a bond is retired early.

Sinking fund   Pool of money accumulated for the eventual repayment of the face value of outstanding bonds.

Feasibility study   Analysis designed to determine the organization's capacity to repay a long-term loan.

✳ SUGGESTED READINGS

Cleverley W, Cleverley J, Song P: *Essentials of health care finance*, ed 7, Sudbury, Mass, 2011, Jones & Bartlett.

Emery D, Finnerty J, Stowe J: *Principles of financial management*, Upper Saddle River, New Jersey, 1998, Prentice Hall.

Finkler S: *Finance & accounting for nonfinancial managers*, ed 4, Chicago, 2011, CCH.

Finkler S, Ward D: *Accounting fundamentals for health care management*, ed 2, Sudbury, Mass, 2012, Jones & Bartlett.

Gapenski L: *Healthcare finance: an introduction to accounting and financial management*, ed 4, Chicago, 2007, Health Administration Press.

Horngren C, Datar S, Foster G: *Cost accounting: a managerial emphasis*, ed 12, Upper Saddle River, New Jersey, 2005, Prentice Hall.

Keown A, Martin J, Petty J: *Foundations of finance*, ed 7, Upper Saddle River, New Jersey, 2010, Prentice Hall.

McLean R: *Financial management in health care organizations*, ed 2, Albany, New York, 2002, Delmar.

Suver J, Neumann B, Boles K: *Management accounting for healthcare organizations*, ed 3, Westchester, Ill, 1992, Pluribus Press.

Zelman W, McCue M, Milikan A, Glick N: *Financial management of health care organizations: an introduction to fundamental tools, concepts, and applications*, ed 3, Cambridge, Mass, 2009, Wiley-Blackwell.

✳ LOOKING TO THE FUTURE

Most nurse managers and executives recognize the importance of financial management. To successfully manage finances, the nurse manager must understand the underlying financial concepts. The preceding chapters described these concepts. In addition to understanding the concepts, it is necessary to have sound financial information on which to base financial decisions. The first step in getting information is to know what to ask for.

In addition to the financial information received from the finance department, nurse managers and executives generate some of the information they need themselves. Other information is readily available in health care organizations; the nurse manager or executive simply needs to ask for it. Still other information is available but not in a format that is useful for the nurse manager. Some information is not available and must be generated either by the nurse manager directly or by other departments in the organization.

The following chapters describe management tools and initiatives that can be used both to generate information and to reconfigure it into a useful format. In addition, the kinds of information that are useful for financial decision making are explored.

Chapter 21 focuses on forecasting using quantitative and qualitative methods. The chapter provides a discussion of data collection and data needs, which are often essential to the various approaches and methods used in forecasting. The use of specific techniques to predict future events, such as patient volume and staffing needs, is explained.

Chapter 22 emphasizes the role of the nurse as entrepreneur. The ideas presented in this chapter reflect the myriad of opportunities available for nurse managers and executives to creatively use financial management to their advantage and to bring sorely needed innovations to health care.

Chapter 23 shifts to focus on current and future issues in nursing, health care, and financial management that provide opportunities for research, growth, and the continued use of financial management techniques to help transform nursing and health care. We believe that nurse managers and executives at all levels must play key roles in leading and managing financial resources in the future. They can do this by influencing policymaking at the levels of clinical practice, health care systems, and society at large.

Forecasting

CHAPTER GOALS

The goals of this chapter are to:

- Explain forecasting techniques used to predict resource use, patient volume, and income
- Discuss the reasons for forecasting

- Discuss the use of computers for forecasting
- Explain the use of qualitative approaches to forecasting
- Explain the expected value technique

✳ INTRODUCTION

The preparation of budgets and other financial decision making requires a number of preliminary steps, including forecasting. A budget cannot be prepared without knowing the types of patients that the organization will likely be treating. A staffing plan to implement a new liver transplant unit cannot be developed without an estimate of the number of patients the unit will serve. And financial decisions cannot be made without knowledge of who the competition is and the actions competitors are likely to take. Similarly, a budget cannot be prepared without information such as how many patients are likely to be treated or how sick they are likely to be. That is where forecasting comes in.

Forecasting techniques allow for prediction of how many patients or patient days the organization or a particular unit or department will treat. Forecasting allows prediction of how sick the patients will be. If a nurse manager were to attempt to prepare an operating budget without some prediction of these elements, there would be no way of determining how much staff is needed. Forecasting can help to estimate how many chest tubes the intensive care unit will need or how many heparin locks a medical-surgical unit will consume. This will enable the nurse manager to plan the supplies portion of the unit's budget.

We are currently entering an era during which hospitals and other health care providers will lose payment if their patients (Medicare patients in particular now, but probably all insured patients as we move forward) have adverse results. For example, payments may be withheld if hospitalized patients develop catheter-associated urinary tract infections, pressure ulcers, ventilator-associated pneumonia, and so on. As pay-for-performance plays a greater role in reimbursement for care, we need the ability to forecast how many adverse results will occur

and what our quality-of-care metrics will show in the future. That will allow us to decide if it makes sense to devote more resources to prevent adverse results and to improve overall quality metrics. Forecasts can be used to provide evidence to justify the need for those resources.

Forecasting is a tool that helps in the preparation not only of the operating budget but also of other budgets. If trends in the demographics of the community can be forecast, it is possible to prepare better long-range and program budgets. If it is forecast that a growing portion of the patient population will be Medicare patients, it can be determined what impact that will have on how quickly the organization gets paid. That will help in preparation of the cash budget.

The range of variables that can be forecast is unlimited. It is possible to predict patients, patient days, various supply items, the percentage of total operations performed by a specific doctor, and so on. Generally, forecasting focuses on predicting values for variables that the manager must respond to, rather than variables that can be controlled. For example, a nursing unit may forecast how sick the patients will be. It cannot control severity of illness, but its budget must be a plan that responds to how sick the patient population is expected to be.

✳ QUANTITATIVE METHODS FOR FORECASTING

Forecasting should be undertaken as an early step in the budget preparation and financial decision-making process. Virtually all managers forecast in some manner. Unsophisticated managers may forecast by simply using their best judgment or by assuming that the previous year's results will occur again the next year. It has been found that more formalized analysis of historical data can yield more accurate predictions than such less sophisticated approaches. These predictions in turn form a basis for many decisions in the planning process.

A formalized forecasting process can be divided into several steps. The first step is collection of historical data. The next step is graphing the data. The third step is analysis of the data to reveal trends or seasonal patterns. The fourth and final step is developing and using formulas to project the variable being forecast into the future.

Before these steps are considered, one point must be stressed: When a forecast is made, it is just an estimate of the future based on probabilities. Sophisticated approaches to forecasting allow the projection to be an educated estimate, but it is still an estimate. An intuitive hunch or gut feeling should not be ignored. Mathematical methods lack the feel for the organization that a manager develops over time. Never accept forecasts on blind faith that if it is mathematical or computer-generated, it must be superior.

Quantitative forecasts are merely aids or supplements that managers should take into consideration along with a number of other factors, many of which often cannot be quantified and entered into formalized predictive models. The best forecasts result from neither naive guessing nor advanced mathematics but from an integration of quantitative methods with the experience and judgment of managers.

Data Collection

The first step in formalized forecasting is collection of historical data. Consider several examples. A nurse manager who wishes to make the most basic of projections—workload—will first have to decide on a workload measure, such as patients or patient days. Then it is necessary to determine what the workload was in the past so it can be projected into the future. This is referred to as a *time-series* approach to forecasting. Historical changes over time are used to help anticipate the likely result in a coming time period.

The method discussed in this section is broadly applicable. To predict diaper usage in the maternity unit, data on the number of diapers used previously can be used. After the number of diapers needed has been predicted, it will probably be necessary to focus on the expected cost per box of diapers. If the purchasing department has a good degree of certainty about the price of diapers for next year (e.g., a purchase contract specifying price), this would be a pretty accurate approach. On the other hand, if it was desired to predict the total cost for diapers directly rather than focusing first on the expected number of diapers, it would be possible to gather information on what total amount was spent on diapers in the past and use that for a direct cost estimate.

In other words, it is possible to first forecast diaper usage and then calculate the projected cost or to forecast diaper cost directly. The preferred choice will depend partly on whether information about the number of diapers to be used in the coming period is considered valuable. Similarly, both the number of patient days and the patient severity of illness can be predicted. Then those data can be used to project the number of nursing hours needed, or historical information about the number of nursing hours consumed can be used to directly forecast nursing hours.

Appropriate Data Time Periods

There is often a tendency to try to "make do" with annual data. In fact, many operating budgets are annual budgets, specifying the total amounts to be spent on each line item for the coming year. However, when a manager is preparing an operating budget, it makes a lot of sense to use monthly rather than annual predictions of costs.

The easiest way to make monthly predictions is to take annual budget information and divide it by 12. In many industries, it would be possible to use such a simple approach; production in one month may be much the same as in any other month. However, in the health care sector, such an expectation is not reasonable. If for no other reason, the weather alone is likely to cause busy and slow periods. Winters are often busier for health care organizations (HCOs) than summers. HCOs must be prepared to have more staff available in busier periods. It is desirable to plan more vacations in slow periods and fewer during peak periods. Thus, it is important to be concerned with month-to-month variations within each year as well as with the predictions for the year as a whole.

Furthermore, the number of days in a month will affect monthly costs. Many HCOs, such as clinics, laboratories, or radiologists' offices, might be open only on weekdays. Some months have as many as 23 weekdays, but other months have as few as 20 weekdays. A 3-day difference on a 20-day base represents a 15% difference. Clearly, a difference that large would have a significant impact on the resources required for the month. Similarly, for a hospital, it is quite likely that the number of weekdays will have an influence, because admissions and discharges tend to be higher on certain days of the week.

Monthly budgets are also important because they can be compared with actual results as they occur. If there is a difference (variance) between the plan and the actual results, the cause can be investigated and perhaps a problem can be corrected immediately. Such variance analysis is the topic of Chapters 16 and 17. Without monthly subdivisions of the budget, it might be necessary to wait until the end of the year to find out if things are going according to plan. By then, of course, it will be too late to do anything about it for this year.

Thus, it is important for most HCOs to have costs broken down on a monthly basis and in a manner that is more sophisticated than simply dividing the year's expected cost or volume by 12. The data collected should generally be historical monthly data. For each type of item to be forecast (patients, chest tubes, diapers, costs), 12 individual data points are needed per year, representing values for the item being forecast for each month.

How far back should the data go? One year seems convenient, and it provides 12 data points. However, one year's worth of data provides only one data point about any single month, such as January, not 12. If this January was unusual (either very costly or unusually low in cost), that would not be readily apparent in a year's worth of data. It is likely that next year would be inaccurately predicted to be like this year. Therefore, more than one year's data are needed.

The use of 10 years of data is often suggested for forecasting, although that has weaknesses as well. It is possible that so much has changed over 10 years that the data are no longer relevant. For that reason, it would seem that 5 years of data (or a total of 60 months) is a reasonable rule of thumb. If a nurse manager knows that things have not changed much on the unit in a long time, using more years of data will make the estimate a better predictor. If there have been drastic changes recently, 5 years might be too long. Judgment is needed; one of the most important things a manager does is exercise judgment. Throughout the budgeting process, as in other managerial functions, a manager can never escape the fact that thoughtful judgment is vital to the process of effective management.

What Data Should Be Collected?

It is necessary to collect historical data on the variables to be forecast. Too often managers stop at that point because those data are sufficient to make a forecast. However, those data points are not all of the data that are really needed to make a good forecast.

Forecasting techniques mindlessly predict the future as an extension of the past, even though many things change over time. Whenever forecasting is done, the manager should question whether factors have changed that will make the future different from the past. Are things changing? For instance, are demographics shifting? When it is predicted that next January will be similar to the previous five Januarys, is the fact that there was a large influx of refugees into the community last July being ignored? Is a sudden shift in population caused by the closing of the town's auto plant being ignored? The forecasting formulas to be developed will not take these recent factors into consideration. Forecasting formulas are based solely on historical information. The manager should collect additional data to use as a judgmental adjustment to forecast results.

For example, the availability of personnel can have a dramatic impact. Suppose an organization had a shortage of available nurses. The result was high overtime payments to staff nurses and high agency charges for per diem nurses. If there has been a noticeable increase in the number of nurses available, a manager should realize that the average hourly cost for nursing can be brought down by the elimination of much overtime and agency cost. A quantitative model for forecasting will not take that into account. Information about nurse availability must be collected, and the manager should give specific consideration to that information.

Note that a unit manager does not have to be a one-person information service. The personnel department can be asked about the outlook for hiring additional staff nurses. Administrators can be asked whether changes in third-party coverage are likely to have any impact. It is unreasonable to expect a home health agency's director of nursing to budget correctly for the coming year if the number of allowable Medicare-reimbursable visits has changed and she or he does not know about it. Most home health agency financial officers would quickly be aware of such a change. That information should promptly be communicated to the chief nursing officer. It is vital to open communication links with other managers throughout the organization to ensure receipt of necessary information that could help in the budget process.

Some changes will not be easy to get information about. For instance, there may be no central clearing person to provide an update on changing technology that will dramatically shift the demand for nursing personnel. Nevertheless, a unit manager must try to get that information and consider its likely impact on the unit. To some extent, nurse managers may have better information on changing technology than the organization's other administrators. First of all, nurse managers have clinical knowledge superior to that of most administrators. Second, nurse managers are likely to know what kinds of changes physicians in their clinical area are planning to implement.

It is also important for nurse managers to be aware of the organization's long-range plan, program budgets, and capital budgets. Many hospitals tend to guard budget data closely, with an "eyes only" attitude. Only people with an immediate need are allowed to see any budget other than their own. It is important that administrators begin to understand that nurse managers do need to see any budget that even indirectly may affect their unit or department. For example, if a new service winds up consuming a significant unplanned amount of nursing time, much of it will likely be at overtime rates or will result in overtime elsewhere in the hospital. Had the nurse managers been involved in the planning for the new service, overtime premiums might have been avoided. If a manager is to be held responsible for overtime, then that manager is entitled to have the information needed to anticipate demands on the unit and to plan for adequate staffing.

Graphing Historical Data

Having collected all of the relevant data that might help predict the future, the next step is to lay out the historical data on a graph. In the forecasting approach discussed here, time is plotted on the horizontal axis. For instance, suppose that the unit manager wants to predict next year's total nursing hours starting with January 2013. Assume that it is currently October 2012 and that historical data from the past 5 years are going to be used. Data for October through December 2012 are not yet available and therefore cannot be used to help forecast what will happen in 2013. Therefore, the horizontal axis begins with October 2007 and goes through September 2012 (Figure 21–1).

The vertical axis provides information on the variable to be forecast. This is nursing hours in Figure 21–1. The forecasting methods discussed later in this chapter allow a manager to predict workload estimates for the future (e.g., the number of patients and the number of patient days), to predict the actual amounts of resource consumption (e.g., the number of nursing hours or the number of rolls of bandage tape), or to predict costs. Depending on the procedures of your specific institution, some of these forecasts may be made by the accounting department rather than by nurse managers.

If costs or some other financial measure expressed in dollars is being predicted directly, the impact of inflation must be considered. If inflation is ignored as forecasting is done, the forecast becomes more complicated, because it must predict not only a workload measure, such as the number of diapers for the coming year, but also the rate of inflation for the coming year.

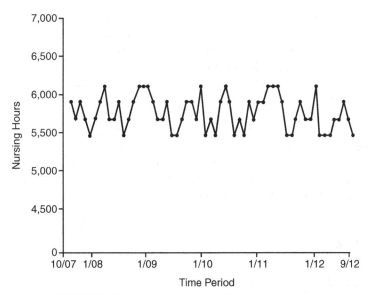

FIGURE 21–1. Basic graph for nursing hours forecast.

The problem of inflation and adjustments that can be made to allow for it are discussed in Chapter 8.

If a prediction is being made for next year's nursing hours (see Figure 21–1), the first point graphed is the number of nursing hours worked in October 2007, the next point is the number of nursing hours in November 2007, and so on. It is important to keep in mind that this forecasting approach is a *time-series* analysis; that is, the variable on the horizontal axis is always time. In time-series analysis, whether the manager is trying to predict workload, resources, or cost, the basic process is to look at how much of that item was used in the past and project that into the future. To make such predictions, the manager will need to be able to analyze the underlying cause of variations in the data that have been graphed.

Analysis of Graphed Data

Before any predictions can be made, it is necessary to assess the basic characteristics of the data that have been graphed. For instance, do the data exhibit *seasonality*? Is there a particular *trend*? Do variations from month to month and year to year appear to be simply random fluctuations? There may be patterns related to the passage of time that can be uncovered.

A visual inspection can usually give a good picture of the type of pattern that exists. Here it is important to focus on a reasonably long period, at least several years, as opposed to several months. By looking at just the past few months, it is possible to get a distorted impression of what is occurring. For instance, see Figure 21–2. (Note: These are not the same data as shown in Figure 21–1.) It appears that the number of nursing

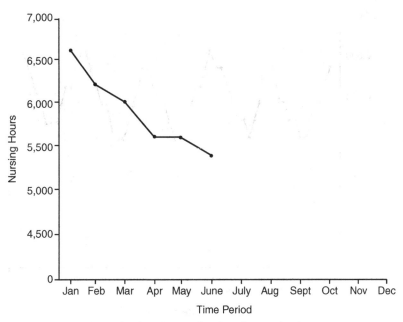

FIGURE 21–2. Six months' data for nursing hours.

hours has a definite downward trend, but this graph covers a period of only 6 months.

Figure 21–3 shows the pattern for the full year. Now the graph gives a totally different impression. The number of nursing hours has not been steadily decreasing over time. For the first half of the year, it was decreasing, and for the second half, it was increasing. The pattern observed is not likely to be indicative of a long-term decline. It is still not possible to tell, however, if some basic change has occurred that caused a downward trend to reverse or if the pattern is seasonal behavior. Will the number of nursing hours continue to rise next year, as it appears to be doing near the end of the current year,

or will it turn downward, as it did at the beginning of the year? To answer that question, it is vital that data for at least several years be graphed.

Now look at Figure 21–4, which covers a period of 5 years. A pattern of falling and then rising hours occurs each year. This is clearly a seasonal pattern rather than a trend. Each year the same pattern repeats itself.

When data for a sufficient number of years are graphed, the pattern that becomes apparent will generally fall into one of four categories: random fluctuations, trend, seasonality, and seasonality and trend together. Each of these patterns will be discussed.

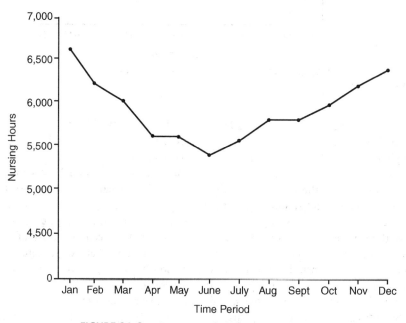

FIGURE 21–3.   One year's data for nursing hours.

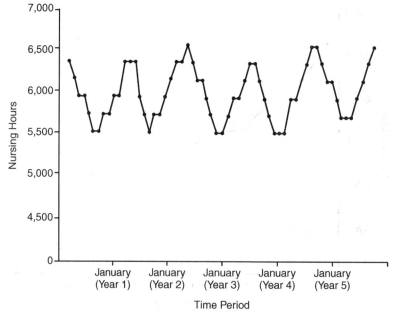

FIGURE 21–4.   Five years' data for nursing hours forecast: seasonality.

Random Fluctuations

It would be quite surprising if a unit or department consumed exactly the same amount of any resource 2 months or 2 years in a row. One year the winter will be a little colder than usual, and more people will get pneumonia. Another year prices will rise a little faster. One year some staff members will take more sick days than another. Yet these events are not likely to be trends—it does not get colder and colder year after year. Nor are they seasonal. They are just random, unpredictable events.

A graph exhibiting random patterns only might look something like that shown in Figure 21–5. As can be seen, there is no clear upward or downward trend. You may also notice that each year there is no discernible seasonal pattern. The month of May is not usually busy or slow. May is a low month in the first year and a high month in the next year relative to the values for the other months in those years.

Seasonality

Seasonal patterns are sometimes visible to the eye, as was the case in Figure 21–4. In health care, one is especially likely to see seasonal patterns because of seasonal disease patterns and as a result of the weather. Winter months bring different ailments than summer months do. For hospitals and home health agencies, this affects overall patient volume. On the other hand, nursing homes may be running at full occupancy year round. Therefore, the number of patient days at a nursing home might not show any seasonality, although the specific care needs of the patients in a nursing home are likely to vary with the different seasons.

However, seasonality may not always be easy to spot. Therefore, it might be a worthwhile exercise to examine certain months that are known as peak or slow periods. Suppose that

January is compared with June for each of the past 5 years and it is found that January almost always has higher levels of the variable being forecast than does June. In that case, seasonality does exist even if it is not readily apparent when the graph is visually inspected.

Trend

In Figure 21–6, although the graph has its ups and downs, there is a clear upward trend. Because nursing hours rather than dollars are being considered here, this is not caused by inflation. Rather, it is probably caused either by an increased number of patient days or by an increased amount of nursing time provided per patient day.

The underlying causes of observed patterns will not be determined in the forecasting process described here. The focus is strictly on projections of past items into the future. Whatever the cause, it appears that a definite trend exists. Unless there is information about expected patient days or a new policy regarding the relative ratio of nurses to patients, it would have to be assumed that this trend will continue. However, managers should try to understand the underlying causes of patterns such as trends. This will better enable them to forecast correctly if something does change the underlying cause of the pattern.

Note further in Figure 21–6 that although the overall trend is upward, there is no discernible seasonal pattern. For example, January does not appear to be consistently high or low each year relative to the other months of those years.

Seasonality and Trend

It is common for HCOs to experience at least some seasonality. At the same time, because of increasing patient volume or the effects of inflation, upward trends are common as well. Downward

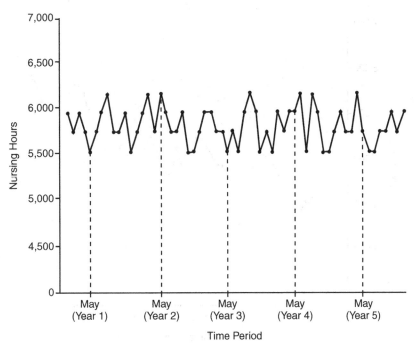

FIGURE 21–5. Five years' data for nursing hours forecast: random fluctuations.

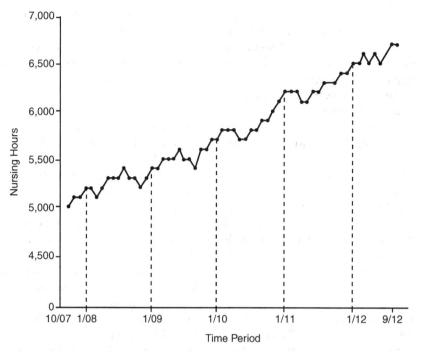

FIGURE 21–6.   Five years' data for nursing hours forecast: trend.

trends may also occur. It is not at all unusual, therefore, for the organization to experience both seasonal influences and trends at the same time. Figure 21–7 shows an example of a historical pattern exhibiting both seasonality and trend.

Often the trend is more obvious than the seasonality in patterns that contain both. In these cases, it becomes especially useful to make several comparisons to see if certain months are always higher or lower than other months. Valid forecasts require an awareness of seasonal patterns if they exist.

Forecasting Formulas

At this point, historical data have been gathered and graphed, and there has been a visual inspection of the graphs for apparent trend or seasonal patterns. It is finally time to begin using the information to make forecasts for the coming year. The approach taken for forecasting depends to a great degree on whether seasonal patterns, trends, both, or neither is present.

An approach to forecasting each of these patterns is discussed next. First, however, it should be noted that the formulas

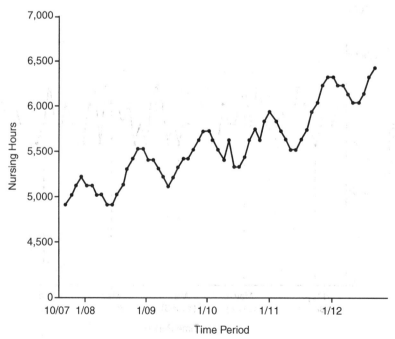

FIGURE 21–7.   Five years' data for nursing hours forecast: seasonality with trend.

assume limited use of computer technology in performing the forecasting function. Much of the tedium and difficulty of the forecasting process is avoided if a computer forecasting program is used. Although the formulas discussed here are valuable in situations in which a computer approach is unavailable, a computer solution is preferred. It takes less management time and can produce superior results. The costs of appropriate software are readily offset by the saved managerial time. A computer approach to forecasting is presented later in this chapter.

Random Fluctuations

The easiest forecasting occurs when there is no seasonal pattern or trend. For example, consider the budget for office supplies for the office of the chief nurse executive (CNE). The need for these supplies may not vary much over time or with the particular workload of nurses who deliver care on patient care units.

The most obvious approach in this case would be to simply add up the 60 monthly data points for the past 5 years and divide by 60. That will give a monthly average. If every month is like every other month in terms of the variable being forecast, this would be a reasonable approximation.

Caution must be exercised, however. Different months have different numbers of days. Even if there is no strong seasonal influence or trend, longer months may consume more of a resource. Months that have more weekdays may consume more of a resource. It may be necessary to adjust for factors such as days in a month or weekdays in a month. For example, if weekdays use much more of a resource than weekends, rather than dividing the total for the last 60 months by 60, the total could be divided by the number of weekdays in the past 60 months. The result is a predicted value per weekday. That value can be multiplied by the specific number of weekdays in each month in the coming year to get the appropriate forecast for each month.

Seasonality

If seasonality exists in the variable being forecast, it means that some months are typically low in the use or consumption of a resource and other months are typically high. If all 60 months for the past 5 years are averaged together, the seasonality becomes lost in the broad average. An approach is needed that is more sensitive to fluctuations within each year. The most obvious approach is to add together the values for a given month for several years and divide by the number of years over which a forecast is being made, to get an average for just that month. For example, the previous five February values can be totaled and then divided by 5. That provides a February average for the past 5 years that can be used as a prediction for next February.

This approach is not always acceptable, however. Suppose that seasonal variations do not repeat in the exact same month each year. For instance, suppose that February is usually the coldest month, causing patient days to peak because of many flu cases. Sometimes, however, January or March is colder. Because of this variation in seasonality from year to year, a better prediction may result from adding January plus February plus March for the last 5 years. Thus, February is based on

January, February, and March. This total is divided by 15 to get a prediction of February for next year. Then March is estimated by adding February plus March plus April for each of the past 5 years and dividing by 15.

The key to this moving-average approach is to add up not only the month in question for the last 5 years, but also the month preceding and the month following the month being predicted. This formula will often give a good prediction. However, there are also problems with this approach. Peaks and valleys in activity will be understated. For instance, what if January is typically the busiest month of the year, and both December and February are less busy? By averaging December and February with January, the slower December and February will cause the busier January to be understated in the forecast.

How can a nurse manager determine whether predictions will be improved by using calculations such as these? Should the manager simply take an average of five Februarys or use January, February, and March information for 5 years to predict next February? One good way to make that determination is to use historical data (excluding data from the most recent past year) to predict the results of the past year. For instance, if 2012 has just ended, take data from 2007 through 2011 and use them to predict 2012. Because the actual results for 2012 are known, the prediction can immediately be compared with the actual results. This is a good way to test any formula or forecasting technique to see if it is a reasonable predictor.

Keep in mind two things, however. First, no forecast can predict the future perfectly. The future is uncertain, and all of the specific events that will occur can never be fully anticipated. Therefore, the prediction should not be expected to match the actual results precisely. Second, the predictions or forecasts using formulas must be adjusted based on the manager's own knowledge about the unit—its patients, staff, and resources—and the future. The formulas just use information about the past. If managers have some information about the future that leads them to believe that the future will not follow the patterns of the past, that information must be used to adjust the predictions of the formulas. The role of an intelligent manager should never be relinquished to the mathematical precision of a formula.

When a formula is tested by seeing how well it predicts what actually happened the year before, the manager should determine whether the predictions based on the formula are closer to what actually happened than the predictions might have been if a different formula was used or in the absence of the formula. If so, then it is a useful tool. Otherwise, the formula should be either modified or discarded.

Trend

If a trend is observed, it is desirable to project that trend into the future. Trends are usually represented by a straight line. However, trends tend to have some random elements within them. If one were to draw a straight line, it would not generally go through each historical point. Some points would be above the line, and some would be below. A manager could just eyeball the points on the graph and try to draw a line that is as close as possible to all of the points and that extends into the future. However, such manual attempts are likely to be inaccurate.

If the line is drawn too high or too low, the estimates for the future will also be too high or too low. Even worse, if the slope of the line is too high or too low, the error will be magnified, as seen in Figure 21–8. In this figure, the solid line represents the best straight line that uses the known data to forecast the future. The dashed line represents a judgmental, eyeball estimate. Note that near the center of the graph, the two lines are relatively close. However, to the extreme right side of the graph, in the area of the forecast for the coming year, the two lines have diverged to the point that the number of nursing hours predicted differs a great deal, depending on which line is used.

One solution to this problem is to use a statistical technique called *regression analysis*. The goal of regression analysis is to find the unique straight line that comes closest to all of the historical data points. Regression analysis can be readily performed by a nurse manager on a computer using statistical software packages, electronic spreadsheet programs, or dedicated forecasting software packages.

Regression analysis, discussed in Chapter 8, is a technique that applies mathematical precision to a scatter diagram. The scatter diagram used in regression analysis is a graph that plots points of information. Each data point represents a dependent variable and one or more independent variables (or casual variables). Each independent variable is responsible for causing variations in the dependent variable.

When making forecasts, time is considered an independent variable, and a second variable is considered a dependent variable. For example, the dependent variable could be the number of patients treated by the organization. As time passes, the organization may have more or fewer patients. The change in the number of patients over time may reflect a random pattern, seasonal effect, trend, or seasonality and trend. If a trend exists, regression analysis will generate a line that is a good predictor of the future.

Regression is a tool that can help managers to manage better. The major difficulty in using regression is simply a fear of the process (and this relates not only to nurse managers but to all managers). However, when a computer program is used, regression analysis does not require the user to do extensive mathematical computation. The computer carries out all of the calculations.[1] Most spreadsheet software programs used to perform the financial calculations discussed throughout this book will also perform simple linear regression and multiple regression computations.

Because regression analysis requires the manager to provide numerical values, months and years cannot be used by their names for the independent variable. An independent variable cannot be referred to as January 2007. Instead, the month names can be replaced by assigned numerical values. The historical months used for the analysis can be identified as 1 through 60 instead of October 2007, November 2007, and so forth to September 2012. Table 21–1 presents the data. After entering the information into a calculator or computer (e.g., in month 1, there were 5,000 nursing hours; in month 2, there were 5,100 nursing hours; and so on through month 60, with 6,700 nursing hours), the calculator or computer is instructed to "run" (compute) the regression. When the computation is complete, it is possible to determine how many nursing hours are expected in months 64 through 75, which represent the 12 months of next year. Note that months 61 through 63 have been intentionally skipped over. There are neither historical data points nor forecast points plotted for those 3 months, because those months represent the remaining months of the current year, for which data are not yet available. The goal is to develop predictions for the months in the coming year.

---

[1]Although regression is easy to perform with a computer, the user should have some familiarity with regression to interpret the regression results and their significance. See the discussion of regression in Chapter 8 or a statistics text.

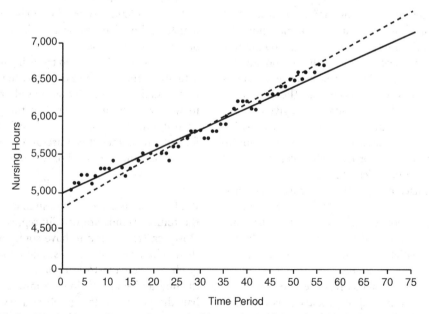

FIGURE 21–8. Nursing hours forecast for trend with no seasonality: judgmental versus regression results.

✳ **TABLE 21–1** *Nursing Hours—Historical Data for Trend with No Seasonality*

Data Point	Date		Nursing Hours	Data Point	Date		Nursing Hours
1	October	2007	5,000	31	April		5,800
2	November		5,100	32	May		5,700
3	December		5,100	33	June		5,700
4	January	2008	5,200	34	July		5,800
5	February		5,200	35	August		5,800
6	March		5,100	36	September		5,900
7	April		5,200	37	October		5,900
8	May		5,300	38	November		6,000
9	June		5,300	39	December		6,100
10	July		5,300	40	January	2011	6,200
11	August		5,400	41	February		6,200
12	September		5,300	42	March		6,200
13	October		5,300	43	April		6,100
14	November		5,200	44	May		6,100
15	December		5,300	45	June		6,200
16	January	2009	5,400	46	July		6,200
17	February		5,400	47	August		6,300
18	March		5,500	48	September		6,300
19	April		5,500	49	October		6,300
20	May		5,500	50	November		6,400
21	June		5,600	51	December		6,400
22	July		5,500	52	January	2012	6,500
23	August		5,500	53	February		6,500
24	September		5,400	54	March		6,600
25	October		5,600	55	April		6,500
26	November		5,600	56	May		6,600
27	December		5,700	57	June		6,500
28	January	2010	5,700	58	July		6,600
29	February		5,800	59	August		6,700
30	March		5,800	60	September		6,700

The results are shown in the scatter diagram in Figure 21–9. The regression results are plotted as a solid line for 2013 and are extended back from 2012 to 2007 with a dashed line. The specific predictions of nursing-hour requirements for 2013, by month, are as follows:

January	6,772
February	6,800
March	6,828
April	6,856
May	6,884
June	6,911
July	6,939
August	6,967
September	6,995
October	7,023
November	7,051
December	7,079

Note in Figure 21–9 that the projections for the next year all fall on the trend line, even though in the past, many actual points are not on the extended (dashed) trend line. Actual results over the coming year are not really expected to fall right on the line either; however, in the absence of any other information, the points on the trend line represent the best prediction that can be made for the actual uncertain outcome. To guess higher than the trend-line value would probably be too high more than half the time; to guess lower than the trend-line value would probably be too low more than half the time.

Seasonality and Trend

Seasonality together with trend poses a more complex problem, yet it is likely to be a common occurrence, so readers should pay special attention to the approach discussed here. This example uses the data provided in Table 21–2. The first step is to use regression analysis to predict a trend line for the coming year. After a set of results for the regression has been plotted for each month in the coming year (January 2013 through December 2013), it should be noted that there is no seasonal appearance to the line predicting next year; it simply shows an upward trend (see Figure 21–10 for 2013).

The next step is to extend the trend backward into the 5 years for which there are historical data. This is fairly straightforward because it simply requires extending backward a straight line that has been already located for the coming year (see the dashed line on Figure 21–11).

After the line has been extended backward, the manager must calculate how much above or below the line the actual value each month was for the past 5 years. Those amounts must then be converted into a percentage. For example, in January 2008 (see Figure 21–11), there were 5,200 nursing hours, but the trend line was at a vertical height of 5,000. The actual value was 200 hours above the trend. Because it is a trend, however, it is necessary to convert it to a percentage. In this case, it is a positive 4%, because 5,200 is 4% above the trend-line point of 5,000.

Now simply revert to the seasonal approach. Add together the percentages that December, January, and February are over

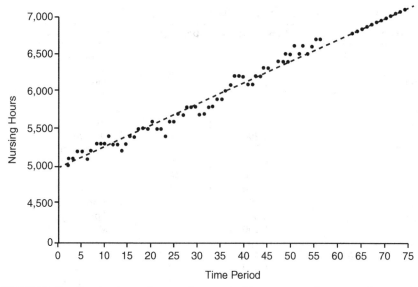

FIGURE 21–9. Nursing hours forecast for trend with no seasonality: regression results.

✳ **TABLE 21–2** *Nursing Hours—Historical Data for Trend with Seasonality*

Data Point	Date		Nursing Hours	Data Point	Date		Nursing Hours
1	October	2007	4,900	31	April		5,500
2	November		5,000	32	May		5,400
3	December		5,100	33	June		5,600
4	January	2008	5,200	34	July		5,300
5	February		5,100	35	August		5,300
6	March		5,100	36	September		5,400
7	April		5,000	37	October		5,600
8	May		5,000	38	November		5,700
9	June		4,900	39	December		5,600
10	July		4,900	40	January	2011	5,800
11	August		5,000	41	February		5,900
12	September		5,100	42	March		5,800
13	October		5,300	43	April		5,700
14	November		5,400	44	May		5,600
15	December		5,500	45	June		5,500
16	January	2009	5,500	46	July		5,500
17	February		5,400	47	August		5,600
18	March		5,400	48	September		5,700
19	April		5,300	49	October		5,900
20	May		5,200	50	November		6,000
21	June		5,100	51	December		6,200
22	July		5,200	52	January	2012	6,300
23	August		5,300	53	February		6,300
24	September		5,400	54	March		6,200
25	October		5,400	55	April		6,200
26	November		5,500	56	May		6,100
27	December		5,600	57	June		6,000
28	January	2010	5,700	58	July		6,000
29	February		5,700	59	August		6,100
30	March		5,600	60	September		6,300

and under the trend line for the past 5 years and divide by 15. The result is a prediction of the percent above or below the trend line January will be next year. Find the point on the trend line next year for January and multiply it by the moving-average percent to find how much above or below the trend line the predicted point is. This process can be repeated for each month of the coming year. For example, Table 21–3 shows the actual number of nursing hours incurred and the extended trend-line information for December, January, and February for 5 years.

The trend-line prediction for January 2013 from Figure 21–11 is 6,204. This is before adjustment for seasonality. In the calculation shown in Table 21–3, it was determined that for January, the moving-average percentage is a positive 3.2%. By adding 3.2% of 6,204 to the trend-line value of 6,204, the resulting prediction adjusted for seasonality is 6,403. That point has been plotted for January 2013 on Figure 21–11. Similarly, to get the 2013 forecast for the entire year, this process should be repeated on a moving-average basis for each month in turn.

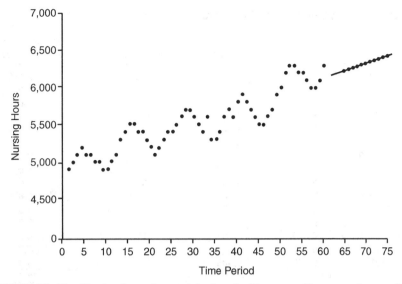

FIGURE 21–10. Nursing hours forecast for trend with seasonality: regression results

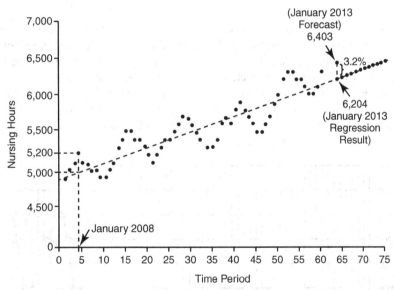

FIGURE 21–11. Nursing hours forecast for trend with seasonality: regression results extended back into historical data.

Using Computers for Forecasting

The previous section on forecasting formulas demonstrates how complicated forecasting can become when historical data are influenced by both trend and seasonality. However, HCOs frequently do have at least seasonality; both trend and seasonality are not uncommon. The ability of nurse managers and executives to deal with such patterns has improved dramatically as a result of personal computers and specially designed computer software. These computer programs make the work of forecasting easier and the results more accurate.

Regression analysis produces a straight-line or linear forecast. When there is seasonality, certain months are always above the regression line, and others are always below it. Seasonal patterns cannot be estimated well with straight lines. Trends and seasonal patterns occurring at the same time increase the complexity further. *Curvilinear* forecasting uses curved lines for making its estimates of the future. Because the

forecast line can curve, it will come closer to the historical points, and therefore its projections are likely to be closer to the results that will actually occur.

Electronic spreadsheet programs such as Excel can do some forecasting analysis. However, this is not their primary function, and using spreadsheet programs for forecasting can be difficult. A number of specialized forecasting programs can perform curvilinear forecasting.[2] Such programs tend to be

---

[2]SmartForecasts for Windows is a trademark of Smart Software, Inc., 4 Hill Road, Belmont, MA 02178; phone: 617-489-2743. Version 4.16 was used for Figures 21–13 and 21–14 and Tables 21–4 and 21–5 in this chapter. This chapter does not attempt to demonstrate all of the capabilities of this software. The software program is used simply as an example of the use of computer forecasting. Permission has been obtained from the vendor for the use of these examples. The use of the examples in this chapter does not represent a formal endorsement of the product.

✳ **TABLE 21–3** *Calculation of Moving-Average Percent for January 2013*

Month	Actual	Trend Line	Difference	Difference as a Percentage of Trend Line
December 2007	5,100	4,980	120	2.4%
January 2008	5,200	5,000	200	4.0
February 2008	5,100	5,020	80	1.6
December 2008	5,500	5,221	279	5.3
January 2009	5,500	5,241	259	4.9
February 2009	5,400	5,261	139	2.6
December 2009	5,600	5,461	139	2.5
January 2010	5,700	5,482	218	4.0
February 2010	5,700	5,502	198	3.6
December 2010	5,600	5,702	(102)*	(1.8)*
January 2011	5,800	5,723	77	1.3
February 2011	5,900	5,743	157	2.7
December 2011	6,200	5,943	257	4.3
January 2012	6,300	5,963	337	5.7
February 2012	6,300	5,983	317	5.3
Total				48.4%
Divided by 15 =				3.2%

*Negative amounts.

much easier to use, generating curvilinear forecasts automatically. This makes the forecasting process something that can be done by managers who are not expert in statistics. These programs provide data entry formats similar to an electronic spreadsheet (e.g., Excel) with columns and rows. Each column represents a time period, and each row represents a variable to be forecast, such as patients or nursing hours.

Reconsider the forecast for the data from Table 21–2. After the data have been entered, one of the first steps is to print a time plot graph to get a visual sense of the data. Figure 21–12 is a time plot that has been generated by one of the specialized software forecasting programs. This time plot quickly alerts the user to the upward trend; closer inspection reveals the seasonal nature of the data.

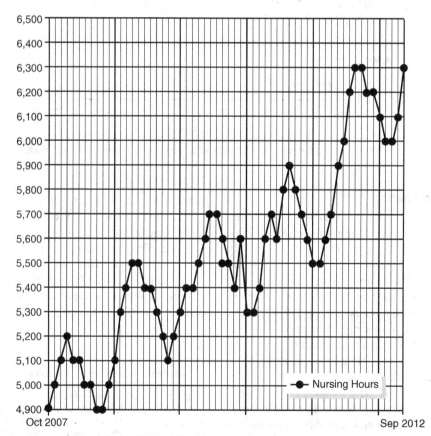

FIGURE 21–12. Time plot graph of historical data.

A number of different forecasting models are available within forecasting software programs. Generally, the user can forecast nursing hours using regression analysis. However, the key advantage of this type of software is that it allows use of a curved line for forecasting. This should remove the necessity to adjust the trend line for seasonality. Furthermore, the program can automatically chose among various forecasting approaches. With the automatic approach, the computer will calculate the forecast with a number of different methods to see which predicts best.

Figure 21–13 is the forecast graph generated by a forecasting software program. What does the graph consist of? The historical data points are connected by a solid line. The forecast during the historical (past) periods is dotted. Compare this dotted line with the regression line shown in Figure 21–11. During the first 5 years in Figure 21–11, the actual points are usually substantially above or below the regression line. Therefore, it is reasonable to assume that as the line is used to project next year, each month's actual result is likely to be substantially above or below the forecast trend line.

Although the statistical theory is complex, effectively, the closer the forecast line comes to the actual results in the past, the more likely the forecast line is to come close to the actual results in the future. When the computer performs forecasting automatically, it examines how close the forecast line is to the actual historical points for each of a series of different forecasting methods. The computer can be given a command to examine the relative accuracy of the different forecasting methods examined. Table 21–4 shows the results of the competition among forecasting methods for this example. The best technique is Winters' multiplicative method. This is a curvilinear approach that works extremely well for seasonal data. The data points are only 1.3% farther away from the forecast line for the next best method, another form of Winters' forecasting. However, using alternatives to the Winters' approaches generates much less accurate results.

In Figure 21–13, it is evident that the dotted forecast line for the first 5 years followed extremely closely the actual results. In some cases, the solid and dotted lines are so close that they cannot be distinguished from each other. Therefore, the forecast line, when projected through 2013, is likely to give a fairly accurate estimate.

In the graph shown in Figure 21–13, there are solid lines above and below (bracketing) the forecast line projected into the future. These lines represent a margin-of-error interval.

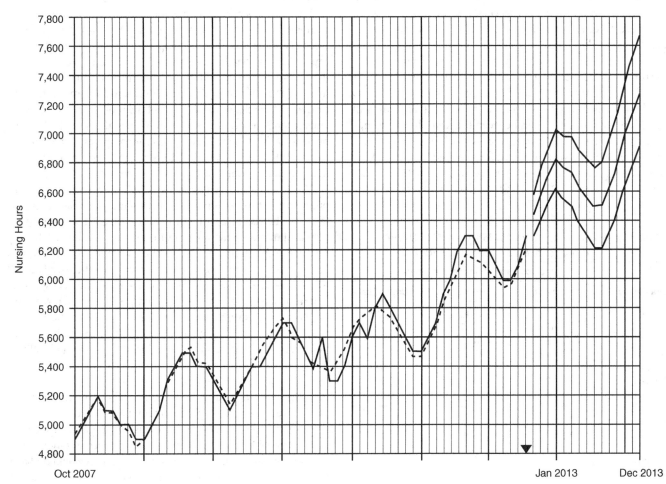

FIGURE 21–13. Forecast of nursing hours.

※ **TABLE 21–4** *Tournament Rankings for AUTOMATIC Forecasts of V1 Nursing Hours*

Rank	Method	% Worse than Winner
1	Winters' multiplicative, weights = 22%, 22%, 22%	(Winner)
2	Winters' additive, weights = 20%, 20%, 20%	1.3
3	Double exponential smoothing, weight = 8%	57.2
4	Linear moving average of 12 periods	65.0
5	Simple moving average of 1 period	118.3
6	Single exponential smoothing, weight = 59%	118.9

Forecasts can never be expected to be exactly correct. It is possible, however, to use statistics to get some idea of how large the difference might be between the forecast and the actual result. In this case, based on the statistical analysis, there is a 90% likelihood that the actual result will fall somewhere between these solid lines. That means that for the variable being forecast by this graph, we would only expect the actual result to be higher than the upper bracketed line once in 20 years, or to be below the lower bracketed line once in 20 years. But graphs, although visually informative, are hard to read when it is time to write the actual forecast. A numerical table of the forecast results can be generated by the software. See Table 21–5 for the forecast results.

Table 21–5 shows not only the forecast but also the margin of error or confidence interval above and below the forecast. If desired, that interval can easily be changed by the software so that there is 95% or 99% confidence that the actual result will fall within the range of values between the lower limit and upper limit estimates. If the percentage is raised to a higher confidence level, the interval around the forecast line becomes wider. For example, for January 2013, the prediction is 6,821 nursing hours, and there is 90% confidence that the actual nursing

hours will not be less than 6,622 or more than 7,020. If a manager wants to be 99% confident that the actual results will not exceed the boundaries of the projection, the lower limit value becomes lower and the upper limit higher.

In practice, it is rarely necessary to be so precise. Although 95% or 99% confidence may be important for academic research studies, in practice, managers tend to have a greater degree of latitude. A 90% confidence interval implies that 9 times out of 10, the actual result will fall within the bounds of the interval. That is an extremely good result for most managers' forecasts.

Compare the result from Winters' multiplicative method (see Table 21–5 and Figure 21–13) with the earlier result obtained by the combined regression analysis–moving-average approach (see January 2013 in Figure 21–11). As can be seen, the results differ. This is because the approach used earlier is less accurate than Winters' method. Earlier, the January 2013 number of nursing hours was projected to be 6,403, but Winters' method predicts it to be approximately 6,821. In fact, the earlier estimate is below the lower limit value of the 90% confidence interval. It is clear that using more sophisticated techniques can generate results that differ markedly from the manual approaches used before computer software was readily available. It is probable that the manual moving-average calculation will be more accurate than simply a judgmental guess. However, the computer-based Winters' solution is likely to be even more accurate.

It is also possible to refine Winters' method even further. The computer makes some general assumptions when it performs forecasts under the automatic approach. If Winters' method was immediately selected as the forecasting method instead of selecting automatic, some additional options would be provided to improve the forecast further. Specifically, the software can be informed of the relative importance of the most recent level, trend, and seasonal factors. If the user knows that the trend is changing because of shifts in the underlying demographics of the community population, it is possible to give more weight to the most recent trend compared with the trend in the earlier years.

Not only can information be supplied to enable the computer forecast to be more accurate, such as the relative importance of the recent trend, but it is also possible to modify the results of the computer analysis. Results can be adjusted directly on the forecast graph, or historical data points can be modified on the basis of some judgment or knowledge the user has that is not reflected in the historical information. This is especially helpful when there is an outlier data point. For example, suppose that a rare event caused data for one month to be atypical. That data point can cause the forecast to be thrown off substantially. A better forecast may be obtained by judgmentally adjusting that data point's value. Judgmental adjustments are also needed because computer-generated forecasts assume that factors that affected nursing hours remain the same in the future as they were in the past. That may not be the case.

Most managers initially use a forecasting program only to forecast one variable at a time. However, as one becomes more adept at using computer-based forecasting, the program would probably be used to generate forecasts on a number of different variables. The user will also want to be able to save the data file, to avoid having to reenter data each time an analysis is to be performed.

※ **TABLE 21–5** *Forecasts of V1 NURSING HOURS Using Multiplicative WINTERS' METHOD*

Time Period	Approximate 90% Forecast Interval		
	Lower Limit	Forecast	Upper Limit
Oct 2012	6,284	6,434	6,584
Nov 2012	6,405	6,572	6,740
Dec 2012	6,520	6,704	6,888
Jan 2013	6,622	6,821	7,020
Feb 2013	6,549	6,766	6,983
Mar 2013	6,502	6,737	6,973
Apr 2013	6,391	6,641	6,891
May 2013	6,306	6,570	6,834
Jun 2013	6,210	6,493	6,775
Jul 2013	6,205	6,507	6,809
Aug 2013	6,311	6,633	6,956
Sep 2013	6,449	6,788	7,126
Oct 2013	6,634	6,996	7,358
Nov 2013	6,769	7,143	7,516
Dec 2013	6,897	7,282	7,666

The most significant aspect of using sophisticated software programs is that they can generate a substantially improved result. The ability of the forecast line to curve in synchronization with the actual historical seasonal pattern decreases the required effort by the manager substantially while enhancing the result.

After a period of time goes by, actual results should be compared with our forecasts to ensure that our forecasting model is working sufficiently for our needs. If our forecasts are not giving reasonable results, we need to consider what other models might provide a better result.

❋ QUALITATIVE METHODS FOR FORECASTING

The discussion in this chapter has assumed that reasonably reliable historical data are available. However, there will be many instances, especially in the case of new ventures, when a forecast will be needed for a budget even though there are no reliable historical data. Subjective estimates will be required. In such cases, regression analysis or even computerized curvilinear forecasting will be inadequate to provide a solution. Two approaches commonly used to aid in making reasonable subjective forecasts are the Delphi and nominal group techniques.

In both approaches, a team or expert panel must be selected to include individuals who are likely to have reasoned insights with respect to the variable being forecast. Although no one may have direct knowledge or experience, an attempt should be made to select a qualified group. Industrial experience has shown that by arriving at a consensus among a team of experts, subjective forecasts can be reasonably accurate.

Nominal Group Technique

The *nominal group technique* is one in which a group of individuals is brought together in a structured meeting. Members write down their forecasts. Then all of the written forecasts are presented to the group by a group leader without discussion. After all of the forecasts have been revealed, the reasoning behind each one is discussed. After the discussions, each member again makes a forecast in writing. Through a repetitive process, eventually a group decision is made.

Obviously, there are weaknesses to the nominal group technique. One problem concerns lack of information. If different forecasts are made based on different assumptions, it may be impossible to reach consensus. Another problem concerns politics and personalities. As members of the group defend their forecasts, extraneous issues having to do with whose idea it is may bias the group decision.

Delphi Technique

With the *Delphi technique*, the group never meets. All forecasts are presented in writing to a group leader, who provides summaries to all group members. For forecasts that differ substantially from the majority's—either high or low—a request is made for the reasoning behind the forecast. That information is also shared with group members. Then a new round of forecasts is made. This process is repeated several times, and a decision is made based on the collective responses.

Delphi has several particular advantages. By eliminating a face-to-face meeting, confrontation is avoided. Decisions are based more on logic than on personality or position. The dissemination of the respondents' underlying reasoning allows erroneous facts or assumptions to be eliminated.

Both the nominal group and the Delphi methods make use of the fact that individual managers cannot be expected to know everything. Different individuals, bringing different expertise and different points of view to bear on the same problem, can create an outcome superior to what any one of them could do individually. It is a cliché to say that two minds are better than one. Nevertheless, it is true that in many forecasting instances, the Delphi and nominal group approaches can substantially improve results.

❋ EXPECTED VALUE

One approach to making decisions in the uncertain world of health care is to estimate the probability that certain events will occur. An *expected value* is a weighted average using the probabilities as weights. For example, assume that the nurse manager of a home health agency is considering two possible approaches to providing nursing care to elderly adults. On the basis of previous experience, reading the literature, and talking with managers of other similar agencies, the manager makes the predictions of cash receipts for care provided under each approach, as shown in Table 21–6. The expected value for each project in Table 21–6 is the weighted average of the possible cash flow outcomes. Each cash flow is weighted by its probability. Therefore, the expected value of Project A, denoted as E(A), is as follows:

$$
\begin{aligned}
E(A) = 0.3 \times 5{,}000 &= \$1{,}500 \\
+ 0.5 \times 8{,}000 &= 4{,}000 \\
+ \underline{0.2 \times 10{,}000} &= \underline{2{,}000} \\
1.0 &= \underline{\underline{\$7{,}500}}
\end{aligned}
$$

The expected value of Project B is:

$$
\begin{aligned}
E(B) = 0.1 \times 3{,}000 &= \$300 \\
+ 0.8 \times 6{,}000 &= 4{,}800 \\
+ \underline{0.1 \times 11{,}000} &= \underline{1{,}100} \\
1.0 &= \underline{\underline{\$6{,}200}}
\end{aligned}
$$

Thus, if the goal of the agency was to choose the option that maximizes revenue, option A offers the greatest likelihood of achieving that goal. Such an option is probably desirable if it has no negative impact on quality.

When using the expected value approach, it is essential to bear in mind that the expected value provides information on the average outcome. Sometimes the results will be better; sometimes they will be worse. Over a large number of decisions, they should average out to the expected value.

For the example just cited, Table 21–6 indicates that the possible outcomes for Project A are $5,000, $8,000, and $10,000. The expected value of the project is $7,500. However, $7,500 is not one of the possible outcomes. When we say that the

❋ **TABLE 21–6** *Projected Cash Receipts for Two Different Projects*

Project A		Project B	
Probability	**Cash Flow**	**Probability**	**Cash Flow**
0.30	$ 5,000	0.10	$ 3,000
0.50	8,000	0.80	6,000
0.20	10,000	0.10	11,000

expected value is $7,500, we recognize that we really expect the outcome to be $5,000 or $8,000 or $10,000. Sometimes the result might turn out to be the low $5,000, sometimes the high $10,000, and sometimes $8,000. Over time, however, we would expect the average cash flow from many projects with similar possible outcomes to be $7,500.

The nurse manager or executive should also remember that expected value is based on the assumed probabilities. The manager should get the best estimate of the probabilities that the event will occur, but this information is not perfect. Often it is based on subjective estimates by managers. Even with the best information, poor outcomes can occur. All decisions must be made on the basis of information available at the time the decision is made. As the probability data indicate, by choosing option A, there is still a 0.30 chance that cash flow will be only $5,000. That may occur, but even if it does, that does not mean that it was a poor decision. Even further, the actual result might be lower than $5,000. It is possible that an unanticipated event may cause actual results to be lower or higher than the manager even believed was probable. However, use of techniques such as expected value should still improve a manager's ability to assess information and make correct decisions.

❋ IMPLICATIONS FOR NURSE MANAGERS AND EXECUTIVES

Forecasting is an essential part of the budgeting process. Some variables, such as number of patients, length of stay, and acuity, are essential ingredients of an operating budget. Preparation of an operating budget cannot begin without some prediction of the values for these variables. The same holds true for other types of budgets.

Managers have great flexibility in selecting the variables that they choose to forecast. They can forecast the number of patients, the patient days, the quantity of a resource that will be consumed (e.g., the number of chest tubes needed or the number of nursing care hours), the amount that will be spent on supplies or personnel, or the acuity level of patients. Any variable for which historical data are available can be forecast using the methods presented.

The forecasting process consists of collecting data, graphing the data, analyzing the graphed data, and preparing prediction formulas. Care must be exercised regarding consideration of things that are changing and that will prevent the future from being like the past. For example, a change in federal regulations concerning types of treatments covered by Medicare might have a dramatic impact on volume. Although managers are aware of such changes, computerized formulas are unlikely to take discrete, recent changes into account. The human role in the forecasting process is critical to generating accurate forecasts.

Analysis of graphed data helps a manager determine whether the variable to be forecast has been exhibiting seasonal or trend behavior, both, or neither. Formulas can then be used to make predictions of the future. Forecasts can be enhanced with the use of computer software. At the same time, one must always bear in mind that the sophisticated quantitative techniques for decision making lack the judgment and experience of managers. Therefore, whether one is using a subjective Delphi technique or a high-powered computer program, the role of the manager in making the final forecast should never be understated.

❋ KEY CONCEPTS

Forecasting   Making a prediction of some future outcome. A great number of management decisions are based on forecasts.

Trend   Patterns related to the passage of time. A trend may be generally upward, constant, or downward over time.

Time series   Approach to forecasting in which historical changes over time are used to help anticipate the likely result in a coming time period.

Seasonality   Variations related to seasons of the year. For example, there may be more communicable diseases in the winter when people are indoors more.

Regression analysis   Mathematical technique to find the unique straight line that comes closest to all of the historical data points. This regression line is used to predict future events.

Curvilinear   Curved line. Sometimes the relationship between the independent variable and dependent variable is not well specified by a straight line. A curvilinear approach to forecasting is especially useful when seasonal patterns exist.

Nominal group technique   Method for qualitative forecasting in which a group of individuals is brought together in a structured meeting. A consensus forecast is developed.

Delphi technique   Method for qualitative forecasting in which the group never meets. A consensus forecast is developed that is less biased by personalities of group members than with the nominal group technique.

Expected value   Method used to estimate the likely value of undertaking an activity that has alternative possible outcomes. It is the weighted average of the value of each possible outcome using probabilities as weights.

❋ SUGGESTED READING

Brockwell P, Davis R: *Introduction to time series and forecasting*, New York, 2003, Springer.

The Nurse as Entrepreneur

CHAPTER GOALS

The goals of this chapter are to:

- Introduce the notion of the nurse as an entrepreneur
- Describe the characteristics of nurse entrepreneurs
- Discuss opportunities for nurse entrepreneurs
- Explain legal and financial issues facing nurse entrepreneurs

- Describe business plans and their relevance
- Identify the steps in developing a business plan
- Discuss pro forma financial statements
- Discuss the use of sensitivity analysis in developing a financial plan

✳ INTRODUCTION

Until recently, there has not been much emphasis on entrepreneurial activity in the nursing literature. Pivotal reports, such as the Institute of Medicine's report, *Future of Nursing: Leading Change, Advancing Health,* as well as national and state-level policies, initiatives, and trends, are converging to provide nurses with opportunities to become entrepreneurs. An *entrepreneur* is someone who starts a new program or venture, often as a for-profit organization, that usually requires some risk. In nursing, entrepreneurship offers the opportunity for nurses to make a profit, provide a new product or service, or develop a new way to deliver a product or service. Entrepreneurial activities need not be profit-driven. Social entrepreneurship applies the entrepreneur's skill to develop new initiatives in not-for-profit and public organizations. Entrepreneurs have been defined as ordinary people who possess an innovative mindset and approach to life that they apply in various undertakings.[1]

Although many think of an entrepreneur as someone who starts an independent venture, the term can also be used to describe a nurse who develops activities within an existing organization. For example, a nurse practitioner (NP) who develops a community diabetes network affiliated with the community hospital where he or she works might be considered an entrepreneur, because some level of risk was involved in the development of the program for the NP and the organization. However, the program provides the opportunity for the NP and the organization to provide a service that is not currently offered in the community. It also offers a new way to educate individuals with diabetes and their families about living with diabetes, monitoring and managing blood sugar levels, staying healthy, and developing connections with resources and others in the community who either have diabetes or have a loved one with diabetes. The NP can charge for the services offered, which enables the organization to realize an income from the venture. Over the long run, this new program might help to keep diabetic patients out of the hospital and provide community-based resources at the time of discharge for patients who are hospitalized. Although this may mean the organization does not generate the same level of revenue as it might for hospitalized diabetic patients, in the future, the organization will likely be rewarded financially for better managing patients' conditions by providing a needed service in the community.

Not many years ago, nursing as a business was almost unthinkable or at least an unpleasant thought to some nurses. Although a few nurses started for-profit home health agencies and employment agencies for temporary and other per diem staff, these nurses were unusual. What was once believed to be disconnected from nursing—and even contrary to nursing's altruistic view of providing care to patients—is becoming commonplace. In fact, there are even websites that provide information and resources for entrepreneurial-minded nurses and a means of connecting with experts or other nurses who share similar experiences.[2]

---

[1]Gergen C, Vanourek G. 2008. *Life Entrepreneurs: Ordinary People Creating Extraordinary Lives.* San Francisco: Jossey-Bass.

[2]See, for example, the Nurse Entrepreneur Network. Accessed November 20, 2011, at http://www.nurse-entrepreneur-network.com.

As health care continues to move in a direction that rewards quality, safety, and patient-centered care, for-profit health care–related organizations such as health care information technology companies will continue to grow. Many nurses will be managers, executives, or clinical leaders in these entrepreneurial ventures. This chapter focuses on the characteristics of successful nurse entrepreneurs, opportunities for nurse entrepreneurs, and related legal and financial issues. It also outlines the development of a business plan, a key component of any entrepreneurial activity. It concludes with specific examples of nurse entrepreneurs.

✳ CHARACTERISTICS OF NURSE ENTREPRENEURS

Business and financial knowledge are consistently identified as skills required for the nurse entrepreneur.[3-5] Beyond those skills, Bhide,[6] who teaches entrepreneurship at the Harvard Business School, states that there is no ideal profile for a successful entrepreneur. Others argue that nurse entrepreneurs are risk takers who are willing to assume financial as well as professional risks with the expectation that they will reap financial and professional success. Additional characteristics of entrepreneurs are imagination and creativity. Parker[7] reported entrepreneurial characteristics that were cited by nurse and health care managers, such as independent, accountable, champions, nontraditional, fast, gutsy, visionary, and courageous. Less flattering characteristics were also cited, such as pushy and irreverent. White and Begun[8] also identified intuition as a characteristic that is important to entrepreneurship.

Having a good idea is not enough to be a successful entrepreneur. Entrepreneurs also need a passion for their undertaking; experience in areas that will inform the idea's development; and a purpose or mission, which often evolves from a desire to "make a difference." Entrepreneurs need business savvy, including knowledge of the market, management and leadership skills, and a solid understanding of financial management. Most entrepreneurial initiatives fail, not because the idea for the business was poor but because the entrepreneur did not have enough capital to keep the business going, a good understanding of how to manage cash flows, or the management skills necessary to run a new venture.

✳ OPPORTUNITIES FOR NURSE ENTREPRENEURS

Nurses are generally involved in one of three broad entrepreneurial categories: an individual who offers a new product or service in the market, a member of a new organizational venture that provides a product or service, or a new venture within an existing organization. Examples are an NP starting a patient care practice, a group of nurses developing a new incontinence product and forming a company to produce and market it, and a nurse who develops a school health program offered through a college of nursing.

Nurses working in a for-profit company or in a business are not necessarily entrepreneurs, although they may be. A nurse can work for a for-profit pharmaceutical corporation explaining new products to physicians and nurses and not be an entrepreneur. The characteristics required for this position could be marketing expertise and loyalty to the corporation. The nurse manager who works to improve productivity on a nursing unit is not an entrepreneur even though the nurse's focus may be to decrease costs. If, on the other hand, nurses work in new business or new product development and there is some financial incentive, they may be entrepreneurs, whether or not they work for a for-profit organization. An example is the nurse developing a community health education program for a tax-exempt, not-for-profit community hospital (such as the diabetes community network described earlier), which will break even financially. Nurse entrepreneurs may also help individuals manage a variety of personal and family health care needs, such as offering case management services for families who live a distance away from a frail parent.[9]

Many sources of information and assistance are available for nurses who wish to pursue entrepreneurship. More and more universities are offering formal or continuing education courses and programs in this field.[10] Numerous articles on nursing entrepreneurship can be found in the nursing literature.[11,12] This issue is not limited to nurses in the United States. Although some of the content in a publication by the Royal Academy of Nursing[13] may not be directly applicable to nurses in the United States, the publication presents a comprehensive overview of the process a nurse would follow to become an entrepreneur.

Starting Your Own Business

Starting a new venture can be an exciting as well as a scary prospect. The new venture can be a completely new idea, a variation on an existing idea, or an existing product or approach in a market that the nurse thinks has room for more providers or in which the nurse believes he or she can provide the product or approach more efficiently. Some ventures require a huge capital investment (e.g., building a new assisted living

[3]See, for example, Ballein K. 1997. Entrepreneurial leadership characteristics of SNEs emerge as their role develops. *Nurs Adm Q* 22(2):60-69; and Gillis CL. 2011. The nurse as social entrepreneur: Revisiting our roots and raising our voices. *Nursing Outlook* 59(6):256-257.

[4]Parker M. 1997. The new entrepreneurial foundation for the nurse executive. *Nurs Adm Q* 22(2):13-21.

[5]Manthey M. 1999. Financial management for nurse entrepreneurs. *Nurs Adm Q* 23(4):81-85.

[6]Bhide A. 1999. *Harvard Business Review on Entrepreneurs*. Cambridge: Harvard Business School Press.

[7]Parker, *Op. cit.*

[8]White K, Begun J. 1997. Nursing entrepreneurship in an era of chaos and complexity. *Nurs Adm Q* 22(2):40-47.

[9]For an example of this service, see *Everybody Needs a Nurse*, described at http://www.everybodyneedsanurse.com. Retrieved November 20, 2011.

[10]For example, the University of Rochester School of Nursing has a Center for Nursing Entrepreneurship. See http://www.son.rochester.edu/welcome/index.html#community.

[11]Ieong S. 2007. Clinical nurse specialist entrepreneurship. *Internet J Adv Nurs Practice* 7(1). Retrieved April 20, 2012 at http://www.ispub.com/journal/the-internet-journal-of-advanced-nursing-practice/volume-7-number-1/clinical-nurse-specialist-entrepreneurship.html.

[12]Sankelo M, Akerblad L. 2009. Nurse entrepreneurs' well-being at work and associated factors. *J Clin Nurs* 18(22):3190-3199.

[13]Royal College of Nursing: Nurse entrepreneurs: turning initiative into independence. December 2007. Retrieved April 20, 2012 at http://www.rcn.org.uk/__data/assets/pdf_file/0018/115632/003215.pdf.

facility).Other ventures like starting a consulting business out of one's home can require almost no capital and may save money because of the possible tax deduction for a home office.

Deciding what to do is only one part of the process. Bhide suggested three guidelines: "(1) Screen opportunities quickly to weed out unpromising ventures. (2) Analyze ideas parsimoniously. Focus on a few important issues. (3) Integrate action and analysis. Don't wait for all the answers, and be ready to change course."[14]

The establishment of a patient care private practice by an NP is an entrepreneurial activity. Two factors have provided the impetus for nurses to provide clinical services on their own, rather than as employees. First, more nurses are educated as advanced practice nurses, and many nurses now have prescriptive privileges. Second, Medicare directly reimburses advanced practice nurses for clinical care, although at a rate less than if "incident to" a physician. When billed as "incident to" a physician, services provided and supplies used are " . . . an integral, although incidental, part of the physician's personal professional services in the course of diagnosis or treatment of an injury or illness."[15] Services and supplies provided "incident to" nonphysician providers (e.g., NPs, physician assistants, clinical nurse specialists, nurse midwives, clinical psychologists) can be billed through Medicare but at a rate that is 85% of the physician fee.

Another example of an entrepreneurial activity is developing a consulting practice. Porter-O'Grady,[16] in describing his career as a consultant, offers practical advice about starting up a consulting business. He provides two mandates: (1) be patient and (2) the client is always right. In the process of developing a consulting practice, he suggests putting away 6 months of income and building a good network of colleagues and potential clients before starting the business. Simpson[17] describes the development of a nursing informatics consulting practice. He identified job satisfaction, flexibility, and income potential as positive aspects of consulting, and tough competition and the ups and downs of running a business as negative aspects.

Although developing a new product or service by a group of people is similar to developing a practice alone, the key difference is in working with others. Porter-O'Grady[18] advises that if one is working with a partner, it is critical to draw up a clear contract. A contract is imperative for any formal arrangement, especially when financial agreements are involved and there are expectations that a service or product will be delivered for an agreed-upon amount. It is best to be clear about financial and work responsibilities and rewards before any issues arise.

For example, when we agreed to write the fourth edition of this book, we signed a contract with the publisher that clearly identified what we would produce, when we would produce it, and what the royalty payment would be.

Developing a product requires skills that few nurses learned in school. Building a prototype, getting a manufacturer, obtaining a patent, obtaining any regulatory approvals, and marketing the product or service usually require outside expertise. Nurses who develop a new continence pad, for example, must realize that the Kimberly-Clark Corporation has been in this business for a long time, has access to capital and accounting and legal expertise, and is a tough competitor. Would it be in the nurses' best interests to compete with Kimberly-Clark or to partner with them? This is the kind of question that must be investigated in product development that usually requires expert help.

Developing a service also requires some of these same skills. However, most nurses have experience in serving patients and working in health care organizations (HCOs), so the leap from nurse employee to nursing service entrepreneur may not be as great as the case in which a product is developed and marketed. For example, a group of nurses seized the opportunity to build a telephone triage business to answer questions from patients cared for by an OB-GYN physician practice outside of normal business hours.[19] This service not only allows patients to get quick answers to their questions but also eliminates the need for physicians to be interrupted at all hours of the night. What ingenuity! Today this service has contracts with numerous physician practices and actively markets its services to physicians via the web.[20]

Developing an entrepreneurial service or product within an organization in many cases is the most risk-free for the nurse entrepreneur. At the same time, the rewards may not be as great as they can be when individuals start their own companies. That does not mean it is simpler to start something new within an existing organization. In fact, this may be the most complicated of the three entrepreneurial approaches. Much depends on the arrangement that the nurse has with the organization. If part of the nurse's job is new product and service development, he or she may not assume any financial risk. A nurse can arrange for the organization to provide all of the start-up funding but to share any profits. An important question is who owns the "intellectual property" of the service or product. If the nurse develops this endeavor as part of his or her job, the intellectual property may be considered to be owned by the organization. However, this issue should be spelled out in a contract so that ownership of intellectual property is understood by the nurse and the organization.

An example of an entrepreneurial activity within an organization is a nurse-managed primary care center. Newland and Rich[21]

[14]Bhide, *Op. cit.*, p. 59.

[15]See *Centers for Medicare and Medicaid Services Medicare Benefit Policy Manual* (07-08-11). Retrieved November 23, 2011, at https://www.cms.gov/manuals/downloads/bp102c15.pdf. See also Incident to Services (September 2011). Retrieved November 23, 2011, at https://www.cms.gov/manuals/downloads/bp102c15.pdf.

[16]Porter-O'Grady T. 1997. The private practice of nursing: The gift of entrepreneurialism. *Nurs Adm Q* 22(1):23-29.

[17]Simpson R. 1997. From nurse to nursing informatics consultant: A lesson in entrepreneurship. *Nurs Adm Q* 22(2):87-90.

[18]Porter-O'Grady, *Op. cit.*

[19]Field A. July 12, 2007. Making a little business look big. *The New York Times*. Retrieved November 20, 2011, at http://www.gazette.com/articles/afshari-6387-hagler-exclusively.html.

[20]For more information about this company, *Exclusively RNs*, see http://www.exclusivelyrns.com/ob-gyn-telephone-triage/index.aspx. Retrieved November 20, 2011.

[21]Newland J, Rich E. 1996. Nurse-managed primary care center. *Nurs Clin North Am* 31(3):471-486.

describe the conception, development, and implementation of Pace University Health Care Unit, a primary care center at Pace University in New York. In 1977, the family NP faculty began a nurse-managed health unit to provide a site for faculty practice and student clinical experience. At that time, this type of arrangement was almost nonexistent. Although foundations provided initial and later additional support, the expectation was that the unit would generate revenue. Pace University paid a portion of the unit's operating expenses. Other revenue comes from Medicaid, private insurance, and self-pay patients. The unit provides primary health care including laboratory services. Today, these types of clinics are much more common. For example, the University of Michigan School of Nursing employs NPs and midwives who offer health promotion and preventive care focused on the care of adults, children, and families.[22]

✳ LEGAL AND FINANCIAL ISSUES

The entrepreneur faces many legal issues, both before starting a business and on an ongoing basis. The entrepreneur is encouraged to obtain legal counsel from an attorney who specializes in business law early in the process.[23,24] Three general legal structures are used in business: sole proprietorship, partnership, and corporation. Corporations can be for profit or not for profit. Lambert and Lambert[25] provide a detailed discussion about the advantages and disadvantages of each legal structure. A proprietorship is the least formal arrangement and simply means that an individual owns the business and is responsible for its taxes and other obligations. An advantage of a partnership includes the availability of additional capital from the partner, but that advantage may be offset by the fact that each partner is responsible for all of the business debts. Earnings of proprietorships and partnerships are taxed as personal income. The primary advantage of a corporation is that the owner's personal assets beyond those invested in the corporation are not at risk if the business fails. However, the corporation pays taxes on profits, and then the nurse pays taxes again on income from the corporation. Small corporations can be set up as "Sub-S" corporations, which have the legal protection of the corporate form but are taxed as if they were partnerships.

Legal issues include problems related to compliance with the numerous laws and regulations that have an impact on how a business operates. Some of these laws may not apply to businesses that have no employees aside from the principal. These laws vary from workers' compensation to the Americans with Disabilities Act. Other laws relate to purchasing or leasing property, borrowing money, and consumer rights. In addition to laws that affect all businesses, specific laws and regulations affect only HCOs. Most nurses are familiar with the regulations about professional practice, including malpractice; however, fewer nurses know about various state and local regulations such as those about care provided in ambulatory care facilities.

By having read up to this chapter in the book, readers have obtained a substantial background in financial management. However, we strongly advise nurse entrepreneurs to contact an accountant early in the entrepreneurial endeavor. The accountant can provide advice on the tax and financial implications of various decisions. Should the nurse lease or buy equipment? Incorporate or start as a proprietorship? Operate locally or from a tax-advantaged location? Prepare the organization's payroll or use an outside service? These are critical questions that should be addressed in collaboration with an accountant.

Obtaining expert advice early in the business development process can save costly mistakes later on. Nurses who develop entrepreneurial activities within an organization will most likely have the benefit of the legal and financial expertise of the organization.

✳ THE BUSINESS PLAN

The creation of a business plan is essential to the development of any entrepreneurial endeavor, whether for a new health services business or for a new venture with an established organization such as a hospital. Understanding the actual costs of doing business is essential to assess the likelihood of success of any new venture. Even nurse managers and executives who abhor the notion that providing health care is a business will recognize that new services cost something. New services cannot be provided to improve the health of the community unless adequate attention has been paid to determining how those services will be paid for. A "business plan" does not necessarily equate to a "business motive." Instead, it reflects a proactive approach to planning, initiating, and managing an enterprise to ensure its success.

A business plan is a detailed strategy that provides an assessment of a proposed program, project, or service based on the market and projections of financial feasibility. Developing a business plan requires an understanding of the "business," the competition in the market, the projected revenue and expenses, and the time frame for achieving a break-even position. Although the business plan is discussed within the context of the nurse entrepreneur, the process is actually useful for developing a variety of different kinds of projects, grants, and initiatives.

Many individuals—including nurses—have ventured into providing a service without a firm understanding of the regulatory environment within which the venture exists (this has been especially true in home care) or without a solid base in financial management. Starting programs that fail because of inadequate financial planning does not serve the health care needs of society. It is more sensible to determine whether a proposed new venture has financial flaws and work to correct them. If business planning shows that a service can be provided only at a loss, then the sources of possible subsidies should be determined before a significant amount of time, effort, and money have been invested. The depth and complexity of the business plan will vary by the venture. For ventures that will require a large capital investment, a business plan is critical. On the other

[22]See, for example, *Nursing Healthcare Centers*. Retrieved November 20, 2011, at http://www.nurse-practitioners.org.

[23]Blouin A, Brent N. 1995. The nurse entrepreneur: Legal aspects of owning a business. *J Nurs Adm* 25(6):13-14.

[24]Lambert V, Lambert C Jr. 1996. Advanced practice nurses: Starting an independent practice. *Nurs Forum* 31(1):11-21.

[25]*Ibid.*

hand, devoting months and months to the business plan may delay entry into the market, and thus a valuable time advantage will be lost.

The plan should define the tactics that are being used to accomplish the organization's goals. It should clearly state the objectives of the proposed project and provide a link showing how the plan's objectives will lead to accomplishment of the organization's goals.

The plan must clearly communicate the concept of the project. It must also communicate the organization's ability to carry out the project. One can think of a business plan as a document that answers the questions one should ask before investing money in a project:

- What exactly is the proposed project?
- To what extent does the organization have the capabilities to undertake the project?
- Where will the organization acquire the capabilities that it lacks?
- Will the project make or lose money?
- How much money?
- Does the organization have the financial resources to undertake the project?
- If not, where can those resources be obtained?
- How will the new product or service be marketed?
- What competitors exist, and how can the proposed product or service be distinguished from them?
- What alternative approaches have been considered?
- Why is the proposed approach considered better than the alternatives?

The Steps in Developing a Business Plan[26]

Project Proposal

The first step in developing a business plan is the preparation of a proposal describing the new product or service or the expansion of an old one. Nursing is often involved in new products and services, either in a support role or as the principal proponent. For example, the addition of a new type of laser surgery would clearly have implications for nursing. Changes would likely occur in the operating room as well as in the postanesthesia care unit and on surgical units that provide postoperative care. The project might be proposed by the surgeons, with the nursing department providing valuable assistance in developing the business plan. On the other hand, the decision to add an outpatient surgical service unit might be suggested by the nursing director of the operating room. As such, it would be primarily a nursing business plan. Nurses can become involved in developing a variety of different programs and innovative services. Developing a new home care agency or additional home care services for an existing agency, developing a nurse staffing agency, and developing an educational or counseling clinic are just a few examples.

Product Definition

After a program has been proposed, the product or service must be carefully defined. What is the specific product, what are the ways it can be provided, and what are the resources needed to provide it? What are the unique benefits of the service? Are the patients homogeneous or mixed in terms of diagnoses or acuity? Are the required resources limited to labor and other operating items, or are capital investments needed as well? How long will it take to get the program up and running? Are there economic or technological trends that could have an impact on patient demand in the future? What are the environmental impacts? Who will comprise the management team? Answering these questions will enable someone unfamiliar with the service to better understand the business aspects of the venture. In this step, the mission of the business should be presented along with the goals and strategies to achieve it.

Market Analysis

Having defined the product, the next step is a market analysis. This component of the plan should address the 4 Ps of marketing (discussed in Chapter 10): product, place (with special attention to competitors), pricing, and promotion. In addressing these areas, a trip to the library or an Internet search is always helpful. For example, a reference librarian can help to ensure that other similar business endeavors are identified and examined. What can you learn from these other businesses? Are these close competitors or are they located across the country? An Internet search may also turn up similar information, but the advantages of engaging a librarian are that librarians are generally familiar with a broader set of keywords to use in the search and a wide array of sources to search.

The market analysis section of the business plan addresses questions such as, are there people who want the product and are willing to pay for it? Can the organization create a market? How many potential buyers are there, and how many other organizations (i.e., competitors) offer the product or service? What *market share* can the organization get? Market share is a percentage of the total demand or volume for the product or service. For example, if there are 10,000 patients in your community who will be treated and your organization gains a 10% market share, it will expect to treat 1,000 patients. The organization or potential investors must be convinced that there will be sufficient demand to justify the investment in this project as opposed to some other project.

As part of the market study, it is necessary to consider change. Is the market likely to grow? That is, will there be a growing number of patients? Will competition grow? Will there be more and more providers competing for the patients? If so, will the organization's market share decline?

The issue of competition is critical. Is there competition? Is there the potential for competition? What will competitors do when they see that the new program or project will be offered? What are the strengths and weaknesses of the competition?

The market analysis must consider who the patients will be and who the payers will be. Is the population largely insured, and if so, who are the primary insurers? What proportion of

---

[26]For additional information on developing a business plan, see: Small Business Association at http://www.sba.gov/category/navigation-structure/starting-managing-business/starting-business/writing-business-plan/essential-elements-good-busines. Retrieved November 20, 2011; and Shirey MR. 2007. The nurse as entrepreneur. *Clin Nurse Spec* 21(3):142-144.

the population served will be indigent? Can the product or service be sold to a managed care organization (MCO), physician practice, insurer, or other provider? Having enough patients or purchasers of the service is the first step. Equally important, however, is knowing the mix of patients or types of providers who might purchase the service.

Mix of patients refers to the different types of ailments or diagnoses that will be the focus of the service or product and the different types of payers who will pay for it. The types of patients with each specific ailment must be known so that the expected costs can be calculated. The mix of payers is also important. What percentage of patients will have their care paid for by Medicare? What percentage by Medicaid? What percentage by private insurers such as an MCO? What percentage are self-pay? The program's revenue can vary dramatically based on who will ultimately be responsible for paying the organization's charges. The charges represent gross revenues. Generally, however, only a portion of total charges is collected, because of government-mandated rates, discounted rates, or because the patients are uninsured and unable to pay. The ultimate cash receipts must be known, in addition to the volume of patients.

Other areas to include are pricing (i.e., common prices for the service in the area), how the product can or will be differentiated from its competitors, and any known competitive advantage the venture might have. Included in this last point would be any specialized knowledge of the service and training the entrepreneur brings. The location of the business is also important, including distance of the enterprise from its competitors. If the market analysis shows little demand or excessive competition, the planning process for this specific program may be discontinued. If it appears that there is demand for the product or service and a reasonable potential market share for the organization, the planning can continue. An overall marketing strategy addressing the 4 Ps of marketing should also be included in this section of the plan.

Rough Financial Plan

After the market analysis is completed and indicates that demand exists for the product, a rough financial plan can be developed. The purpose of this rough plan is to determine whether the project warrants further attention. The rough financial plan revolves around an operating budget.

The operating budget includes preliminary estimates of both revenues and expenses. The revenues can be calculated based on the demand projections from the market analysis. The expenses can be based on rough approximations of the types and amounts of various resources needed.

The results of a rough financial plan are imprecise. The purpose of the plan is to arrive at one of three findings. The first possible finding is that the cost of the program will far exceed the revenues under any reasonable set of assumptions. In that case, managers should save their time by discontinuing the planning process if the project is being evaluated solely on financial merit. A second finding is that the program looks as if it will definitely be profitable. In that case, the manager can proceed with the substantial time investment required to develop a fully detailed plan.

A third finding is that it is unclear whether the project will be profitable. This result creates some difficulty for entrepreneurs. A major potential danger in program planning is that the manager working on the data collection, having invested so much time in the analysis, will begin to push harder and harder for the project. The more time entrepreneurs invest, the greater their psychological need to justify that investment by having the plan indicate that the project is favorable. This could result in a bias in the collection and interpretation of data concerning project feasibility.

Given the unknowns encountered in putting any new program into place, there should be a healthy degree of skepticism about the project. "If it's such a good project, why isn't someone else already doing it?" is a reasonable thought. Therefore, one should always continue with analysis cautiously. Plans should be discontinued unless factors lead the entrepreneur to believe that a more detailed analysis may in fact produce information in the project's favor.

Detailed Operations Plan

Assuming that planning for the project is still continuing after the rough financial plan, the next step is to develop a detailed operations plan. This element of the plan should consider detailed information on the physical location, structure, and size required by the program or project. Next, one must consider the specific human resources required. Equipment and supplies must also be taken into account. These are all direct costs of the project.

Detailed Financial Plan

After a thorough analysis has been made concerning the various components of the proposed plan, a detailed and thorough financial plan can be developed. This financial plan incorporates all of the information from the operations plan and should include the financial impact of the resources to be used. This information will ultimately be used to determine whether it is possible to go ahead with the new project.

The financial plan has three critical elements: a break-even analysis, a cash-flow analysis, and the development of a set of *pro forma* financial statements. The break-even analysis (discussed in Chapter 8) provides information on the minimum volume of patients that must be achieved for the new program not to lose money. Many new programs or projects start with low volume and gradually attract more patients. The pattern of growth in the volume of patients is predicted as part of the market analysis. Break-even analysis is valuable because combined with the volume projection, it can help give the entrepreneur a sense of how long it will take before the new program stops losing money.

The cash-flow analysis provides information on how much cash the program or project will spend each year and how much cash will be received. This information is not available from the operating budget for the program. That budget will focus on revenues and expenses. However, revenues are generally received some time after the patients are treated. In many cases, it takes payers (including Medicare, Medicaid, insurers, and others) weeks or months to pay for the services provided.

On the other hand, cash outlays at the beginning of the project may be substantial. In addition to paying salaries on a current basis, the organization may need to acquire supplies, equipment, office or clinic space, and (in some cases) buildings. The nurse entrepreneur should also include a salary for him- or herself and the repayment of any loans made from personal funds to the company. Otherwise, there may be no way to recoup these investments.

In the case of salaries and supplies, the time between cash payment and cash receipt may be a matter of months. In the case of buildings and equipment, substantial amounts of money may be needed to start the project, but the receipt of cash from the use of the buildings and equipment may stretch out over a period of years. Therefore, it is important to know the amount of cash required. That information will allow one to decide if there is sufficient cash available to undertake the project. Cash budgeting is discussed further in Chapters 12 and 19.

Pro forma financial statements are predictions of what the financial statements for the project or program will look like at some point in the future. These financial statements present a more comprehensive summary of the financial implications of the plan than is provided by the operating budget developed as part of the rough financial plan.

Pro Forma Financial Statements

Every organization has a set of financial statements that are summaries used to indicate the financial position of the organization at a point in time, as well as the financial results of its activities for a period of time. Often financial statements are used to indicate the organization's financial position at the end of its fiscal year as well as its revenues and expenses and cash receipts and payments for an entire fiscal year. The most typically used financial statements are the balance sheet (also called the *statement of financial position*), the operating statement (also called the *activity statement* or the *income statement*), and the statement of cash flows (or the *cash flow statement*). (See Chapters 6 and 7 for a more detailed discussion of these financial statements.)

When a business plan is prepared, an operating budget is developed. The operating budget provides some basic information used for developing the pro forma statements. Using the planned operating budget and the various projections and assumptions about the proposed program or project, the key financial statements are projected for each year into the future, usually for 3 to 5 years. Any predictions beyond 5 years are generally considered unreliable. Any predictions for fewer than 3 years fail to give a picture of what the financial impact of the program is likely to be when it is fully up and running.

Pro forma statements allow the user to determine some basic financial information about the proposed program or project. The pro forma balance sheets will indicate for each future year what the year-end obligations are likely to be relative to the resources. One would want to always have sufficient resources to be able to pay obligations as they become due. The pro forma statements of revenues and expenses will tell the project's expected profitability for each future year. The pro forma cash flow statements provide a summary of the information from the cash-flow analysis.

Forecasting and Capital Budgeting

The detailed financial plan, as noted previously, includes a break-even analysis, a cash-flow analysis, and a set of pro forma financial statements. To get the information needed for these elements, the business plan relies heavily on several aspects of budgeting. Two critical areas of budgeting are forecasting and capital budgeting.

To prepare a cash-flow analysis and to generate pro forma financial statements, a great number of items must be forecast. These include, but are not limited to, inflation, regulation, revenues, wage rates, availability of personnel, detailed expenses, cash flows, and patient volumes. To make these forecasts, the techniques discussed in Chapter 21 are used.

Program budgets frequently require the acquisition of capital assets. Such assets, however, require special attention because of their multiyear life and frequently high costs. The techniques of capital budgeting, which are discussed in Chapter 12, must be taken into account in preparing this part of the business plan.

Sensitivity Analysis

In developing the detailed financial plan, a helpful technique is sensitivity analysis. Sensitivity analysis is concerned with the fact that often a number of assumptions and predictions are made in calculating the financial aspects of a business plan. The number of expected patients used to develop pro forma financial statements is the result of a forecast, which may not be exactly correct. The revenues are based on a stated average charge, which is an assumption. The actual rates charged may be higher or lower. Sensitivity analysis is a process whereby the financial results are recalculated under a series of varying assumptions and predictions. This is often referred to as "what-if" analysis.

Suppose the pro forma financial statements lead one to believe that the proposed project will be a reasonable financial success. Using sensitivity analysis, one could then ask, "What if managed care penetration increases by 10%? What if there are 5% fewer patients than expected? 10% fewer? What if there are 5% more patients than expected? 10% more? What if the average amount charged is raised by 10%? What if the number of staff nurses needed is three full-time equivalents (FTEs) greater than anticipated? What if the construction costs are $30,000 more than expected?" These estimations are easy to make using a spreadsheet program.

Essentially, sensitivity analysis provides recognition of uncertainty. Uncertainty creates risk. Before a final business plan is put together and accepted, one needs to have some idea of the magnitude of risk involved. By going through the what-if analysis, one can get a sense of how unfavorable the financial results would be if some things do not occur just as hoped for or expected. If a project can show an expected favorable financial result over a range of what-if questions, it can provide an extra degree of assurance. If that is not the case, one must carefully question whether the potential benefits are worth the risk that must be undertaken. The nurse manager or executive may find that sensitivity analysis is a useful tool for a variety of financial activities, including the development of a unit or organizational budget.

Examination of Alternatives

A final consideration in the development of a detailed financial plan is the examination of alternatives. There is often more than one way to implement a new service. The alternatives consider factors such as the capacity of the service, the approach to providing the service, and the quality of the service. The business plan should be based on having selected one specific approach after having considered a wide variety of potential alternatives. Calculations regarding the costs and benefits of the various alternatives that have been considered become part of the final business plan package.

The Elements of a Business Plan Package

With business plans, as with great cooking, presentation of the finished product is an essential component of the process. Business plan development requires a significant amount of time and effort. The finished result is often a very long document. Unless carefully presented in a final package, the benefits of much of the work may be lost. When preparing a business plan for oneself, this is not critical. However, when preparing a business plan for prospective funders, the packaging of the finished product is crucial.

The first and most critical element is a concise executive summary. The executive summary outlines the mission of the endeavor, names the founders or partners, provides an overview of the expected number of employees, specifies the location, presents a description of the location, identifies specific services to be provided or products to be offered, indicates key investors or banking relationships, and includes a summary of profit and growth potential, as well as a summary of future plans or implementation. The executive summary should be brief—ideally, no more than one to three pages. The summary should convey what the project is, why it is being proposed, and what the most likely projected results are. This should be presented in just a few brief sentences. If the information in the summary indicates that the project is worth pursuing, the reader will read further.

The next part of a business plan should be a detailed abstract, generally about 20 or 30 pages long. The abstract should provide much greater detail than the executive summary. However, it still is a summary or abstract. It does not include all the specific documentation for the calculations that underlie the plan.

If the program is developed under the auspices of an organization, the abstract should describe the mission of the organization and the way the proposed program fits in with the mission. It should briefly describe the founders or principals, the product or service to be provided and its potential consumers, the expected number of employees, the location, key investors or banking relationships, a summary of growth potential, and a summary of future plans or implementation. The abstract should explain how the new product fits in with the organization's existing services. It should explain why there is a belief that the organization has a competitive edge for this product or service that will allow it to gain and maintain a certain level of market share. The profitability of the program should be discussed in greater detail than that provided in the executive summary. The pro forma financial statements should be included.

It is essential that the abstract identify potential risks. Regulation and other elements that would impede the project should be discussed as well. Finally, the abstract should include some estimate of the requirement for management time needed to implement the program and a statement of commitment by the manager who will bear primary responsibility for the implementation of the program.

The final part of the business plan package is the detailed analysis of each element. At this point, all remaining data are included—detailed descriptions of the product and service; a detailed market research plan indicating market potential and competition; a detailed timeline for implementation of the plan; a detailed marketing plan for attracting patients; and a detailed financial plan, including the analyses used to develop the pro forma statements. Some of the data may be organized into appendixes to the detailed analysis.

By grouping the business plan into these three sections—executive summary, detailed abstract, and full detailed analysis—the entrepreneur allows others less familiar with the project to understand it. This will allow the project to get a fair examination and should lead to a reasoned final decision on whether to implement the proposed program. The business plan package should be accompanied by a cover page that provides the name of the business and any pertinent contact information for the entrepreneur. Exhibit 22–1 provides a summary of the steps used in the development of a business plan, and Exhibit 22–2 provides a summary of the basic elements of the business plan.

✱ **EXHIBIT 22–1** *Steps in Developing a Business Plan*

1. Develop a project proposal.
   a. Include a cover page and executive summary.
2. Define the product.
3. Analyze the market.
4. Conduct a market analysis.
   a. Address the 4 "Ps" of marketing: product, place (especially competitors), pricing, and promotion.
5. Develop a rough financial plan.
6. Develop a detailed operations plan.
7. Develop a detailed financial plan based on:
   a. Break-even analysis
   b. Cash-flow analysis
   c. Pro forma financial statements

✱ **EXHIBIT 22–2** *Elements of the Business Plan*

- Cover letter
- Executive summary
- Detailed abstract
- Full detailed analysis
- Appendixes

❋ EXAMPLES OF ENTREPRENEURS

As discussed previously, entrepreneurs take a variety of approaches to the development of their ventures and face multiple problems. Preventing potential problems is easier than solving problems when they occur. This section describes composites of nursing entrepreneurial experiences.

Example 1

Carol Aspiria expected to graduate from a master's program and become certified as a gerontological NP. She worked as a staff nurse on a medical-surgical unit, where she earned about $60,000 per year. Her dream was to have her own practice. After she was certified, she decided to rent an office. Carol made an arrangement with a physician colleague to use a portion of her space and agreed to pay $1,200 per month for rent. Carol calculated that if she charged $60 per visit and saw 20 patients a day, her revenue would be $300,000 per year. This was more than enough money.

What Carol failed to recognize on the revenue side was that most insurers do not pay providers for at least 90 days and that not all of them pay the full amount charged. She had also allowed herself no vacation. Carol would need income for herself during the time she waited for insurers to pay, *and* she would have to pay rent. In addition, at least for the first year, it would be unlikely that she would see 20 patients per day. It would take time to build her client load, and this would take at least a year from the start of her practice. Although Carol knew that she would have to pay for a phone, she failed to take into account that she would need to buy a computer and software, mobile phone, fax machine, answering service, paper, supplies, and many other items. Finally, Carol had planned initially to schedule her own appointments, thus saving the expense of office staff time. This meant she needed to complete all of the insurance forms, deal with insurance companies to get payment, and answer questions about billing from patients. All of this took time, reducing the number of patients she could see each day unless she worked extra hours. She found that she had to work 2 days a week as a staff nurse to earn additional money. She also needed time to build her patient load, because this does not begin on day 1!

Example 2

Before Martha Spade graduated from her geriatric NP program, she realized that start-up costs for a private practice would be extensive. She decided to work in a clinic as an NP for 1 year to gain experience, to save money for start-up expenses, and to learn how to run a practice. After that year, she started her own practice but continued to work 2 days a week in the clinic to be sure she had an income while the practice got off the ground. In terms of space, she made an arrangement with a physician colleague to lease space to see patients 3 days per week and to pay the physician's office staff to schedule her appointments. She also had a good relationship with the physician, so they referred patients to one another when appropriate. At the end of her first year, she

earned a profit, and her business was doing so well that she planned to quit her clinic job in a few months.

Example 3

John Munchkin is a psychiatric-mental health advanced practice nurse. With a PhD in nursing, he works at a university and earns a full-time salary. He sees clients in his home 3 evenings and 1 day per week. He has few additional expenses. He obtained a separate telephone line for the practice and increased his malpractice and homeowner's insurance. He also obtained life insurance to cover the practice if anything happened to him. He engaged an accountant to prepare his taxes. In addition, because he has a room in his house that is used only for his practice, the cost of a home office could be counted as a business expense for tax purposes.

Example 4

Margaret Milton is the dean of a small college of nursing. Over the past several years, it has become increasingly difficult to find clinical placements for both undergraduate and graduate students. Placing NP students was particularly difficult. At the same time, she realized that the federal government had grant money to set up clinics for underserved populations who had limited access to care. Dr. Milton's grant application to set up an NP-run clinic in a housing project was funded, providing the start-up capital needed as well as 50% of the salary for a part-time NP to get the program started. This clinic served as a training site for adult and pediatric NPs and undergraduate community health nurses. The final year of funding is next year, and Dr. Milton now realizes that the clinic's expenses continue to exceed the clinic's revenue. It is not clear that the clinic can ever break even, because of the state reductions in Medicaid payments, the many uninsured people for whom the clinic cares, and the quality of care that the faculty strive to provide. She is faced with the decision of whether to close the clinic or to find other sources of funding.

Each of these cases reflects different degrees of entrepreneurial "savvy." Any one of these nurse entrepreneurs would have benefited from the development of a well-thought-out business plan to help address uncertainties. By developing such a plan, nurse entrepreneurs can take into account factors such as the economy and local conditions that might impact ventures.

Good mentors and counselors are essential to help nurse entrepreneurs think through their ideas, determine how to best develop and present their ideas into a cohesive plan, and identify resources needed to develop their plan and gain support for their ideas. Advice from a seasoned mentor can save a nurse entrepreneur from making costly mistakes that may prevent him or her from offering a truly needed and innovative service.

❋ IMPLICATIONS FOR NURSE MANAGERS AND EXECUTIVES

The 21st century is an exciting time for nursing. It is intriguing how many people on the *Forbes* magazine annual list of billionaires are in businesses that were complete unknowns a few decades ago. Thinking back only 25 years, personal computers were rare, and regular use of the Internet was unheard of. Cellular telephones and digital televisions were dreams. The technological and communications explosion that has had such an incredible impact on the way nurses provide care was in many ways unimaginable. For example, home health nurses today carry laptop computers or tablets and mobile phones, and increasing numbers of patients are treated with telehealth capabilities. One does not have to invent technology to have great success. In fact, it is often the simple service such as nurse telephone triage offered to minimize the work of physicians and their office staff that can make a difference. Creative, risk-taking nurses and nurse managers and executives who can think about how new technologies can be used to provide new or better programs and services have the opportunity to participate in and profit from the developments of the next 25 years. More importantly, they have the opportunity to lead the way in developing new care delivery innovations that better meet the needs of patients and society.

✳ KEY CONCEPTS

Entrepreneur   Person who starts a venture that involves risk but that also offers the opportunity to make a profit or provide a new product or service or a new way to deliver a product or service.

Business plan   Detailed plan for a proposed program, project, or service, including information to be used to assess the venture's financial feasibility. The plan should clearly state the objectives of the proposed project and provide a link that shows how the plan's objectives will lead to accomplishment of the organization's goal.

Sensitivity analysis   Process whereby financial results are recalculated with a series of varying assumptions and predictions.

✳ SUGGESTED READINGS

Abrams R: *Business plan in a day: get it done right, get it done fast!* Palo Alto, Calif, 2005, Planning Shop.

Abrams R: *The successful business plan: secrets & strategies*, ed 4, Palo Alto, Calif, 2003, Planning Shop.

Ballein K: Entrepreneurial leadership characteristics of SNEs emerge as their role develops, *Nurs Adm Q* 22(2):60–69, 1997.

Bhide A: *Harvard Business Review on entrepreneurs*, Cambridge, 1999, Harvard Business School Press.

Blouin A, Brent N: The nurse entrepreneur: legal aspects of owning a business, *J Nurs Adm* 25(6):13–14, 1995.

Caffrey R: The rural community care gerontologic nurse entrepreneur: role development strategies, *J Gerontol Nurs* 31(10):11–16, 2005.

Campbell K: Intravenous nursing services: strategies for success, *J Intraven Nurs* 19(1):35–37, 1996.

Campbell M: Nurse entrepreneur gives new face to care, *Nursingmatters* 15(5):14, 22, 2004.

Campbell S: The newest gatekeepers: nurses take on the duties of primary care physicians, *Health Care Strat Manage* 15(3):14–15, 1997.

Crow G: The entrepreneurial personality: building a sustainable future for self and the profession, *Nurs Adm Q* 22(2):30–35, 1997.

Eaton D: Perinatal home care: one entrepreneur's experience, *J Obstet Gynecol Neonat Nurs* 23(8):726–730, 1994.

Gergen C, Vanourek G: *Life entrepreneurs: ordinary people creating extraordinary lives*, San Francisco, 2008, Jossey-Bass.

Gillis CL: The nurse as social entrepreneur: revisiting our roots and raising our voices, *Nursing Outlook* 59(6), 256–257, 2011.

Haag A: Writing a successful business plan, *J Am Assoc Occupat Health Nurs* 45(1):25–32, 33–34, 1997.

Holman E, Branstetter E: An academic nursing clinic's financial survival, *Nurs Econ* 15(5):248–252, 1997.

Hupalo P: *Thinking like an entrepreneur: how to make intelligent business decisions that will lead to success in building and growing your own company*, West Saint Paul, Minn, 2004, HCM Publishing. Available at http://www.hcmpublishing.com.

Ieong S: Clinical nurse specialist entrepreneurship, *Internet J Adv Nurs Pract* 7(1), 2007. Retrieved April 20, 2012 at http://www.ispub.com/journal/the-internet-journal-of-advanced-nursing-practice/volume-7-number-1/clinical-nurse-specialist-entrepreneurship.html.

Johnson J: Developing an effective business plan, *Nurs Econ* 8(3):152–154, 1990.

Lachman V: Care of the self for the nurse entrepreneur, *Nurs Adm Q* 22(2): 48–59, 1997.

Lamb G, Zazworsky D: The Carondelet model, *Nurs Manage* 28(3):27–28, 1997.

Lambert V, Lambert C Jr: Advanced practice nurses: starting an independent practice, *Nurs Forum* 31(1):11–21, 1996.

Langton P: Obstetricians' resistance to independent, private practice by nurse-midwives in Washington, D.C. hospitals, *Women Health* 22(1): 27–48, 1994.

Manthey M: Financial management for nurse entrepreneurs, *Nurs Adm Q* 23(4):81–85, 1999.

McNiel N, Mackey T: The consistency of change in the development of nursing faculty practice plans, *J Prof Nurs* 11(4):220–226, 1995.

Newland J, Rich E: Nurse-managed primary care center, *Nurs Clin North Am* 31(3):471–486, 1996.

Parker M: The new entrepreneurial foundation for the nurse executive, *Nurs Adm Q* 22(2):13–21, 1997.

Pastula P: *Successful business planning in 30 days: a step-by-step guide for writing a business plan and starting your own business*, ed 3, Edmonton, Alberta, Canada, 2004, Patsula Media. Retrieved at http://www.patsula.com.

Porter-O'Grady T: The private practice of nursing: the gift of entrepreneurialism, *Nurs Adm Q* 22(1):23–29, 1997.

Puszko GB: An interview with nurse entrepreneur Barbara Puszko, *Gastroenterol Nurs* 24(2):75–76, 2001.

Rainer S, Papp E: The self employed occupational and environmental health nurse: maximizing business success by managing financial resources, *AAOHN J* 48(4):185–196, 2000.

Royal College of Nursing: Nurse entrepreneurs: turning initiative into independence. December 2007. Retrieved April 20, 2012 at http://www.rcn.org.uk/__data/assets/pdf_file/0018/115632/003215.pdf.

Sankelo M, Akerblad L: Nurse entrepreneurs' well-being at work and associated factors, *J Clin Nurs* 18(22), 3190–3199, 2009.

Shames K: Holistic nurse entrepreneur. Exemplary leadership for the new millennium, *Beginnings* 20(2):7, 9, 2000.

Shames K: Holistic nurse entrepreneur. Insurance reimbursement, *Beginnings* 19(3):3–5, 1999.

Shames K: Holistic nurse entrepreneur. What is your style? *Beginnings* 20(5):10, 2000.

Shirey, MR: The nurse as entrepreneur, *Clin Nurse Spec* 21(3):142–144, 2007.

Simpson R: From nurse to nursing informatics consultant: a lesson in entrepreneurship, *Nurs Adm Q* 22(2):87–90, 1997.

Tiffany P, Peterson S: *Business plans for dummies*, ed 2, Hoboken, New Jersey, 2005, Wiley.

Walker P, Chiverton P: The University of Rochester experience, *Nurse Manage* 28(3):29–31, 1997.

White K, Begun J: Nursing entrepreneurship in an era of chaos and complexity, *Nurs Adm Q* 22(2):40–47, 1997.

Wilson A, Averis A, Walsh K: The influences on and experiences of becoming nurse entrepreneurs: a Delphi study, *Int J Nurs Pract* 9(4):236–245, 2003.

Wilson C: Mentoring the entrepreneur, *Nurs Adm Q* 22(2):1–12, 1997.

Zeier J: Leading a rural clinic toward financial stability, *J Nurse Pract* 2(5): 318–322, 2006.

Nursing and Financial Management: Current Issues and Future Directions

CHAPTER GOALS

The goals of this chapter are to:

- Review the current nursing literature on financial management
- Discuss the skills required for nurse managers and executives to assume expanded roles in financial management

- Discuss the differences in financial responsibility for varying levels of nurse managers and executives
- Discuss the role of the nurse manager and executive in policymaking

✳ INTRODUCTION

Nurse managers and executives perform a variety of functions related to financial management. To perform these functions as efficiently as possible, they must be aware of current issues in the fields of financial management and nursing, and they must understand where the two intersect. This chapter reviews current issues identified in the nursing literature followed by a discussion of the future role of nurse managers and executives in financial management. By having a sense of the current issues and future directions in nursing as it relates to health care, financial management, and nursing, nurse managers and executives will be in a better position to "work smarter, not harder." The most important thing for managers and executives to avoid is complacency. The role of a manager or executive includes innovation. Innovation, however, is only occasionally the result of inspiration; often it is the product of careful attention to the changing world and what others have done to cope with changing realities.

Throughout nursing's history, there has been tension about whether the management of nursing-related financial resources resides in the domain of nursing or financial management. We believe that nursing financial management is a blend of both fields and as such is a subset of nursing. Some nursing leaders argue that only studies about patients (clients) and the nursing interventions associated with these clients are the purview of nursing. We believe that this view is extremely short-sighted and places nursing in a vulnerable position, subject to greater external control. Thus, we propose that nursing encompasses the organization, delivery, and financing of nursing care. This view acknowledges that nursing financial management is an integral part of nursing care delivery.

✳ NURSING FINANCIAL MANAGEMENT RESEARCH

National health expenditures were more than $2.6 trillion in 2010, or more than $8,300 per person, representing almost 18% of the U.S. gross domestic product (GDP).[1] Health care spending is forecast to grow to over $13,000 per person and to almost 20% of GDP by 2020.[2] Thus, the importance of efficiently and effectively using valuable health care resources should be of great interest to nurse managers, executives, and the nursing profession at large.

Nurse researchers can play a key role in helping nurse managers and executives understand the financial management of organizations, the financial implications of various programs or interventions, and the development of organizational and public policies that impact the financial management of organizations. If research can give us a greater understanding of the way the world works in general, then research can be used to understand both the financial implications of various decisions and the way we manage nursing financial resources. Studies about the costs of care can influence the way care is actually delivered, as well as clinical practice, health care systems, and government policymaking.

Review of a profession's body of research and associated literature can provide insights into current issues in the field. Although research can be described as a continuum from theoretical to applied, most people think of research as the development or testing of theory. Nursing financial

---

[1] Keehan SP, Sisko AM, Truffer CJ, et al. 2011. National health spending projections through 2020: Economic recovery and reform drive faster growth. *Health Aff* 30(8):1-12.

[2] *Ibid.*

management research includes studies such as those that look at:

- market behaviors (e.g., how nurses respond to recruitment and retention efforts, how organizations respond to the availability of nursing resources within a geographic area),
- management science (e.g., the relationship between chief executive officers' [CEOs'] or chief nursing officers' leadership style and the impact of allocating nursing resources or decentralizing unit-level financial decision making to nurse managers), or
- nursing science (e.g., comparing the cost-effectiveness of two nursing interventions to prevent patient falls).

The application of research in areas such as these has been included in discussions throughout the book.

There is very little research that advances theory development in the area of nursing financial management. Most theory-based financial management research takes place within the strict disciplines of accounting and finance. Nursing financial management research, on the other hand, tends to apply theoretical developments in accounting or finance to nursing or health management in general.

Despite this lack of theory development in nursing financial management, there is a growing body of literature in applied nursing financial management research. Some studies fall under the general rubric of policy and evaluation research. These studies describe how resources are allocated within organizations and explore relationships between the cost and financing of nursing care. A few of these studies examine the cost-effectiveness of various approaches to provide nursing care or assess the impact of various nursing practice innovations on nursing costs. Comparative effectiveness research is also being used to compare two or more care delivery approaches or interventions and in turn help decision makers evaluate the usefulness of the approaches or interventions. Some studies also develop instruments to measure the cost of providing care. Many of the cost studies use economic or organizational theory or both as the framework to answer research questions. Others use no theoretical framework at all; rather, they describe the relationships among cost and related variables of interest.

In addition to the policy and evaluation research literature, increasing numbers of articles in nursing journals focus on the application and evaluation of financial techniques in nursing. Almost every issue of the major nursing management journals has at least one article on the financial consequences of nursing practices or policies. It is likely that future trends in nursing financial management can be assessed from this applied research.

There have been calls for more targeted research in the area of nursing financial management. Using a Delphi technique to identify nursing administration research priorities, Lynn et al.[3] recognized five priorities (of 44) that directly pertain to nursing financial management (e.g., examine the effects

of downward substitution of workers on organizational costs and quality of care); several others indirectly pertained to nursing financial management (e.g., the creation of databases that enable cross-institutional analysis of effectiveness and efficiency of care). These financial management research priorities still exist today.

A conference on nursing and health services research also identified research needs in five domains, one of which was the cost and cost-effectiveness of care.[4] Within this category, research recommendations were made to address policymaking in clinical nursing practice, health care systems, and public policy. Examples of research recommendations included the development of a theoretically relevant production function for nursing, the identification of direct and indirect costs and benefits of maintaining adequate nurse staffing levels, and the impact of changing reimbursement policies on the quality of nursing care.

The mandate for evidence-based nursing practice has brought about a concomitant interest in evidence-based management (EBM) for nursing. Kovner[5] introduced this notion for managing health care services in general, and Finkler[6] has called for the incorporation of evidence-based financial management in health administration practice and education. EBM has great potential for nurse managers and executives. In a review of the literature, Young[7] reported that the benefits of EBM for nursing include motivating nursing staff, justifying management decisions, and contributing to management science. The 2004 Institute of Medicine (IOM) report *Keeping Patients Safe*[8] specifically called for the use of EBM to build trust within nursing and to recognize nursing's voice in patient care delivery. Much work is yet needed to develop an evidence base upon which to base nursing financial management decisions and to incorporate evidence-based financial management in nursing administration educational programs and practice. However, it is highly likely that the incorporation of EBM—including evidence from nursing and financial management research—will provide a stronger foundation for decision making that relates to the allocation of scarce nursing resources and in turn potentially improve organizational performance.

To meet these challenges, there is a dire need for nurses prepared with advanced knowledge of financial management. It is also critical for nurse managers, executives, and researchers to collaborate with financial management researchers to

[3] Lynn M, Layman E, Richard S. 1999. Research priorities. The final chapter in the nursing administration research priorities saga: the state of the state. *J Nurs Adm* 29(5):5-9.

[4] See Jones C, Mark B. 2005. The intersection of nursing and health services research: Overview of an agenda-setting conference. *Nurs Outlook* 53(6):270-273; and Jones C, Mark B. 2005. The intersection of nursing and health services research: An agenda to guide future research. *Nurs Outlook* 53(6):324-333.

[5] Kovner A, Elton J, Billings J, et al. 2000. Evidence-based management/commentaries/reply. *Front Health Serv Manage* 16(4):3-46. See also Kovner AR, Rundall TG. 2006. Evidence-based management reconsidered. *Front Health Serv Manage* 22(3):3-22.

[6] Finkler S. 2005. Evidence based financial management—what are we waiting for? *Res Healthc Financ Manage* 9(1):1-3.

[7] Young S. 2002. Evidence-based management: A literature review. *J Nurs Manage* 10:145-161.

[8] Page A. 2004. *Keeping Patients Safe: Transforming the Work Environment of Nurses*. Institute of Medicine. Washington, DC: National Academies Press.

apply and test financial theories, principles, and techniques in studying nursing care delivery and the financial consequences of innovations in nursing practice. Through such partnerships, the knowledge and experiences of both nursing and financial experts can be brought to bear on the challenges facing health care organizations (HCOs) today.

✳ CURRENT AND FUTURE ISSUES IN FINANCIAL MANAGEMENT IN NURSING

The broad categories of nursing financial management that have been the focus of recent literature include (1) allocation of nursing resources, (2) financial compensation and incentives, (3) cost-benefit ratio or cost-effectiveness and application of other financial analysis tools, and (4) approaches to decreasing the cost of care.

The allocation of nursing resources continues to be a major topic in the literature for two primary reasons. First, the rate of increase in reimbursement has been quite constrained, and HCOs often look for ways to find efficiencies in the delivery of care. Because nursing represents the largest professional group in most HCOs, it is often perceived to be expensive, and nursing resources are often scrutinized as a source of cost-cutting. Second, because HCOs have difficulty recruiting and retaining nurses during recurring nursing shortages, there is often a focus on how to more effectively deploy scarce nursing resources. These two needs have generated research focusing on the impact of nurse staffing levels on patient outcomes, effective and efficient levels of staffing, differentiated nursing practice, and the impact of nurse staffing on organizational performance. Several unresolved issues remain, such as determining the most appropriate level of manager to make nurse staffing decisions and the appropriate number of nursing hours, visits, or staff mix that is required for delivering care to certain groups of patients in different settings.

Financial compensation for nurses continues to be an issue. For example, Medicare reimbursement for advanced practice nurses and per-visit payments to home health nurses have been ongoing concerns. Answers are needed to a number of questions, such as: How should nurses be compensated? Should nurses be salaried or hourly wage earners? What is the impact of compensation (e.g., salaries, bonuses) on productivity? What are the policy implications of various models of nurse reimbursement?

The cost and benefits or cost-effectiveness of nursing care is an important area of focus, particularly in light of the IOM's *Future of Nursing Report* (2011). The cost-effectiveness of specific nursing interventions such as pain and symptom management and the cost-effectiveness of nursing care delivery models will continue to be the focus of future research. We still lack sufficient evidence about the cost-effectiveness of unlicensed assistive personnel, many nursing interventions, and nurse practitioners relative to other types of providers. We also need research that examines the impact of implementing recommendations made in the *Future of Nursing Report*.[9] For example,

what are the financial implications of expanding or amending Medicare requirements for reimbursing advanced practice nurses? What are the financial implications of expanding nurses' scope of practice? What are the financial implications of implementing nurse residency programs, including the costs and benefits or the cost-effectiveness of these programs? What are the financial costs and benefits of increasing the proportion of nurses with baccalaureate degrees—or doubling the number of nurses with doctoral degrees—by 2020? These are critical policy issues that nurse managers and executives must address because they could have great financial consequences that must be considered.

Finally, although minimizing the cost of nursing care is an ongoing theme, there is still little research on financial models for increasing nursing revenues. Nurse managers and executives make decisions on a daily basis that have the potential to impact nursing costs. Their use of approaches to address such issues as nurse scheduling and assignment, setting nurse-patient ratios, varying the staffing mix, implementing a particular model of care delivery, and using supplies all have cost implications. Often, however, these decisions are not balanced by adequate consideration of how nursing revenues might be recognized and increased in existing programs or generated through innovations in service delivery.

✳ THE EVOLVING ROLE OF THE NURSE EXECUTIVE IN FINANCIAL MANAGEMENT

Health care organizations are dynamic and in a constant state of flux. To maximize opportunities in such a situation, managers and executives must be flexible in defining their role. Two decades ago, nurse managers and executives might have been astonished to be asked to participate in the development of a business or strategic plan. Yet today, nurse managers and executives have become key players in business and strategic plan development in a variety of HCOs. The roles of nurse managers and executives clearly have been changing and likely will continue to change.

Along with this evolving and constantly changing role, the responsibility of nurse managers and executives in the area of financial management has expanded. Although in the past, a nurse executive might have gone to the CEO and asked for a budget of $50 million for "her" department, more often than not the nurse executive now attends board meetings, sits on the executive committee of the organization, and is an active voice in the decision-making process for the allocation of all the system's resources to all organizational entities, not just nursing. In home health agencies, the management team may consist almost entirely of nurses.

Numerous reports point to the challenges faced by nurse executives. The *Future of Nursing Report*[10] even goes so far as to say that nurse executives are "losing ground." This report notes that these executives are increasingly reporting to chief operating officers rather than the top organizational executive, the CEO, which potentially limits the nurse executive's ability

---

[9] Institute of Medicine. 2011. *The Future of Nursing: Leading Change, Advancing Health.* Washington, DC: The National Academies Press.

---

[10] *Ibid.*

to advocate for patient care and nursing resources or affect organizational decision making. At the same time, nurse executives are held accountable for patient care quality as nursing resources have come under increasing budget pressures and scrutiny.[11] And despite the increase in nurse executive participation on organizational and community boards, they are still woefully underrepresented.[12]

In the future, the need for nurses to assume responsibility and authority for financial management is likely to expand at all organizational levels. It does not require extraordinary imagination to realize that the roles of nurse managers and executives must expand to include participation in such decisions as issuing bonds to finance new buildings, merging with competitors, or launching new initiatives to gain market share. The delivery of health care in the future through entities such as accountable care organizations and patient-centered medical homes, both emphasized in health care reform, present opportunities and challenges for nurses. The areas recognized as being particularly relevant to nursing include team-based care; interdisciplinary communication, coordination, and collaboration; infrastructures and technologies to support nursing; and payment incentives that support value-based care (i.e., payment based on quality).[13] It will be critical for nurse managers and executives to be knowledgeable about these opportunities and challenges and be at the table when related decisions and organizational policies are made.

Chapters throughout this book contain useful tools that are necessary for nurse manager and executive practice today and in the future. It is critical for current and future nurse managers and executives to appreciate the value of the entire interdisciplinary administrative team in making organizational budgetary decisions and for them to become actively engaged in the process. As the role of the top nursing leader expands, so too will the roles of midlevel and first-line nurse managers to include ever-increasing responsibilities for financial management. It will be up to the nurse executive to create an environment that values the engagement of nurse managers and frontline staff in financial matters and encourages collaboration across disciplines to achieve the ultimate goal of delivering quality care to patients in a fiscally responsible manner.

Setting Organizational Policy

The roles of nurse managers and executives will likely expand to include greater involvement in setting organizational policy about financial matters. As more nurse executives participate in board meetings, board members will look to them for explanations about rising costs and, more important, options for

restraining costs and increasing revenues. Often tactics may require reorganization of the way services are provided and the consideration of new models of care. The nurse executive can play a key role in proposing, developing, implementing, and evaluating such strategies.

A generation of nurse managers and executives has emerged who are better prepared academically to actively participate in financial management. Courses in budgeting and finance are required in almost every graduate program focusing on nursing management or administration and nursing and health care systems. Some nurse managers and executives are choosing joint MBA-MSN programs, and others are choosing graduate study in health management, or a joint MHA-MSN. As these nurse managers and executives seek information on the financial operation of the organization and make informed observations, many senior financial managers will embrace them as members of the executive team. Others will be threatened by the newfound knowledge of nurse managers and executives and will put up subtle barriers to their full involvement in financial decision making.

Concerns about the rising costs of care delivery and cost restraints will be ever-present in the future of health care delivery. In an effort to achieve and maintain fiscal solvency, it is likely that CEOs and boards will hold nurse managers and executives accountable for high-quality care at a cost that will position the organization to survive and compete in the marketplace. The informed manager or executive must know the financial condition of the organization to know what costs the organization can in fact survive without and where cuts might be made without detrimental effects on care delivery. As information generation improves within HCOs, the nurse manager or executive will have the information readily available that is necessary to look at the financial management of specific units and care teams within the organization.

Continuing Organizational Responsibility for Nursing Expenses

The nurse executive in virtually all HCOs is currently responsible for the direct operating expense budget for all of nursing services. In many organizations, the nurse executive is also responsible for other departments, such as the operating room or the emergency department. In most cases, the nurse executive has a high degree of control over the budget in the area of his or her responsibility. On occasion, the nurse executive may be asked to cut, for example, 3% off the budget, but in most organizations, how those actions are taken is based on a departmental decision under the nurse executive's direction. In most HCOs, salary increases are set by top management, with the nurse executive being a leader in making these decisions, whether the raise is part of an organized labor settlement or not.

In some organizations, the nurse executive has less control over indirect expenses and the allocation of those expenses to the nursing department. The nurse executive also has less control over the capital budget than over direct departmental expenses. The CEO and the chief financial officer (CFO) generally control the expenses of the other departments and the

[11] See, for example, Ballein Search Partners and AONE (American Organization of Nurse Executives). 2003. *Why Senior Nursing Officers Matter: A National Survey of Nursing Executives.* Oak Brook, IL: Ballein Search Partners; and Jones CB, Havens DS, Thompson PA. 2008. Chief nursing officer retention and turnover: A crisis brewing? Results of a national survey. *J Healthc Manage* 53(2):89-105; discussion 105-106.

[12] Prybil L, Levey S, Peterson R, et al. 2009. *Governance in High-Performing Community Health Systems: A Report on Trustee and CEO Views.* Chicago, IL: Grant Thornton LLP.

[13] Korda H, Eldridge GN. 2011. ACOs, PCMHs, and health care reform: Nursing's next frontier? *Policy Polit Nurs Pract* 12(2):100-103.

allocation of these expenses to nursing. Various departments and key members of the medical staff in hospitals compete for capital. Often capital decisions are made by the CEO and the board. Because few nurses are actual voting members of the board and only slightly more are on board committees, the voice of nursing has been historically less strong in hospital capital expenditure decision making.

As more nurse executives understand capital financing, they will be in a stronger position to lobby more forcefully for capital expenditures. Moreover, nurse executives with a strong understanding of the economic laws of supply and demand will be able to argue regarding the likely positive organizational effects of investments in nursing. As more nurses understand the allocation of indirect expenses and begin to question these allocations, the nurse executive's voice in these decisions will be heard.

Assuming Organizational Responsibility for Nursing Revenues

Accountability for revenue is the likeliest growth area in expectations for nurse managers and executives. The focus in the past has been to maintain costs with no reduction in quality. Many organizations focus marketing efforts on product lines, and organizational survival has been linked to the ability to attract a sufficient volume of patients within those product lines. With the wider adoption of formal structured nursing or interdisciplinary plans of patient care, the nurse manager or executive will be asked to identify those patients the organization wants to attract and the nurse's role in that revenue generation. In home health care, nurse managers and executives almost always have this responsibility.

As patients continue to take on larger portions of their health care bills, they will seek more "caring" and personal attention in the services provided by health care facilities. As they do so, patients will also recognize that nursing is a key service provided, and HCOs will come to value the quality of nursing care as a marketing strategy. Nurses are already viewed among the most highly trusted health care professionals. This will enhance the power of nurse managers and executives as key managers of a highly regarded service.

Assuming an Organizational Role in New Ventures

As organizations seek alternatives to balancing expenses and revenues, the nurse manager and executive will likely be more involved in new ventures. Whereas in the past, the nurse manager or executive was told that the hospital was opening a new transplant unit and that adequate staff would need to be provided, in the future, the financially adept nurse manager or executive will participate in the decision making about new ventures from the beginning. The nurse managers and executives who are familiar with business plan development and skilled at financial projections will be seen by organizational executives as a valuable asset in the decision-making process.

Responding to Extra-Organizational Changes

Along with financial responsibilities within the organization, the nurse manager and executive will increasingly be involved with extra-organizational financial issues, particularly those related to reimbursement. Nurse managers and executives will be faced with the conflict about what the professional benefit is to nursing, what is in the best interest of the nursing department, and what is in the best interest of the organization and its patients.

Cross-training of health workers and the use of assistive staff are two areas in which the nurse manager or executive will continue to face potential conflict. Nurse managers and executives with their roots in the profession of nursing will continue to share the values associated with the profession. As they face future nurse shortages and increasing salaries for professional nurses, they will likely be asked to train less-educated workers to perform activities formerly within the purview of professional nurses. In this scenario, the nurse executive will be confronted with an ethical dilemma: how to provide the safest possible care under conditions of scarce human and financial resources. This may, indeed, be one of the nurse executive's greatest challenges in the foreseeable future.

Government Relations

Although professional associations such as the American Nurses Association and many nurse leaders have a long history of involvement with the government, many nurse managers and executives in smaller health organizations do not. Given that many reimbursement decisions are regulated by government, nurse managers and executives of the 21st century must be able to interact with government officials in the executive branch as well as with legislators to influence how reimbursement decisions are made. To do so, the nurse manager or executive must understand the payment system, current health care policies, and the financial implications of reimbursement and regulatory decisions for the HCOs where they practice. With the growing emphasis on pay-for-performance and value-based care, nurse managers and executives also need to understand how the system will impact nurses so they can effectively interact with government officials to ensure that, for example, information systems are built to include nurses and nursing care, and to make their concerns about policy changes known. This interaction can occur via letters and e-mails, during in-person meetings with government officials, and informally at a variety of social and professional meetings. It behooves nurse managers and executives to become engaged with their professional colleagues through associations such as the American Organization of Nurse Executives (AONE) to form coalitions for more effective and strategic lobbying efforts.

Payer Relations

Although much of the reimbursement system is regulated by government, reimbursement decisions for individual patients are made by private insurers, a fiscal intermediary, or the government directly. Bills denied payment or for which payment is delayed cost health organizations a substantial amount of money.

The organizational entity responsible for collections is usually the finance office. Clearly, nurse managers and executives do not want to become financial analysts or bill collectors. However, unless they understand issues of cash flow, they will not be able to assume a role in helping the organization solve cash-flow problems. The promptness and completeness with which records are generated affect the cash flow of the organization. The nurse manager or executive who understands cash flows will realize the benefit to the organization of working with the nursing staff to document care and diminish the claims that are denied or delayed. In home health care, denied claims and delayed payment are major issues threatening the fiscal viability of many agencies.

The capitation of payments for health services will continue to be a major issue facing HCOs. Home health agencies have capitated arrangements. Whether in home care, ambulatory care, or hospitals, capitation changes organizational incentives. Today's nurse managers and executives must know these incentives and be prepared to deal with them.

In all of these areas, there is a trade-off between nurse manager or executive involvement in financial management and having others in the organization make these decisions. In practice, nurse managers and executives may be asked to provide a comparison of departmental or unit-level data with regional or national benchmark data on financial issues such as budgeted and actual hours per patient day, overtime use, and nonproductive hours (see Chapter 18 for a discussion of benchmarking). They might also be asked to examine departmental or unit-level financial trends across time. Nurse managers and executives should consider the value of these activities to determine whether an investment of time to develop fiscal skills produces positive financial outcomes for nursing. In some cases, it may be more advantageous to engage financial staff rather than nurse managers or executives to produce needed information. This is the "value-added" question: to what extent should nurse managers and executives be engaged in financial management activities to add value to the organization? We believe that the days of the nurse manager and nurse executive getting a budget from the CEO or CFO are over. However, each nurse manager or executive must decide the amount of information needed to effectively manage the nursing department, decide the time that should be invested by nurse managers and executives in the process, and actively engage nurses at all levels and others within the organization to produce the information needed.

❋ FUTURE ROLE OF FIRST-LINE AND MIDLEVEL NURSE MANAGERS IN FINANCIAL MANAGEMENT

As the nurse executive assumes greater responsibility for financial matters in both the nursing department and the organization, first-line and midlevel managers can also expect to have expanded responsibilities over their areas of accountability. In most HCOs, the first-line managers have budget responsibility for one or more patient care units, and midlevel managers and above are generally responsible for multiple patient care units or service lines. In a home health agency, it might include responsibility for a geographic area where care is provided by a set number of nurses or nursing teams. Increasingly, advanced practice nurses are also setting up their own practices. In such

cases, a nurse may be responsible for the budget of a small business.

In decentralizing fiscal accountability, the nurse executive must balance the cost of having a nurse manager devote time to fiscal management against the potential benefits of increased control of unit and department resources. It is likely that midlevel nurse managers and first-line managers will have increasing authority for staffing allocations. Patient care units and service lines will be run more like small businesses than parts of large bureaucratic organizations. Some nurse managers may elect to hire more support staff; others may think that an all–registered nurse (RN) staff provides the highest quality of care and is also most cost-effective. At the same time, these managers will have greater responsibility for controlling their expenditures, and they must be prepared to defend the decisions they make. In an environment of constrained resources, decisions about hiring support staff or additional RNs must be well supported by drawing on research and other available resources to support their decisions.

HCOs are developing new approaches for paying nurses, such as salary rather than an hourly wage. Organizations commonly pay a premium to nurses who work off-shifts, weekends, or holidays, and many offer nurses premium pay as they advance to higher levels on clinical ladders (discussed in Chapter 3). Issues of productivity and accountability under such payment structures will challenge nurse managers. Some organizations may consider contracting with entrepreneurial groups of nurses to provide nursing care for all patients on a unit or in a particular service, similar to the way that HCOs contract with physicians to provide certain medical services such as emergency care. Many home care agencies are paying nurses on a per-visit rather than a salary basis. Managers who use these approaches believe that financial incentives increase the productivity of nurses. Nurse managers and executives at all levels will need to address the financial implications of such changes. It is not enough to know whether the staff would prefer to be salaried. Nurse managers must be able to assess the market to determine competitive payment structures and calculate and understand the financial impact of any such change on the areas they manage and their organizations.

As they gain proficiency in affecting financial indicators, midlevel and first-line managers will have increased accountability for revenue as well. Historically, nurse managers were held accountable for the fixed nursing personnel cost per year or, more progressively, the nursing personnel costs per patient day of care. As reimbursement moves to an episode or capitation basis, nurse managers are being held accountable for the episode of care and covered lives. This means that they are accountable for both the nursing cost associated with an episode of care or the group of patients as well as for providing an acceptable level of quality nursing care.

❋ THE NURSE AS A POLICYMAKER FOR FINANCING HEALTH CARE

The focus of this book has been on financial management in HCOs. Although this is the role most nurses will assume in financial management, there is a role for nurses in developing the external financing and regulatory systems that have an impact on organizations. Nurses can work in a variety of non-provider settings that have a dramatic impact on people's health.

Lobbyist

Nurses serve as lobbyists to both the legislative and executive branches of all levels of government. Lobbyists often work for professional organizations such as national or state nurses' associations or for special interest groups such as those concerned with a particular disease or cause. Many decisions about the provision of care are directly related to the payment for that care. Given that many of the payment decisions are now made by federal and state governments, the nurse who understands financial management can be a formidable lobbyist. For example, if the state is planning to require that all Medicaid patients be part of managed care programs, what implications does this have for nursing? How can advanced practice nurses become recognized as care providers in these programs?

Many policy decisions affecting the financial management of HCOs are made in industry. For example, pharmaceutical companies set pricing levels for drugs, and insurance companies set reimbursement policy. Other policies are made outside of health care altogether in the business sector. Major industries such as the auto industry decide which health care benefits will be provided to their employees and covered in their plans. Financial consulting organizations, including some of the largest accounting firms, employ nurses to help their clients improve operations. Nurses possessing finance skills along with their understanding of clinical care are viewed as invaluable employees in these organizations.

Policymaker

Nurses can also work in government and help develop government policies for financing health care. There is a small but growing group of nurses that is knowledgeable about financial matters working for government in financial policy development. They work at all levels of government, developing and implementing the financial policies that affect the provision of patient care. Rather than continuing to complain about the decisions government makes about financing care that affects nursing, the profession needs nurses who are knowledgeable about financing to make those decisions for and with us.

Many nurses say about colleagues who work in industry or government, "They've left nursing" or "They are no longer nurses." Although working in industry or for government may not be providing direct patient care to individuals, we believe that nursing encompasses caring for the community and society at large, as well as individuals. Nurse theorists debate what nursing is and what the role of nurses should be in determining the health of people. Is developing policy to change health care reimbursement for nurses part of nursing? Are actions to address compassion fatigue among nurses, who in turn care for patients, part of nursing? Are efforts to redesign care delivery—the direct, hands-on delivery of care, or creating community models to meet clients' needs—nursing? However

nursing is defined, it cannot be done without the provision of the resources to do so. Providing resources cannot be done without a firm understanding of the intricate relationship between financial management and public policymaking.

❋ IMPLICATIONS FOR NURSE MANAGERS AND EXECUTIVES

As the functions of nurse executive and midlevel and first-line nurse managers expand in the future, possession of financial skills will remain critical. Although historically, many nurse managers and executives obtained financial knowledge through on-the-job training, this is no longer the case. Today's nurse manager and executive must have formal knowledge of the principles and conceptual foundations of financial management and budgeting to survive in their roles.

Some academic programs prepare nurses for executive practice; others prepare midlevel or first-line nurse managers (or both). Regardless of whether the focus is on executive versus first-line or midlevel nurse managers, nursing educational programs must prepare graduates to meet the challenges facing nurse leaders of the future. Nurse executives have reported that they spend about 20% of their time on managing nursing resources, including the establishment of balanced nursing budgets and resource management systems, and the development of cost reduction programs.[14] Thus, acquiring these skills should be central to their educational preparation.

Scoble and Russell[15] identified educational priorities and content that should be required in graduate programs preparing nurse administrators by surveying nurse executives and managers from a variety of practice settings along with faculty, deans, nurse consultants and graduate students. Financial management ranked third in curriculum content needs for future nurse managers and executives, just after content in business administration and leadership. They concluded that finance should be a fundamental component of content to meet the growing need for nurse managers and executives to have core competencies in financial management. This focus will also better equip nurse managers and executives with nursing and financial management research upon which to base nursing resource allocation decisions.

Historically, nursing graduate programs focused almost exclusively on preparing nurses for clinical nursing practice. As practicing nurse managers and executives recognized that management skills, including financial management, were necessary to be an effective manager, schools of nursing began to include this content in their programs. Although budgeting and financial management may not be required in all programs, these skills are necessary for practicing nurses today. In addition to their nursing education, nurse managers and executives need to obtain the conceptual foundations and principles of finance to have a good grasp of content that will enable them to develop and apply these skills in practice. Many

---

[14] Arnold L, Drenkard K, Ela S, et al. 2007. Strategic positioning for nursing excellence in health systems. *Nurs Adm Q* 30(1):11-20.

[15] Scoble K, Russell G. 2003. Vision 2020, part 1: Profile of the future nurse leader. *J Nurs Adm* 33(6):324-330.

managers currently working in health organizations may not have these skills but will be expected to obtain them through formal academic programs, workshops, or on-the-job training.

Over the past several decades, we have seen a renewed focus on preparing nurses with advanced clinical expertise, and most graduate programs now offer advanced practice nursing programs. These nurses must also understand financial management to meet the challenges they will face throughout their careers, yet few get exposure to the depth of content needed to prepare them for the financial management issues they will be facing upon graduation. There is a growing movement to prepare advanced practice nurses with doctorate degrees in nursing practice. These degrees combine knowledge of advanced practice *clinical* nursing with advanced practice *leadership* skills. The impetus behind this movement is partially the acknowledgement that advanced practice nurses simply need greater skills in organizational, financial, and quality management to function in today's constantly changing and complex

health care system. We hope this book will serve as just the beginning of nurses' efforts to learn about financial management and to bring that knowledge into nursing. We have provided the foundations. Nurse managers and executives who have studied this book should feel confident about holding conversations and interacting with financial managers and other administrators. Nurse managers and executives who have studied this book are prepared to apply the concepts of financial management in HCOs.

We hope, however, that this is only the beginning of nurses' interest in learning about and integrating nursing and health care financial management concepts and principles in their practice. We encourage nurse managers and executives to continue reading, studying, and learning about nursing financial management, a field still in its infancy. Nurse managers and executives have the opportunity to participate in and lead the innovations still to come as well as to bring about lasting changes that improve the overall delivery of health care.

✳ KEY CONCEPTS

Nursing financial management research   Research can be described as a continuum from theoretical to applied. Research in this area is primarily applied and focuses on nursing resource use, costing nursing care, and cost-benefit analysis.

Role of nurse executive in financial management   This role is expanding to include participation in the major financial decisions of health organizations and setting organizational policy.

Role of midlevel nurse manager in financial management   This role is expanding in direct relation to the nurse executive; the midlevel manager contributes to financial decision making in HCOs by leading and carrying out their financial responsibilities for a service line(s).

Role of first-line nurse manager in financial management   This role is expanding relative to the midlevel nurse manager and the nurse executive; the first-line manager contributes to the service line and the overall HCO by leading and providing financial responsibility for one or more patient care units within a service line.

Government relations   Interaction with government officials in the executive and legislative branches. The nurse manager and executive must understand the payment system and its financial implications for reimbursement and regulatory decisions.

Payer relations   Relationship with payers is critical for the fiscal health of the organization. Nurse managers and executives must understand payer policies about reimbursement, particularly those that affect denial of claims.

Policymaker   Nurse managers and executives can affect health care delivery as lobbyists or financial policymakers in government.

✳ SUGGESTED READINGS

Aiken L, Clarke S, Cheung R, et al: Educational levels of hospital nurses and surgical patient mortality, *JAMA* 290(12):1617–1623, 2003.

Aiken L, Clarke S, Silber J, Sloane D: Hospital nurse staffing, education, and patient mortality, *LDI Issue Brief* 9(2):1–4, 2003.

Aiken L, Clarke S, Sloane D, et al: Hospital nurse staffing and patient mortality, nurse burnout, and job dissatisfaction, *JAMA* 288(16):1987–1993, 2002.

Arnold L, Drenkard K, Ela S, et al: Strategic positioning for nursing excellence in health systems, *Nurs Adm Q* 30(1):11–20, 2007.

Ballein K: Entrepreneurial leadership characteristics of SNEs emerge as their role develops, *Nurs Adm Q* 22(2):60–69, 1997.

Ballein Search Partners, American Organization of Nurse Executives: *Why senior nursing officers matter: a national survey of nursing executives*, Oak Brook, Ill, 2003, Ballein Search Partners.

Bloom J, Alexander J, Nichols B: Nurse staffing patterns and hospital efficiency in the United States, *Soc Sci Med* 44(2):147–155, 1997.

Blouin A, Brent N: The nurse entrepreneur: legal aspects of owning a business, *J Nurs Adm* 25(6):13–14, 1995.

Borromeo A: The professional salary model: meeting the bottom lines, *Nurs Econ* 14(4):241–244, 1996.

Brennan T, Hinson N, Taylor M: Nursing and finance: MAKING the connection, *Healthc Financ Manage* 62(1):90–94, 2008.

Burke R: Hospital restructuring, workload, and nursing staff satisfaction and work experiences, *Health Care Manage* 22(2):99–107, 2003.

Campbell S: The newest gatekeepers: nurses take on the duties of primary care physicians, *Health Care Strat Manage* 15(3):14–15, 1997.

Caroselli C: Economic awareness of nurses: relationship to budgetary control, *Nurs Econ* 14(5):292–298, 1996.

Cho S, Ketefian S, Barkauskas V, Smith D: The effects of nurse staffing on adverse events, morbidity, mortality, and medical costs, *Nurs Res* 52:71–79, 2003.

Crowell D: Organizations *are* relationships: a new view of management, *Nurs Manage* 29(5):28–29, 1998.

Ervin N, Chang W, White J: A cost analysis of a nursing center's services, *Nurs Econ* 16(6):307–312, 1998.

Finkler S: Evidence based financial management—what are we waiting for? *Res Healthc Financ Manage* 9(1):1–3, 2004.

Finkler S: Teaching future healthcare financial managers to use evidence, *J Health Adm Educ* 20(4):243–261, 2003.

Finkler S, Henley R, Ward D: Evidence based financial management, *Healthc Financ Manage* 57(10):64–68, 2003.

Finkler S, Kovner C, Knickman J, Hendrickson G: Innovation in nursing: a benefit/cost analysis, *Nurs Econ* 12(1):25–29, 1994.

Grandinetti D: Will patients choose NPs over doctors? *Med Econ* 74(14):134–151, 1997.

Holman E, Branstetter E: An academic nursing clinic's financial survival, *Nurs Econ* 15,(5):248–252, 1997.

Huston C: Unlicensed assistive personnel: a solution to dwindling health care resources or the precursor to the apocalypse of registered nursing, *Nurs Outlook* 44(2):67–73, 1996.

Institute of Medicine: *The future of nursing: leading change, advancing health,* Washington, DC, 2011, National Academies Press.

Jones C, Mark B: The intersection of nursing and health services research: an agenda to guide future research, *Nurs Outlook* 53(6):324–333, 2005.

Jones C, Mark B: The intersection of nursing and health services research: overview of an agenda-setting conference, *Nurs Outlook* 53(6):270–273, 2005.

Jones CB, Havens DS, Thompson PA: Chief nursing officer retention and turnover: a crisis brewing? Results of a national survey, *J Healthc Manage* 53(2):89–105; discussion 105–106, 2008.

Keehan SP, Sisko AM, Truffer CJ, et al: National health spending projections through 2020. economic recovery and reform drive faster growth, *Health Aff* 30(8):1–12, 2011.

Kirk R: *Managing outcomes, process, and cost in a managed care environment,* Gaithersburg, Maryland, 1997, Aspen.

Korda H, Eldridge GN: ACOs, PCMHs, and health care reform: nursing's next frontier? *Policy Polit Nurs Pract* 12(2):100–103, 2011.

Kovner A, Elton J, Billings J, et al: Evidence-based management/commentaries/reply, *Front Health Serv Manage* 16(4):3–46, 2000.

Kovner AR, Rundall TG: Evidence-based management reconsidered, *Front Health Serv Manage* 22(3):3–22, 2006.

Kovner C, Gergen P: Nurse staffing levels and adverse events following surgery in U.S. hospitals, *Image* 30(4):315–321, 1998.

Kovner C, Jones C, Zahn C, et al: Nurse staffing and post surgical adverse events: an analysis of administrative data from a sample of U.S. hospitals, 1990–1996, *Health Serv Res* 37(3):611–629, 2002.

Kovner C, Schore J: Differentiated levels of nursing workforce demand, *J Prof Nurs* 14:242–253, 1998.

Lambert V, Lambert C Jr: Advanced practice nurses: starting an independent practice, *Nurs Forum* 31(1):11–21, 1996.

Lynn M, Layman E, Richard S: Research priorities. The final chapter in the nursing administration research priorities saga: the state of the state, *J Nurs Adm* 29(5):5–9, 1999.

Mark B, Harless D, McCue M, Xu Y: A longitudinal examination of hospital registered nurse staffing and quality of care, *Health Serv Res* 39:279–301, 2004.

Needleman J, Buerhaus P, Mattke S, et al: Nurse staffing levels and the quality of care in hospitals, *N Engl J Med* 346(22):1715–1722, 2002.

Needleman J, Buerhaus P, Stewart M, et al: Nurse staffing in hospitals: is there a business case for quality? *Health Aff* 25(1):204–211, 2006.

Page A, Institute of Medicine: *Keeping patients safe: transforming the work environment of nurses,* Washington, DC, 2004, The National Academies Press.

Pappas I, Rushenberg J: Help students see dollars, *Nursing Manage* 40(6):37–42, 2009.

Prescott P, Soeken K, Griggs M: Identification and referral of hospitalized patients in need of home care, *Res Nurs Health* 18(2):85–95, 1995.

Prybil L, Levey S, Peterson R, et al: *Governance in high-performing community health systems: a report on trustee and CEO views,* Chicago, Ill, 2009, Grant Thornton LLP.

Scoble K, Russell G: Vision 2020, part 1: profile of the future nurse leader, *J Nurs Adm* 33(6):324–330, 2003.

Seago J: Nurse staffing, models of care delivery, and interventions. In Shojania K, Duncan B, McDonald K, Wachter R, editors: *Making health care safer: a critical analysis of patient safety practices.* Rockville, Maryland, 2001, Agency for Healthcare Research and Quality. Evidence Report/Technology Assessment(43), AHRQ Publication No. 01–E058.

Vahey D, Aiken L, Sloane D, et al: Nurse burnout and patient satisfaction, *Med Care* 42(Suppl 2):II57–II66, 2004.

Young S: Evidence-based management: a literature review, *J Nurs Manage* 10:145–161, 2002.

Glossary

A

ABC *See* activity-based costing.

access to care The availability of care that is appropriate and adaptable to patients' health needs, acceptable to the patient, and affordable.

accounting System for keeping track of the financial status of an organization and the financial results of its activities.

accounting controls Methods and procedures for the authorization of transactions, safeguarding of assets, and accuracy of accounting records.

accounting cost Measurement of cost based on a number of simplifications, such as an assumed useful life for a piece of equipment.

accounting cycle Period of time from when cash is spent to acquire resources to provide care until cash is received in payment for the services provided.

accounting rate of return (ARR) Profitability of an investment calculated by considering the profits it generates compared with the amount of money invested.

accounts payable Amounts owed to suppliers (e.g., a per diem agency or a medical supply company).

accounts receivable Money owed to an organization or individual in exchange for goods and services provided.

accrual accounting Accounting system that matches revenues and related expenses in the same fiscal year by recording revenues in the year in which they are earned (whether received or not) and the expenses related to generating those revenues in the same year.

accrue Increase or accumulate.

accumulated depreciation Total amount of depreciation related to a fixed asset that has been recorded over the years the organization has owned that asset.

activity accounting Method of tracking costs and other information by focusing on the activities undertaken to produce the good or service.

activity-based costing (ABC) Approach to determining the cost of products or product lines using multiple overhead allocation bases that relate to the activities that generate overhead costs.

activity report Measures key statistics concerning current operations; centers on the number of units of service and the relative proportion of the organization's capacity being used.

acuity Measurement of a patient's severity of illness related to the amount of nursing care resources required to care for the patient.

acuity subcategory Amount that would have been budgeted for the actual output level if the actual acuity level had been correctly forecast.

acuity system System to assess the amount of care required by patients; may be developed for a particular hospital or can be purchased.

acuity variance Variance resulting from the difference between the actual acuity level and the budgeted level; the difference between the flexible budget and the value of the acuity subcategory.

ADC *See* average daily census.

adjusted occupied beds Measure that combines both inpatient days and outpatient care by using a formula for the number of outpatient visits considered to be the equivalent of 1 inpatient day.

administration Management.

administrative control Plan of organization (e.g., formal organization chart concerning who reports to whom) and all methods and procedures that enable management planning and control of operations.

adverse event Harm to a patient that results from the health care received.

adverse selection "A tendency for utilization of health services in a population group to be higher than average. From an insurance perspective, adverse selection occurs when persons with poorer-than-average life expectancy or health status apply for or continue insurance coverage to a greater extent than do persons with average or better health expectations."[1]

age-of-plant ratio *See* plant-age ratio.

aging schedule Management report that shows how long receivables have been outstanding since a bill was issued.

algebraic distribution Cost-allocation approach that uses simultaneous equations to allocate nonrevenue cost center costs to both nonrevenue and revenue cost centers in a manner that does not create distortions.

allowance for bad debts *See* allowance for uncollectible accounts.

allowance for uncollectible accounts Estimated portion of total accounts receivable that is not expected to be collected because of bad debts; sometimes called allowance for bad debts.

allowances Discounts from the amount normally charged for patient care services. These discounts are sometimes negotiated (e.g., with HMOs or Blue Cross) and are other times mandated by law (e.g., Medicare, Medicaid).

all-payer system System of payment in which all payers use the same payment method for paying for health care services.

ALOS *See* average length of stay.

alternative workers Workers who perform tasks and activities that augment the care delivered by professional

---

[1]The definition for this term has been quoted from Bartlett L, Hitz P, Simon R. 1996. Appendix A—Glossary of common managed care terms. In *Assessing Roles, Responsibilities, and Activities in a Managed Care Environment: A Workbook for Local Health Officials*. Rockville, MD: Agency for Health Care Policy and Research, Department of Health and Human Services, AHCPR Publication No. 96–0057.

nurses. These may include workers such as unit hostesses, who orient patients and their families to the hospital and the unit, thereby freeing up nurses to focus on care delivery.

ambulatory care "All types of health services that are provided on an outpatient basis in contrast to services provided in the home or to persons who are inpatients. Although many inpatients may be ambulatory, the term *ambulatory care* usually implies that the patient must travel to a location to receive services that do not require an overnight stay."[2]

amortization Allocation of cost of an intangible asset over its lifetime.

annuity Series of payments or receipts, each in the same amount and spaced evenly over time (e.g., $127.48 paid monthly for 3 years).

annuity payments *See* annuity.

any willing provider law "Laws that require managed care plans to contract with all health care providers that meet their terms and conditions."[3]

ARR *See* accounting rate of return.

assets Valuable resources; they may be either physical, having substance and form such as a table or building, or intangible, such as the reputation the organization has gained for providing high-quality health care services.

audit Examination of the financial records of an organization to discover material errors, evaluate the internal control system, and determine if financial statements have been prepared in accordance with generally accepted accounting principles.

auditor Person who performs an audit.

audit trail Set of references that allows an individual to trace back through accounting documents to the source of each number used.

average cost Full cost divided by volume of service units.

average daily census (ADC) Average number of inpatients on any given day; patient days in a given time period divided by number of days in the time period.

average length of stay Average number of patient days for each patient discharged; number of patient days in a given time period divided by number of discharges in that time period.

axiom Unproven but accepted assertion that is either self-evident or a mutually accepted principle.

B

bad debts Operating expenses related to care provided to patients who ultimately do not pay the provider, although they were expected to pay. Amounts included in revenues but never paid are balanced by the charge to bad debts.

balance sheet Financial report that indicates the financial position of the organization at a specific point in time; officially referred to as the statement of financial position.

balanced scorecard Internal organizational report card used by organizations for strategic management purposes to examine performance. Typically, performance is monitored in four areas: customer perspective, financial perspective, internal processes (including human resources), and learning and growth.[4]

benchmarking Technique aimed at finding the best practices of other organizations and incorporating those practices within an organization.

benefit-cost ratio The benefits of a proposed project divided by its costs. If the ratio is greater than 1, the project is financially attractive.

Blue Cross Major provider of hospitalization insurance to both individuals and groups; for most hospitals, one of the largest sources of revenue.

board designated Portion of the net assets or fund balance that the board has identified and a corresponding amount of assets that the board has restricted for a specific purpose; sometimes called board restricted.

board of directors *See* board of trustees.

board of trustees Governing body that has the ultimate responsibility for decisions made by the organization.

board restricted *See* board designated.

bondholder Owner of one or more of an organization's outstanding bonds payable.

bonding of employees Insurance policy that protects the organization against embezzlement and fraud by employees.

bond payable Formal borrowing arrangement in which a transferable paper or electronic certificate represents the debt. The holder of the bond may sell it, in which case the liability is owed to the new owner.

bonds Formal paper or electronic certificates of indebtedness. The certificate indicates a promise to pay interest, usually semiannually, and the face value of the bond at a future specified maturity date.

bond sinking fund Pool of segregated assets to be used for the eventual repayment of outstanding bonds.

bonus system Method to provide incentives for employees to improve performance. Employees receive financial payment, shares of stock, or other remuneration if certain targets are achieved or exceeded.

break-even analysis Technique for determining the minimum volume of output (e.g., patient days of care) necessary for a program or service to be financially self-sufficient.

break-even point *See* break-even volume.

break-even time (BT) Amount of time before the present value of cash inflows is at least equal to the present value of cash outflows.

break-even volume Volume needed to just break even. Losses are incurred at lower volumes and profits at higher volumes.

budget Plan that provides formal, quantitative expression of management's plans and intentions or expectations.

---

[2]*Ibid.*
[3]*Ibid.*

[4]Oliveira J. 2001. The balanced scorecard: An integrative approach to performance evaluation. *Healthc Financ Manage* 55(5):42-46.

budgeting Process whereby plans are made and then an effort is made to meet or exceed the goals of the plans.

building fund Restricted fund containing assets that can be used only to acquire buildings and equipment.

business case Position on whether or not an investment should be made in a project or initiative based on a systematic evaluation of the worth or value of the project or initiative. Involves the calculation of rates of return on investments, break-even points, costs and benefits, and other financial indices.[5]

business plan Detailed plan for a proposed program, project, or service, including information to be used to assess the venture's financial feasibility.

C

cafeteria plan Method of providing fringe benefits in which the employee chooses from a variety of options those fringe benefits that the employee wants.

call provisions Elements of a loan agreement between the bond issuer and purchaser indicating the rights of the bond issuer to call in and pay off the bonds early; specifies penalties that must be paid if a bond is retired early.

capital acquisitions *See* capital assets.

capital assets Buildings or equipment with useful lives extending beyond the year in which they are purchased or put into service; also referred to as long-term investments, capital items, capital investments, or capital acquisitions.

capital budget Plan for the acquisition of buildings and equipment that will be used by the organization for 1 or more years beyond the year of acquisition. Often a minimum dollar cutoff must be exceeded for an item to be included in the capital budget.

capital budgeting Process of proposing the purchase of capital assets, analyzing the proposed purchases for economic or other justification, and encompassing the financial implications of accepted capital items into the master budget.

capital equipment Equipment with an expected life beyond the year of purchase. Such equipment must generally be included in the capital budget.

capital investments *See* capital assets.

capitalism *See* market economy.

capital items *See* capital assets.

capitation "A method of payment for health services in which an individual or institutional provider is paid a fixed amount for each person served without regard to the actual number or nature of services provided to each person in a set period of time. Capitation is the characteristic payment method in certain health maintenance organizations. It also refers to a method of federal support of health professional schools. Under these authorizations, each eligible school receives a fixed payment, called a *capitation grant*, from the federal government for each student enrolled."[6]

career ladder Approach to promotion and compensation that allows a worker to progress in an organization or a field.

carrying costs of inventory Capital costs and out-of-pocket costs related to holding inventory. Capital cost represents the lost interest because money is tied up in inventory. Out-of-pocket costs include such expenses as insurance on the value of inventory, annual inspections, and obsolescence of inventory.

carve out "Regarding health insurance, an arrangement whereby an employer eliminates coverage for a specific category of services (e.g., vision care, mental health or psychological services, or prescription drugs) and contracts with a separate set of providers for those services according to a predetermined fee schedule or capitation arrangement. *Carve out* may also refer to a method of coordinating dual coverage for an individual."[7]

case management "The monitoring and coordination of treatment rendered to patients with a specific diagnosis or requiring high-cost or extensive services."[8]

case mix "A measure of the mix of cases being treated by a particular health care provider that is intended to reflect the patients' different needs for resources. Case-mix is generally established by estimating the relative frequency of various types of patients seen by the provider in question during a given time period and may be measured by factors such as diagnosis, severity of illness, utilization of services,"[9] and patient characteristics.

case-mix index Measurement of average complexity or severity of illness of patients treated by a health care organization.

cash Money on hand plus cash equivalents such as savings and checking accounts and short-term certificates of deposit.

cash basis Accounting system under which revenues are recorded when cash is received a expenses are recorded when cash is paid. This system does not meet the standards of generally accepted accounting principles because it does not adequately match revenues and related expenses in the same year.

cash budget Plan for the cash receipts and cash disbursements of the organization. The cash budget includes the starting cash balance plus expected cash receipts less expected cash payments.

cash budgeting Process of planning the cash budget.

cash disbursement Outflow of cash from the organization.

cash equivalents Savings and checking accounts and short-term certificates of deposit; items that are quickly and easily convertible into cash.

cash flow Measure of the amount of cash received or disbursed at a given point in time, as opposed to revenues or income, which frequently are recorded at a time other than when the actual cash receipt or payment occurs.

cash management Active process of planning for borrowing and repayment of cash or investing excess cash on hand.

cash payment *See* cash disbursement.

[5]Jones CB. 2005. The costs of nursing turnover, part 2: Application of the Nursing Turnover Cost Calculation Methodology. *J Nurse Adm* 35(1):41-49.
[6]Bartlett et al., *Op. cit.*
[7]*Ibid.*
[8]*Ibid.*
[9]*Ibid.*

cash receipt Inflow of cash into the organization.

census Number of patients occupying beds at a specific time of day (usually midnight).

Centers for Medicare and Medicaid Services (CMS) Federal agency that administers the Medicare and Medicaid programs.

CFO *See* chief financial officer.

charge master List of an organization's prices for each of its services.

charity care Care provided to patients who are not expected to pay because of limited personal financial resources.

chart of accounts Accounting document that assigns an identifying number to each cost center and each type of revenue or expense. These code numbers are assigned to all financial transactions. By looking at any code number and referring to the chart of accounts, one would know exactly which cost center was involved and the specific type of revenue or expense.

chief financial officer (CFO) Manager responsible for all financial functions of an organization.

chief nurse executive (CNE) Top-level nurse manager responsible for all nursing functions in the organization. This includes all nursing care provided to clients.

clinical ladder Approach to promotion and compensation based on the achievement of clinical excellence.

CNE *See* chief nurse executive.

coefficient of determination Measure of the goodness of fit of a regression; generally referred to as the *R-squared*.

coinsurance Percentage of a patient's health services charge that must be paid by the patient.

collaborative benchmarking Finding information within your industry that is based on industry-wide statistics.

collateral Specific asset pledged to a lender as security for a loan.

collection period Time from when a patient bill is issued until cash is collected.

commercial paper Form of short-term borrowing in which the borrower issues a financial security that can be traded by the lender to someone else.

committed costs Costs that cannot be changed in the short run.

common size ratios Class of ratios that allow evaluation of each number on a financial statement relative to the size of the organization. This is accomplished by dividing each financial statement number by a key number from that statement, such as total assets or total revenues.

comparative effectiveness research (CER) "The generation and synthesis of evidence that compares the benefits and harms of alternative methods to prevent, diagnose, treat, and monitor a clinical condition or to improve the delivery of care. The purpose of CER is to assist consumers, clinicians, purchasers, and policy makers to make informed decisions that will improve health care at both the individual and population levels."[10]

competitive benchmarking Finding specific information about individual organizations providing the same services as your organization.

competitive strategy Organization's plan for achieving its goals, specifically, what will be sold and to whom.

compound interest Method of calculating interest that accrues not only on the amount of the original investment but also on the interest earned in interim periods.

congruent goals *See* goal congruence.

conservatism principle Financial statements must give adequate consideration to the risks faced by the organization.

constant dollars Dollar amounts that have been adjusted for the effects of inflation.

consumer Person who receives services from a health care provider.

contingency Event that may or may not occur.

continuous budgeting System in which a budget is prepared each month for a month 1 year in the future. For example, after the actual results for this January are known, a budget for January of next year is prepared.

continuous quality improvement (CQI) A philosophy concerning the production of an organization's goods and services that proposes that there should be a constant focus on improvement in the quality of the product or service.

contractual allowances Discounts from full charges that are given to large payers of health care services, such as the government and other third-party payers.

contribution from operations Contribution margin from the routine annual operations of the organization.

contribution margin Amount by which the price exceeds the variable cost. If the contribution margin is positive, each extra unit of activity makes the organization better off by that amount.

control Attempt to ensure that actual results come as close to planned results as possible.

control chart Graph of variances that indicates upper and lower limits. A variance should be investigated if either of the limits is exceeded.

controllable Items over which a manager can exercise a degree of control.

control limit Amount beyond which a variance should be investigated.

cooperative benchmarking Seeking information from organizations in other industries that can be adapted to the health care industry to improve health care practices.

co-payment Dollar amount that must be paid by individuals each time a health service is used.

corporation Business owned by a group of persons (shareholders or stockholders) who have limited liability; owners are not liable for more than the amount invested in the firm.

cost Amount spent on something. Costs have two stages: acquisition cost and expired cost. When an asset or service is purchased, it has an acquisition cost. If the item is an asset, it will appear on the balance sheet at its cost until it is used up. When the asset is used up, it becomes an expired cost, or an expense.

---

[10]Committee on Comparative Effectiveness Research Prioritization, Institute of Medicine. 2009. *Comparative Effectiveness Research*. Washington, DC: National Academies, p 29.

cost accounting A subset of accounting related to measuring costs to generate cost information for reporting and making management decisions.

cost accounting system Any coherent system designed to gather and report cost information to the management of an organization.

cost allocation Process of taking costs from one area or cost objective and allocating them to others.

cost base Statistic used as a basis for allocation of overhead (e.g., patient days, labor hours).

cost-based price Charge that reflects the exact cost of providing a service.

cost-based reimbursement Payments made to providers based on reimbursement to the provider for the cost incurred in providing care.

cost behavior Way that costs change in reaction to events within the organization.

cost-benefit analysis (CBA) Measurement of the relative costs and benefits associated with a particular project or task.

cost center (or expense center) Unit or department in an organization for which a manager is assigned responsibility for costs. These organizational units are not responsible for generating a budgeted amount of revenue because they are only accountable for controlling their expenses.

cost driver Activity that causes costs to be incurred.

cost-effective Approach that provides care as good as any other approach but at a lower cost or an approach that provides the best possible care for a given level of cost.

cost-effectiveness Measure of whether costs are minimized for the desired outcome.

cost-effectiveness analysis (CEA) Technique that measures the cost of alternatives that generate the same outcome. *See also* cost effective.

cost estimation Process of using historical cost information to segregate mixed costs into their fixed and variable components and then using that information to estimate future costs.

cost finding Process that finds the costs of units of service (e.g., lab tests, radiographs, routine patient days) based on allocation of nonrevenue cost center costs to revenue centers.

cost measurement Process of assessing resources consumed and assigning a value to those resources.

cost objective Any particular item, program, or organizational unit for which we wish to know the cost.

cost of capital Cost to the organization of the money used for capital acquisitions; often represented by the interest rate that the organization pays on borrowed money.

cost of product What the organization must pay for the product; can be affected by quantity discounts.

cost pass-through Payment by a third party that reimburses the health care organization for the amount of costs it incurred in providing care to patients.

cost-per-hire ratio Personnel recruiting costs related to advertising vacancies, using placement firms, interviewing and processing potential candidates, traveling, and moving, all divided by the number of individuals hired.

cost pool Any grouping of costs.

cost reimbursement Revenue based on paying the organization for the costs incurred in providing care to patients.

cost reporting Process of conveying information about the cost of resources consumed relative to a specific cost objective.

cost-volume-profit relationship The associations among costs, volume, and profits.

costing out nursing services Process of determining the cost of providing nursing care for different patients. This cost has traditionally been included in the room and board charge.

CPM *See* critical path method.

CQI *See* continuous quality improvement.

cr. Credit.

credit Bookkeeping term for an increase in an item on the right side of the fundamental equation of accounting or a decrease in an item on the left side.

creditors People or organizations to whom the organization owes money.

cross-subsidization of costs Situation in which some patients are assigned more costs than they cause the organization to incur and others are assigned less.

current assets Resources the organization has that either are cash or can be converted to cash within 1 year or that will be used up within 1 year. Current assets are often referred to as *short-term* or *near-term assets*.

current liabilities Obligations that are expected to be paid within 1 year.

current ratio Current assets divided by current liabilities.

curvilinear Curved line. Statistical methods that create forecasts taking into account curved line relationships between the variables.

curvilinear forecasting Forecasting using curved lines to make estimates of future values.

customary and reasonable charges Limits set by insurers on the amount that they will consider for payment based on surveys of typical charges in the community.

D

database Compilation of related information systematically organized.

days receivable ratio Accounts receivable divided by patient revenue per day; a measure of how long it takes on average until revenues are collected.

debit Bookkeeping term for an increase in an item on the left side of the fundamental equation of accounting or a decrease in an item on the right side.

debt Borrowed money, or liability. Interest is generally paid on the debt.

debt service Required interest and principal repayments on money owed.

debt service coverage ratio Cash available to pay interest and principal repayments divided by required interest and principal repayments; a measure of the ability of the organization to meet required debt service.

debt-to-equity ratio *See* total debt-to-equity ratio.

decentralization Delegation of decision-making autonomy downward within the organization.

decision package Zero-based budgeting term referring to a package of all the information to be used in ranking alternatives and making a final decision.

decision variables Factors controllable by the organization that can affect volume.

decreasing returns to scale Extremely large volume may lead to increasing cost per unit produced because of capacity constraints or shortages of labor or supplies.

deductible Amount that must first be paid by an insured individual before insurance covers any costs; usually the first several hundred dollars (e.g., $100 or $200 or $500) consumed per year for health insurance.

deferred revenues Amounts that will become revenue in the future when the organization provides goods or services. These are liabilities until the goods or services are provided.

deficit Excess of expenses over revenues. This term sometimes is used to refer to just the current year or budgeted year and sometimes to the deficit accumulated over a period of years.

Delphi technique Technique sometimes used for forecasting that uses an expert group, which never meets, to generate written information as the basis for making a decision. When used in forecasting, each member's written forecast, along with the reasoning behind it, is distributed. This process is repeated several times, and eventually a group decision is made.

demand Amount of the good or service that consumers are willing to acquire at any given price.

demand curve Quantity (horizontal axis) desired by consumers for any given price (vertical axis).

demographics Characteristics of the human population, including age, sex, growth, density, distribution, and other vital statistics.

dependent variable Item whose value is being predicted.

depreciate Decline in value or productive capability.

depreciation Allocation of a portion of the cost of a capital asset into each of the years of the item's expected useful life.

depreciation expense Amount of the original cost of a fixed asset allocated as an expense each year.

Diagnosis Related Groups (DRGs) System that categorizes patients into specific groups based on their medical diagnosis and other characteristics, such as age and type of surgery, if any. Payment for each patient within a specific group is the same. The payment is a predetermined fixed amount and is not dependent on the costs incurred in treating the patient. Currently used by Medicare and some other hospital payers as a basis for payment.

differential advantage Characteristic that provides the organization with a distinct advantage over a competitor; advantages might include location, cost, services offered, and other factors.

differential costs *See* incremental costs.

direct costs (1) Costs incurred within the organizational unit for which the manager has responsibility are referred to as the direct costs of the unit; (2) costs of resources used for direct care of patients are referred to as the direct costs of patient care.

direct distribution Allocation of nonrevenue center costs directly and only to revenue centers.

direct expenses Expenses that can be specifically and exclusively related to the activity within the cost center; *see also* direct costs.

direct labor Labor that is a direct cost element.

direct labor cost The amount spent on direct labor.

direct labor dollars *See* direct labor cost.

direct labor hours Number of hours of direct labor consumed in making a product or providing a service.

disbursement Cash payment.

discount rate Interest rate used in discounting.

discounted cash flow Method that allows comparisons of amounts of money paid at different times by discounting all amounts to the present.

discounting Reverse of compound interest; process in which interest that could be earned over time is deducted from a future payment to determine how much the future payment is worth at the present time.

discretionary costs Costs for which there is no clear-cut relationship between inputs and outputs. The treatment of more patients does not necessarily require more of this input; use of more of this input does not necessarily allow for treatment of more patients.

disequilibrium Condition under which the quantity demanded at the current price is not the same as the quantity suppliers want to provide at that price. In such a situation, there is pressure to either raise or lower the price until equilibrium is achieved.

divergent goals *See* goal divergence.

dividend Distribution of profits to owners of the organization.

double distribution Allocation approach in which all nonrevenue centers allocate their costs to all other cost centers once; then a second allocation takes place using either stepdown or direct distribution.

double-entry accounting Whenever a change is made to the accounting equation, at least one other change must be made as well, to keep the equation in balance.

dr. Debit.

DRGs *See* Diagnosis Related Groups.

E

economic goods Goods or services acquired by consumers to provide physical or psychological benefit.

economic order quantity (EOQ) Approach to determine the optimal quantity for each order. It is based on creating a balance between ordering costs and carrying costs.

economics Study of how scarce resources are allocated among possible uses.

economies of scale Cost of providing a good or service falls as quantity increases because fixed costs are shared by the larger volume.

effectiveness A measure of the degree to which the organization accomplishes its desired goals.

efficiency "Mix of health care resource inputs that produce optimal quantity and quality of health and health care outputs."[11] Inputs can be direct costs (e.g., labor, capital, equipment) or indirect costs (e.g., time). Efficiency can be expressed as output divided by input.

efficiency ratios Class of ratios that examines the efficiency with which the organization uses its resources in providing care and generating revenues.

efficiency variance *See* quantity variance.

elasticity of demand Degree to which demand increases in response to a price decrease or degree to which demand decreases in response to a price increase.

electronic data Data that are computerized.

employee benefits *See* fringe benefits.

employees per occupied bed (EPOB) Total number of paid full-time equivalents (FTEs) divided by the average daily census.

endowment fund Restricted fund that contains the endowment assets that belong to the organization; only earnings may be removed from this fund under normal conditions.

engineered costs Costs for which there is a specific input-output relationship.

entity Specific individual, organization, or part of an organization that is the focus of attention; accounting must be done from the perspective of the relevant entity.

entrepreneur Person who starts a venture that involves risk but that also offers the opportunity to make a profit or provide a new product or service or a new way to deliver a product or service.

environmental scan Critical review of the external organizational environment that considers the impact on the organization of such factors as the economy, inflation, growth, employment, interest rates, competition, and so on.

environmental variables Factors that can affect an organization but that are not controllable by the organization.

EOQ *See* economic order quantity.

EPOB *See* employees per occupied bed.

equilibrium Condition under which the quantity of a good or service offered at the stated price is the same as the quantity that buyers want to purchase at that price.

equity (1) Fairness. (2) Ownership; for example, the share of a house that is owned by the homeowner free and clear of any mortgage obligations is the homeowner's equity in the house.

evaluative budgeting Approach to allocating resources based on the idea that each proposed element of expenditure for each unit or department is explained and justified.

exception report List of only individual items, such as variances, that exceed a specified limit.

expected value Weighted average of possible outcomes using known or subjective probabilities as weights.

expenditure Payment; often used interchangeably with expense.

expense budget Budget for all expenses under a manager's direction, generally within a cost center. Generally divided into personnel expenses and expenses for other than personnel services (OTPS) (includes both direct unit or department expenses and indirect overhead expenses).

expense centers *See* cost centers.

expenses Costs of services provided; expired cost.

expired cost *See* expenses.

external accountant Accountant hired by an organization to consult or to perform an audit of the organization's financial records.

external costs Costs imposed on individuals and organizations resulting from the actions of an unrelated individual or organization. *See also* externality.

externality Secondary effect of an action by an individual or organization that presents additional costs or benefits to those affected.

F

factoring Selling the organization's accounts receivable, usually for less than their face value.

favorable variance Variance in which expenses were less than the budgeted amount, or revenues were more than the budgeted amount.

feasibility study Analysis designed to determine the organization's capacity to repay a long-term loan; assessment of whether a venture is likely to be financially successful.

feedback Information about actual results. Used to avoid repeating past mistakes and improve future plans.

fee-for-service System in which there is an additional charge for each additional type and unit of service provided (as opposed to a prepaid system, in which all services are included in exchange for one flat payment).

fiduciary Relating to holding something in trust; a fiduciary is a trustee, who maintains assets in trust.

FIFO *See* first-in, first-out.

financial accounting System that records historical financial information, summarizes it, and provides reports of what financial events have occurred and the financial impact of those events.

financial ratios Ratios developed using data from the organization's financial statements.

financial statements Reports that convey information about the organization's financial position and the results of its activities.

financing accounts receivable Borrowing money and using the organization's accounts receivable as security or collateral for the loan.

first-dollar coverage Insurance coverage that has no deductible or co-payment; the insurance company pays all costs starting from the "first dollar."

first-in, first-out (FIFO) Method of accounting for inventory that assumes the oldest inventory is always used up first.

first-line manager Person responsible for one patient care unit, area, or group of nursing staff.

---

[11]Committee on Redesigning Health Insurance Performance Measures, Payment, and Performance Improvement Programs. 2006. *Performance Measurement: Accelerating Improvement. Institute* of Medicine. Washington, DC: National Academies Press.

fiscal Financial.

fiscal year One-year period defined for financial purposes. A fiscal year may start at any point during the calendar year and ends 1 year later; for example, fiscal year 2014 with a June 30 year end refers to the period from July 1, 2013, through June 30, 2014.

fixed assets Assets that will not be used up or converted to cash within 1 year; sometimes referred to as long-term assets.

fixed costs Costs that do not change in total as volume changes within the relevant range.

fixed staff Employees on the unit whose wages or salary does not vary with patient volume.

flexible budget Budget that is adjusted for volume of output.

flexible budgeting Process of developing a budget based on different workload levels. Often used after the fact to calculate the amount that would have been budgeted for the actual workload levels attained. Depends heavily on the existence of variable costs.

flexible budget variance Difference between actual results and the flexible budget.

flexible budget variance analysis Process that expands upon traditional variance analysis by dividing the total variance into price, quantity, and volume variances.

float (1) Interim period from when a check is written until the check is cashed and clears the bank. (2) Movement of staff from one unit or department to another.

forecast Prediction of some future value such as patient days, chest tubes used, or nursing care hours per patient day (HPPD).

forecasting Process of making predictions.

forecast interval Range of values surrounding a forecast for which there is a specified probability that the actual result will fall within the range.

for-profit organization Organization whose mission includes earning a profit that may be distributed to its owners.

free enterprise *See* market economy.

fringe benefits Compensation provided to employees in addition to their base salary (e.g., health insurance, life insurance, vacation and holiday pay).

FTE *See* full-time equivalent.

full cost Total of all costs associated with an organizational unit or activity; includes direct and indirect costs.

full-time equivalent (FTE) Equivalent of one full-time employee working for 1 year. This is generally calculated as 40 hours per week for 52 weeks or a total of 2,080 paid hours. This includes both productive and nonproductive (e.g., vacation, sick, holiday, education) time. Two employees each working half-time for 1 year are the same as 1 FTE.

fund accounting System of separate financial records and controls; assets of the organization are divided into distinct funds with separate bank accounts and a complete separate set of financial records.

fundamental equation of accounting Assets equal liabilities plus fund balance.

fund balance Owner's equity in a governmental or not-for-profit organization. Also called net assets.

future value (FV) Amount a sum of money will grow to be worth at some point in the future.

G

GAAP *See* generally accepted accounting principles.

general journal First place that financial transactions are entered into the accounting records; chronological listing of all financial transactions.

generally accepted accounting principles (GAAP) Set of rules that must be followed for the organization's financial statements to be deemed a fair presentation of the organization's financial position and results of operations.

general operating fund Unrestricted fund used for the day-to-day operations of the organization.

goal congruence When the goals, desires, and needs of the organization are aligned with those of its employees.

goal divergence Differences between the goals, desires, and needs of the organization and those of its employees.

goals Broad, timeless ends of the organization meant to aid in accomplishing the mission.

going-concern principle Assumption that the numbers reported on a financial statement are those of an organization that will continue in business for the foreseeable future. If the organization is not a going concern, that must be noted in the auditor's letter that accompanies audited financial statements.

goodwill Intangible asset that represents a measure of the value of the organization that goes beyond its specific physical assets.

government grants Direct payments by governmental bodies to health care organizations, usually to finance construction.

gross patient revenues Charges for health care services provided. Note that most providers do not collect this gross amount, because of discounts, bad debts, charity care, and other allowances to customers and third-party payers.

group rated Price charged for insurance based on the experience of the group.

H

health insurance Insurance that pays part or all of the costs of specified health care services.

health maintenance organization (HMO) "An entity with four essential attributes: (1) an organized system providing health care in a geographic area, which accepts the responsibility to provide or otherwise assure the delivery of (2) an agreed-upon set of basic and supplemental health maintenance and treatment services to (3) a voluntarily enrolled group of persons, (4) for which services the entity is reimbursed through a predetermined fixed, periodic prepayment made by, or on behalf of, each person or family unit enrolled. The payment is fixed without regard to the amounts of actual services provided to an individual enrollee. Individual practice associations involving groups or independent physicians can be included under the definition."[12]

---

[12]Bartlett et al., *Op. cit.*

Health Plan Employer Data and Information Set (HEDIS) "A core set of comparable performance measures of managed care plans on quality, access, patient satisfaction, membership, utilization, finance, and descriptive information on health plan management and activities. HEDIS was developed by the National Committee for Quality Assurance (NCQA) to enable employers to compare the value of their health care dollar across a variety of health care plans."[13]

HEDIS *See* Health Plan Employer Data and Information Set.

hierarchy Structure that establishes the authority and responsibility of various persons within an organization.

HMO *See* health maintenance organization.

Hospital-acquired conditions (HAC) High-cost or high-volume conditions that are not "present on admission," result in the assignment of a higher-paying DRG as a secondary diagnosis, and could have been prevented through the application of evidence-based guidelines.

hourly rate Allocation method that assigns costs to units of service based on the amount of time required to provide a treatment or procedure.

hours per patient day (HPPD) Paid hours divided by patient days.

HPPD *See* hours per patient day.

hurdle rate *See* required rate of return.

I

incentives Activities, rewards, or punishments that make it in the individual's interest to act in a desired manner.

income Excess of revenues over expenses for a specific period.

income statement Financial statement that presents the financial results of the organization's revenue and expense activities for a specific period of time.

increasing returns to scale *See* economies of scale.

incremental budgeting Approach to resource allocation that simply adds an additional percentage or amount onto the prior year's budget allocation without investigation of whether the continuation of the amounts authorized in the prior year's budget are warranted.

incremental costs Additional costs that will be incurred if a decision is made that would not otherwise be incurred by the organization.

indemnity Compensation for losses incurred, usually a dollar amount.

independent audit Examination of an organization's financial statements and supporting documents by an outside independent auditor.

independent variable Variable used to predict the dependent variable.

indexing for inflation Adjustment of historical information for the impact of changes in price levels.

indirect costs (1) Costs assigned to an organizational unit from elsewhere in the organization are indirect costs for the unit. (2) Costs within a unit that are not incurred for direct patient care are indirect costs of patient care.

indirect expenses *See* indirect costs.

indirect method Method for measuring cash flows that starts with the excess of operating revenues over expenses and reconciles to actual cash flows.

inputs Resources used for treating patients or otherwise producing output; examples include paid nursing hours, chest tubes, and IV solutions.

institutional cost report Document prepared by many health care organizations for submission, as required, to third-party payers such as Medicare, Medicaid, and Blue Cross.

intangible asset Asset without physical substance or form, for example a patent or trademark.

integrated services network (ISN) "A network of organizations, usually including hospitals and physician groups, that provides or arranges to provide a coordinated continuum of services to a defined population and is held both clinically and fiscally accountable for the outcomes of the populations served."[14]

interest coverage ratio Cash available to pay interest divided by interest; a measure of the organization's ability to meet its required interest payments.

internal accountant Accountant who works for an organization, recording financial information throughout the year.

internal control System of accounting checks and balances designed to minimize both clerical errors and the possibility of fraud or embezzlement; the process and systems that ensure that decisions made in the organization are appropriate and receive appropriate authorization. Requires a system of accounting and administrative controls.

internal rate of return (IRR) Discounted cash-flow technique that calculates the rate of return earned on a specific project or program.

inventory Materials and supplies held for use in providing services or making a product.

inventory carrying costs *See* carrying costs of inventory.

inventory costing Process of determining the cost to be assigned to each unit of inventory, generally for financial statement purposes.

inventory management The appropriate ordering and storage of supplies, considering the product cost, ordering costs, stockout costs, carrying costs, and quality costs.

inventory ordering costs *See* ordering costs.

inventory valuation Process of determining the cost of inventory used and the value of inventory assets.

investment center A responsibility center that controls not only its revenues and expenses but the level of capital investment as well.

investments Stocks and bonds that the organization does not intend to sell within 1 year.

IRR *See* internal rate of return.

issuance of corporate stock Sale of ownership interests in the organization; available only to for-profit organizations.

[13]*Ibid.*

[14]*Ibid.*

J

job-cost sheet Management document used to accumulate all of the materials and labor used for a specific job.

job-order costing Approach to product costing that directly associates the specific resources used for each job with that job.

joint costs Fixed costs required for the treatment of several types of patients; elimination of any one of those types of patients would have no effect on these costs.

journal Book or computer file in which the financial events of the organization are recorded in chronological order.

journal entry Financial notation made in the general journal or a subsidiary journal.

justification Explanation used in defending a proposed budget or in explaining variances that have occurred.

just-in-time (JIT) inventory Approach to inventory management that calls for the arrival of inventory just as it is needed, resulting in zero inventory levels.

L

last-in, first-out (LIFO) Inventory valuation method that accounts for inventory as if the most recent acquisitions are always used before inventory acquired at an earlier date and still on hand.

lease Agreement providing for the use of an asset in exchange for rental payments.

ledger Accounting book for keeping track of increases, decreases, and the balance in each asset, liability, revenue, expense, and fund balance account.

length of stay (LOS) Number of days a patient is an inpatient; generally measured by the number of times the patient is an inpatient at midnight; *see* average length of stay.

liabilities Legal financial obligations an organization has to outsiders; essentially, money the organization owes to someone.

LIFO *See* last-in, first-out.

linearity Straight-line relationship.

line function Element of running an organization that implies direct authority, in contrast with the staff function, which is consultative and without direct authority. Nursing is a line department.

line item Any resource listed separately on a budget; for example, all nursing labor for a unit may appear in aggregate (one line item), or nurse manager costs may appear separately from RN costs and from LPN costs (resulting in three line items). Further subdivisions of nursing costs create additional line items.

line manager Manager of a line department or unit of the organization; *see also* line function.

lines of authority Formal lines of authority may be either direct (full authority), such as the associate director of nursing reporting to the chief nurse executive, or indirect (limited authority), such as the director of dietary reporting to the chief of the medical staff.

liquid assets Cash or other assets that can quickly be converted to cash to meet the short-term liabilities of the organization.

liquidate Convert into cash.

liquidity ratios Class of ratio that examines the ability of the organization to meet its obligations in the coming year.

lock box Post office box that is emptied directly by the bank. The bank removes the receipts and credits them directly to the organization's account.

long-range budget Plan that covers a period of time longer than 1 year, typically 3, 5, or 10 years.

long-range planning Planning process that focuses on general objectives to be achieved by the organization over a period of typically 3 to 5 years; often referred to as strategic planning.

long run *See* long term.

long term Period longer than 1 year.

long-term assets *See* capital assets.

long-term debt Borrowed sources of financing that don't have to be repaid in the coming year, including mortgages, long-term notes, leases, and bonds.

long-term financing Sources of money that the organization can use for longer than 1 year.

long-term investment *See* capital assets.

long-term liabilities Obligations that are not expected to be paid for more than 1 year.

LOS *See* length of stay.

lower of cost or market Marketable securities and investments are recorded on financial statements at their cost or the market value, whichever is lower. This treatment results from the principle of conservatism.

M

managed care "Systems that integrate the financing and delivery of health care services to covered individuals by means of arrangements with selected providers to furnish comprehensive services to members; explicit criteria for the selection of health care providers; significant financial incentives for members to use providers and procedures associated with the planned and formal programs for quality assurance and utilization review."[15]

managed care organization (MCO) Insurance and provider organization that adheres to principles of managed care. *See also* managed care.

management by objectives (MBO) Technique in which a supervising manager and the subordinate manager agree upon a common set of objectives whereby performance will be measured.

management control system Complete set of policies and procedures designed to keep operations going according to plan.

management letter Letter from the certified public accountant (CPA) to the management of an organization discussing weaknesses in the internal control system that were revealed as part of an audit.

management role Three of the most essential elements are planning, control, and decision making.

---

[15]*Ibid.*

managerial accounting Subset of accounting that generates any financial information that can help managers to manage better.

managerial hierarchy *See* hierarchy.

managerial reports Reports that provide information to help managers run the organization more efficiently.

margin At the edge; usually refers to the effects of adding one more patient.

marginal benefit *See* marginal utility.

marginal cost Additional amount that must be spent to acquire or produce one more unit, or the additional costs related to the impact of a specific decision, such as contracting with a managed care organization.

marginal cost analysis Process for making decisions about changes should be based on the marginal costs of the change rather than on the full or average costs.

marginal costs Change in cost related to a change in activity; includes variable costs and any additional fixed costs incurred because the volume change exceeds the relevant range for existing fixed costs.

marginal utility Additional benefit or utility gained from the purchase of one more unit of a particular item.

market Potential customers for a product or an organization.

marketable investments Investments that are bought and sold in financial markets, making them readily convertible to cash.

marketable securities Investments in stocks and bonds that the organization intends to sell within 1 year.

market-based prices Prices that are set based on a survey of what others in the community are charging for the same services.

market economy System in which individuals can choose whether to invest their wealth or capital in a business venture, workers can choose whether to work for that venture at the wages offered, and consumers can choose whether to buy the products of the venture at the seller's price.

market efficiency In a fully functioning free market economy, resources are optimally allocated and used as a result of the supply-and-demand mechanism.

market failure Situations in which the free market does not operate efficiently. A market failure can occur for several reasons in health care, such as government intervention, lack of full information for decision making, lack of direct payment for health care services, monopoly or monopsony power, or government-induced inefficiencies.

market share Portion or percentage of the overall market that a specific organization controls. If half of all patients with leg fractures go to a particular hospital's emergency department, that hospital has a 50% share of the market for leg fractures.

market size variance Variance caused by the existence of a greater or smaller number of patients in the community than was expected.

markup Certain percentage added to the cost of a product or service to establish its selling price.

markup-based prices Prices that reflect the cost of care plus a certain percentage.

master budget Set of all of the major budgets of an organization; generally includes the operating budget, long-range budget, program budgets, capital budget, and cash budget.

material Amount of money substantial enough that an error of that magnitude in the financial statements would cause a user of the statements to make a decision different from one based on the correct information.

matrix distribution *See* algebraic distribution.

matrix management System in which a manager has responsibility that cuts across department lines.

MBO *See* management by objectives.

MCO *See* managed care organization.

Medicaid (Title XIX) "A Federally aided, State-operated and administered program which provides medical benefits for certain indigent or low-income persons in need of health and medical care. The program, authorized by Title XIX of the Social Security Act, is basically for the poor. It does not cover all of the poor, however, but only persons who meet specified eligibility criteria. Subject to broad Federal guidelines, States determine the benefits covered, program eligibility, rates of payment for providers, and methods of administering the program."[16] Medicaid is administered through the Centers for Medicare and Medicaid Services and state governments.

Medicare Federal program administered by the Centers for Medicare and Medicaid Services that pays providers for care delivered to the aged and permanently disabled.

Medicare cost report Institutional cost report prepared for Medicare.

Medical loss ratio Amount of the health care premium that is spent on medical care, as opposed to health plan administration and profits.

Medicare risk contract Contract between the Medicare program and a health maintenance organization (HMO) to provide all medically necessary benefits to any Medicare beneficiary who is enrolled in the plan in exchange for a monthly capitated payment.

microcosting Process of closely examining the actual resources consumed by a particular patient or service. Microcosting tends to be extremely costly and is generally done only for special studies.

midlevel nurse manager Person responsible for nursing functions on more than one nursing unit or area.

mission Set of primary goals that justify an organization's existence, such as providing high-quality hospital care to the surrounding community or providing research and education.

mission statement Statement of the purpose or reason for existence of an organization, department, or unit. Provides direction regarding the types of activities that the organization should undertake.

mixed costs Costs that contain an element of fixed costs and an element of variable costs, such as electricity. A unit or department budget as a whole represents a mixed cost.

---

[16]*Ibid.*

monitoring and control ratios Cost accounting ratios that can be used to generate information to aid managers in monitoring and controlling various aspects of the organization's operations.

monopoly Sole seller who therefore has the power to set prices at a higher-than-equilibrium level.

monopsony Market condition in which there is only one buyer.

moral hazard Fact that people behave differently if they are insured than if they are not. Patients are more likely to consume more health care services if they have health insurance.

mortgage payable Loan that is secured by a specific asset.

moving average Method of averaging out the roughness caused by random variation in a historical series of data points.

multiple distribution The double distribution and the algebraic or matrix distribution approaches to cost allocation.

multiple regression analysis Form of regression analysis that uses more than one independent, or causal, variable. This can yield a better result than using only one variable.

N

near term *See* current assets.

negotiated price Agreement between provider and payer for the payment of services that can include a flat fee for service, percent discounts for services, or payments per episode of service.

negotiative budgeting Approach to resource allocation in which the amount allocated to a unit or department is based on a process of negotiation.

net assets *See* fund balance.

net cash flow Net difference between cash receipts and cash payments.

net income Revenue less expense; profit.

net patient revenues Gross revenues less contractual allowances, bad debts, and charity care.

net present cost Aggregate present value of a series of payments to be made in the future.

net present value (NPV) Present value of a series of receipts less the present value of a series of payments.

networking Internal and external relationships used to build coalitions for influencing goals and resource allocation decisions. External relationships formed through professional and social networking opportunities provide a broader context for understanding issues that affect health care.

net working capital Current assets less current liabilities.

nominal group technique Forecasting technique in which a group of individuals are brought together in a structured meeting and arrive at a group consensus forecast.

noncontrollable Item a manager does not have the authority or ability to control.

nonoperating revenue Categorization that no longer appears on the statement of revenues and expenses. All revenues are operating unless they are incidental and peripheral to the organization, in which case they are shown as gains.

nonproductive time Sick, vacation, holiday, and other paid nonworked time. Time paid to staff as a benefit that is not spent delivering care to patients.

nonrevenue cost center Cost center that does not charge directly for its services; its costs must be allocated to a revenue center to be included in the organization's rates.

nonroutine decisions Management decisions that are not made on a routine, regularly scheduled basis.

normality Element of specification analysis that requires that there be a normal distribution of historical points around the regression line.

not-for-profit organization Organization whose mission does not include earning a profit for distribution to owners. A not-for-profit organization may earn a profit, but such profit must be reinvested for replacement of facilities and equipment or for expansion of services offered.

note payable Written document representing a loan.

NPV *See* net present value.

NRG *See* nursing resource grouping.

nurse councils Components of a shared governance structure that aim to give staff nurses a voice in decision making. Common councils are nursing practice, quality of care, education or professional development, and research; an executive council provides a central function to coordinate, facilitate, and integrate the activities of all other councils.

nurse executive Senior nurse responsible for managing the nursing services of an entire organization; *see also* chief nurse executive.

nurse manager Person responsible for an organizational unit, program, or department.

nursing financial management research Research that is primarily applied to and focuses on nursing resource use, costing nursing care, and cost-benefit analysis.

nursing intensity weights (NIWs) Approach developed to cost out nursing care that allocates costs based on the amount of nursing care needed by patients in each DRG for each day of their hospital stay. NIWs take into account five scoring dimensions: assessment, teaching, emotional support, medical, and physical assistance.

nursing resource grouping (NRG) Classification of patients into homogeneous groups based on nursing care consumed. Any patient in an NRG consumes a set of nursing resources similar to those of any other patient in that NRG.

O

objective function Equation that states the relationship between the objective in a linear programming problem and the other variables in the process. The objective is the item, the value of which we wish to optimize.

objectives Specific targets to be achieved to attain goals.

occupancy rate Percentage of total beds filled on a patient care unit or in an entire organization (i.e., the number of beds filled divided by the total number of beds available).

one-shot budget Budget that is prepared one time only, rather than on a regular basis (e.g., monthly or annually).

operating Related to the normal routine activities of the organization in providing its goods or services.

operating budget Plan for the day-to-day operating revenues and expenses of the organization. It is generally prepared for 1 year.

operating expenses Costs of the organization related to its general operations.

operating margin Operating income (revenues less expenses before other gains or losses) divided by revenue; a profitability measure.

operating revenues Revenues earned in the normal course of providing the organization's goods or services.

operating statement *See* income statement.

operations Routine activities of the organization related to its mission and the provision of goods or services.

opinion letter Letter from the CPA to users of the organization's audited financial statements providing expert opinion on whether the financial statements are a fair presentation of the financial position and results of operations of the organization in accordance with generally accepted accounting principles (GAAP).

opportunity cost A measure of cost based on the value of the alternatives that are given up in order to use the resource as the organization has chosen.

opportunity costs of inventory Carrying costs or costs of having money tied up in inventory rather than in a revenue-producing endeavor such as an interest-bearing bank account.

ordering costs Costs associated with an order of inventory (e.g., clerk time for preparation of a purchase order).

organizational structure *See* hierarchy.

other than personnel services (OTPS) Expenses included in the budget for non-personnel expenses such as supplies or minor equipment.

outcome Result; can be affected by management actions, in contrast with events, which are defined as occurrences beyond the control of managers. Outcomes are also one of Donabedian's three aspects of quality. In this case, outcomes are the consequences or results of care, such as condition-specific results of care and patient satisfaction.[17]

out-of-pocket expense Money an individual must expend directly for health care services not covered by insurance or other third-party sources.

outputs Product or service being produced (e.g., patients, patient days, visits, operations).

overapplied or underapplied overhead Amount by which the actual overhead costs differ from the amount of overhead applied to units of service.

overhead Indirect costs. Often cannot be easily associated with individual patients, even by a job-order type of detailed observation and measurement. Overhead costs therefore require some form of aggregation and then allocation to units, departments, and ultimately patients or other units of service.

overhead application Process of charging overhead costs to units of service based on a standard overhead application rate.

overhead application rate Amount charged per unit of service for overhead; calculated using a cost base.

overhead costs *See* overhead.

owner's equity Residual value after the liabilities of an organization are subtracted from the assets. Represents the portion of the assets owned by the organization itself or its owners.

---

[17]*Ibid.*

P

partial productivity A portion of the total productivity; total outputs divided by some subpart of total inputs.

partnership Business owned by a group of persons (partners) who have unlimited liability; partners may be sued for all liabilities of the firm. *See also* corporation.

pass-through costs *See* cost pass-through.

patient classification System for distinguishing among different patients based on their acuity, functional ability, or resource needs.

patient day One patient occupying one bed for 1 day.

patient mix *See* case mix.

patient mix variance Variance from the organization's expected patient case mix.

patient revenue per day Total patient revenue divided by the number of days in the year.

patient revenues *See* gross patient revenues *and* net patient revenues.

payback Capital budgeting approach that calculates how many years it takes for a project's cash inflows to equal or exceed its cash outflows.

payer Individual or organization that provides money to pay for health care.

pay-for-performance System of paying hospitals and health care providers based on quality performance rather than on the costs incurred to provide specific services for patients with a particular diagnosis. Also known as *value-based purchasing*.

per diem Daily charge. Refers to (1) the charge per day for routine care and (2) agency nurses who work day to day.

per diem method Approach used to allocate department costs to units of service if the surcharge, hourly rate, and relative value unit methods do not reasonably apply.

performance budget Plan that relates the various objectives of a cost center with the planned costs of accomplishing those activities.

period costs Costs that are treated as expenses in the accounting period when they are incurred regardless of when the organization's goods or services are sold.

periodic inventory *See* perpetual versus periodic inventory.

perpetual versus periodic inventory Under the perpetual inventory method, the organization keeps a record of each inventory acquisition and sale, so it always knows how much has been sold and how much is supposed to be in inventory; under the periodic method, the organization records only purchases and uses a count of inventory to determine how much has been sold and how much is on hand.

personnel Persons employed by an organization.

philanthropy Gifts and donations made to the organization.

PHO *See* physician-hospital organization.

physician-hospital organization (PHO) "A legal entity formed by a hospital and a group of physicians to further mutual interests and to achieve market objectives. A PHO generally combines physicians and a hospital into a single organization for the purpose of obtaining payer contracts. Doctors maintain ownership of their practices and agree to accept managed care patients according to the terms of a professional services agreement with the PHO. The PHO serves as a collective negotiating and contracting unit. It is typically owned and governed jointly by a hospital and shareholder physicians."[18]

planning Deciding on goals and objectives, considering alternative options for achieving those goals and objectives, and selecting a course of action from the range of possible alternatives.

plant Building.

plant-age ratio Accumulated depreciation of buildings and equipment divided by annual depreciation expense; widely used as an approximation for the average age of physical facilities.

point-of-service organization Managed care organization that offers members either in-network, HMO-type coverage with low coinsurance and deductible rates but limited choice or out-of-network care with greater choice but higher deductible and coinsurance rates.

policy statements Limiting statements indicating what managers can or cannot do as they work to carry out the organization's mission by attainment of goals and objectives.

position One person working for the organization for any number of hours per week occupies a position.

posting Process of transferring all parts of a journal entry to the specific ledger accounts that are affected by the entry.

PPO *See* preferred provider organization.

PPS *See* prospective payment system.

preferred provider organization (PPO) "Formally organized entity generally consisting of hospital and physician providers. The PPO provides health care services to purchasers usually at discounted rates in return for expedited claims payment and a somewhat predictable market share. In this model, consumers have a choice of using PPO or non-PPO providers; however, financial incentives are built in to benefit structures to encourage utilization of PPO providers."[19]

premium Payment to an insurance company for coverage for a set period of time.

prepaid assets Assets that have been paid for and not yet used but that will be used within 1 year. This includes items such as fire insurance premiums or rent paid in advance.

prepaid group plan *See* health maintenance organization.

present cost *See* net present cost.

present on admission (POA) A health condition that exists at the time a patient is admitted to the hospital.

present value Value of future receipts or payments discounted to the present.

preventive controls *See* accounting controls.

price Amount charged for a particular service. Prices can be market based, cost based, markup based, or negotiated.

price variance Portion of the total variance for any line item that is caused by spending a different amount per unit of resource than had been anticipated (e.g., higher or lower salary rates, higher or lower supply prices).

principal The amount of money borrowed.

private insurers Insurance companies that are not part of the government.

probability Likelihood of an event's occurring. The probability of future events can be estimated based on data from historical events.

process One of Donabedian's three aspects of quality. Process refers to activities involved in providing care, such as models of care delivery, and organizational policies and procedures.[20]

process costing Approach to product costing based on broad averages of costs over a large volume of units of service.

product costing Determination of the cost per unit of service. Whereas job-order costing separately measures the cost of producing each job, process costing is based on costs averaged across a large number of units of service. An individual patient or group of patients of a similar type may be considered a job.

product costs Costs that are treated as part of the product and that do not become expenses until the product is sold.

production function Financial implications of making and distributing a product.

productive time Straight time and overtime worked. Includes time spent by staff delivering care to patients, communicating with other staff about patients, obtaining supplies needed by patients, and engaging in other patient care–related activities.

productivity Ratio of any given measure of output to any given measure of input over a specified period.

productivity improvement Learning to do things more efficiently without requiring increased and often unsustainable individual efforts by employees.

productivity measurement Process of assessing and quantifying productivity.

productivity standards Use of some criterion (e.g., broad industry average experience, best industry practice, the organization's budget, or the productivity percent) to evaluate organizational productivity.

product line Group of patients who have some commonality (e.g., a common diagnosis) that allows them to be grouped together.

product-line budget Budget for a group of patients with some commonality that allows them to be grouped together, such as a common diagnosis.

product-line costing "Determination of the cost of providing care to specific types of patients. This approach is sometimes aided by the use of standard cost techniques, such as Cleverley's model of standard treatment protocols."[21]

profit Amount by which an organization's revenues exceed its expenses.

profitability analysis Analysis of the profits related to a specific program, project, or service under existing conditions or under a specific set of assumptions.

profitability ratios Class of ratios that evaluates the profitability of the organization.

profit center *See* revenue center.

[18]*Ibid.*

[19]*Ibid.*

[20]*Ibid.*

[21]Cleverley WO. 1987. Product costing for health care firms. *Health Care Manage Rev* 12(4):39-48.

profit margin Excess of revenue over expense divided by total revenue; an indication of the amount of profits generated by each dollar of revenue.

profit-sharing plan Incentive arrangement under which executives receive a portion of an organization's profits that exceed a certain threshold.

pro forma financial statements Financial statements that predict what the financial statements for a project, program, or organization will look like at some point in the future.

program Project or service that cuts across departments.

program budget Plan that looks at all aspects of a program across departments and over the long term.

programming Process of deciding what major programs the organization will commence in the future.

property, plant, and equipment Land, buildings, and pieces of equipment owned by an organization.

proprietary *See* for-profit organization.

proprietorship Business owned by one individual.

prospective payment Payment made to providers based on a predetermined price for each particular category of patient (e.g., a particular DRG) as opposed to reimbursement based on the costs of care provided to the patient.

prospective payment system (PPS) Approach to paying for health care services based on predetermined prices.

provider Health care worker or health care organization that dispenses health care to people.

Q

quality "The degree to which health care services for individuals and populations increase the likelihood of desired health outcomes and are consistent with current professional knowledge."[22] Includes consideration of structures, processes, and outcomes of health care.[23]

quality costs Costs incurred to ensure that a product is of the required quality; may include costs such as inspection or replacement or harm to the patient created by providing inferior-quality care.

quality driver Factor that is critical to the level of quality of a product or service.

quantity variance Portion of the total variance for any line item that is caused by using more input per unit of output (e.g., patient day) than had been budgeted.

quick ratio Cash plus marketable securities plus accounts receivable, all divided by current liabilities.

R

R² (R squared) Regression analysis statistic that can range from a low of zero to a high of 1.0. The closer it is to 1.0, the more of the variability in the dependent variable has been explained by the independent variable(s).

rate setting Process of assigning prices to the units of service of the revenue centers. Prices must be set high enough to recover the organization's total financial requirements.

rate variance Price variance that relates to labor resources. In such cases, it is typically the hourly rate that has varied from expectations. *See also* price variance.

ratio One number divided by another.

ratio analysis Widely used managerial tool that compares one number with another to gain insights that would not arise from looking at either of the numbers separately.

ratio of cost to charges (RCC) Method used to convert a patient's bill to the patient's costs by applying the ratio of the organization's costs to its charges.

RCC *See* ratio of cost to charges.

reciprocal distribution *See* algebraic distribution.

recruitment Efforts directed at hiring potential employees.

regression analysis Statistical model that measures the average change in a dependent variable associated with a one-unit change in one or more independent variables.

regulation Government rule that has the force of law.

relative value unit (RVU) scale Arbitrary unit scale in which each patient is assigned a number of relative value units based on the relative costs of different types of patients. For example, if nursing care costs twice as much for type A patients as for type B patients, then type A patients will be assigned a number of relative value units twice as high as that assigned to type B patients.

relevant costs Only those costs that are subject to change as a result of a decision.

relevant range Range of activity that might reasonably be expected to occur in the budget period; range of activity within which fixed costs do not vary.

report card Quality reporting strategy that grades health care providers on measures of quality and performance to provide individuals, payers, and other decision makers with information upon which to base health care decisions.[24]

repurchase agreement Flexible bank-related financial investment instrument; can be for periods as short as 1 day.

required rate of return Interest rate that must be achieved for a capital project to be considered financially worthwhile; also called hurdle rate.

residual Portion left over; when liabilities are subtracted from assets, the leftover or residual value is the fund balance or owner's equity.

residual income (RI) Profits from a project in excess of the amount necessary to provide a desired minimum rate of return.

responsibility accounting Accounting approach that attempts to measure financial outcomes and assign those outcomes to the individual or department responsible for them.

responsibility center Part of the organization, such as a department or a unit, for which a manager is assigned responsibility. Health care organization responsibility centers generally have cost centers and revenue centers.

[22]Institute of Medicine. 1990. *Medicare: A Strategy for Quality Assurance.* Lohr KN, editor. Washington, DC: National Academies Press.

[23]Donabedian A. 1966, suppl. Evaluating the quality of medical care. *Milbank Mem Fund Q* 44(3):166-206.

[24]RAND. 2002. *Research Highlights: Report Cards for Health Care.* Retrieved September 3, 2006, at http://www.rand.org/pubs/research_briefs/RB4544/index1.html.

restricted funds Funds whose assets are limited as to their use. If the restriction is placed by the donor, it can be removed only by the donor; however, if the assets are restricted by the board, the restriction may be removed by the board.

retained earnings Profits earned by the organization and retained in the organization to finance future operations.

retention Continued employment; often conceptualized as the converse of turnover or staff leaving an organization.

retrospective patient classification Categorization of patients into a patient classification based on the nursing care needs that were met.

return on assets (ROA) Profit divided by total assets; a measure of the amount of profit earned for each dollar invested in the organization's assets.

return on investment (ROI) Ratio that divides the amount of profit by the amount of investment. Just as an individual would measure the success of a personal investment, so an organization would use ROI to measure the yield received relative to an amount of money invested.

revenue Amounts of money an organization has received or is entitled to receive in exchange for goods or services provided.

revenue budget Component of the operating budget that outlines expected revenues for a revenue center. Includes the price charged for each service provided by the unit multiplied by the number of units of service provided.

revenue center Unit or department that is responsible and accountable not only for costs of providing services but also for the revenues generated by those services. These units have revenue budgets. They are often called *profit centers* in other industries and generally have responsibility for expenses as well as revenues.

revenue variances Assessment of how much of the variance between expected and actual revenues results from changes in the total health care organization demand in a given geographic region, a health care organization's share of that total demand, its mix of patients, and the prices for each class of patient.

RI *See* residual income.

risk pools Money withheld from the capitation payment that would normally be due to each provider. The withheld amount, used as an incentive, is eventually paid to the provider if certain utilization targets are achieved.

risk sharing "The distribution of financial risk among parties furnishing a service. For example, if a hospital and a group of physicians from a corporation provide health care at a fixed price, a risk-sharing arrangement would entail both the hospital and the physician group being held liable if expenses exceed revenues."[25]

ROA *See* return on assets.

ROI *See* return on investment.

rolling budget System in which a budget is prepared each month for a month 1 year in the future. For example, after the actual results for this January are known, a budget for January of next year is prepared.

RVU *See* relative value unit scale.

---

[25]Bartlett et al., *Op. cit.*

S

safety stock Minimum inventory that an organization attempts always to maintain on hand; would be dipped into only when an event arises that would, in the absence of a safety stock, have resulted in a stockout.

seasonality Predictable pattern of monthly, quarterly, or other periodic variation in historical data within each year.

seasonalization Adjustment of the annual budget for month-to-month seasonality.

self-pay patients Patients who are responsible for payment of their own health care bills because they do not have private insurance and are not covered by either Medicare or Medicaid.

semi-fixed cost *See* step-fixed.

semi-variable cost *See* mixed cost.

sensitivity analysis Process whereby financial results are recalculated under a series of varying assumptions and predictions. This is often referred to as "what if" analysis.

service unit (SU) Basic measure of an item being produced by an organization (e.g., patient days, home care visits, hours of operations).

short run *See* short term.

short term Period of time shorter than the long term; *see also* long term.

short-term assets *See* current assets.

short-term debt Unsecured short-term loans.

simple linear regression Regression analysis that uses one dependent variable and one independent variable and produces predictions along a straight line.

simulation Mathematical approach that processes a number of different estimates a large number of times and projects the likelihood of various aggregate outcomes.

sinking fund Segregated assets to be used for replacement of plant and equipment, or to repay a bond or other long-term debt.

skimming Charging a high price knowing that market share will be low but planning to make a high profit on the volume achieved.

social costs *See* external costs.

solvency Ability to meet current and future obligations.

solvency ratios Class of ratios that evaluate the organization's ability to meet its obligations as they come due over a time frame longer than 1 year.

special purpose budget Any plan that does not fall into one of the other specific categories of budgets.

special purpose funds Assets restricted to a particular purpose (e.g., government grant research projects, student loans, establishment of a new burn care unit).

specific identification Inventory valuation method that identifies each unit of inventory and tracks which specific units are on hand and which have been sold.

spending variance Equivalent of the price or rate variance for fixed and variable overhead costs.

spreadsheet Large ledger sheet often used by accountants for financial calculations. Spreadsheets are often computerized today and are prepared using programs such as Excel or LOTUS 1–2–3.

staff function Provision of auxiliary assistance or service to the line managers and their departments. Finance is a staff function. Units designated to provide staff functions do not provide direct patient care.

staff manager Manager with no direct line responsibility for running the organization. Most nurse managers are line managers; the director of nursing education and the director of nursing recruitment are examples of staff manager positions.

standard cost Expectation of what it should cost to produce a good or service, usually on a per-unit basis. Such costs are targets, often established based on industrial engineering studies.

standard cost profile Costs, fixed and variable, direct and indirect, of producing each service unit (SU); *see also* standard treatment protocol.

standard treatment protocol Set of intermediate products or service units (SUs) consumed by a patient in each product line.

statement of cash flows Financial statement that shows where the organization's cash came from and how it was used over a specific period.

statement of changes in net assets Financial statement that summarizes items that affect the organization's unrestricted, temporarily restricted, and permanently restricted net assets.

statement of financial position Financial report that indicates the financial position of an organization at a specific point in time; often referred to as the balance sheet.

step-down Method of cost allocation in which nonrevenue centers allocate their costs to all cost centers, both revenue and nonrevenue, that have not yet been allocated. After a nonrevenue center allocates its costs, no costs can be allocated to it.

step-fixed Cost that is fixed over short ranges of volume but varies within the relevant range; sometimes referred to as step-variable.

step-variable *See* step-fixed.

stock option plan *See* stock plan.

stockout costs Costs incurred when supply is needed but not available. If the supply is needed for patient care, it often must be purchased at a higher price from a local vendor.

stock plan Bonus arrangement that provides shares of stock as part of an executive incentive system.

stop-loss coverage "Insurance coverage purchased by a health plan from an insurance company to reimburse the plan for the cost of benefits paid out to an individual or account that has exceeded what the plan expected to pay out. It stops the insurance company's loss. It is also known as reinsurance or risk-control insurance."[26]

strategic budget *See* long-range budget.

strategic business unit Approach to product-line management in which managers look not only at marketing but also at allocation of resources and profitability.

strategic management Process of setting the goals and objectives of an organization, determining the resources to be allocated to achieving those goals and objectives, and establishing policies concerning getting and using those resources.

strategic planning Process of setting long-term goals and designing a plan to achieve those goals; often referred to as long-term planning.

strategies Broad plans for the attainment of goals.

structure One of Donabedian's three aspects of quality. Structure includes the resources used in the provision of care (e.g., physicians, nurses, and other care providers), as well as the characteristics of organizations.[27]

SU *See* service unit.

subcategory Device to allow separation of the flexible budget variance into the price variance and the quantity variance. The actual quantity of input per unit of output multiplied by the budgeted price of the input times the actual output level.

subsidiary journal Detailed journals in which original entries are first made, with only a summary total entry being made to the general journal. For example, a sales journal would list each patient bill, with only a summary of total of revenue recorded in the general journal.

subsidiary ledger Ledgers in which detailed information is recorded, with only a summary being posted to the general ledger. For example, a subsidiary accounts receivable ledger would keep track of each patient's receivable separately, and the general ledger would show only the total increase or decrease in receivables.

substitute Economic good that can be used as an alternative to another economic good.

sunk costs Costs that already have been incurred and will not be affected by future actions.

suppliers Manufacturers and distributors of supplies, equipment, pharmaceuticals, and technologies used by health care providers.

supply Amount of a good or service that all suppliers in aggregate would like to provide for any given price.

supply curve Quantity that would be offered by suppliers at any given price.

support cost center Cost center that is not a revenue center.

surcharge method Approach to cost allocation in which a revenue center compares its costs, excluding inventory, with the inventory cost and determines a proportional surcharge.

surplus *See* profit.

T

tactics Specific activities undertaken to carry out a strategy.

taxes payable Taxes owed to local, state, or federal government.

third-party payer "Any organization, public or private, that pays or insures health or medical expenses on behalf of beneficiaries or recipients. An individual pays a premium for such coverage in all private and in some public programs; the payer organization then pays bills on the individual's behalf. Such payments are called third-party

---

[26]*Ibid.*

[27]Donabedian, *Op. cit.*

payments and are distinguished by the separation among the individual receiving the service (the first party), the individual or institution providing it (the second party), and the organization paying for it (third party)."[28]

time and motion studies Industrial engineering observations of the specific time and resources consumed for some activity.

time series analysis Use of historical values of a variable to predict future values for that variable without the use of any other variable other than the passage of time.

time value of money Recognition that money can earn compound interest and therefore a given amount of money paid at different points in time has a different value; the further into the future an amount is paid, the less valuable it is.

Title XIX (Medicaid) "The title of the Social Security Act which contains the principal legislative authority for the Medicaid program and therefore a common name for the program."[29]

total costs Sum of all costs related to a cost objective.

total debt-to-equity ratio Total liabilities divided by fund balance. The higher this ratio, the less borrowing capacity the organization has left.

total financial requirements (TFR) Financial resources needed to provide for the present and future health care needs of the population served by the organization.

total productivity Ratio of total outputs to total inputs; amount of output per unit of input.

total quality management (TQM) A philosophy that prevention of defects is less costly than correcting them; TQM focuses on doing things right initially and avoiding having to do them a second time.

total variance Sum of the price, quantity, and volume variances; the difference between the actual results and the original budgeted amount.

TQM *See* total quality management.

trade credit Accounts payable; generally no interest is charged for a period of time, such as one month.

traditional variance analysis Process of comparing the budget with actual results for the most recent month and year to date for each line item in each cost center.

transfer prices Amounts charged to one responsibility center for goods or services acquired from another responsibility center in the same organization.

trend Patterns related to the passage of time. For example, although there are daily fluctuations in the census, the pattern of the census is relatively stable.

true costs Actual resources consumed. Measurement of unique true costs is rarely possible; no matter how accurate accounting information is, there always will be different assessments of cost in different situations. Even beyond this, however, true costs do not exist, because accounting can never do more than approximate economic cost.

turnover rate The number of employees who leave an organization's employment during a specified time period, divided by the average number of organizational employees during that same period. A turnover rate can be calculated for certain categories of employees, such as RNs, or for larger groups of employees, such as unit staff, division staff, or all organizational employees.

U

uncontrollable *See* noncontrollable.

unfavorable variance Variance in which more is spent than the budgeted amount.

uniform reporting Approach to have health care organizations improve comparability of financial information from organization to organization by completing uniform accounting reports.

unit costing Process of estimating costs based on the amount of effort (e.g., labor, supplies) involved in producing one unit of service. Also called cost per unit of service.

unit of service *See* service unit.

unlicensed assistive personnel (UAP) Employees who are less skilled than professional nurses and do not hold licensure. They may be able to assume some activities traditionally performed by registered nurses.

unrestricted funds Funds whose assets may be used for any normal purpose; usually only the general operating fund is unrestricted.

unsecured note Loan secured without collateral.

use variance Another name for quantity variance; so called because the quantity variance focuses on how much of a resource has been used; *see also* quantity variance.

utility Physical or psychological benefit one receives from goods or services.

V

value Relationship between costs and quality, or quality divided by cost.[30]

value-added Costs that directly affect the quality of patient care. Many total quality management (TQM) initiatives focus on identifying value-added costs as opposed to non-value-added costs.

value-based purchasing *See* pay-for-performance.

variable billing System in which the amount billed to each patient for nursing care per patient day varies based on the differing resource consumption of different patients.

variable costs Costs that vary in direct proportion with volume.

variable staff Staff needed to provide the required number of care hours, whose time and work vary with volume or service.

variance Difference between budget and actual results.

variance analysis Comparison of actual results compared with the budget followed by investigation to determine why variances occurred.

---

[28]*Ibid.*
[29]*Ibid.*

[30]Folland S, Goodman AC, Stano M. 2006. *The Economics of Health and Health Care,* 5th edition. Upper Saddle River, NJ: Prentice-Hall.

vendor Supplier, such as a pharmaceutical company or hospital supply company.

volume The number of different types of patients cared for, surgeries performed, or procedures completed.

volume variance Amount of variance in any line item that is caused simply because the workload level changed.

W

wages payable Amounts owed to employees.

wealth Value of all resources a consumer currently owns.

weighted average method Inventory valuation method that accounts for inventory as if the inventory gets mixed together and each unit is unidentifiable.

weighted procedure method Approach to allocating a cost center's costs to units of service based upon a special study that establishes the relative costliness of each type of service the center performs.

Winters' forecasting method Statistical forecasting method that predicts seasonal patterns particularly well.

working capital Current assets and current liabilities of an organization.

working capital management Management of current assets and current liabilities of an organization.

working capital method Method for measuring cash flows that focuses on working capital.

workload Volume of work for a unit or department. There should be a direct relationship between the workload and the amount of resources needed; therefore, a workload measure such as patient days is inferior to one such as patient days adjusted for average patient acuity.

workload budget Budget that indicates the amount of work performed by a unit or department measured in terms of units of service.

work measurement Technique that evaluates what a group of workers is doing and attempts to assess the number of workers needed to accomplish the tasks efficiently.

work sampling Approach to determining time and resources used for an activity based on observations at intervals of time rather than continuous observation.

Y

year-to-date Sum of the budget or of actual values for all months from the beginning of the year through the most recent period for which data are available, or of both.

Z

ZBB See zero-base budgeting.

zero balance accounts System in which separate accounts are maintained at a bank for each major source of cash receipt and for major types of payments; at the close of each day, the bank, using computer technology, automatically transfers all balances, positive or negative, into one master concentration account. Any borrowing or investing of cash can then be done against that one account.

zero-base budgeting (ZBB) Program budgeting approach that requires an examination and justification of all costs rather than just the incremental costs and that requires examination of alternatives rather than just one approach.

Index

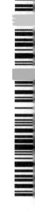

Edwards Brothers Inc.
Ann Arbor MI. USA
January 10, 2018